D1314233

Physician Characteristics and Distribution in the US 2012

Derek R. Smart

Division of Survey and Data Resources

AMA
AMERICAN
MEDICAL
ASSOCIATION

Executive Vice President, Chief Executive Officer: James L. Madara, MD

Chief Operating Officer: Bernard L. Hengesbaugh

Senior Vice President, Publishing and Business Services: Robert A. Musacchio, PhD

Vice President, Business Operations: Vanessa Hayden

Vice President, Publications and Clinical Solutions: Mary Lou White

Continuity Editor: Carol Brockman

Manager, Book and Product Development and Production: Nancy Baker

Senior Developmental Editor: Michael Ryder

Production Specialist: Meghan Anderson

Director, Sales, Marketing and Strategic Relationships: Joann Skiba

Director, Sales and Business Products: Mark Daniels

Manager, Marketing and Strategic Planning: Erin Kalitowski

Marketing Manager: Lori Hollacher

Physician Characteristics and Distribution in the US, 2012 Edition

Internet address: www.ama-assn.org

Additional copies of this book may be ordered by calling 800 621-8335.
Mention product number OP390212.
Secure online orders can be taken at www.amabookstore.com.

ISBN 978-1-60359-609-1

BP64:11-P-022:10/11

Preface

Physician Characteristics and Distribution in the US has been published since 1963. As in previous editions of this volume, the 2012 Edition presents extensive statistical information on all physicians located in the United States and possessions. The growth in physician supply and the focus on primary care physicians coupled with the emphasis on health systems reform have contributed to the rapidly changing health care environment. The current and future supply of physicians has become a significant component in planning for the nation's health care needs. Changes in size and composition of the physician population affect the organization of the US health care system.

To provide necessary statistical data about physician supply, this edition presents a series of summary and detailed tabulations on the professional characteristics of physicians, which can be used as a basis of comparison essential for health manpower planning, policy development, and research studies. In addition, the tabulations in this volume serve as guides for comparing census regions and divisions, states, counties, and metropolitan areas with respect to the distribution of physicians by their specialty and major professional activity.

As in past years, the 2012 edition includes physician/population ratios for the nation, state of location, and specialty of practice. Also presented are comparative data on the activity, specialty, and location of physicians from 1975 through 2010, along with information on the school and year of graduation, specialty board certification, and age and sex. The book contains summary and detailed tabulations in six separate chapters of physician data — Physician Characteristics, Physician Distribution, Analysis of Professional Activity by Self-Designated Specialty and Geographic Region, Primary Care Specialties, Osteopathic Physicians, and Physician Trends. The Introduction describes these chapters in more detail and also describes the overall format of the book.

New in recent editions is a chapter on Doctors of Osteopathic Medicine. As this segment of the physician populace grows, it becomes more and more important to understand their impact on the overall question of physician supply, as well as how their characteristics compare to their Allopathic colleagues, an issue this chapter strives to address.

As a basic and comprehensive source of data related to the specialty, activity, location, and other characteristics of physicians, this publication serves a wide audience. Hospitals, medical societies, medical schools, specialty boards, government agencies, associations, as well as other health-related organizations have found earlier editions of this book to be significant data sources when conducting research on health care issues, trends in physician supply, and the availability of physician services.

All data in this volume are derived from the American Medical Association's (AMA) Physician Masterfile and represent the collection, management, and validation efforts of several departments within the Division of Survey and Data Resources.

Table of Contents

List of Tables

Mini-Tables

List of Figures

Introduction

Physician Characteristics and Distribution in the US, 2012 Edition, is the latest in a series begun in 1963 as the *Distribution of Physicians.* It contains historical and current data on the US physician population that provide a basis for comparison essential for health services research, program planning, and policy development. All summary and detailed data on physicians in this edition have been compiled as of December 31, 2010, from the American Medical Association's (AMA) Physician Masterfile, maintained by the Division of Survey and Data Resources. A historical and developmental overview of the Physician Masterfile is provided in the next part of this book. Included in this overview is a description of the structure of the Masterfile, as well as data collection and management procedures.

Data in this publication are presented in six separate chapters: Physician Characteristics, Physician Distribution, Analysis of Professional Activity by Specialty and Geographic Region, Primary Care Specialties, Osteopathic Physicians, and Physician Trends.

Chapter 1 — Physician Characteristics — presents key professional and individual characteristics of the physician population. Cross-tabulations include physicians by age, sex, major professional activity, specialty, and race/ethnicity. The section provides separate tabulations for women physicians and International Medical Graduates (IMGs), for physicians by country, school, and year of graduation, and data on specialty and board certification status.

Chapter 2 — Physician Distribution — focuses on the geographical location of physicians. Tabulations are presented for the states, including statistics for IMG physicians and physicians by age and sex.

Chapter 3 — Analysis of Professional Activity by Specialty and Geographic Region—accents specialty and activity data for the nation, as well as for states, census regions and divisions, MSAs, and counties, including separate tabulations by gender and IMG physicians.

Chapter 4 — Primary Care Specialties — presents data in two groups: (1) the general primary care specialties of Family Medicine, General Practice, Internal Medicine, Obstetrics and Gynecology, and Pediatrics, *excluding* the subspecialties within these general specialties and (2) the primary care subspecialties *including only* the subspecialties of those listed in group one. This section presents detailed tabulations about primary care physicians, including the data variables of activity, age, sex, board certification, school and year of graduation, IMGs, state of location, and metropolitan area.

Chapter 5 — Osteopathic Physicians — presents key data on Osteopathic Physicians with table formats taken from each of the first four chapters, allowing for an understanding of what the Osteopathic population looks like both on its own, and when compared to the Allopathic population.

Chapter 6 — Physician Trends — presents data from 1975 through 2010 on the physician characteristics of specialty, major professional activity, age, and sex. National trend data are also displayed for Metropolitan Statistical Areas (MSAs), female physicians, and international medical graduates (IMGs). Physician population ratios for selected years 1965–2010 are included, as are ratios by state and specialty.

Five appendices provide easy access to information on geographical locations and categories and include lists of divisions, regions, and the county composition for Metropolitan and Micropolitan Statistical Areas. Also provided is information on the American Specialty Boards. A sample of the Physicians' Practice Arrangements questionnaire, which is sent to physicians in order to update the AMA Physician Masterfile, is included as well.

Although this publication was designed to address and meet many of the anticipated data requirements concerning the physician population, various users may have specific requests for information from the AMA Physician Masterfile. Such inquiries regarding data contained in this publication, in earlier publications, or from the AMA Physician Masterfile should be directed to the AMA Division of Survey and Data Resources.

This publication is copyrighted, and any use of data contained within this publication is to be referenced as follows: *Physician Characteristics and Distribution, 2012 Edition*, Division of Survey and Data Resources, American Medical Association, 2012.

AMA Physician Masterfile

The American Medical Association (AMA) has continued to develop a unique and comprehensive database of physician and medical student information since the establishment of the Masterfile in 1906. Although initially the Masterfile was primarily used by the Association as a record-keeping device for membership and mailing purposes, today the Masterfile is widely considered to be the most complete and extensive source of physician-related information in the United States.

Current and Historical Information

The Masterfile contains current and historical data on all physicians, including members and nonmembers of the AMA, and graduates of foreign medical schools who are in the United States and meet educational standards for recognition as physicians. International Medical Graduates (IMGs), comprising graduates of foreign medical schools residing in the United States, are included in the Masterfile, generally upon entry into graduate medical training programs accredited by the Accreditation Council on Graduate Medical Education (ACGME). Included also in the Masterfile are IMGs who have been granted a state license to practice medicine but may not have entered ACGME training programs. The Masterfile also includes physicians licensed to practice in the United States but temporarily located abroad.

A record is started on each individual upon entry into medical school or, in the case of international or Canadian medical graduates, upon entry into the United States. A physician's record includes medical school and year of graduation, sex and birthdate. As the physician's training and career develop, additional information is added, such as residency training, state licensure data, and board certification. This information, which comprises the historical portion of the Masterfile, facilitates studies of trends in geographic mobility and medical education.

In addition, the current professional activities portion of each physician's record identifies geographical location and current address, type of practice (Patient Care or Nonpatient Care), specialties (primary and secondary), and present employment (solo, partnership, group practice, medical schools, hospitals, government, and other organizations). These data are particularly useful in manpower planning and research. By definition, the current portion of the record is subject to constant change and must be updated continually through extensive monitoring and data collection activities. Over time, the objectives, collection techniques, and need assessments undergo regular review and change. Quality control, Masterfile expansion, and upgrading of the information collected and analyzed continue to be the major focus of the AMA's Division of Survey and Data Resources.

Data Collection and Updating

A major source of data collection is the Census of Physicians (PPA Questionnaire), which the AMA designed in 1968 in order to collect data under a new classification of physician activities based on "hours worked" criteria. The PPA Questionnaire was sent every four years between 1969 and 1985 to all physicians residing in the United States, as well as to US physicians residing temporarily overseas. Between 1985 and 2006, the PPA Questionnaire evolved into a rotating census in which approximately one third to one fourth of all physicians were surveyed via mail each year. Since then, the AMA has employed a more diversified survey approach in which more than 500,000 active physicians are targeted each year via mail, telephone and Web-based surveys.

Each physician is asked to choose among the categories in each of the following items:

- Professional Activity — Direct Patient Care or Nonpatient Care activities (i.e., Administrative Activities, Medical Education, Medical Research, Other Medical Activities)
- Specialization — primary and secondary specialties selected from the AMA list of over 200 Self-Designated Practice Specialties
- Present Employment — type of employer (i.e., Self-Employed, Solo Practice, Two-Physician Practice, Group Practice, HMO, Medical School, Non-Government Hospital, City/County/State Government, US Government, Locum Tenens, Other Patient Care, and Other Nonpatient Care)

All data obtained through the surveys are loaded to the AMA Masterfile and major professional activity, specialty, and employment classifications are assigned to physicians' records.

In addition to the professional activity, specialty, and employment categories, the Census also captures mailing and primary office addresses, hospital affiliations, group affiliations, telephone numbers, and other data.

While the data collected from the Census represent a major source of information to the Masterfile, data also are obtained from many organizations and institutions. Some of these sources and the data they provide include:

- Medical schools — name, address, birthdate, birthplace, school, and year of graduation
- Training Institutions — physicians in graduate medical training, including IMGs entering US training
- Group Practices — group practice address, telephone number, organizational structure and physician affiliations.
- Medical societies — address, communications and membership information
- State licensing agencies — licensure status of physicians
- Educational Commission for Foreign Medical Graduates (ECFMG) — IMGs who are certified or have applied for certification by the ECFMG
- American Board of Medical Specialties (ABMS) — physicians certified by ABMS Member Boards

Data are also extracted from the AMA Masterfile for use by some of these agencies. In addition, the data that is maintained in the Masterfile is to communicate with physicians, segment physician markets, draw samples for health-related research, perform workforce analysis, and track professional trends.

Definitions

The following material provides definitions and explanations of the specific physician attributes included in the tabulations of this publication. These materials are presented as a common reference base to facilitate analysis and interpretation of the data.

Major Professional Activity

Major professional activity (MPA) classifications are reported by physicians in the Physicians' Practice Arrangements (PPA) questionnaire. The physician's professional activity is shown in the two categories of Patient Care and Nonpatient care, the latter category being referred to as Other Professional Activity. Patient Care activities include Office-Based practice and Hospital-Based practice. Physicians in Residency training (including Clinical Fellows) and full time members of Hospital Staffs comprise Hospital-Based practice. Other Professional Activity includes Administration, Medical Teaching, Research, and Other Activities. The subcategory Clinical Fellows is no longer tabulated; physicians formerly counted as Clinical Fellows are now in the category Residents/Fellows and are tabulated as Residents.

Physicians who are retired, semi-retired, working part-time, temporarily not in practice, or not active for other reasons are classified as Inactive. Physicians are categorized as Not Classified if the American Medical Association (AMA) has not received any recent information as to their type of practice and present employment.

Following are definitions of each of the MPA categories.

Office-Based Practice includes physicians engaged in seeing patients. Physicians may be in solo practice, group practice, two-physician practice, or other patient care employment. This category also includes physicians in patient services such as those provided by pathologists and radiologists.

Hospital-Based Practice includes physicians employed under contract with hospitals to provide direct patient care.

Residents — All Years includes any physician in supervised practice of medicine among patients in a hospital or in its outpatient department, with continued instruction in the science and art of medicine by the staff of the facility. This category also includes clinical fellows in advanced training in the clinical divisions of medicine, surgery, and other specialty fields preparing for practice in a given specialty. These physicians are engaged primarily in patient care.

Medical Teaching includes physicians with teaching appointments in medical schools, hospitals, nursing schools, or other institutions of higher learning.

Medical Research includes physicians in activities (funded or non-funded) performed to develop new medical knowledge, potentially leading to publication. This category also includes physicians in research fellowship programs distinct from an accredited residency program and those primarily engaged in nonpatient care.

Administration includes physicians in administrative activities in a hospital, health facility, health agency, clinic, group, or any similar organization.

Other Activity includes physicians employed by insurance carriers, pharmaceutical companies, corporations, voluntary organizations, medical societies, associations, grants, foreign countries, and the like.

Inactives include physicians who are retired, semi-retired, working part-time, temporarily not in practice, or not active for other reasons and who indicated they worked 20 hours or less per week.

Not Classified includes physicians who did not provide information on their type of practice or their present employment.

Self Designated Practice Specialty[1]

A physician's self designated practice specialty (SDPS) is determined, like major professional activity, by the physician from a list of codes included with the PPA Questionnaire. Tables 1.8 and 1.9 provide all specialties listed on the PPA Questionnaire and maintained on the Masterfile for which there is at least one physician designating it as their area of practice. Specialty classifications based on the 40 specialties used by the AMA for statistical purposes are listed in Appendix A.

In the specialty tabulations presented in the Physician Trends, Physician Characteristics (except Tables 1.8 and 1.9), Physician Distribution, and Analysis of Activity by Specialty chapters of the book, the specialties of Family Medicine (FM), General Practice (GP), Internal Medicine (IM), Obstetrics/Gynecology (OBG), and Pediatrics (PD) include both the general primary care specialties and their respective subspecialties as listed in the specialty abbreviations appearing in Appendix A. However, in the primary care chapter, the data are presented separately for the general primary care specialties and the primary care subspecialties.

Primary Care Specialties

As just mentioned in reference to the primary care chapter, detailed statistical data are presented in two separate specialty groupings: (1) the general primary care specialties of Family Medicine, General Practice, Internal Medicine, Obstetrics and Gynecology, and Pediatrics *excluding* the subspecialties associated with these general specialties and (2) the primary care subspecialties *including only* the subspecialties of the general specialties listed in group one. The primary care subspecialties are listed in the footnote to Tables 4.5, 4.7-4.9, 4.11-4.13, and 4.15 and include the following:

- FM Subspecialties

Geriatric Medicine (Family Medicine) (FPG) and Sports Medicine (Family Medicine) (FSM)

- IM Subspecialties

Adolescent Medicine (AMI), Critical Care Medicine (CCM), Diabetes (DIA), Endocrinology, Diabetes, & Metabolism (END), Hematology (HEM), Hepatology (HEP), Hematology/Oncology (HO), Cardiac Electrophysiology (ICE), Infectious Diseases (ID), Clinical & Laboratory Immunology (Internal Medicine) (ILI), Geriatric Medicine (Internal Medicine) (IMG), Sports Medicine (Internal Medicine) (ISM), Nephrology (NEP), Nutrition (NTR), Medical Oncology (ON), Pulmonary Critical Care Medicine (PCC), and Rheumatology (RHU)

- OBG Subspecialties

Gynecological Oncology (GO), Gynecology (GYN), Maternal & Fetal Medicine (MFM), Obstetrics (OBS), Critical Care Medicine (Obstetrics & Gynecology) (OCC), and Reproductive Endocrinology (REN)

- PD Subspecialties

Adolescent Medicine (ADL), Pediatric Critical Care Medicine (CCP), Pediatrics/Internal Medicine (MPD), Neonatal-Perinatal Medicine (NPM), Pediatric Allergy (PDA), Pediatric Cardiology (PDC), Pediatric Endocrinology (PDE), Pediatric Infectious Disease (PDI), Pediatric Pulmonology (PDP), Medical Toxicology (Pediatrics), (PDT), Pediatric Emergency Medicine (PEM), Pediatric Gastroenterology (PG), Pediatric Hematology/Oncology (PHO), Clinical & Laboratory Immunology (Pediatrics) (PLI), Pediatric Nephrology (PN), Pediatric Rheumatology (PPR), and Sports Medicine (Pediatrics) (PSM)

The tables in Chapter 4 also include separate statistics for All Other specialties and the Not Classified physicians. In the chapter on primary care, the specialty of Pediatric Cardiology is included in the Pediatrics subspecialty grouping while in the Physician Trends, Physician Characteristics, Physician Distribution, and Analysis of Activity by Specialty, it is listed separately.

Board Certification

Board certification by one or more of the 24 American Specialty Boards listed in Appendix B represents a voluntary effort on the part of the physician. The process of certification entails a complex and rigid series of requirements, including examination and successful completion of an approved residency training program. A licensed physician may practice in any specialty, however, regardless of board certification status. Tables in this publication indicate board certification in the corresponding specialty in which the physician is classified. Although the attainment of certification demonstrates proficiency within a chosen discipline, "Medical specialty board certification is an additional process to receiving a medical degree, completing residency training, and receiving a license to practice medicine."[2]

The terms *corresponding board* and *non-corresponding board* in this publication (Tables 1.14 through 1.16) are used to describe the appropriate board certification status of physicians in relation to their SDPS as follows:

- Certified by Corresponding Board Only

Includes physicians in an SDPS who are certified by the respective board having authority to grant certification for that specialty (for example, a physician in the specialty of Family Medicine certified only by the American Board of Family Medicine)

- Certified by Corresponding Board and Non Corresponding Board(s)

Includes physicians in a specialty SDPS who hold two or more certifications: one from the respective board having authority to grant certification in the physicians' SDPS and another from a different board that does not grant certification in the physicians' SDP (for example, a physician in the specialty of Internal Medicine certified by the American Board of Internal Medicine and also the American Board of Surgery)

- Certified by Non Corresponding Board Only

Includes physicians in an SDPS who are certified by a board that does not grant certification in the physicians' SDPS (for example, a physician in the specialty of Emergency Medicine certified by the American Board of Internal Medicine)

- Not Certified

Includes physicians who are not certified by any board

A listing of the American Specialty Boards and information regarding general certification and subspecialty certification are provided in Appendix B.

Residency Training Data

Neither SDPS nor certification by a member board of ABMS should be confused with the fact that a physician has successfully completed a program (or programs) of accredited graduate medical education. Accreditation is the process whereby the Accreditation Council for Graduate Medical Education (ACGME) grants public recognition to a specialized program that meets certain established educational standards as determined through initial and subsequent periodic evaluation by one of the 27 Residency Review committees. AMA collects physicians' residency training data through an annual census of all ACGME accredited residency training programs.

Other Physician Characteristics

The medical education of physicians is grouped into four graduation classifications: (1) US active schools, (2) US inactive schools, (3) Canadian schools, and (4) international schools. Schools of basic medical sciences as well as undeveloped medical schools which, although operational, have not graduated any physicians and therefore are not yet eligible for approval, are excluded from the tabulations. In February 1990, the AMA began using the term *International Medical Graduates (IMGs)* in place of *Foreign Medical Graduates* when referring to physicians who graduated from a medical school located outside of the United States, Possessions (Puerto Rico, Virgin Islands, and Pacific Islands), or Canada. Data in prior editions of *Physician Characteristics and Distribution* refer to this population as Foreign Medical Graduates.

Physician distribution by age is presented in 10 year intervals on a continuum from younger than 35 to 65 and older. Also included are distributions by sex.

Metropolitan Statistical Area Definition

Beginning in this year's edition, we are using an updated set of Metropolitan and Micropolitan Statistical Area codes commonly referred to as Core Based Statistical Areas (CBSA).

The United States Office of Management and Budget (OMB) defines Metropolitan and Micropolitan Statistical Areas according to published standards that are applied to Census Bureau data. The general concept of a Metropolitan or Micropolitan Statistical Area is that of a core area containing a substantial population nucleus, together with adjacent communities having a high degree of economic and social integration with that core.

The standards provide that each CBSA must contain at least one urban area of 10,000 or more population. Each Metropolitan Statistical Area must have at least one urbanized area of 50,000 or more inhabitants. Each Micropolitan Statistical Area must have at least one urban cluster of at least 10,000 but less than 50,000 population.

Under the standards, the county (or counties) in which at least 50 percent of the population resides within urban areas of 10,000 or more population, or that contain at least 5,000 people residing within a single urban area of 10,000 or more population, is identified as a "central county" (counties). Additional "outlying counties" are included in the CBSA if they meet specified requirements of commuting to or from the central counties. Counties or equivalent entities form the geographic "building blocks" for Metropolitan and Micropolitan Statistical Areas throughout the United States and Puerto Rico.[3]

County Data

Beginning with the 1993 edition, the independent cities of Virginia are listed separately from the individual counties in Virginia and are designated with the suffix (ic), as shown in Table 3.11. In addition, the independent cities of Baltimore, Maryland, and St. Louis, Missouri, are listed separately from the counties of Baltimore and St. Louis.

The Alaskan Boroughs/Census Areas are listed in Table 3.11 instead of the four Judicial Divisions appearing in editions prior to 1993. Table 3.11 lists only the 23 Boroughs/Census Areas having at least one physician rather than the entire 26 defined by the US Census Bureau. The Boroughs/Census Areas not listed are Denali, Lake and Peninsula, and Wade Hampton.

Endnotes

1. The Self-Designated Practice Specialties (SDPS) appearing on the AMA Physician Masterfile and in this publication do not imply recognition or endorsement of any field of medical practice by the AMA.
2. *Graduate Medical Education Directory, 1995-1996.* Accreditation Council for Graduate Medical Education, American Medical Association; p. 934.
3. Population Division, US Census Bureau; *About Metropolitan and Micropolitan Statistical Areas;* Last Revised: August 19, 2008 <http://www.census.gov/population/www/metroareas/aboutmetro.html>

Acknowledgments

The Physician Characteristics and Distribution in the US publication is the result of the combined efforts and participation of a number of staff members within the American Medical Association (AMA).

The publication was greatly improved by Dave Doty, who made sure that the tables were in proper order and incorporated all the figures in the text.

The annual publication of *Physician Characteristics and Distribution in the US* represents the support, commitment, and dedicated efforts of the departments within the Division of Survey and Data Resources that manage ongoing data collection activities of physician-related information, and the planning, survey, and dissemination activities for the AMA Physician Masterfile and other supplementary data files, with particular thanks going to the Department of Database Licensing.

Derek Smart, Manager
Information Management and Data Release
AMA Division of Survey and Data Resources

Chapter 1

Physician Characteristics

This chapter provides statistics on several key characteristics of the physician population in the US as of December 31, 2010. These include information regarding (1) major professional activity, (2) primary specialty, (3) specialty board certification status, (4) age and sex, and (5) country, school, and year of graduation. Also presented are separate tabulations for female physicians and International Medical Graduates (IMGs) by their specialty and activity.

Activity by Age and Sex

Table 1.1 indicates that in 2010, nearly two fifths of US physicians were younger than 45 years of age (38.6%). The 45 to 54 age interval accounted for the highest percentage of total physicians (22.4%). Of all Office-Based physicians (565,024), the highest percentage was indicated for the 45 to 54 age group — 30.6%. Within the Administration total of 14,009, the largest proportion of physicians comprised the 55 to 64 age group — more than one third or 40.0%. Physicians 65 and older numbered 194,857 or 19.8% of the physicians in the US. Within this group, Patient Care accounted for two-fifths (38.2%), with half (54.7%) listed as Inactive.

Of total female physicians (296,907), the highest percent (29.0%) were 35 to 44 years of age. Only 7.6% were 65 or older. Approximately one tenth (11.6%) of Office-Based female physicians were younger than 35, compared to 4.9% of Office-Based male physicians. Over one third (34.5%) of all male physicians in Other Professional Activity were in Administration. Administration accounted for 28.9% of all female physicians in Other Professional Activity. The age interval 35 to 44 comprised nearly one fifth (18.4%) of female physicians in Medical Teaching but less than one tenth (8.2%) of male physicians. The 45 to 54 age interval contained the highest percentages of both male (31.0%) and female (32.6%) physicians working in hospitals as full-time staff. Figure 1.1 displays a percentage distribution of the total US physician population by age and sex.

Self Designated Specialty by Age and Sex

An analysis of Table 1.2 indicates that at the end of 2010, three fifths (58.1%) of all physicians (572,862) were in the following ten specialty fields:

Internal Medicine (161,276)

Family Medicine (87,618)

Pediatrics (76,401)

Anesthesiology (43,359)

Obstetrics/Gynecology (42,797)

Psychiatry (39,738)

General Surgery (37,100)

Emergency Medicine (33,278)

Diagnostic Radiology (26,054)

Orthopedic Surgery (25,241)

These same specialties (but replacing Diagnostic Radiology with Cardiovascular Diseases) were also highest for all male physicians (Table 1.3), representing 54.6% of the male population. The five disciplines with the most male physicians younger than 35 were Internal Medicine (19.3% of males younger than 35), Family Medicine (6.9%), General

Figure 1.1

Percent Distribution of Total US Physicians by Age and Sex, 2010

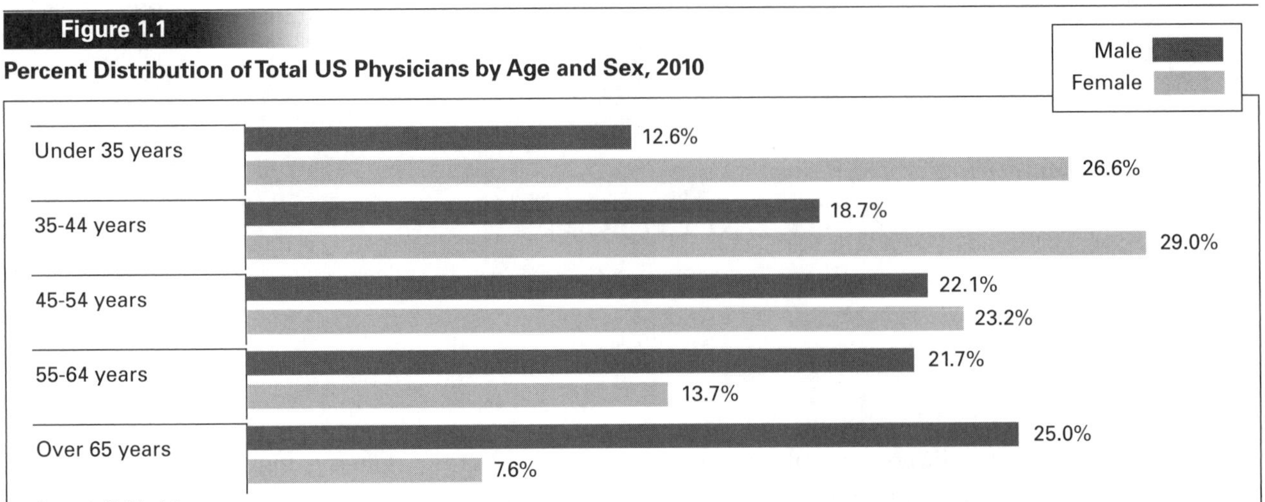

Source: Table 1.1

Surgery (6.2%), Pediatrics (5.4%), and Emergency Medicine (5.4%).

For female physicians, the specialties demonstrating the highest numbers differed from the male and overall physician populations. The top 10 disciplines for female physicians (Table 1.4) consisted of the following:

Internal Medicine (54,182)

Pediatrics (43,079)

Family Medicine (32,376)

Obstetrics/Gynecology (20,820)

Psychiatry (14,264)

Anesthesiology (10,437)

Emergency Medicine (8,300)

Pathology (7,013)

General Surgery (6,640)

Diagnostic Radiology (6,135)

For these specialties, the highest percentages of female physicians younger than 35 were found in Internal Medicine (17.8% of those females younger than 35), Pediatrics (14.8%), Family Medicine (9.8%), Obstetrics/Gynecology (7.1%), and Emergency Medicine (3.8%).

Table A illustrates, for the highest 10 specialties ranked by size, the percent distribution of total male and female IMG physicians by age. As Table A indicates, Internal Medicine and Family Medicine had the highest proportions of male physicians younger than 35. For female physicians, the disciplines with the highest proportions younger than 35 included General Practice, Neurology, and Obstetrics/Gynecology.

Distribution of Detail Specialties by Activity

Detailed specialty data are reported by physicians on the Census of Physicians (PPA Questionnaire) and included on the AMA Physician Masterfile. To meet user needs and requests for more detailed specialty information, Table 1.9 lists those specialties reported by at least one physician. However, care must be exercised in comparing the specialty data displayed in Table 1.9 with the other tables in this publication because it is the *only table* in this publication that presents the entire list of detail specialties with one or more physicians. For all other tables in this volume, the detail specialties are aggregated into the more generalized specialty categories. The List of Detailed Self-Designated Practice Specialty Codes appearing in Appendix A presents the grouping of the detail specialties into the general specialty categories used throughout this publication.

The 10 specialties showing highest counts of physicians in 2010, in the detail specialties in Table 1.9, included: Internal Medicine (113,591), Family Medicine (86,155), Pediatrics (57,830), Anesthesiology (40,636), Obstetrics/Gynecology (38,520), Psychiatry (37,684), Emergency Medi-

Table A

Percent Distribution of International Medical Graduates by Age and Self-Designated Specialty Ranked by Size, 2010

Specialty	*Rank*	*Total*	*Under 35*	*35-44*	*45-54*	*55-64*	*65 & Over*
Total Male IMG's		**173,007**	**11.99%**	**19.79%**	**21.29%**	**20.73%**	**26.21%**
Anesthesiology	4	8,453	5.42%	19.38%	29.54%	26.97%	18.69%
Cardiovascular Diseases	6	6,395	9.07%	18.67%	30.35%	26.47%	15.43%
Family Medicine	2	11,971	16.82%	24.60%	23.76%	22.38%	12.45%
General Surgery	7	6,086	13.56%	13.70%	14.11%	28.06%	30.56%
Internal Medicine	1	40,624	18.17%	26.10%	27.16%	19.01%	9.56%
Neurology	9	3,729	12.58%	22.58%	30.22%	23.22%	11.40%
Obstetrics/Gynecology	8	4,566	6.77%	11.54%	15.13%	35.26%	31.30%
Pathology	10	3,440	6.34%	14.56%	30.32%	20.67%	28.11%
Pediatrics	3	9,564	11.17%	17.63%	29.40%	26.39%	15.41%
Psychiatry	5	7,913	6.96%	15.53%	24.15%	28.18%	25.17%
Total Female IMG's		**81,389**	**20.45%**	**29.19%**	**21.07%**	**15.28%**	**14.02%**
Anesthesiology	5	2,970	8.01%	23.47%	25.96%	25.93%	16.63%
Child Psychiatry	9	1,156	9.08%	32.09%	28.63%	18.94%	11.25%
Family Medicine	10	1,113	1.89%	5.21%	16.53%	38.54%	37.83%
General Practice	3	8,134	26.97%	35.37%	21.81%	11.14%	4.71%
Internal Medicine	8	1,472	20.18%	33.08%	27.51%	14.27%	4.96%
Neurology	1	20,311	26.53%	35.67%	23.19%	10.72%	3.88%
Obstetrics/Gynecology	7	2,415	22.11%	23.44%	13.46%	21.82%	19.17%
Pathology	6	2,717	9.02%	22.23%	30.33%	21.60%	16.82%
Pediatrics	2	10,878	16.33%	24.03%	27.01%	22.44%	10.19%
Psychiatry	4	4,678	11.20%	20.27%	27.26%	26.06%	15.22%

Note: Percentages may not always add to 100 due to rounding.
Source: Tables 1.6 & 1.7

cine (32,683), General Surgery (29,505), Diagnostic Radiology (26,036), and Cardiovascular Disease (22,888). Considering only the category Residents/Fellows, the percentages of Residents/Fellows to total physicians in each of these specialties are Internal Medicine (16.7%), Family Medicine (9.2%), Pediatrics (12.3%), Anesthesiology (12.8%), Obstetrics/Gynecology (11.7%), Psychiatry (11.3%), Emergency Medicine (14.0%), General Surgery (25.2%), Diagnostic Radiology (18.6%), and Cardiovascular Disease (10.9%).

Mean Age by Detail Specialty and Activity

Table 1.8 shows the mean age of physicians in the detail specialties. The 10 specialties with the highest mean ages include the following:

Psychoanalysis (71.7)

Hospice and Palliative Medicine (Pediatrics) (69.0)

Hospice and Palliative Medicine (68.0)

Hospice & Palliative Medicine (Obstetrics & Gynecology) (65.7)

Neuromuscular Medicine (Physical Medicine & Rehabilitation)(65.0)

Critical Care Medicine (Obstetrics & Gynecology) (64.8)

Immunology (64.4)

Allergy (64.4)

General Practice (64.3)

Clinical Pharmacology (64.2)

The table also shows that within the category of Patient Care, Hospital Based physicians are an average of more than one year older than their Office Based counterparts, while physicians in Administration are an average of ten years older than the physician population as a whole.

International Medical Graduates (IMGs)

Activity by Specialty

In 2010, IMGs accounted for 25.8% of the total physician population and 25.5% of the total physicians in Patient Care (Tables 1.10 and 1.1). Within the IMG population itself, 75.5% of physicians were in Patient Care. Of this group of 192,046 physicians, nearly three quarters (73.0%) were in Office-Based practice, representing 24.8% of all Office-Based physicians in the US and Possessions. IMGs accounted for 26.3% of all physicians in residency/fellowship training and nearly one third (29.4%) of all Hospital-Based full-time physician staff. Almost one fifth of all physicians in Research (19.9%) and one out of six physicians in Medical Teaching (16.7%) were IMGs. Only 12.9% of all physicians in Administration were graduates of international medical schools.

Nearly three fifths (57.4%) of all IMGs were in the specialties of Internal Medicine (60,935), Pediatrics (20,442), Family Medicine (20,105), Psychiatry (12,591), Anesthesiology (11,423), Cardiovascular Disease (7,089), Obstetrics/Gynecology (6,981), and General Surgery (6,580). More than half (53.8%) of all IMGs in residency/fellowship training were concentrated in the Medical Specialties, while 24.8% were in Other Specialties. General/Family Medicine comprised one eighth of all IMG residents (12.5%), while the Surgical Specialties represented 8.9%.

Activity by Age and Sex

The highest percentage of IMGs (Table 1.11) were in the 35-44 age group in 2010 (22.8%). Female IMGs comprised 32.0% of the IMG complement. Age distribution for female IMGs indicated the highest percentage in the 35 to 44 age group (29.2%), followed by 21.1% between ages 45 and 54. Over one fifth of male IMGs (21.3%) were in the 45 to 54 age group, and nearly as many (20.7%) were in the 55 to 64 age group. Figure 1.2 illustrates the distribution of total IMGs by age and activity.

Female Physicians by Self-Designated Specialty and Activity

Representation of female physicians in medicine continues to show steady increases. In 1980, female physicians comprised 11.6% of the physician workforce, but by 2010, they accounted for 30.1% of the total physician population. Female physicians represented two fifths (45.4%) of all residents/fellows in 2010 compared to 21.5% of the resident total in 1980 (Tables 1.13 and 1.1). Of the total female physician population of 296,907, more than four fifths (80.5%) were in Patient Care. Within Patient Care, nearly three quarters (69.3%) were in Office-Based practice. The specialties of Internal Medicine, Pediatrics, Family Medicine, Obstetrics/Gynecology, Psychiatry, and Anesthesiology accounted for more than three fifths (59.0%) of all female physicians in 2010. Percentages of women in residency training in these specialties are displayed in Table B.

Other Professional Activity, which includes Administration, Medical Teaching, Research, and Other, accounted for 3.5% of the total female physician population. Female physicians represented 28.0% of all physicians in Medical Teaching, 21.2% of all physicians in Administration, and 22.5% of total physicians in Research (Tables 1.13 and 1.1).

Self-Designated Specialty by Board Certification

Table 1.14 presents data on the specialty board certification status of physicians in the following four categories:

Table B

Female Physicians by Self-Designated Specialty and Residency Training, 2010

Specialty	*Total Female Physicians*	*Total Female Residents*	*Percentage of Total*
Internal Medicine	54,182	10,915	20.1%
Pediatrics	43,079	7,874	18.3%
Family Medicine	32,376	4,480	13.8%
Obstetrics/Gynecology	20,820	3,661	17.6%
Psychiatry	14,264	2,420	17.0%
Anesthesiology	10,437	2,067	19.8%

Source: Table 1.13

Figure 1.2

International Medical Graduates by Age and Major Professional Activity, 2010

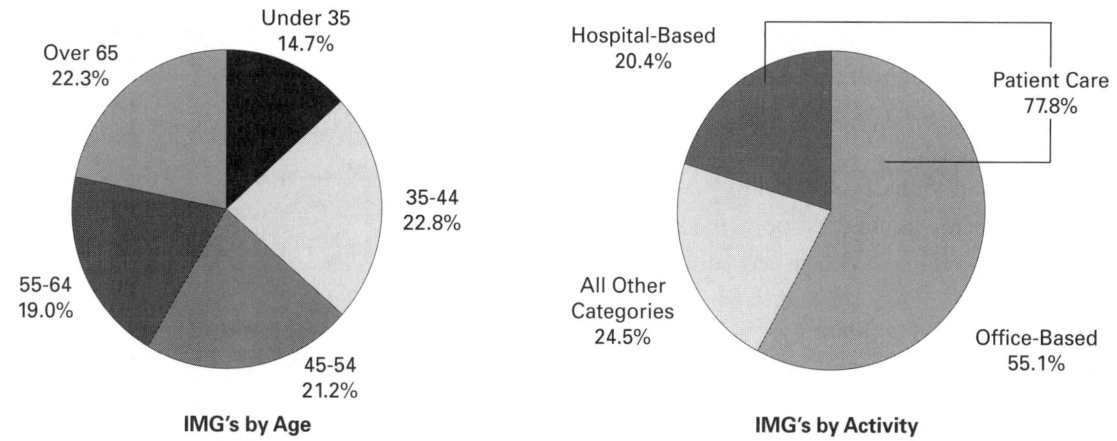

Source: Table 1.11

- Certified by Corresponding Specialty Board Only
- Certified by Corresponding Specialty Board and Other Boards
- Certified by Non-Corresponding Board
- Not Board Certified

These categories can best be illustrated by an example. If a physician reports a specialty of Allergy and Immunology and is certified only by the specialty board of Allergy and Immunology, then the physician falls into the category of Certified by Corresponding Specialty Board Only. If a physician reports the same specialty but is certified by the specialty board of Internal Medicine as well as Allergy and Immunology, then the physician falls into the category of Certified by Corresponding Specialty Board and Others. If a physician reports the same specialty but is certified by the specialty board of Internal Medicine only, then the physician falls into the category of Certified by Other than Board of Corresponding Specialty. See Appendix D for a listing of specialty boards and the subspecialties certified.

In 2010, more than one half (65.7%) of all physicians were certified by their corresponding specialty board only, while another 3.9% of physicians were certified by their corresponding specialty board and others. Physicians certified only by a board other than that corresponding to their specialty totaled 50,552 or 5.1% of all physicians. One quarter (25.3%) of all physicians were not board certified. The greatest proportion of physicians who were board certified (including certification by corresponding board only, certification by corresponding board and others, and certification by non-corresponding board) were physicians in the following 10 specialties:

Pulmonary Disease (95.4%)

Pediatric Cardiology (94.9%)

Gastroenterology (94.6%)

Colon/Rectal Surgery (93.8%)

Cardiovascular Disease (93.7%)

Radiology (93.1%)

Allergy/Immunology (91.8%)

Thoracic Surgery (91.7%)

Medical Genetics (90.5%)

Vascular Medicine (90.0%)

Nearly two thirds of male physicians (71.1%) were certified by a board corresponding to their specialties or certified by a corresponding board and other boards (Table 1.15). The ratio of female physicians similarly accredited was 66.1% (Table 1.16).

Female physicians who were not board certified represented nearly one third (29.4%) of all female physicians. Almost one quarter (23.5%) of male physicians were without board certification. The five specialties having the highest percentages of female physicians who were board certified included Transplant Surgery (100%), Vascular Medicine (100%), Pulmonary Disease (94.7%), Gastroenterology (94.5%), and Pediatric Cardiology (93.6%). The five specialties with the highest percentages of male physicians who were board certified consisted of Pulmonary Diseases (95.5%), Pediatric Cardiology (95.4%), Gastroenterology (94.6%), Colon & Rectal Surgery (93.8%), and Radiology (93.8%).

School of Graduation by Year of Graduation

Table 1.17 indicates that US active medical schools accounted for 72.9% of all physicians in the US and Possessions. Of the total of 985,375 physicians, more than three fifths (66.1%) received their MD degrees since 1980.

The 10 highest schools, ranked by total number of graduates, included University of Illinois (14,476), Jefferson Medical College (14,185), Indiana University (12,938), University of Minnesota (11,900), Wayne State University (10,800), University of Michigan (10,738), SUNY at Brooklyn (10,727), Ohio State University (10,345), Medical College of Pennsylvania (9,851), and New York Medical College (9,611). These schools graduated 115,571 physicians, who represented one in six (16.1%) of all graduates of US active medical schools.

Tables 1.18 and 1.19 reveal that within the composite physician population, nearly nine tenths (83.7%) of all female physicians graduated from medical schools between 1980 and 2010, while 58.5% of male physicians did so. Of the 252,097 IMGs in the US and Possessions in 2010, the highest proportion (23.4%) graduated between 1980 to 1989 (Table 1.17). Figure 1.3 illustrates these patterns in the data.

Self-Designated Specialty by Race/Ethnicity

Race/Ethnicity was known for over three fourths (79.9%) of all physicians, 78.6% for male physicians and 82.9% for female physicians (Tables 1.20 through 1.22). The 10 specialties of all physicians for whom race/ethnicity was known in greatest proportions were Colon/Rectal Surgery (90.6%), Forensic Pathology (88.7%), Dermatology (87.7%), Plastic Surgery (87.3%), Pediatric Cardiology (87.1%), Otolaryngology (86.7%), Medical Genetics (86.6%), Radiation Oncology (86.4%), Physical Medicine and Rehabilitation (86.0%), and Neurological Surgery (85.5%).

Whites accounted for the largest proportion of all physicians with known ethnicity (69.3%), followed by Asians (17.4%), Hispanics (6.5%), and Blacks (4.8%). The five specialties having the highest proportions of white physicians among those for whom an ethnicity was known were Vascular Medicine (88.0%), Aerospace Medicine (87.8%), Orthopedic Surgery (84.5%), Public Health & General Preventive Medicine (83.1%), and Occupational Medicine (82.9%). For Asians, the specialties were Internal Medicine (26.7%), Nuclear Medicine (25.6%), General Practice (25.3%), Physical Medicine and Rehabilitation (24.4%), and Gastroenterology (22.8%). For Hispanics, the specialties were General Practice (13.0%), Pediatrics (8.3%), Colon and Rectal Surgery (8.1%), Child Psychiatry (8.1%), and Nuclear Medicine (7.7%). For Blacks, the specialties were General Preventative Medicine (11.5%), Obstetrics/Gynecology (9.3%), Child Psychiatry (7.3%), Public Health & General Preventive Medicine (6.5%), and Pediatrics (6.3%).

Figure 1.3

Percent Distribution of International Medical Graduates Compared with Total Physicians by Sex and Year of Graduation, 2010

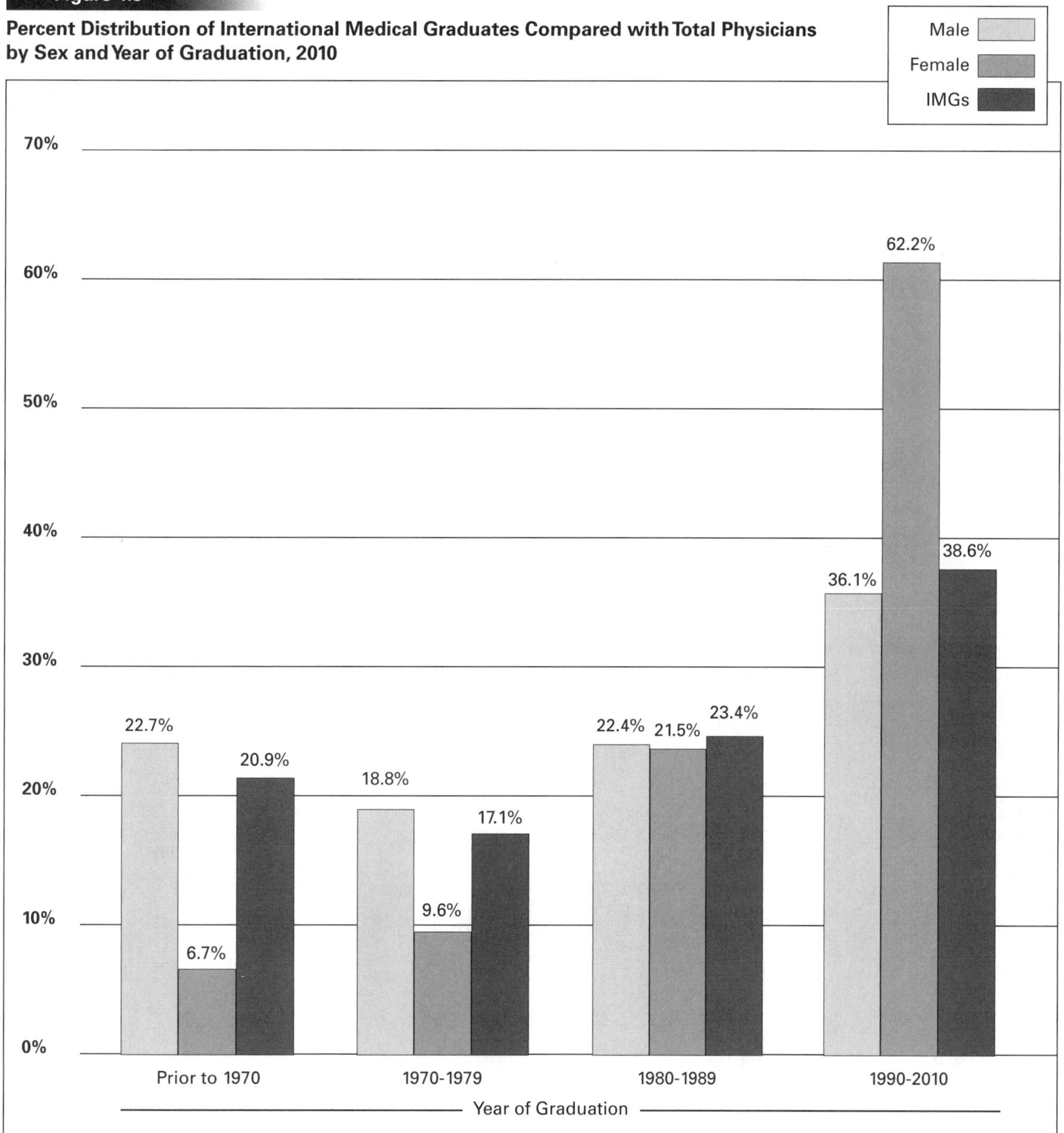

Source: Tables 1.17 through 1.19

Table 1.1

Total Physicians by Age, Activity, and Sex, 2010

Activity	Total Physicians	< 35	35-44	45-54	55-64	≥ 65
			Both Sexes			
Total Physicians	985,375	165,544	214,468	220,858	189,648	194,857
Patient Care	752,572	136,881	183,279	199,436	158,576	74,400
Office-Based Practice	565,024	38,994	151,232	173,113	137,668	64,017
Hospital-Based Practice	187,548	97,887	32,047	26,323	20,908	10,383
Residents	109,065	91,023	16,106	1,767	154	15
Full-Time Staff	79,406	3,470	19,769	25,009	20,789	10,369
Other Professional Activity	42,290	417	3,520	10,135	15,984	12,234
Administration	14,009	59	608	3,060	5,606	4,676
Medical Teaching	9,909	191	1,094	2,575	3,530	2,519
Research	13,755	111	1,313	3,404	5,290	3,637
Other	4,617	56	505	1,096	1,558	1,402
Inactive	125,928	168	1,461	4,749	12,919	106,631
Not Classified	64,153	28,076	26,203	6,538	2,124	1,212
Address Unknown	432	2	5		45	380
			Male			
Total Physicians	688,468	86,505	128,445	152,102	149,078	172,338
Patient Care	513,592	72,441	110,808	138,796	126,115	65,432
Office-Based Practice	399,429	19,759	91,298	120,992	110,471	56,909
Hospital-Based Practice	114,163	52,682	19,510	17,804	15,644	8,523
Residents	59,089	50,862	7,411	738	65	13
Full-Time Staff	55,074	1,820	12,099	17,066	15,579	8,510
Other Professional Activity	32,010	201	1,922	6,773	12,370	10,744
Administration	11,036	24	362	2,075	4,432	4,143
Medical Teaching	7,134	90	583	1,644	2,637	2,180
Research	10,661	57	742	2,410	4,207	3,245
Other	3,179	30	235	644	1,094	1,176
Inactive	107,072	42	489	2,404	9,108	95,029
Not Classified	35,498	13,820	15,224	4,129	1,449	876
Address Unknown	296	1	2		36	257
			Female			
Total Physicians	296,907	79,039	86,023	68,756	40,570	22,519
Patient Care	238,980	64,440	72,471	60,640	32,461	8,968
Office-Based Practice	165,595	19,235	59,934	52,121	27,197	7,108
Hospital-Based Practice	73,385	45,205	12,537	8,519	5,264	1,860
Residents	49,053	43,555	4,867	576	54	1
Full-Time Staff	24,332	1,650	7,670	7,943	5,210	1,859
Other Professional Activity	10,280	216	1,598	3,362	3,614	1,490
Administration	2,973	35	246	985	1,174	533
Medical Teaching	2,775	101	511	931	893	339
Research	3,094	54	571	994	1,083	392
Other	1,438	26	270	452	464	226
Inactive	18,856	126	972	2,345	3,811	11,602
Not Classified	28,655	14,256	10,979	2,409	675	336
Address Unknown	136	1	3		9	123

Table 1.2

Total Physicians by Age and Self-Designated Specialty, 2010

Specialty	Total Physicians	< 35	35-44	45-54	55-64	≥ 65
			Both Sexes			
Total Physicians	985,375	165,544	214,468	220,858	189,648	194,857
Aerospace Medicine	413	10	36	121	143	103
Allergy/Immunology	4,312	478	820	1,121	1,171	722
Anesthesiology	43,359	7,068	8,993	14,670	9,013	3,615
Cardiovascular Disease	22,888	2,466	4,170	6,939	6,281	3,032
Child Psychiatry	7,438	838	1,758	2,182	1,708	952
Colon/Rectal Surgery	1,491	158	480	409	309	135
Dermatology	11,316	2,065	2,670	2,706	2,513	1,362
Diagnostic Radiology	26,054	5,189	5,847	7,094	5,646	2,278
Emergency Medicine	33,278	7,641	9,343	7,513	7,092	1,689
Family Medicine	87,618	13,640	25,065	24,153	19,160	5,600
Forensic Pathology	670	47	144	216	160	103
Gastroenterology	13,210	1,671	2,986	3,931	3,323	1,299
General Practice	8,591	61	310	1,290	2,920	4,010
General Preventive Medicine	2,227	213	581	716	489	228
General Surgery	37,100	8,321	8,125	8,541	7,314	4,799
Internal Medicine	161,276	30,813	41,003	42,280	33,843	13,337
Medical Genetics	597	72	148	156	143	78
Neurological Surgery	5,781	1,117	1,361	1,443	1,088	772
Neurology	15,850	2,646	3,379	4,286	3,843	1,696
Nuclear Medicine	1,456	112	279	341	423	301
Obstetrics/Gynecology	42,797	6,848	10,383	10,987	9,712	4,867
Occupational Medicine	2,426	16	138	738	1,003	531
Ophthalmology	18,457	2,337	3,991	5,148	4,438	2,543
Orthopedic Surgery	25,241	4,796	5,437	6,427	5,368	3,213
Otolaryngology	10,326	1,929	2,341	2,605	2,076	1,375
Pathology-Anatomic/Clinical	19,027	2,458	3,299	5,305	4,693	3,272
Pediatric Cardiology	2,101	402	536	609	334	220
Pediatrics	76,401	16,383	20,751	18,788	14,384	6,095
Physical Medicine & Rehabilitation	9,045	1,718	2,364	2,847	1,497	619
Plastic Surgery	7,418	877	1,629	2,170	1,777	965
Psychiatry	39,738	4,497	6,283	10,209	10,804	7,945
Public Health & General Preventive Medicine	1,283	4	40	278	470	491
Pulmonary Diseases	11,126	1,485	2,867	3,133	2,725	916
Radiation Oncology	4,698	767	1,038	1,453	955	485
Radiology	9,386	898	2,447	2,221	1,697	2,123
Thoracic Surgery	4,605	198	895	1,445	1,194	873
Transplant Surgery	191	4	55	91	34	7
Urological Surgery	10,701	1,523	2,276	2,633	2,448	1,821
Vascular Medicine	30		7	8	10	5
Other Specialty	5,482	795	641	965	1,467	1,614
Unspecified	9,458	4,737	1,883	1,403	892	543
Inactive	125,928	168	1,461	4,749	12,919	106,631
Not Classified	64,153	28,076	26,203	6,538	2,124	1,212
Address Unknown	432	2	5		45	380

Table 1.3

Male Physicians by Age and Self-Designated Specialty, 2010

Specialty	Total Physicians	< 35	35-44	45-54	55-64	≥ 65
			Male			
Total Physicians	688,468	86,505	128,445	152,102	149,078	172,338
Aerospace Medicine	378	6	28	113	130	101
Allergy/Immunology	2,956	182	437	767	927	643
Anesthesiology	32,922	4,516	6,662	11,533	7,241	2,970
Cardiovascular Disease	20,294	1,903	3,396	6,186	5,879	2,930
Child Psychiatry	3,843	311	789	1,045	1,022	676
Colon/Rectal Surgery	1,245	108	357	348	297	135
Dermatology	6,385	698	1,192	1,435	1,849	1,211
Diagnostic Radiology	19,919	3,718	4,190	5,272	4,660	2,079
Emergency Medicine	24,978	4,649	6,765	5,879	6,160	1,525
Family Medicine	55,242	5,933	13,248	15,821	15,309	4,931
Forensic Pathology	440	25	87	133	109	86
Gastroenterology	11,359	1,139	2,382	3,452	3,120	1,266
General Practice	6,735	31	182	893	2,191	3,438
General Preventive Medicine	1,334	86	308	437	320	183
General Surgery	30,460	5,375	6,330	7,326	6,722	4,707
Internal Medicine	107,094	16,710	23,921	28,193	26,486	11,784
Medical Genetics	314	26	65	92	73	58
Neurological Surgery	5,351	960	1,241	1,336	1,044	770
Neurology	11,315	1,389	2,154	3,091	3,154	1,527
Nuclear Medicine	1,134	80	192	255	339	268
Obstetrics/Gynecology	21,977	1,203	3,519	5,891	7,135	4,229
Occupational Medicine	1,900	13	88	509	812	478
Ophthalmology	14,561	1,392	2,822	4,031	3,892	2,424
Orthopedic Surgery	23,804	4,226	5,050	6,118	5,215	3,195
Otolaryngology	8,779	1,350	1,893	2,251	1,929	1,356
Pathology-Anatomic/Clinical	12,014	1,140	1,775	3,198	3,287	2,614
Pediatric Cardiology	1,458	244	328	429	275	182
Pediatrics	33,322	4,691	7,485	8,418	8,435	4,293
Physical Medicine & Rehabilitation	6,036	1,073	1,552	1,932	1,017	462
Plastic Surgery	6,389	646	1,315	1,884	1,609	935
Psychiatry	25,474	2,035	3,445	6,046	7,391	6,557
Public Health & General Preventive Medicine	879	1	25	143	332	378
Pulmonary Diseases	9,248	1,034	2,216	2,596	2,532	870
Radiation Oncology	3,500	515	728	1,085	743	429
Radiology	7,819	701	2,013	1,801	1,365	1,939
Thoracic Surgery	4,384	164	816	1,379	1,154	871
Transplant Surgery	171	3	47	80	34	7
Urological Surgery	9,911	1,179	2,023	2,497	2,396	1,816
Vascular Medicine	23		4	5	9	5
Other Specialty	4,112	374	426	680	1,212	1,420
Unspecified	6,143	2,813	1,234	989	679	428
Inactive	107,072	42	489	2,404	9,108	95,029
Not Classified	35,498	13,820	15,224	4,129	1,449	876
Address Unknown	296	1	2		36	257

Table 1.4

Female Physicians by Age and Self-Designated Specialties, 2010

Specialty	Total Physicians	< 35	35-44	45-54	55-64	≥ 65
			Female			
Total Physicians	296,907	79,039	86,023	68,756	40,570	22,519
Aerospace Medicine	35	4	8	8	13	2
Allergy/Immunology	1,356	296	383	354	244	79
Anesthesiology	10,437	2,552	2,331	3,137	1,772	645
Cardiovascular Disease	2,594	563	774	753	402	102
Child Psychiatry	3,595	527	969	1,137	686	276
Colon/Rectal Surgery	246	50	123	61	12	
Dermatology	4,931	1,367	1,478	1,271	664	151
Diagnostic Radiology	6,135	1,471	1,657	1,822	986	199
Emergency Medicine	8,300	2,992	2,578	1,634	932	164
Family Medicine	32,376	7,707	11,817	8,332	3,851	669
Forensic Pathology	230	22	57	83	51	17
Gastroenterology	1,851	532	604	479	203	33
General Practice	1,856	30	128	397	729	572
General Preventive Medicine	893	127	273	279	169	45
General Surgery	6,640	2,946	1,795	1,215	592	92
Internal Medicine	54,182	14,103	17,082	14,087	7,357	1,553
Medical Genetics	283	46	83	64	70	20
Neurological Surgery	430	157	120	107	44	2
Neurology	4,535	1,257	1,225	1,195	689	169
Nuclear Medicine	322	32	87	86	84	33
Obstetrics/Gynecology	20,820	5,645	6,864	5,096	2,577	638
Occupational Medicine	526	3	50	229	191	53
Ophthalmology	3,896	945	1,169	1,117	546	119
Orthopedic Surgery	1,437	570	387	309	153	18
Otolaryngology	1,547	579	448	354	147	19
Pathology-Anatomic/Clinical	7,013	1,318	1,524	2,107	1,406	658
Pediatric Cardiology	643	158	208	180	59	38
Pediatrics	43,079	11,692	13,266	10,370	5,949	1,802
Physical Medicine & Rehabilitation	3,009	645	812	915	480	157
Plastic Surgery	1,029	231	314	286	168	30
Psychiatry	14,264	2,462	2,838	4,163	3,413	1,388
Public Health & General Preventive Medicine	404	3	15	135	138	113
Pulmonary Diseases	1,878	451	651	537	193	46
Radiation Oncology	1,198	252	310	368	212	56
Radiology	1,567	197	434	420	332	184
Thoracic Surgery	221	34	79	66	40	2
Transplant Surgery	20	1	8	11		
Urological Surgery	790	344	253	136	52	5
Vascular Medicine	7		3	3	1	
Other Specialty	1,370	421	215	285	255	194
Unspecified	3,315	1,924	649	414	213	115
Inactive	18,856	126	972	2,345	3,811	11,602
Not Classified	28,655	14,256	10,979	2,409	675	336
Address Unknown	136	1	3		9	123

Table 1.5

International Medical Graduates by Age and Self-Designated Specialty, 2010

Specialty	Total Physicians	< 35	35-44	45-54	55-64	≥ 65
			Both Sexes			
Total Physicians	254,396	37,385	57,994	53,973	48,295	56,749
Aerospace Medicine	32		2	5	13	12
Allergy/Immunology	1,000	49	158	336	290	167
Anesthesiology	11,423	696	2,335	3,268	3,050	2,074
Cardiovascular Disease	7,089	740	1,435	2,106	1,775	1,033
Child Psychiatry	2,231	183	659	626	472	291
Colon/Rectal Surgery	281	17	71	58	82	53
Dermatology	605	38	101	132	154	180
Diagnostic Radiology	2,871	314	526	526	892	613
Emergency Medicine	2,843	482	442	472	928	519
Family Medicine	20,105	4,207	5,822	4,618	3,585	1,873
Forensic Pathology	144	4	16	46	38	40
Gastroenterology	3,675	413	985	1,072	796	409
General Practice	4,308	36	145	604	1,511	2,012
General Preventive Medicine	320	28	79	103	63	47
General Surgery	6,580	1,023	979	922	1,768	1,888
Internal Medicine	60,935	12,771	17,848	15,745	9,899	4,672
Medical Genetics	154	22	52	45	23	12
Neurological Surgery	749	86	136	125	210	192
Neurology	5,201	766	1,329	1,532	1,076	498
Nuclear Medicine	559	52	110	130	151	116
Obstetrics/Gynecology	6,981	843	1,093	1,016	2,137	1,892
Occupational Medicine	349	1	20	88	148	92
Ophthalmology	1,343	83	214	294	380	372
Orthopedic Surgery	1,512	117	153	196	504	542
Otolaryngology	811	35	57	91	320	308
Pathology-Anatomic/Clinical	6,157	463	1,105	1,867	1,298	1,424
Pediatric Cardiology	507	79	144	151	68	65
Pediatrics	20,442	2,844	4,300	5,750	4,965	2,583
Physical Medicine & Rehabilitation	2,629	290	637	653	655	394
Plastic Surgery	804	49	113	143	291	208
Psychiatry	12,591	1,075	2,177	3,186	3,449	2,704
Public Health & General Preventive Medicine	142		6	21	35	80
Pulmonary Diseases	3,926	662	1,313	1,047	630	274
Radiation Oncology	727	12	71	175	280	189
Radiology	1,679	123	367	211	404	574
Thoracic Surgery	953	39	160	207	234	313
Transplant Surgery	56	2	14	29	9	2
Urological Surgery	1,412	32	103	163	585	529
Vascular Medicine	5		3		2	
Other Specialty	1,052	167	160	147	218	360
Unspecified	3,771	835	927	959	616	434
Inactive	29,608	49	282	778	2,774	25,725
Not Classified	25,748	7,656	11,341	4,330	1,516	905
Address Unknown	86	2	4		1	79

Table 1.6

Male International Medical Graduates by Age and Self-Designated Specialty, 2010

Specialty	Total Physicians	< 35	35-44	45-54	55-64	≥ 65
			Male			
Total Physicians	173,007	20,739	34,238	36,827	35,861	45,342
Aerospace Medicine	30		2	5	12	11
Allergy/Immunology	649	18	70	224	208	129
Anesthesiology	8,453	458	1,638	2,497	2,280	1,580
Cardiovascular Disease	6,395	580	1,194	1,941	1,693	987
Child Psychiatry	1,075	78	288	295	253	161
Colon/Rectal Surgery	263	15	61	52	82	53
Dermatology	380	13	49	75	101	142
Diagnostic Radiology	2,176	207	341	380	717	531
Emergency Medicine	2,361	324	342	421	814	460
Family Medicine	11,971	2,013	2,945	2,844	2,679	1,490
Forensic Pathology	99	2	9	32	27	29
Gastroenterology	3,192	298	784	960	751	399
General Practice	3,195	15	87	420	1,082	1,591
General Preventive Medicine	201	12	43	66	44	36
General Surgery	6,086	825	834	859	1,708	1,860
Internal Medicine	40,624	7,382	10,604	11,034	7,721	3,883
Medical Genetics	88	12	24	33	12	7
Neurological Surgery	724	81	124	119	208	192
Neurology	3,729	469	842	1,127	866	425
Nuclear Medicine	394	36	61	97	103	97
Obstetrics/Gynecology	4,566	309	527	691	1,610	1,429
Occupational Medicine	266	1	11	62	119	73
Ophthalmology	1,045	50	137	205	317	336
Orthopedic Surgery	1,485	113	147	192	498	535
Otolaryngology	757	29	47	86	294	301
Pathology-Anatomic/Clinical	3,440	218	501	1,043	711	967
Pediatric Cardiology	357	48	84	112	57	56
Pediatrics	9,564	1,068	1,686	2,812	2,524	1,474
Physical Medicine & Rehabilitation	1,698	174	400	435	419	270
Plastic Surgery	745	46	94	130	277	198
Psychiatry	7,913	551	1,229	1,911	2,230	1,992
Public Health & General Preventive Medicine	89		6	9	20	54
Pulmonary Diseases	3,337	518	1,082	904	580	253
Radiation Oncology	528	9	43	120	202	154
Radiology	1,328	84	263	179	308	494
Thoracic Surgery	935	34	155	204	230	312
Transplant Surgery	56	2	14	29	9	2
Urological Surgery	1,401	32	100	162	581	526
Vascular Medicine	5		3		2	
Other Specialty	792	103	111	110	179	289
Unspecified	2,514	478	562	665	469	340
Inactive	22,940	14	113	478	1,811	20,524
Not Classified	15,099	4,019	6,579	2,807	1,052	642
Address Unknown	62	1	2		1	58

Table 1.7

Female International Medical Graduates by Age and Self-Designated Specialty, 2010

Specialty	Total Physicians	< 35	35-44	45-54	55-64	≥ 65
			Female			
Total Physicians	81,389	16,646	23,756	17,146	12,434	11,407
Aerospace Medicine	2				1	1
Allergy/Immunology	351	31	88	112	82	38
Anesthesiology	2,970	238	697	771	770	494
Cardiovascular Disease	694	160	241	165	82	46
Child Psychiatry	1,156	105	371	331	219	130
Colon/Rectal Surgery	18	2	10	6		
Dermatology	225	25	52	57	53	38
Diagnostic Radiology	695	107	185	146	175	82
Emergency Medicine	482	158	100	51	114	59
Family Medicine	8,134	2,194	2,877	1,774	906	383
Forensic Pathology	45	2	7	14	11	11
Gastroenterology	483	115	201	112	45	10
General Practice	1,113	21	58	184	429	421
General Preventive Medicine	119	16	36	37	19	11
General Surgery	494	198	145	63	60	28
Internal Medicine	20,311	5,389	7,244	4,711	2,178	789
Medical Genetics	66	10	28	12	11	5
Neurological Surgery	25	5	12	6	2	
Neurology	1,472	297	487	405	210	73
Nuclear Medicine	165	16	49	33	48	19
Obstetrics/Gynecology	2,415	534	566	325	527	463
Occupational Medicine	83		9	26	29	19
Ophthalmology	298	33	77	89	63	36
Orthopedic Surgery	27	4	6	4	6	7
Otolaryngology	54	6	10	5	26	7
Pathology-Anatomic/Clinical	2,717	245	604	824	587	457
Pediatric Cardiology	150	31	60	39	11	9
Pediatrics	10,878	1,776	2,614	2,938	2,441	1,109
Physical Medicine & Rehabilitation	931	116	237	218	236	124
Plastic Surgery	59	3	19	13	14	10
Psychiatry	4,678	524	948	1,275	1,219	712
Public Health & General Preventive Medicine	53			12	15	26
Pulmonary Diseases	589	144	231	143	50	21
Radiation Oncology	199	3	28	55	78	35
Radiology	351	39	104	32	96	80
Thoracic Surgery	18	5	5	3	4	1
Urological Surgery	11		3	1	4	3
Other Specialty	260	64	49	37	39	71
Unspecified	1,257	357	365	294	147	94
Inactive	6,668	35	169	300	963	5,201
Not Classified	10,649	3,637	4,762	1,523	464	263
Address Unknown	24	1	2			21

Table 1.8

Physicians' Mean Age by Self-Designated Specialty and Activity (236 Specialties), 2010

		Patient Care				Other Professional Activity			
				Hospital Based					
Specialty	Total Physicians	Total Patient Care	Office Based	Resid./ Fellows	Phys. Staff	Admin.	Med. Teach.	Research	Other
Total Physicians	51.0	47.7	50.4	30.2	51.7	61.1	57.7	58.6	58.9
A	64.4	64.3	64.2		65.5	60.5	63.5	67.2	70.3
ACA	32.9	32.7	33.6	32.0	35.0				63.0
ADL	49.8	47.9	50.2	32.5	53.2	61.8	57.0	53.3	50.0
ADM	59.6	59.6	59.3		60.9	59.1	65.0	55.2	63.3
ADP	45.9	45.4	46.5	36.6	50.6	53.8	53.0	52.7	
AI	48.8	48.3	50.1	31.7	48.5	59.9	60.0	56.9	53.1
ALI	51.2	50.7	51.3		49.0	46.0	66.0	54.5	
AM	57.6	55.5	58.8		52.2	60.4	65.4	59.0	61.7
AMF	49.7	49.7	42.5		64.0				
AMI	55.0	55.8	57.6		47.3	49.5	72.0	36.0	
AN	48.2	47.9	50.5	29.8	51.8	59.2	58.4	57.9	58.2
APM	44.2	44.2	44.2	31.0	44.4	36.0	45.5	48.0	
AR	36.7	36.4	37.6	33.5	38.5	70.0			38.0
AS	63.2	63.1	63.9		59.9	72.8	60.3	57.0	56.0
ATP	57.9	57.1	56.6	28.0	58.5	61.1	64.7	58.3	58.7
BBK	52.1	49.1	49.8	33.4	54.2	61.5	56.4	57.1	58.8
CAP	45.3	47.5	45.7		53.0	48.0	41.0	38.0	
CBG	54.3	49.9	50.8		49.0		74.0	57.4	
CCA	43.1	42.9	44.6	33.2	45.1	53.2	50.4	43.5	44.0
CCG	54.1	54.0	55.5		48.0			54.0	54.3
CCM	46.9	46.0	47.3	33.4	49.9	59.2	58.1	56.5	55.5
CCP	42.0	41.6	44.7	32.2	46.1	56.7	50.0	46.7	
CCS	42.0	41.7	43.4	34.6	45.3	63.3	44.9	59.5	52.0
CD	51.2	50.6	53.0	32.1	54.0	64.2	62.2	59.9	61.1
CFS	40.7	40.7	43.8	32.5	43.3				
CG	57.9	57.1	58.3		55.1	60.0	61.8	60.5	61.0
CHN	48.4	47.3	51.5	31.8	52.6	61.7	60.5	57.1	58.8
CHP	50.1	49.5	50.9	33.4	53.7	60.6	60.0	57.4	62.8
CHS	40.3	40.3	46.0	37.0	51.0				
CLP	60.9	60.0	60.2	30.0	60.0	63.6	59.7	60.0	61.7
CMG	47.0	52.0	52.0				54.0	44.8	41.0
CN	39.0	38.7	40.1	33.7	41.8	43.0	35.7	42.6	67.4
CPP	31.4	31.4	38.8	29.2	43.0			33.0	
CRS	48.5	48.3	49.2	32.7	49.3	58.3	55.6	54.8	58.0
CS	52.3	52.3	52.3		52.5	40.0			
CTR	41.5	41.9	45.2	32.0	39.0		38.0		

A	Allergy
ACA	Adult Cardiothoracic Anesthesiology (Anesthesiology)
ADL	Adolescent Medicine (Pediatrics)
ADM	Addiction Medicine
ADP	Addiction Psychiatry
AI	Allergy And Immunology
ALI	Clinical Laboratory Immunology (Allergy & Immunology)
AM	Aerospace Medicine
AMF	Adolescent Medicine (Family Medicine)
AMI	Adolescent Medicine (Internal Medicine)
AN	Anesthesiology
APM	Pain Medicine (Anesthesiology)
AR	Abdominal Radiology
AS	Abdominal Surgery
ATP	Anatomic Pathology
BBK	Blood Banking/Transfusion Medicine
CAP	Child Abuse Pediatrics
CBG	Clinical Biochemical Genetics
CCA	Critical Care Medicine (Anesthesiology)
CCG	Clinical Cytogenetics
CCM	Critical Care Medicine (Internal Medicine)
CCP	Pediatric Critical Care Medicine
CCS	Surgical Critical Care (Surgery)
CD	Cardiovascular Disease
CFS	Craniofacial Surgery
CG	Clinical Genetics
CHN	Child Neurology
CHP	Child & Adolescent Psychiatry
CHS	Congenital Cardiac Surgery (Thoracic Surgery)
CLP	Clinical Pathology
CMG	Clinical Molecular Genetics
CN	Clinical Neurophysiology
CPP	Pediatrics/Psychiatry/Child & Adolescent Psychiatry
CRS	Colon And Rectal Surgery
CS	Cosmetic Surgery
CTR	Cardiothoracic Radiology

Table 1.8

Physicians' Mean Age by Self-Designated Specialty and Activity (236 Specialties), 2010, continued

		Patient Care				Other Professional Activity			
				Hospital Based					
Specialty	Total Physicians	Total Patient Care	Office Based	Resid./ Fellows	Phys. Staff	Admin.	Med. Teach.	Research	Other
D	48.4	48.2	50.6	29.9	49.0	61.1	59.2	57.6	57.2
DBP	39.8	39.0	45.1	34.3	43.7	60.5	55.0	40.0	
DDL	56.0								56.0
DIA	63.9	62.8	62.9		62.3	69.0	66.5	65.6	61.0
DMP	44.6	43.8	44.9	33.2	49.9	56.0	60.8	59.0	50.5
DR	47.2	46.9	50.5	30.2	52.6	60.9	58.2	58.9	55.7
DS	49.7	49.7	49.7		48.3				
EFM	45.4	45.4	50.5	29.5	53.8				
EM	45.2	44.8	46.6	29.2	49.9	57.7	53.8	51.2	55.8
EMP	30.4	30.4	36.8	29.0					
END	49.0	47.3	49.1	32.1	51.2	63.6	60.1	59.0	59.8
ENR	36.0	36.0		36.0					
EP	56.2	55.2	53.3	55.0	61.0	53.8	48.0	59.7	51.9
ES	37.0	37.0	37.0						
ESM	41.5	40.9	46.3	29.5	35.0		54.0		
ESN	40.3	40.2	43.2	32.8	42.3		43.0		
ETX	39.1	38.0	41.3	33.2	40.3	58.0	53.5		52.8
FM	47.2	46.9	48.6	30.9	49.4	57.0	53.1	53.4	56.0
FMP	36.3	36.3	34.0	35.0	40.0				
FOP	51.8	48.8	49.8	35.4	51.0	60.9	68.6	66.3	57.8
FPG	45.6	44.9	46.1	33.7	49.3	59.1	53.0	46.6	57.3
FPP	33.4	33.0	38.9	29.6	55.0				60.0
FPS	50.4	50.4	50.5	30.0	48.6	45.0	52.0		55.0
FSM	37.4	37.4	38.4	31.8	39.9	51.0			
GE	49.4	48.9	50.9	31.8	51.1	63.0	59.6	58.9	62.1
GO	54.0	53.3	53.8	33.5	51.0	63.9	61.2	58.9	58.0
GP	64.3	64.3	64.4		63.6	65.4	66.0	62.8	62.6
GPM	49.6	47.5	49.3	35.6	49.9	58.4	57.3	57.6	51.9
GS	47.2	46.7	52.6	29.5	53.5	65.8	61.4	60.7	65.3
GYN	60.8	60.7	60.8		59.5	64.8	63.3	59.3	65.7
HEM	56.6	54.7	55.0	32.4	57.3	66.8	63.9	62.0	56.7
HEP	53.0	51.8	53.2		48.3	61.3	58.8	58.5	49.0
HMP	43.2	42.6	43.6	35.2	47.7	59.5	53.4	51.7	49.7
HNS	57.4	57.6	57.5		58.2	59.3	55.5	35.0	46.0
HO	41.3	41.0	43.8	32.6	44.5	59.0	52.7	48.8	54.1
HOS	43.2	43.1	43.3	29.5	43.2	47.0	53.0	39.0	

D Dermatology
DBP Developmental-Behavioral Pediatrics
DDL Clinical & Laboratory Dermatological Immunology
DIA Diabetes
DMP Dermatopathology (Pathology)
DR Diagnostic Radiology
DS Dermatologic Surgery
EFM Emergency Medicine/Family Medicine
EM Emergency Medicine
EMP Pediatrics/Emergency Medicine
END Endocrinology, Diabetes & Metabolism
ENR Endovascular Surgical Neuroradiology (Neurology)
EP Epidemiology
ES Endovascular Surgical Neuroradiology (Neurological Surgery)
ESM Sports Medicine (Emergency Medicine)
ESN Endovascular Surgical Neuroradiology (Radiology)
ETX Medical Toxicology (Emergency Medicine)
FM Family Medicine
FMP Family Medicine/Preventive Medicine
FOP Forensic Pathology
FPG Geriatric Medicine (Family Medicine)
FPP Psychiatry/Family Medicine
FPS Facial Plastic Surgery
FSM Sports Medicine (Family Practice)
GE Gastroenterology
GO Gynecological Oncology
GP General Practice
GPM General Preventive Medicine
GS General Surgery
GYN Gynecology
HEM Hematology (Internal Medicine)
HEP Hepatology
HMP Hematology (Pathology)
HNS Head And Neck Surgery
HO Hematology/Oncology
HOS Hospitalist

Table 1.8

Physicians' Mean Age by Self-Designated Specialty and Activity (236 Specialties), 2010, continued

		Patient Care				Other Professional Activity			
				Hospital Based					
Specialty	Total Physicians	Total Patient Care	Office Based	Resid./ Fellows	Phys. Staff	Admin.	Med. Teach.	Research	Other
HPD	68.0	68.0			68.0				
HPE	53.0	53.0	53.0						
HPF	51.2	49.4	49.4			54.8			
HPI	52.2	54.1	54.5		52.8	49.3	35.0	45.0	61.0
HPM	37.2	36.3	41.9	34.0	45.3	54.4			
HPN	60.0					60.0			
HPO	65.7	65.7	68.5		60.0				
HPP	69.0	69.0			69.0				
HPR	47.0	47.0	47.0						
HS	49.9	49.7	49.7		49.2	62.4	58.3	59.6	67.3
HSO	34.2	34.2	34.9	32.9	36.3				
HSP	35.6	35.6	37.2	33.2	37.5				
HSS	34.5	34.5	35.9	32.4					
IC	40.9	40.8	41.6	34.7	44.2	60.0	49.6	43.0	
ICE	42.7	42.5	43.7	34.4	45.5	46.0	48.3	56.9	50.7
ID	48.0	45.7	47.3	32.4	50.0	59.8	58.7	57.4	54.5
IEC	33.8	33.8	44.5	31.1					
IFP	38.6	38.6	45.6	30.3	66.5				
IG	64.4	59.2	59.0		59.8	70.3	66.6	65.6	64.4
ILI	64.2	77.0	74.0		80.0	48.0	66.0	58.5	
IM	46.5	46.0	49.5	29.2	49.6	58.8	55.0	56.9	56.4
IMD	28.8	28.8	31.7	28.3	31.0				
IMG	46.5	45.5	45.9	34.3	49.5	58.3	56.8	54.7	61.5
INM	40.0	40.0	40.0						
IPM	37.8	37.1	48.4	30.3	38.0	58.0	50.0		
ISM	44.4	44.2	43.9		47.3		49.0	50.0	
LM	61.5	60.0	61.1		54.8	62.1	69.0	56.0	61.4
MBG	32.0	32.0		32.0					
MDG	29.6	29.6		29.6					
MDM	59.9	62.3	62.5		61.0	59.8	72.0	57.0	59.1
MEM	30.2	30.2	35.8	29.2	32.0				
MFM	54.2	53.6	54.2	34.8	52.6	61.9	56.8	56.4	66.0
MG	47.7	45.1	48.8	34.2	47.8	59.0	61.3	55.2	56.2
MGG	49.0							49.0	
MGP	38.0	37.9	40.4	36.6	52.0	48.0			35.0
MM	52.3	46.8	46.5	32.4	59.4	61.6	77.5	63.7	55.7
MN	33.0	29.7	39.0	28.5			63.0		
MP	33.1	32.7	37.8	31.0	50.0	53.5			

HPD Hospice and Palliative Medicine (Radiology)
HPE Hospice & Palliative Medicine (Emergency Medicine)
HPF Hospice & Palliative Medicine (Family Medicine)
HPI Hospice & Palliative Medicine (Internal Medicine)
HPM Hospice & Palliative Medicine
HPN Hospice & Palliative Medicine (Psychiatry & Neurology)
HPO Hospice & Palliative Medicine (Obstetrics & Gynecology)
HPP Hospice and Palliative Medicine (Pediatrics)
HPR Hospice and Palliative Medicine (Physical Medicine & Rehabilitation)
HS Hand Surgery
HSO Hand Surgery (Orthopedics)
HSP Hand Surgery (Plastic Surgery)
HSS Hand Surgery (Surgery)
IC Interventional Cardiology
ICE Clinical Cardiac Electrophysiology
ID Infectious Disease
IEC Internal Med/Emergency Med/Critical Care Med
IFP Internal Medicine/Family Practice
IG Immunology
ILI Clinical And Laboratory Immunology (Internal Medicine)
IM Internal Medicine
IMD Internal Medicine/Dermatology
IMG Geriatric Medicine (Internal Medicine)
INM Internal Medicine/Nuclear Medicine
IPM Internal Medicine/Preventive Medicine
ISM Sports Medicine (Internal Medicine)
LM Legal Medicine
MBG Medical Biochemical Genetics
MDG Internal Medicine/Medical Genetics
MDM Medical Management
MEM Internal Medicine/Emergency Medicine
MFM Maternal And Fetal Medicine
MG Medical Genetics
MGG Molecular Genetic Pathology (Medical Genetics)
MGP Molecular Genetic Pathology (Pathology And Medical Genetics)
MM Medical Microbiology
MN Internal Medicine/Neurology
MP Internal Med/Psychiatry

Table 1.8

Physicians' Mean Age by Self-Designated Specialty and Activity (236 Specialties), 2010, continued

		Patient Care				Other Professional Activity			
				Hospital Based					
Specialty	Total Physicians	Total Patient Care	Office Based	Resid./ Fellows	Phys. Staff	Admin.	Med. Teach.	Research	Other
MPD	36.4	36.3	39.5	28.8	40.1	42.8	40.3	42.1	46.1
MPM	64.0	64.0	64.0						
MSR	37.2	37.0	37.8	32.9	40.1	50.0	49.0		
N	49.6	48.8	52.2	30.5	52.4	62.1	60.5	57.9	60.3
NC	51.0	51.0	52.0		48.0				
NDN	37.9	37.9	47.8	34.2	47.0				
NDP	52.9	53.7	53.3		55.3	52.0	48.0	46.0	
NEP	47.4	46.4	48.1	31.9	51.1	63.3	60.3	58.5	61.2
NM	53.5	52.4	54.0	34.7	57.0	61.6	62.1	63.8	63.3
NMN	35.8	35.8	39.1	32.8	38.0				
NMP	65.0	65.0	65.0						
NO	50.6	50.6	53.3	33.8	51.1		55.0		
NP	54.7	50.9	52.9	36.2	57.9	61.1	65.9	61.0	65.0
NPM	48.8	47.9	50.0	32.3	52.4	60.2	59.0	56.8	60.4
NR	48.4	47.8	49.1	35.0	49.8		56.0	64.5	59.0
NRN	54.7	52.3	52.6		51.1	67.0	56.0	74.0	67.0
NS	48.0	47.7	52.2	30.4	51.4	66.2	60.1	61.9	65.5
NSP	52.3	52.3	52.3		52.2				
NTR	61.7	58.9	59.1		57.5	67.8	58.5	66.0	63.0
NUP	53.8	53.6	54.5		51.0		53.0	50.0	63.0
OAR	43.0	42.9	44.1	33.2	42.7		52.7	52.0	
OBG	47.5	47.2	49.6	29.0	50.5	62.1	57.8	56.8	58.1
OBS	58.9	58.5	58.8		57.1	59.4	63.0	68.8	49.0
OCC	64.8	54.5	54.5			72.0		71.5	
OFA	42.5	42.5	43.0	32.5	50.6		35.0		
OM	58.4	57.5	57.7	38.0	56.7	60.8	58.4	61.1	61.4
OMF	42.7	42.3	42.8	31.6	41.4	64.5	54.8		
OMM	54.8	54.8	54.8						
OMO	43.0	42.7	43.7	35.1	44.7		55.0		
ON	55.2	54.5	55.0	32.8	55.2	63.9	61.9	57.7	60.3
OP	47.1	46.8	47.6	32.7	49.9	63.0	59.8		
OPH	50.1	49.9	51.9	29.3	50.2	60.7	56.0	59.6	61.1
OPR	36.0	36.0	36.0						
ORS	49.3	49.0	53.0	29.3	52.7	64.7	61.2	62.1	68.3
OS	54.9	46.9	56.7	27.3	59.1	69.2	70.9	70.0	63.1
OSM	40.9	40.8	41.5	32.4	45.2	47.5	43.5	54.0	
OSS	46.8	46.7	47.3	32.5	46.1	49.0	47.2	59.5	64.5
OTO	48.3	48.1	51.6	29.1	50.5	60.3	56.0	61.2	62.5

MPD Internal Medicine/Pediatrics
MPM Internal Med/Phys Med And Rehabilitation
MSR Musculoskeletal Radiology
N Neurology
NC Nuclear Cardiology
NDN Neurodevelopmental Disabilities (Psychiatry & Neurology
NDP Neurodevelopmental Disabilities (Pediatrics)
NEP Nephrology
NM Nuclear Medicine
NMN Neuromuscular Medicine (Neurology)
NMP Neuromuscular Medicine (Physical Medicine & Rehabilitation)
NO Neurotology (Otolaryngology)
NP Neuropathology
NPM Neonatal-Perinatal Medicine
NR Nuclear Radiology
NRN Neurology/Diagnostic Radiology/Neuroradiology
NS Neurological Surgery
NSP Pediatric Surgery (Neurology)
NTR Nutrition
NUP Neuropsychiatry
OAR Adult Reconstructive Orthopedics
OBG Obstetrics & Gynecology
OBS Obstetrics
OCC Critical Care Medicine (Obstetrics & Gynecology)
OFA Foot And Ankle Orthopedics
OM Occupational Medicine
OMF Oral & Maxillofacial Surgery
OMM Osteopathic Manipulative Medicine
OMO Musculoskeletal Oncology
ON Medical Oncology
OP Pediatric Orthopedics
OPH Ophthalmology
OPR Ophthalmic Plastic and Reconstructive Surgery
ORS Orthopedic Surgery
OS Other Specialty
OSM Sports Medicine (Orthopedic Surgery)
OSS Orthopedic Surgery Of The Spine
OTO Otolaryngology

Table 1.8

Physicians' Mean Age by Self-Designated Specialty and Activity (236 Specialties), 2010, continued

		Patient Care				Other Professional Activity			
				Hospital Based					
Specialty	Total Physicians	Total Patient Care	Office Based	Resid./ Fellows	Phys. Staff	Admin.	Med. Teach.	Research	Other
OTR	44.8	44.5	46.5	32.2	46.8		50.2		
P	53.1	52.5	55.1	31.5	56.8	62.3	59.3	58.1	63.4
PA	64.2	59.7	59.6		59.9	69.6	66.1	63.8	70.4
PAN	39.0	38.8	40.6	32.4	42.0	55.0	46.8	39.0	
PCC	39.7	39.5	42.0	32.2	42.8	53.8	45.1	43.6	45.2
PCH	59.6	55.7	55.7	39.0	72.0	62.6	58.0	57.0	67.8
PCP	43.6	43.3	44.6	35.9	46.0	62.0	56.8	55.8	44.9
PCS	50.5	50.2	50.1		50.6	65.0			
PD	46.9	46.4	48.9	28.5	50.0	60.6	57.0	56.9	56.9
PDA	61.1	60.7	61.3		54.8	55.5	59.7	65.8	68.5
PDC	47.2	46.3	49.8	31.7	50.9	66.9	60.1	58.6	58.2
PDD	44.2	44.2	42.9		55.0				
PDE	45.4	44.0	48.0	31.7	49.3	61.0	62.4	53.9	57.6
PDI	40.1	38.4	42.0	31.9	45.8	53.1	48.3	48.6	47.0
PDM	31.3	31.3	33.0	29.5					
PDO	45.5	45.2	47.0	31.1	46.0		53.2		
PDP	45.3	44.6	47.0	32.2	50.3	55.6	55.2	51.1	65.0
PDR	48.8	48.3	49.0	33.9	53.4	66.8	57.1	63.8	54.3
PDS	50.8	50.0	51.7	33.7	51.7	67.4	64.9	59.1	60.5
PDT	62.0	62.0	62.0						
PE	38.3	37.9	41.1	32.2	41.6	47.3	45.0	52.0	
PEM	39.7	39.1	42.8	31.2	45.6	56.2	52.6	50.3	48.0
PFP	42.7	41.3	42.4	35.5	42.8	49.6	48.0	51.3	61.8
PG	42.4	41.8	45.8	31.6	46.8	57.3	58.0	50.2	65.5
PHL	53.2	53.2	53.4		48.3	56.0		40.0	
PHM	54.2	53.2	53.2			51.8	38.0	55.8	53.0
PHO	45.7	44.4	48.2	31.7	49.3	63.4	52.3	53.4	54.5
PHP	62.9	60.7	61.3	42.5	59.8	65.8	65.6	59.7	59.1
PLI	63.0	63.0	63.0						
PLM	52.9	52.4	52.9	38.0	51.6	56.4	59.5	48.3	56.3
PM	47.2	46.8	48.5	30.6	52.7	59.1	61.3	52.7	61.0
PME	53.5	53.3	53.3		52.8	56.5	56.0	67.4	64.0
PMG	33.4	33.4	52.8	29.8	43.0				
PMM	39.7	39.5	41.3	33.3	47.2	61.5	58.6	47.0	49.5
PMN	48.7	48.7	47.5		51.0				
PMP	47.6	47.1	47.3		44.0				56.0

OTR Orthopedic Trauma
P Psychiatry
PA Clinical Pharmacology
PAN Pediatric Anesthesiology (Anesthesiology)
PCC Pulmonary & Critical Care Medicine
PCH Chemical Pathology
PCP Cytopathology
PCS Pediatric Cardiothoracic Surgery
PD Pediatrics
PDA Pediatric Allergy
PDC Pediatric Cardiology
PDD Pediatric Dermatology
PDE Pediatric Endocrinology
PDI Pediatric Infectious Disease
PDM Pediatrics/Dermatology
PDO Pediatric Otolaryngology
PDP Pediatric Pulmonology
PDR Pediatric Radiology
PDS Pediatric Surgery (Surgery)
PDT Medical Toxicology (Pediatrics)
PE Pediatric Emergency Med (Emergency Med)
PEM Pediatric Emergency Medicine (Pediatrics)
PFP Forensic Psychiatry
PG Pediatric Gastroenterology
PHL Phlebology
PHM Pharmaceutical Medicine
PHO Pediatric Hematology/Oncology
PHP Public Health And General Preventive Medicine
PLI Clinical & Laboratory Immunology (Pediatrics)
PLM Palliative Medicine
PM Physical Medicine And Rehabilitation
PME Pain Management
PMG Pediatrics/Medical Genetics
PMM Pain Medicine
PMN Pain Medicine (Neurology)
PMP Pain Medicine (Physical Medicine & Rehabilitation)

Table 1.8

Physicians' Mean Age by Self-Designated Specialty and Activity (236 Specialties), 2010, continued

		Patient Care				Other Professional Activity			
				Hospital Based					
Specialty	Total Physicians	Total Patient Care	Office Based	Resid./ Fellows	Phys. Staff	Admin.	Med. Teach.	Research	Other
PN	46.4	44.6	48.5	31.3	51.5	61.7	55.4	54.3	57.5
PO	52.3	52.2	51.9		55.9	58.0	56.0		
PP	48.9	48.0	49.5	34.9	49.9		57.4	67.0	56.0
PPM	33.0	32.6	43.6	29.4				41.0	
PPN	55.2	55.0	55.0			56.0			
PPR	40.1	38.3	43.6	31.9	46.1		58.0	50.4	47.0
PRD	34.0	34.0	35.3	31.7	37.0				
PRO	49.0	49.0	49.0						
PRS	41.6	41.7	45.5	30.3	44.0			39.0	
PS	51.2	51.1	52.6	32.0	50.8	61.0	62.1	63.9	62.6
PSH	45.0	45.0	47.0		35.0				
PSI	29.3	29.3		29.3					
PSM	38.1	38.1	39.1	30.5	45.7			36.0	
PSO	37.0	37.0	37.0						
PSP	57.7	57.7	57.7						
PTH	52.4	51.0	54.4	31.6	58.1	64.6	64.9	65.0	59.1
PTX	44.4	40.3	45.9	32.3	38.0	56.0		65.5	
PUD	56.3	55.6	55.9	32.9	56.4	62.4	62.8	59.7	63.2
PYA	71.7	71.6	71.5		73.7	76.5	75.3	86.5	
PYG	46.6	46.1	46.1	36.3	49.1	62.9	53.2	54.0	
PYM	37.0	37.0	41.0	34.7	36.8				
PYN	37.7	37.7	56.3	29.4	48.0				
R	62.6	62.4	62.3	31.8	63.0	67.5	64.2	64.1	64.6
REN	54.6	54.1	54.2		53.5	60.5	59.1	54.2	63.8
RHU	50.2	49.2	51.0	32.4	51.0	63.2	59.5	58.1	60.2
RNR	42.5	42.3	43.3	33.4	46.1	49.0	52.6	56.0	45.2
RO	48.2	48.0	50.6	30.4	51.3	63.1	56.8	59.6	50.9
RP	50.0							50.0	
RPM	40.2	39.4	46.8	33.0	44.6			57.0	
SCI	41.6	41.4	41.6	30.5	51.1	48.0			49.0
SME	42.9	42.2	45.6	34.2	46.6	61.6	61.7	47.4	66.5
SMI	54.7	54.5	53.8		62.0		61.0		
SMN	55.4	55.4	55.7		51.0				
SMO	41.0	41.0	41.0						
SMP	59.0							59.0	
SO	51.3	51.0	51.6	32.0	49.3	62.4	56.2	53.1	67.0

PN Pediatric Nephrology
PO Pediatric Opthalmology
PP Pediatric Pathology
PPM Pediatrics/Physical Medicine And Rehabilitation
PPN Pain Medicine (Psychiatry)
PPR Pediatric Rheumatology
PRD Procedural Dermatology
PRO Proctology
PRS Sports Medicine (Physical Medicine & Rehabilitation)
PS Plastic Surgery
PSH Plastic Surgery Within The Head & Neck
PSI Plastic Surgery-Integrated
PSM Sports Medicine (Pediatrics)
PSO Plastic Surgery within the Head and Neck (Otolaryngology)
PSP Plastic Surgery Within the Head & Neck (Plastic Surgery)
PTH Anatomic/Clinical Pathology
PTX Medical Toxicology (Preventive Medicine)
PUD Pulmonary Disease
PYA Psychoanalysis
PYG Geriatric Psychiatry
PYM Psychosomatic Medicine
PYN Psychiatry/Neurology
R Radiology
REN Reproductive Endocrinology And Infertility
RHU Rheumatology
RNR Neuroradiology
RO Radiation Oncology
RP Radiological Physics
RPM Pediatric Rehabilitation Medicine
SCI Spinal Cord Injury Medicine
SME Sleep Medicine
SMI Sleep Medicine (Internal Medicine)
SMN Sleep Medicine (Psychiatry & Neurology)
SMO Sleep Medicine (Otolaryngology)
SMP Sleep Medicine (Pediatrics)
SO Surgical Oncology

Table 1.8

Physicians' Mean Age by Self-Designated Specialty and Activity (236 Specialties), 2010, continued

		Patient Care				Other Professional Activity			
				Hospital Based					
Specialty	Total Physicians	Total Patient Care	Office Based	Resid./ Fellows	Phys. Staff	Admin.	Med. Teach.	Research	Other
SP	40.0	39.9	42.5	34.4	42.2		47.0	43.0	45.8
THP	35.2	35.2	38.4	33.8					
TRS	53.2	52.6	52.6		52.7	61.7	51.9	60.1	61.5
TS	53.7	53.3	54.4	34.3	54.2	66.2	61.8	64.5	64.0
TSI	30.3	30.3		30.3					
TTS	48.9	48.7	49.3	40.0	47.1	57.7	55.8	45.4	42.0
U	50.6	50.4	52.9	29.9	54.2	64.8	58.5	56.8	68.9
UCM	54.6	54.7	54.7		54.5	48.4	59.0		52.0
UM	53.6	53.7	54.6	38.0	52.7	53.5		53.0	
UME	41.6	41.6	40.7	42.7					
UP	47.7	47.3	49.3	33.1	48.2	62.3	55.0		53.5
US	40.2	39.6	49.4	29.4	50.2	61.0	55.1	58.5	50.0
VIR	42.9	42.7	43.6	33.6	44.8	55.8	55.8	59.3	
VM	53.9	53.5	53.3		54.2			64.0	
VN	34.6	34.5	38.2	32.6	37.5		49.0		
VS	49.0	48.6	50.5	32.6	50.8	64.5	59.9	57.8	61.4
Inactive	75.0								
Not Class	37.7								
Addr Unkn	79.8								

SP Selective Pathology
THP Transplant Hepatology (Internal Medicine)
TRS Traumatic Surgery
TS Thoracic Surgery
TSI Thoracic Surgery-Integrated
TTS Transplant Surgery
U Urology
UCM Urgent Care Medicine
UM Underseas Medicine (Preventive Medicine)
UME Underseas Medicine (Emergency Medicine)
UP Pediatric Urology
US Unspecified
VIR Vascular And Interventional Radiology
VM Vascular Medicine
VN Vascular Neurology
VS Vascular Surgery

Table 1.9

Physicians by Self-Designated Specialty and Activity (236 Specialties), 2010

		Patient Care				Other Professional Activity			
				Hospital Based					
Specialty	Total Physicians	Total Patient Care	Office Based	Resid./ Fellows	Phys. Staff	Admin.	Med. Teach.	Research	Other
Total Phys	985,375	752,572	565,024	108,142	79,406	14,009	9,909	13,755	4,617
A	592	548	537		11	10	4	26	4
ACA	184	183	76	103	4				1
ADL	482	390	258	61	71	37	34	16	5
ADM	227	181	144		37	25	4	9	8
ADP	355	336	224	58	54	9	7	3	
AI	3,425	3,257	2,786	299	172	17	24	115	12
ALI	37	33	24		9	1	1	2	
AM	413	243	121		122	116	8	24	22
AMF	3	3	2		1				
AMI	21	17	14		3	2	1	1	
AN	40,636	39,642	29,574	5,212	4,856	261	457	200	76
APM	1,444	1,440	1,301	1	138	1	2	1	
AR	114	111	70	35	6	1			2
AS	95	85	68		17	4	3	2	1
ATP	1,023	739	510	1	228	32	54	127	71
BBK	502	364	248	37	79	83	7	22	26
CAP	7	4	3		1	1	1	1	
CBG	14	8	4		4		1	5	
CCA	543	526	355	81	90	5	9	2	1
CCG	9	5	4		1			1	3
CCM	1,510	1,400	942	181	277	39	43	24	4
CCP	1,436	1,368	725	373	270	22	21	25	
CCS	765	747	445	170	132	3	8	6	1
CD	22,888	21,640	17,454	2,502	1,684	236	301	639	72
CFS	22	22	13	6	3				
CG	116	91	59		32	6	5	13	1
CHN	1,408	1,277	794	282	201	16	37	74	4
CHP	7,438	6,962	5,367	720	875	192	135	118	31
CHS	7	7	1	5	1				
CLP	462	239	164	1	74	105	22	78	18
CMG	10	1	1				2	6	1
CN	923	904	647	207	50	2	3	7	7
CPP	115	114	24	89	1			1	
CRS	1,488	1,459	1,272	78	109	6	14	5	4
CS	135	134	130		4	1			
CTR	18	16	11	3	2		2		

A	Allergy
ACA	Adult Cardiothoracic Anesthesiology (Anesthesiology)
ADL	Adolescent Medicine (Pediatrics)
ADM	Addiction Medicine
ADP	Addiction Psychiatry
AI	Allergy And Immunology
ALI	Clinical Laboratory Immunology (Allergy & Immunology)
AM	Aerospace Medicine
AMF	Adolescent Medicine (Family Medicine)
AMI	Adolescent Medicine (Internal Medicine)
AN	Anesthesiology
APM	Pain Medicine (Anesthesiology)
AR	Abdominal Radiology
AS	Abdominal Surgery
ATP	Anatomic Pathology
BBK	Blood Banking/Transfusion Medicine
CAP	Child Abuse Pediatrics
CBG	Clinical Biochemical Genetics
CCA	Critical Care Medicine (Anesthesiology)
CCG	Clinical Cytogenetics
CCM	Critical Care Medicine (Internal Medicine)
CCP	Pediatric Critical Care Medicine
CCS	Surgical Critical Care (Surgery)
CD	Cardiovascular Disease
CFS	Craniofacial Surgery
CG	Clinical Genetics
CHN	Child Neurology
CHP	Child & Adolescent Psychiatry
CHS	Congenital Cardiac Surgery (Thoracic Surgery)
CLP	Clinical Pathology
CMG	Clinical Molecular Genetics
CN	Clinical Neurophysiology
CPP	Pediatrics/Psychiatry/Child & Adolescent Psychiatry
CRS	Colon And Rectal Surgery
CS	Cosmetic Surgery
CTR	Cardiothoracic Radiology

Table 1.9

Physicians by Self-Designated Specialty and Activity (236 Specialties), 2010, continued

		Patient Care				Other Professional Activity			
				Hospital Based					
Specialty	Total Physicians	Total Patient Care	Office Based	Resid./ Fellows	Phys. Staff	Admin.	Med. Teach.	Research	Other
D	11,223	10,977	9,218	1,249	510	45	78	102	21
DBP	144	136	48	75	13	2	4	2	
DDL	1								1
DIA	261	176	154		22	12	11	59	3
DMP	637	580	446	77	57	2	5	7	43
DR	26,036	25,289	17,492	4,837	2,960	137	230	113	267
DS	154	154	151		3				
EFM	22	22	12	6	4				
EM	32,683	31,531	20,264	4,591	6,676	692	297	95	68
EMP	35	35	6	29					
END	5,628	4,851	3,815	577	459	99	127	528	23
ENR	1	1		1					
EP	51	5	3	1	1	5	3	26	12
ES	1	1	1						
ESM	24	23	15	6	2		1		
ESN	19	18	10	5	3		1		
ETX	101	94	42	36	16	1	2		4
FM	86,155	82,908	68,794	7,930	6,184	1,370	1,428	207	242
FMP	3	3	1	1	1				
FOP	670	473	373	39	61	33	8	7	149
FPG	643	594	465	73	56	14	25	7	3
FPP	63	62	20	41	1				1
FPS	421	417	401	1	15	2	1		1
FSM	802	801	626	137	38	1			
GE	13,210	12,603	10,466	1,338	799	110	157	311	29
GO	482	440	361	2	77	14	18	8	2
GP	8,591	8,243	7,202		1,041	192	30	43	83
GPM	2,155	1,691	1,184	238	269	208	40	148	68
GS	29,505	28,687	18,490	7,444	2,753	328	249	156	85
GYN	2,276	2,176	2,080		96	43	28	19	10
HEM	2,048	1,563	1,226	51	286	72	71	333	9
HEP	117	96	68		28	3	6	11	1
HMP	695	657	448	118	91	4	7	11	16
HNS	207	193	166		27	6	6	1	1
HO	5,922	5,749	3,824	1,474	451	24	31	102	16
HOS	239	234	120	2	112	2	2	1	

D Dermatology
DBP Developmental-Behavioral Pediatrics
DDL Clinical & Laboratory Dermatological Immunology
DIA Diabetes
DMP Dermatopathology (Pathology)
DR Diagnostic Radiology
DS Dermatologic Surgery
EFM Emergency Medicine/Family Medicine
EM Emergency Medicine
EMP Pediatrics/Emergency Medicine
END Endocrinology, Diabetes & Metabolism
ENR Endovascular Surgical Neuroradiology (Neurology)
EP Epidemiology
ES Endovascular Surgical Neuroradiology (Neurological Surgery)
ESM Sports Medicine (Emergency Medicine)
ESN Endovascular Surgical Neuroradiology (Radiology)
ETX Medical Toxicology (Emergency Medicine)
FM Family Medicine
FMP Family Medicine/Preventive Medicine
FOP Forensic Pathology
FPG Geriatric Medicine (Family Medicine)
FPP Psychiatry/Family Medicine
FPS Facial Plastic Surgery
FSM Sports Medicine (Family Practice)
GE Gastroenterology
GO Gynecological Oncology
GP General Practice
GPM General Preventive Medicine
GS General Surgery
GYN Gynecology
HEM Hematology (Internal Medicine)
HEP Hepatology
HMP Hematology (Pathology)
HNS Head And Neck Surgery
HO Hematology/Oncology
HOS Hospitalist

Table 1.9

Physicians by Self-Designated Specialty and Activity (236 Specialties), 2010, continued

		Patient Care				Other Professional Activity			
				Hospital Based					
Specialty	Total Physicians	Total Patient Care	Office Based	Resid./ Fellows	Phys. Staff	Admin.	Med. Teach.	Research	Other
HPD	1	1			1				
HPE	1	1	1						
HPF	12	8	8			4			
HPI	22	15	11		4	4	1	1	1
HPM	154	146	34	106	6	8			
HPN	1					1			
HPO	3	3	2		1				
HPP	1	1			1				
HPR	1	1	1						
HS	1,519	1,482	1,396		86	5	19	7	6
HSO	300	300	178	116	6				
HSP	35	35	19	14	2				
HSS	27	27	16	11					
IC	1,841	1,833	1,472	256	105	1	5	2	
ICE	1,316	1,293	1,003	183	107	3	9	8	3
ID	6,942	5,670	4,054	770	846	262	226	729	55
IEC	10	10	2	8					
IFP	38	38	16	20	2				
IG	258	58	44		14	16	11	168	5
ILI	6	2	1		1	1	1	2	
IM	113,591	108,179	77,990	18,950	11,239	2,101	1,230	1,594	487
IMD	30	30	3	26	1				
IMG	3,322	3,009	2,246	268	495	134	67	99	13
INM	1	1	1						
IPM	48	46	17	28	1	1	1		
ISM	46	44	40		4		1	1	
LM	127	33	27		6	34	6	2	52
MBG	1	1		1					
MDG	9	9		9					
MDM	266	12	11		1	239	2	5	8
MEM	116	116	16	98	2				
MFM	623	535	393	5	137	23	47	16	2
MG	446	344	192	83	69	11	17	69	5
MGG	1							1	
MGP	57	55	11	42	2	1			1
MM	66	44	26	8	10	7	2	10	3
MN	10	9	1	8			1		
MP	115	113	24	87	2	2			

HPD Hospice and Palliative Medicine (Radiology)
HPE Hospice & Palliative Medicine (Emergency Medicine)
HPF Hospice & Palliative Medicine (Family Medicine)
HPI Hospice & Palliative Medicine (Internal Medicine)
HPM Hospice & Palliative Medicine
HPN Hospice & Palliative Medicine (Psychiatry & Neurology)
HPO Hospice & Palliative Medicine (Obstetrics & Gynecology)
HPP Hospice and Palliative Medicine (Pediatrics)
HPR Hospice and Palliative Medicine (Physical Medicine & Rehabilitation)
HS Hand Surgery
HSO Hand Surgery (Orthopedics)
HSP Hand Surgery (Plastic Surgery)
HSS Hand Surgery (Surgery)
IC Interventional Cardiology
ICE Clinical Cardiac Electrophysiology
ID Infectious Disease
IEC Internal Med/Emergency Med/Critical Care Med
IFP Internal Medicine/Family Practice
IG Immunology
ILI Clinical And Laboratory Immunology (Internal Medicine)
IM Internal Medicine
IMD Internal Medicine/Dermatology
IMG Geriatric Medicine (Internal Medicine)
INM Internal Medicine/Nuclear Medicine
IPM Internal Medicine/Preventive Medicine
ISM Sports Medicine (Internal Medicine)
LM Legal Medicine
MBG Medical Biochemical Genetics
MDG Internal Medicine/Medical Genetics
MDM Medical Management
MEM Internal Medicine/Emergency Medicine
MFM Maternal And Fetal Medicine
MG Medical Genetics
MGG Molecular Genetic Pathology (Medical Genetics)
MGP Molecular Genetic Pathology (Pathology And Medical Genetics)
MM Medical Microbiology
MN Internal Medicine/Neurology
MP Internal Med/Psychiatry

Table 1.9

Physicians by Self-Designated Specialty and Activity (236 Specialties), 2010, continued

		Patient Care				Other Professional Activity			
				Hospital Based					
Specialty	Total Physicians	Total Patient Care	Office Based	Resid./ Fellows	Phys. Staff	Admin.	Med. Teach.	Research	Other
MPD	4,433	4,350	2,720	1,324	306	16	36	24	7
MPM	1	1	1						
MSR	126	124	93	24	7	1	1		
N	13,385	12,276	9,054	1,955	1,267	163	202	672	72
NC	8	8	6		2				
NDN	22	22	5	16	1				
NDP	19	16	13		3	1	1	1	
NEP	8,355	7,740	6,226	920	594	124	120	354	17
NM	1,456	1,301	863	153	285	40	31	57	27
NMN	54	54	24	28	2				
NMP	1	1	1						
NO	170	169	131	22	16		1		
NP	343	233	157	39	37	7	31	59	13
NPM	4,442	4,050	2,600	605	845	83	100	195	14
NR	151	145	114	14	17		1	4	1
NRN	34	28	21		7	2	1	1	2
NS	5,730	5,601	3,966	1,147	488	37	40	35	17
NSP	31	31	21		10				
NTR	130	71	61		10	9	6	36	8
NUP	22	19	14		5		1	1	1
OAR	285	281	234	29	18		3	1	
OBG	38,520	37,540	30,526	4,509	2,505	336	395	176	73
OBS	220	198	171		27	7	9	5	1
OCC	5	2	2			1		2	
OFA	122	121	100	12	9		1		
OM	2,426	1,755	1,438	1	316	455	35	78	103
OMF	336	329	295	11	23	2	5		
OMM	6	6	6						
OMO	66	64	46	9	9		2		
ON	5,079	4,370	3,748	102	520	142	51	497	19
OP	374	368	265	31	72	1	5		
OPH	18,256	17,880	15,539	1,493	848	82	121	140	33
OPR	1	1	1						
ORS	21,822	21,437	16,565	3,601	1,271	102	114	71	98
OS	3,645	2,346	1,239	803	304	473	100	607	119
OSM	1,453	1,448	1,239	137	72	2	2	1	
OSS	688	677	607	26	44	1	6	2	2
OTO	9,970	9,810	7,695	1,493	622	54	68	24	14

MPD Internal Medicine/Pediatrics
MPM Internal Med/Phys Med And Rehabilitation
MSR Musculoskeletal Radiology
N Neurology
NC Nuclear Cardiology
NDN Neurodevelopmental Disabilities (Psychiatry & Neurology
NDP Neurodevelopmental Disabilities (Pediatrics)
NEP Nephrology
NM Nuclear Medicine
NMN Neuromuscular Medicine (Neurology)
NMP Neuromuscular Medicine (Physical Medicine & Rehabilitation)
NO Neurotology (Otolaryngology)
NP Neuropathology
NPM Neonatal-Perinatal Medicine
NR Nuclear Radiology
NRN Neurology/Diagnostic Radiology/Neuroradiology
NS Neurological Surgery
NSP Pediatric Surgery (Neurology)
NTR Nutrition
NUP Neuropsychiatry
OAR Adult Reconstructive Orthopedics
OBG Obstetrics & Gynecology
OBS Obstetrics
OCC Critical Care Medicine (Obstetrics & Gynecology)
OFA Foot And Ankle Orthopedics
OM Occupational Medicine
OMF Oral & Maxillofacial Surgery
OMM Osteopathic Manipulative Medicine
OMO Musculoskeletal Oncology
ON Medical Oncology
OP Pediatric Orthopedics
OPH Ophthalmology
OPR Ophthalmic Plastic and Reconstructive Surgery
ORS Orthopedic Surgery
OS Other Specialty
OSM Sports Medicine (Orthopedic Surgery)
OSS Orthopedic Surgery Of The Spine
OTO Otolaryngology

Table 1.9

Physicians by Self-Designated Specialty and Activity (236 Specialties), 2010, continued

		Patient Care				Other Professional Activity			
				Hospital Based					
Specialty	Total Physicians	Total Patient Care	Office Based	Resid./ Fellows	Phys. Staff	Admin.	Med. Teach.	Research	Other
OTR	125	119	85	17	17		6		
P	37,684	34,822	24,268	4,243	6,311	1,262	537	811	252
PA	276	49	36		13	42	9	168	8
PAN	780	764	473	183	108	3	12	1	
PCC	5,186	5,055	3,345	1,305	405	19	31	76	5
PCH	27	12	10	1	1	5	3	2	5
PCP	795	760	542	132	86	3	13	4	15
PCS	54	53	39		14	1			
PD	57,830	55,046	42,832	7,142	5,072	1,003	808	716	257
PDA	131	113	103		10	2	3	11	2
PDC	2,101	1,976	1,243	398	335	23	29	68	5
PDD	9	9	8		1				
PDE	1,019	898	523	231	144	6	17	93	5
PDI	490	411	199	166	46	15	19	40	5
PDM	4	4	2	2					
PDO	184	178	136	18	24		6		
PDP	752	694	482	131	81	12	12	33	1
PDR	736	703	505	71	127	5	18	4	6
PDS	845	796	579	74	143	11	23	13	2
PDT	2	2	2						
PE	152	146	66	54	26	3	1	2	
PEM	805	769	290	292	187	12	16	6	2
PFP	426	388	256	67	65	8	3	4	23
PG	825	787	448	228	111	9	8	19	2
PHL	121	118	115		3	2		1	
PHM	88	5	5			10	1	48	24
PHO	1,925	1,663	918	408	337	28	24	200	10
PHP	1,283	252	182	2	68	584	62	273	112
PLI	1	1	1						
PLM	162	137	91	1	45	17	2	3	3
PM	7,993	7,708	5,751	977	980	153	38	46	48
PME	552	538	513		25	4	4	5	1
PMG	33	33	4	27	2				
PMM	897	886	617	230	39	2	5	2	2
PMN	3	3	2		1				
PMP	20	19	18		1				1

OTR	Orthopedic Trauma
P	Psychiatry
PA	Clinical Pharmacology
PAN	Pediatric Anesthesiology (Anesthesiology)
PCC	Pulmonary & Critical Care Medicine
PCH	Chemical Pathology
PCP	Cytopathology
PCS	Pediatric Cardiothoracic Surgery
PD	Pediatrics
PDA	Pediatric Allergy
PDC	Pediatric Cardiology
PDD	Pediatric Dermatology
PDE	Pediatric Endocrinology
PDI	Pediatric Infectious Disease
PDM	Pediatrics/Dermatology
PDO	Pediatric Otolaryngology
PDP	Pediatric Pulmonology
PDR	Pediatric Radiology
PDS	Pediatric Surgery (Surgery)
PDT	Medical Toxicology (Pediatrics)
PE	Pediatric Emergency Med (Emergency Med)
PEM	Pediatric Emergency Medicine (Pediatrics)
PFP	Forensic Psychiatry
PG	Pediatric Gastroenterology
PHL	Phlebology
PHM	Pharmaceutical Medicine
PHO	Pediatric Hematology/Oncology
PHP	Public Health And General Preventive Medicine
PLI	Clinical & Laboratory Immunology (Pediatrics)
PLM	Palliative Medicine
PM	Physical Medicine And Rehabilitation
PME	Pain Management
PMG	Pediatrics/Medical Genetics
PMM	Pain Medicine
PMN	Pain Medicine (Neurology)
PMP	Pain Medicine (Physical Medicine & Rehabilitation)

Table 1.9

Physicians by Self-Designated Specialty and Activity (236 Specialties), 2010, continued

		Patient Care				Other Professional Activity			
				Hospital Based					
Specialty	Total Physicians	Total Patient Care	Office Based	Resid./ Fellows	Phys. Staff	Admin.	Med. Teach.	Research	Other
PN	581	492	277	127	88	15	26	46	2
PO	200	197	183		14	1	2		
PP	127	117	74	13	30		5	2	3
PPM	23	22	5	17				1	
PPN	5	4	4			1			
PPR	185	161	68	76	17		4	19	1
PRD	92	92	54	36	2				
PRO	3	3	3						
PRS	26	25	16	6	3			1	
PS	6,474	6,374	5,618	443	313	24	39	19	18
PSH	6	6	5		1				
PSI	340	340		340					
PSM	60	59	40	12	7			1	
PSO	1	1	1						
PSP	7	7	7						
PTH	13,924	12,256	7,834	2,219	2,203	410	230	391	637
PTX	20	16	9	6	1	2		2	
PUD	5,940	5,233	4,501	78	654	170	171	340	26
PYA	356	346	340		6	4	4	2	
PYG	775	740	547	50	143	13	10	12	
PYM	93	93	32	53	8				
PYN	24	24	6	16	2				
R	4,168	3,811	3,112	10	689	55	114	61	127
REN	668	597	548		49	20	21	24	6
RHU	4,819	4,349	3,560	425	364	79	97	268	26
RNR	2,180	2,138	1,637	274	227	6	20	6	10
RO	4,698	4,600	3,379	610	611	35	22	33	8
RP	1							1	
RPM	21	20	5	10	5			1	
SCI	73	71	44	13	14	1			1
SME	432	411	265	124	22	5	3	9	4
SMI	25	24	22		2		1		
SMN	14	14	13		1				
SMO	1	1	1						
SMP	1							1	
SO	402	378	285	1	92	5	6	11	2

PN Pediatric Nephrology
PO Pediatric Opthalmology
PP Pediatric Pathology
PPM Pediatrics/Physical Medicine And Rehabilitation
PPN Pain Medicine (Psychiatry)
PPR Pediatric Rheumatology
PRD Procedural Dermatology
PRO Proctology
PRS Sports Medicine (Physical Medicine & Rehabilitation)
PS Plastic Surgery
PSH Plastic Surgery Within The Head & Neck
PSI Plastic Surgery-Integrated
PSM Sports Medicine (Pediatrics)
PSO Plastic Surgery within the Head and Neck (Otolaryngology)
PSP Plastic Surgery Within the Head & Neck (Plastic Surgery)
PTH Anatomic/Clinical Pathology
PTX Medical Toxicology (Preventive Medicine)
PUD Pulmonary Disease
PYA Psychoanalysis
PYG Geriatric Psychiatry
PYM Psychosomatic Medicine
PYN Psychiatry/Neurology
R Radiology
REN Reproductive Endocrinology And Infertility
RHU Rheumatology
RNR Neuroradiology
RO Radiation Oncology
RP Radiological Physics
RPM Pediatric Rehabilitation Medicine
SCI Spinal Cord Injury Medicine
SME Sleep Medicine
SMI Sleep Medicine (Internal Medicine)
SMN Sleep Medicine (Psychiatry & Neurology)
SMO Sleep Medicine (Otolaryngology)
SMP Sleep Medicine (Pediatrics)
SO Surgical Oncology

Table 1.9

Physicians by Self-Designated Specialty and Activity (236 Specialties), 2010, continued

		Patient Care				Other Professional Activity			
				Hospital Based					
Specialty	Total Physicians	Total Patient Care	Office Based	Resid./ Fellows	Phys. Staff	Admin.	Med. Teach.	Research	Other
SP	369	359	218	116	25		3	2	5
THP	27	27	8	19					
TRS	273	240	154		86	11	13	7	2
TS	4,574	4,410	3,600	245	565	61	40	55	8
TSI	24	24		24					
TTS	191	175	133	1	41	3	5	7	1
U	10,468	10,263	8,436	1,170	657	73	64	42	26
UCM	304	293	259		34	7	3		1
UM	52	47	31	1	15	4		1	
UME	13	13	7	6					
UP	233	224	170	26	28	3	4		2
US	8,661	8,359	3,606	4,123	630	69	40	112	81
VIR	1,909	1,892	1,501	190	201	4	9	4	
VM	30	29	23		6			1	
VN	115	114	37	75	2		1		
VS	2,896	2,808	2,230	302	276	31	31	17	9
Inactive	125,928								
Not Class	64,153								
Addr Unkn	432								

SP	Selective Pathology
THP	Transplant Hepatology (Internal Medicine)
TRS	Traumatic Surgery
TS	Thoracic Surgery
TSI	Thoracic Surgery-Integrated
TTS	Transplant Surgery
U	Urology
UCM	Urgent Care Medicine
UM	Underseas Medicine (Preventive Medicine)
UME	Underseas Medicine (Emergency Medicine)
UP	Pediatric Urology
US	Unspecified
VIR	Vascular And Interventional Radiology
VM	Vascular Medicine
VN	Vascular Neurology
VS	Vascular Surgery

Table 1.10

International Medical Graduates by Self-Designated Specialty and Activity, 2010

		Patient Care				Other Professional Activity			
				Hospital Based					
Specialty	Total Physicians	Total Patient Care	Office Based	Resid./ Fellows	Phys. Staff	Admin.	Med. Teach.	Research	Other
Total Physicians	254,396	192,046	140,246	28,434	23,366	1,812	1,654	2,462	980
FM/GP	24,413	23,992	18,522	3,562	1,908	199	120	36	66
Family Medicine	20,105	19,806	14,988	3,562	1,256	126	111	27	35
General Practice	4,308	4,186	3,534		652	73	9	9	31
Medical Specialties	98,179	95,384	70,138	15,304	9,942	614	694	1,285	202
Allergy and Immunology	1,000	932	840	49	43	5	10	49	4
Cardiovascular Disease	7,089	6,869	5,407	943	519	21	61	125	13
Dermatology	605	581	490	46	45	3	8	12	1
Gastroenterology	3,675	3,551	2,854	437	260	21	34	65	4
Internal Medicine	60,935	59,386	42,611	10,423	6,352	368	349	710	122
Pediatric Cardiology	507	488	324	97	67	4	6	9	
Pediatrics	20,442	19,770	14,795	2,642	2,333	175	196	244	57
Pulmonary Disease	3,926	3,807	2,817	667	323	17	30	71	1
Surgical Specialties	21,426	20,848	16,284	2,522	2,042	147	189	177	65
Colon and Rectal Surgery	281	276	240	13	23		3	2	
General Surgery	6,580	6,400	4,403	1,180	817	52	62	42	24
Neurological Surgery	749	726	510	124	92	5	8	8	2
Obstetrics & Gynecology	6,981	6,803	5,522	752	529	59	56	49	14
Ophthalmology	1,343	1,306	1,132	88	86	4	10	20	3
Orthopedic Surgery	1,512	1,473	1,207	141	125	8	12	13	6
Otolaryngology	811	784	679	41	64	7	7	10	3
Plastic Surgery	804	786	681	60	45	2	2	8	6
Thoracic Surgery	953	921	730	71	120	2	9	20	1
Urology	1,412	1,373	1,180	52	141	8	20	5	6
Other Specialties	54,936	51,822	35,302	7,046	9,474	852	651	964	647
Aerospace Medicine	32	18	8		10	4	2	4	4
Anesthesiology	11,423	11,142	8,581	742	1,819	45	145	66	25
Child & Adolescent Psychiatry	2,231	2,141	1,558	252	331	31	22	26	11
Diagnostic Radiology	2,871	2,742	1,845	391	506	14	41	25	49
Emergency Medicine	2,843	2,768	1,637	406	725	45	19	5	6
Forensic Pathology	144	93	74	7	12	6	3	2	40
General Preventive Medicine	320	282	206	49	27	13	4	14	7
Medical Genetics	154	131	71	32	28	2	4	16	1
Neurology	5,201	4,988	3,568	928	492	24	53	116	20
Nuclear Medicine	559	520	305	93	122	5	10	14	10
Occupational Medicine	349	295	248		47	35	4	4	11
Anatomic/Clinical Pathology	6,157	5,403	3,349	883	1,171	146	128	204	276
Physical Medicine and Rehabilitation	2,629	2,549	1,832	319	398	36	18	11	15
Psychiatry	12,591	12,024	7,703	1,484	2,837	265	94	166	42
Public Health and General Preventive Medicine	142	43	29	1	13	62	7	17	13
Radiation Oncology	727	707	549	19	139	6	5	9	
Radiology	1,679	1,549	1,045	164	340	14	40	34	42
Transplant Surgery	56	51	34	1	16		2	2	1
Vascular Medicine	5	5	4		1				
Other Specialty	1,052	744	435	196	113	66	25	183	34
Unspecified	3,771	3,627	2,221	1,079	327	33	25	46	40
Inactive	29,608								
Not Classified	25,748								
Address Unknown	86								

Subspecialties in this table are condensed into major specialties. See Appendix A.

Table 1.11

International Medical Graduates by Age, Activity, and Sex, 2010

Activity	Total Physicians	< 35	35-44	45-54	55-64	≥ 65
			Both Sexes			
Total Physicians	254,396	37,385	57,994	53,973	48,295	56,749
Patient Care	192,046	29,623	45,798	47,480	41,799	27,346
Office-Based Practice	140,246	7,794	34,503	40,545	35,325	22,079
Hospital-Based Practice	51,800	21,829	11,295	6,935	6,474	5,267
Residents	28,434	21,034	6,481	859	53	7
Full-Time Staff	23,366	795	4,814	6,076	6,421	5,260
Other Professional Activity	6,908	55	569	1,385	2,205	2,694
Administration	1,812	5	69	319	608	811
Medical Teaching	1,654	27	208	352	487	580
Research	2,462	17	200	503	810	932
Other	980	6	92	211	300	371
Inactive	29,608	49	282	778	2,774	25,725
Not Classified	25,748	7,656	11,341	4,330	1,516	905
Address Unknown	86	2	4		1	79
			Male			
Total Physicians	173,007	20,739	34,238	36,827	35,861	45,342
Patient Care	129,866	16,674	27,218	32,583	31,399	21,992
Office-Based Practice	97,654	4,176	20,496	28,014	26,958	18,010
Hospital-Based Practice	32,212	12,498	6,722	4,569	4,441	3,982
Residents	16,303	12,015	3,746	504	32	6
Full-Time Staff	15,909	483	2,976	4,065	4,409	3,976
Other Professional Activity	5,040	31	326	959	1,598	2,126
Administration	1,325	3	40	219	445	618
Medical Teaching	1,179	15	120	248	332	464
Research	1,902	9	120	370	622	781
Other	634	4	46	122	199	263
Inactive	22,940	14	113	478	1,811	20,524
Not Classified	15,099	4,019	6,579	2,807	1,052	642
Address Unknown	62	1	2		1	58
			Female			
Total Physicians	81,389	16,646	23,756	17,146	12,434	11,407
Patient Care	62,180	12,949	18,580	14,897	10,400	5,354
Office-Based Practice	42,592	3,618	14,007	12,531	8,367	4,069
Hospital-Based Practice	19,588	9,331	4,573	2,366	2,033	1,285
Residents	12,131	9,019	2,735	355	21	1
Full-Time Staff	7,457	312	1,838	2,011	2,012	1,284
Other Professional Activity	1,868	24	243	426	607	568
Administration	487	2	29	100	163	193
Medical Teaching	475	12	88	104	155	116
Research	560	8	80	133	188	151
Other	346	2	46	89	101	108
Inactive	6,668	35	169	300	963	5,201
Not Classified	10,649	3,637	4,762	1,523	464	263
Address Unknown	24	1	2			21

Table 1.12

Male Physicians by Self-Designated Specialty and Activity, 2010

		Patient Care				Other Professional Activity			
				Hospital Based					
Specialty	Total Physicians	Total Patient Care	Office Based	Resid./ Fellows	Phys. Staff	Admin.	Med. Teach.	Research	Other
Total Physicians	688,468	513,592	399,429	59,089	55,074	11,036	7,134	10,661	3,179
FM/GP	61,977	59,333	50,677	3,661	4,995	1,227	1,036	172	209
Family Medicine	55,242	52,846	44,946	3,661	4,239	1,089	1,016	139	152
General Practice	6,735	6,487	5,731		756	138	20	33	57
Medical Specialties	192,116	178,780	139,723	21,473	17,584	3,789	2,770	6,052	725
Allergy and Immunology	2,956	2,633	2,398	105	130	36	28	248	11
Cardiovascular Disease	20,294	19,177	15,750	1,953	1,474	214	274	569	60
Dermatology	6,385	6,206	5,447	470	289	33	57	75	14
Gastroenterology	11,359	10,826	9,245	922	659	102	133	273	25
Internal Medicine	107,094	99,143	75,463	13,263	10,417	2,416	1,485	3,608	442
Pediatric Cardiology	1,458	1,362	886	243	233	20	18	54	4
Pediatrics	33,322	30,908	23,831	3,570	3,507	795	596	881	142
Pulmonary Disease	9,248	8,525	6,703	947	875	173	179	344	27
Surgical Specialties	126,861	123,470	99,996	14,171	9,303	1,147	1,169	720	355
Colon and Rectal Surgery	1,245	1,221	1,079	54	88	4	14	3	3
General Surgery	30,460	29,469	21,204	5,164	3,101	386	323	188	94
Neurological Surgery	5,351	5,224	3,775	990	459	36	40	34	17
Obstetrics & Gynecology	21,977	21,057	18,592	855	1,610	342	347	177	54
Ophthalmology	14,561	14,248	12,743	865	640	73	101	115	24
Orthopedic Surgery	23,804	23,398	18,537	3,460	1,401	102	137	71	96
Otolaryngology	8,779	8,625	7,035	1,040	550	51	68	22	13
Plastic Surgery	6,389	6,297	5,421	593	283	22	35	17	18
Thoracic Surgery	4,384	4,227	3,462	232	533	58	38	53	8
Urology	9,911	9,704	8,148	918	638	73	66	40	28
Other Specialties	164,648	152,009	109,033	19,784	23,192	4,873	2,159	3,717	1,890
Aerospace Medicine	378	220	110		110	108	8	22	20
Anesthesiology	32,922	32,151	25,021	3,330	3,800	221	329	163	58
Child & Adolescent Psychiatry	3,843	3,539	2,775	280	484	136	81	69	18
Diagnostic Radiology	19,919	19,319	13,601	3,476	2,242	122	178	93	207
Emergency Medicine	24,978	23,958	15,802	2,794	5,362	636	243	82	59
Forensic Pathology	440	302	247	20	35	23	5	5	105
General Preventive Medicine	1,334	1,033	717	110	206	153	23	90	35
Medical Genetics	314	218	129	33	56	13	17	63	3
Neurology	11,315	10,293	7,851	1,337	1,105	144	198	620	60
Nuclear Medicine	1,134	1,011	692	96	223	32	24	47	20
Occupational Medicine	1,900	1,379	1,123	1	255	360	24	60	77
Anatomic/Clinical Pathology	12,014	10,136	6,880	1,298	1,958	492	257	569	560
Physical Medicine and Rehabilitation	6,036	5,843	4,439	781	623	104	29	33	27
Psychiatry	25,474	23,186	16,732	2,067	4,387	1,024	397	659	208
Public Health and General Preventive Medicine	879	156	113	2	41	400	49	203	71
Radiation Oncology	3,500	3,423	2,556	412	455	30	18	24	5
Radiology	7,819	7,440	5,928	473	1,039	65	128	64	122
Transplant Surgery	171	158	120	1	37	3	4	5	1
Vascular Medicine	23	22	18		4			1	
Other Specialty	4,112	2,310	1,617	354	339	757	115	752	178
Unspecified	6,143	5,912	2,562	2,919	431	50	32	93	56
Inactive	107,072								
Not Classified	35,498								
Address Unknown	296								

Subspecialties in this table are condensed into major specialties. See Appendix A.

Table 1.13

Female Physicians by Self-Designated Specialty and Activity, 2010

		Patient Care				Other Professional Activity			
				Hospital Based					
Specialty	Total Physicians	Total Patient Care	Office Based	Resid./ Fellows	Phys. Staff	Admin.	Med. Teach.	Research	Other
Total Physicians	296,907	238,980	165,595	49,053	24,332	2,973	2,775	3,094	1,438
FM/GP	34,232	33,227	26,421	4,480	2,326	354	447	85	119
Family Medicine	32,376	31,471	24,950	4,480	2,041	300	437	75	93
General Practice	1,856	1,756	1,471		285	54	10	10	26
Medical Specialties	110,514	105,636	73,615	21,354	10,667	1,238	1,290	1,896	454
Allergy and Immunology	1,356	1,263	993	194	76	8	12	63	10
Cardiovascular Disease	2,594	2,463	1,704	549	210	22	27	70	12
Dermatology	4,931	4,863	3,825	815	223	12	21	27	8
Gastroenterology	1,851	1,777	1,221	416	140	8	24	38	4
Internal Medicine	54,182	51,578	35,149	10,915	5,514	697	622	1,042	243
Pediatric Cardiology	643	614	357	155	102	3	11	14	1
Pediatrics	43,079	41,315	29,223	7,874	4,218	472	550	570	172
Pulmonary Disease	1,878	1,763	1,143	436	184	16	23	72	4
Surgical Specialties	37,056	36,434	25,086	8,866	2,482	154	252	145	71
Colon and Rectal Surgery	246	241	196	24	21	2		2	1
General Surgery	6,640	6,532	3,123	2,855	554	21	40	32	15
Neurological Surgery	430	427	223	162	42	1	1	1	
Obstetrics & Gynecology	20,820	20,434	15,491	3,661	1,282	102	171	73	40
Ophthalmology	3,896	3,830	2,980	628	222	10	22	25	9
Orthopedic Surgery	1,437	1,423	788	518	117	4	2	4	4
Otolaryngology	1,547	1,534	929	493	112	3	7	2	1
Plastic Surgery	1,029	1,016	759	205	52	5	5	2	1
Thoracic Surgery	221	214	139	42	33	3	2	2	
Urology	790	783	458	278	47	3	2	2	
Other Specialties	67,458	63,683	40,473	14,353	8,857	1,227	786	968	794
Aerospace Medicine	35	23	11		12	8		2	2
Anesthesiology	10,437	10,178	6,798	2,067	1,313	50	143	45	21
Child & Adolescent Psychiatry	3,595	3,423	2,592	440	391	56	54	49	13
Diagnostic Radiology	6,135	5,986	3,902	1,364	720	15	54	20	60
Emergency Medicine	8,300	8,143	4,852	1,899	1,392	67	61	15	14
Forensic Pathology	230	171	126	19	26	10	3	2	44
General Preventive Medicine	893	721	507	135	79	61	17	61	33
Medical Genetics	283	232	131	51	50	4	8	32	7
Neurology	4,535	4,296	2,696	1,183	417	38	45	133	23
Nuclear Medicine	322	290	171	57	62	8	7	10	7
Occupational Medicine	526	376	315		61	95	11	18	26
Anatomic/Clinical Pathology	7,013	6,279	3,808	1,506	965	167	125	146	296
Physical Medicine and Rehabilitation	3,009	2,903	2,015	473	415	52	14	16	24
Psychiatry	14,264	13,584	8,958	2,420	2,206	273	165	174	68
Public Health and General Preventive Medicine	404	96	69		27	184	13	70	41
Radiation Oncology	1,198	1,177	823	198	156	5	4	9	3
Radiology	1,567	1,485	1,104	145	236	7	35	16	24
Transplant Surgery	20	17	13		4		1	2	
Vascular Medicine	7	7	5		2				
Other Specialty	1,370	1,052	533	395	124	108	18	129	63
Unspecified	3,315	3,244	1,044	2,001	199	19	8	19	25
Inactive	18,856								
Not Classified	28,655								
Address Unknown	136								

Subspecialties in this table are condensed into major specialties. See Appendix A.

Table 1.14

Total Physicians by Self-Designated Specialty and Corresponding Board Certification, 2010

Primary Specialty	Total Physicians	Total Certified	By Corresponding Board Only	By Corresponding Board and Other Boards	By Non-Corresponding Board	Not Board Certified
Total Physicians	985,375	736,142	647,329	38,261	50,552	249,233
Aerospace Medicine	413	306	172	69	65	107
Allergy/Immunology	4,312	3,958	28	2,795	1,135	354
Anesthesiology	43,359	32,226	29,453	1,815	958	11,133
Cardiovascular Disease	22,888	21,441	20,820	375	246	1,447
Child Psychiatry	7,438	5,428	5,107	240	81	2,010
Colon/Rectal Surgery	1,491	1,398	41	1,183	174	93
Dermatology	11,316	9,645	8,213	1,124	308	1,671
Diagnostic Radiology	26,054	20,874	19,407	1,257	210	5,180
Emergency Medicine	33,278	24,882	19,639	2,661	2,582	8,396
Family Medicine	87,618	73,115	71,087	1,135	893	14,503
Forensic Pathology	670	536	521	12	3	134
Gastroenterology	13,210	12,496	12,291	71	134	714
General Practice	8,591	1,240			1,240	7,351
General Preventive Medicine	2,227	1,662	810	466	386	565
General Surgery	37,100	25,334	21,284	869	3,181	11,766
Internal Medicine	161,276	125,291	113,728	3,191	8,372	35,985
Medical Genetics	597	540	84	378	78	57
Neurological Surgery	5,781	3,809	3,693	37	79	1,972
Neurology	15,850	11,967	10,214	1,477	276	3,883
Nuclear Medicine	1,456	1,213	500	586	127	243
Obstetrics/Gynecology	42,797	33,024	32,128	514	382	9,773
Occupational Medicine	2,426	1,849	842	585	422	577
Ophthalmology	18,457	15,394	14,832	314	248	3,063
Orthopedic Surgery	25,241	19,125	17,583	107	1,435	6,116
Otolaryngology	10,326	7,982	7,901	56	25	2,344
Pathology-Anatomic/Clinical	19,027	15,416	14,499	452	465	3,611
Pediatric Cardiology	2,101	1,993	1,910	74	9	108
Pediatrics	76,401	61,284	55,889	1,463	3,932	15,117
Physical Medicine & Rehabilitation	9,045	6,963	6,070	283	610	2,082
Plastic Surgery	7,418	6,025	2,810	2,434	781	1,393
Psychiatry	39,738	26,341	24,982	784	575	13,397
Public Health & General Preventive Medicine	1,283	902	397	162	343	381
Pulmonary Diseases	11,126	10,613	5,461	107	5,045	513
Radiation Oncology	4,698	3,817	3,487	300	30	881
Radiology	9,386	8,742	7,801	648	293	644
Thoracic Surgery	4,605	4,225	23	3,791	411	380
Transplant Surgery	191	147			147	44
Urological Surgery	10,701	8,766	8,701	48	17	1,935
Vascular Medicine	30	27			27	3
Other Specialty	5,482	3,198			3,198	2,284
Unspecified	9,458	905			905	8,553
Inactive	125,928	85,943	74,412	5,176	6,355	39,985
Not Classified	64,153	36,066	30,481	1,222	4,363	28,087
Address Unknown	432	34	28		6	398

Table 1.15

Male Physicians by Self-Designated Specialty and Corresponding Board Certification, 2010

Primary Specialty	Total Physicians	Total Certified	By Corresponding Board Only	By Corresponding Board and Other Boards	By Non-Corresponding Board	Not Board Certified
Total Physicians	688,468	526,469	458,550	30,649	37,270	161,999
Aerospace Medicine	378	285	160	64	61	93
Allergy/Immunology	2,956	2,692	27	1,881	784	264
Anesthesiology	32,922	25,390	23,145	1,465	780	7,532
Cardiovascular Disease	20,294	19,016	18,475	317	224	1,278
Child Psychiatry	3,843	2,853	2,682	138	33	990
Colon/Rectal Surgery	1,245	1,168	39	996	133	77
Dermatology	6,385	5,623	4,749	690	184	762
Diagnostic Radiology	19,919	16,170	14,928	1,069	173	3,749
Emergency Medicine	24,978	19,319	14,876	2,312	2,131	5,659
Family Medicine	55,242	46,870	45,271	909	690	8,372
Forensic Pathology	440	353	342	10	1	87
Gastroenterology	11,359	10,747	10,581	62	104	612
General Practice	6,735	1,043			1,043	5,692
General Preventive Medicine	1,334	999	495	290	214	335
General Surgery	30,460	21,999	18,438	807	2,754	8,461
Internal Medicine	107,094	84,415	76,525	2,304	5,586	22,679
Medical Genetics	314	285	54	196	35	29
Neurological Surgery	5,351	3,618	3,510	36	72	1,733
Neurology	11,315	8,918	7,612	1,126	180	2,397
Nuclear Medicine	1,134	971	370	510	91	163
Obstetrics/Gynecology	21,977	18,574	17,995	342	237	3,403
Occupational Medicine	1,900	1,439	637	464	338	461
Ophthalmology	14,561	12,525	12,095	273	157	2,036
Orthopedic Surgery	23,804	18,360	16,937	104	1,319	5,444
Otolaryngology	8,779	7,051	6,978	51	22	1,728
Pathology-Anatomic/Clinical	12,014	10,110	9,528	315	267	1,904
Pediatric Cardiology	1,458	1,391	1,327	57	7	67
Pediatrics	33,322	27,781	24,834	855	2,092	5,541
Physical Medicine & Rehabilitation	6,036	4,705	4,019	179	507	1,331
Plastic Surgery	6,389	5,294	2,403	2,205	686	1,095
Psychiatry	25,474	17,569	16,661	505	403	7,905
Public Health & General Preventive Medicine	879	627	281	113	233	252
Pulmonary Diseases	9,248	8,835	4,891	101	3,843	413
Radiation Oncology	3,500	2,907	2,642	245	20	593
Radiology	7,819	7,334	6,549	563	222	485
Thoracic Surgery	4,384	4,035	23	3,642	370	349
Transplant Surgery	171	127			127	44
Urological Surgery	9,911	8,328	8,264	48	16	1,583
Vascular Medicine	23	20			20	3
Other Specialty	4,112	2,440			2,440	1,672
Unspecified	6,143	598			598	5,545
Inactive	107,072	74,755	64,521	4,676	5,558	32,317
Not Classified	35,498	18,910	15,669	729	2,512	16,588
Address Unknown	296	20	17		3	276

Table 1.16

Female Physicians by Self-Designated Specialty and Corresponding Board Certification, 2010

Primary Specialty	Total Physicians	Total Certified	By Corresponding Board Only	By Corresponding Board and Other Boards	By Non-Corresponding Board	Not Board Certified
Total Physicians	296,907	209,673	188,779	7,612	13,282	87,234
Aerospace Medicine	35	21	12	5	4	14
Allergy/Immunology	1,356	1,266	1	914	351	90
Anesthesiology	10,437	6,836	6,308	350	178	3,601
Cardiovascular Disease	2,594	2,425	2,345	58	22	169
Child Psychiatry	3,595	2,575	2,425	102	48	1,020
Colon/Rectal Surgery	246	230	2	187	41	16
Dermatology	4,931	4,022	3,464	434	124	909
Diagnostic Radiology	6,135	4,704	4,479	188	37	1,431
Emergency Medicine	8,300	5,563	4,763	349	451	2,737
Family Medicine	32,376	26,245	25,816	226	203	6,131
Forensic Pathology	230	183	179	2	2	47
Gastroenterology	1,851	1,749	1,710	9	30	102
General Practice	1,856	197			197	1,659
General Preventive Medicine	893	663	315	176	172	230
General Surgery	6,640	3,335	2,846	62	427	3,305
Internal Medicine	54,182	40,876	37,203	887	2,786	13,306
Medical Genetics	283	255	30	182	43	28
Neurological Surgery	430	191	183	1	7	239
Neurology	4,535	3,049	2,602	351	96	1,486
Nuclear Medicine	322	242	130	76	36	80
Obstetrics/Gynecology	20,820	14,450	14,133	172	145	6,370
Occupational Medicine	526	410	205	121	84	116
Ophthalmology	3,896	2,869	2,737	41	91	1,027
Orthopedic Surgery	1,437	765	646	3	116	672
Otolaryngology	1,547	931	923	5	3	616
Pathology-Anatomic/Clinical	7,013	5,306	4,971	137	198	1,707
Pediatric Cardiology	643	602	583	17	2	41
Pediatrics	43,079	33,503	31,055	608	1,840	9,576
Physical Medicine & Rehabilitation	3,009	2,258	2,051	104	103	751
Plastic Surgery	1,029	731	407	229	95	298
Psychiatry	14,264	8,772	8,321	279	172	5,492
Public Health & General Preventive Medicine	404	275	116	49	110	129
Pulmonary Diseases	1,878	1,778	570	6	1,202	100
Radiation Oncology	1,198	910	845	55	10	288
Radiology	1,567	1,408	1,252	85	71	159
Thoracic Surgery	221	190		149	41	31
Transplant Surgery	20	20			20	
Urological Surgery	790	438	437		1	352
Vascular Medicine	7	7			7	
Other Specialty	1,370	758			758	612
Unspecified	3,315	307			307	3,008
Inactive	18,856	11,188	9,891	500	797	7,668
Not Classified	28,655	17,156	14,812	493	1,851	11,499
Address Unknown	136	14	11		3	122

Table 1.17

Country and School of Graduation of Total Physicians by Year of Graduation, 2010

Country School	Total Physicians	Prior 1950	1950-1959	1960-1969	1970-1979	1980-1989	1990-1999	2000-Present
Total Physicians	985,375	21,910	54,358	100,073	157,998	217,816	211,266	221,954
US Active Schools	718,521	17,481	38,138	64,044	112,122	155,324	155,918	175,494
AL-U Of Alabama	6,847	29	257	591	1,106	1,548	1,566	1,750
" -U Of So Alabama	2,071				184	603	607	677
AZ-U Of Arizona	3,424				597	818	882	1,127
AR-U Of Arkansas	6,163	156	354	638	1,010	1,241	1,274	1,490
CA-Loma Linda U	7,206	275	548	720	1,213	1,279	1,478	1,693
" -Stanford U	4,331	190	386	418	778	754	844	961
" -U Of Cal (Davis)	3,367				592	891	889	995
" -U Of Cal (Irvine)	4,852			1,482	649	855	879	987
" -U Of Cal (LA)	7,215		126	536	1,288	1,705	1,768	1,792
" -U Of Cal (San Diego)	4,033				476	1,107	1,164	1,286
" -U Of Cal (SF)	7,449	266	472	877	1,294	1,442	1,470	1,628
" -U Of So Cal (LA)	6,913	131	380	571	1,003	1,495	1,547	1,786
CO-U Of Colorado	6,185	145	390	665	1,097	1,215	1,251	1,422
CT-U Of Connecticut	2,857				395	822	800	840
" -Yale U	5,210	208	436	659	874	970	975	1,088
DC-George Wash U	7,349	220	490	791	1,212	1,454	1,485	1,697
" -Georgetown U	9,020	237	582	860	1,550	2,010	1,913	1,868
" -Howard U	5,027	163	360	620	909	1,023	886	1,066
FL-Florida St U	336							336
" -U Of Florida	4,694			405	777	1,114	1,124	1,274
" -U Of Miami	6,693		109	555	1,262	1,692	1,459	1,616
" -U Of So Florida	3,138				287	815	905	1,131
GA-Emory U	5,468	167	386	567	902	1,146	1,083	1,217
" -Med Coll Of Georgia	7,910	140	405	721	1,285	1,728	1,725	1,906
" -Mercer U	1,086					84	412	590
" -Morehouse U	867					118	302	447
HI-U Of Hawaii	2,082				287	621	539	635
IL-Chgo Med School	7,022	117	429	568	900	1,407	1,613	1,988
" -Loyola U/Stritch	6,424	210	444	660	1,228	1,196	1,250	1,436
" -Northwestern U	9,082	385	864	1,141	1,531	1,704	1,656	1,801
" -Rush Med Coll	4,227	71			513	1,186	1,164	1,293
" -Southern Illinois U	2,300				233	631	672	764
" -U Of Chgo/Pritzker	5,232	182	410	580	851	1,031	1,029	1,149
" -U Of Illinois	14,476	582	923	1,542	2,357	3,046	2,850	3,176
IN-Indiana U	12,938	310	701	1,377	2,380	2,757	2,517	2,896
IA-U Of Iowa	8,032	250	574	921	1,412	1,618	1,642	1,615
KS-U Of Kansas	8,321	236	550	841	1,520	1,689	1,685	1,800
KY-U Of Kentucky	3,995			281	852	962	877	1,023
" -U Of Louisville	6,472	255	428	675	1,078	1,294	1,226	1,516
LA-Lsu (New Orleans)	8,174	218	540	924	1,328	1,671	1,654	1,839
" -Lsu (Shreveport)	3,237				298	926	926	1,087
" -Tulane U	7,906	355	687	1,002	1,321	1,454	1,441	1,646
MD-Johns Hopkins	5,995	263	440	687	1,041	1,146	1,159	1,259
" -U Of Maryland	7,804	359	547	849	1,403	1,614	1,454	1,578
" -Uniformed Services U	4,510					1,174	1,581	1,755
MA-Boston U	6,693	171	395	582	1,026	1,437	1,452	1,630
" -Harvard U	9,286	557	940	1,211	1,555	1,559	1,655	1,809

Table 1.17

Country and School of Graduation of Total Physicians by Year of Graduation, 2010, continued

Country School	Total Physicians	Prior 1950	1950-1959	1960-1969	1970-1979	1980-1989	1990-1999	2000-Present
" -Tufts U	8,143	331	645	934	1,402	1,459	1,530	1,842
" -U Of Massachusetts	3,245				256	958	968	1,063
MI-Michigan State U	3,709				576	991	1,026	1,116
" -U Of Michigan	10,738	388	989	1,531	2,079	2,096	1,860	1,795
" -Wayne State U	10,800	200	370	831	1,790	2,471	2,475	2,663
MN-Mayo Medical School	1,353				155	376	389	433
" -U Of Minnesota	11,900	463	766	1,190	2,223	2,642	2,259	2,357
MS-U Of Mississippi	4,847		76	498	965	1,307	929	1,072
MO-St Louis U	7,461	288	614	842	1,248	1,449	1,402	1,618
" -U Of Mo (Columbia)	4,629		57	586	934	1,068	988	996
" -U Of Mo (Kansas City)	2,841				211	805	867	958
" -Washington U	6,393	287	584	718	1,110	1,253	1,180	1,261
NE-Creighton U	5,455	167	393	551	900	1,077	1,122	1,245
" -U Of Nebraska	6,393	215	466	655	1,289	1,300	1,176	1,292
NV-U Of Nevada	1,487					449	478	560
NH-Dartmouth Med School	2,169				272	562	637	698
NJ-N Jersey Med Sch (Newark)	6,510			580	1,012	1,465	1,657	1,796
" -N Jersey Med Sch (Rutgers)	4,524				294	1,191	1,429	1,610
NM-U Of New Mexico	2,678			31	490	694	685	778
NY-Albany Med Coll	5,733	119	283	501	914	1,241	1,288	1,387
" -Albert Einstein Coll Of Med	7,481		39	774	1,447	1,695	1,642	1,884
" -Columbia U	8,068	430	747	1,017	1,299	1,458	1,466	1,651
" -Cornell U	5,619	278	539	732	929	1,062	1,000	1,079
" -Mt Sinai School Of Med	4,414				634	1,249	1,297	1,234
" -New York Med Coll	9,611	333	681	1,020	1,646	1,930	1,898	2,103
" -New York U	8,899	560	858	1,112	1,460	1,674	1,473	1,762
" -Suny (Brooklyn)	10,727	334	842	1,306	1,941	2,154	2,026	2,124
" -Suny (Buffalo)	6,846	226	422	708	1,187	1,382	1,429	1,492
" -Suny (Stony Brook)	3,218				177	793	1,067	1,181
" -Suny (Syracuse)	6,918	149	402	704	1,066	1,463	1,466	1,668
" -U Of Rochester	5,002	191	435	595	822	968	956	1,035
NC-Bowman Gray	4,700	90	285	420	719	1,015	1,024	1,147
" -Duke University	5,482	206	455	706	980	1,081	1,016	1,038
" -East Carolina U	1,875					439	678	758
" -U Of No Carolina	6,437		227	534	990	1,512	1,524	1,650
ND-U Of No Dakota	1,721				151	441	524	605
OH-Case Western Res	6,923	237	450	692	1,115	1,455	1,404	1,570
" -Northeastern Ohio U	2,780					664	969	1,147
" -Ohio State U	10,345	195	675	1,165	1,988	2,086	2,053	2,183
" -U Of Cincinnati	7,672	264	504	741	1,212	1,817	1,477	1,657
" -U of Toledo	4,394				464	1,176	1,259	1,495
" -Wright State U	2,576					762	852	962
OK-U Of Oklahoma	6,975	144	391	721	1,197	1,615	1,356	1,551
OR-U Of Oregon	5,167	200	383	608	943	1,013	894	1,126
PA-Jefferson Med Coll	14,185	446	927	1,328	1,894	2,138	2,384	5,068
" -Med Coll Of Penn	9,851	489	781	1,155	2,031	2,869	2,526	
" -Pennsylvania State U	3,751				585	909	972	1,285
" -Temple U	9,099	375	705	1,097	1,529	1,728	1,685	1,980
" -U Of Pennsylvania	8,441	471	799	1,147	1,421	1,514	1,444	1,645
" -U Of Pittsburgh	6,720	259	506	750	1,103	1,275	1,293	1,534

Table 1.17

Country and School of Graduation of Total Physicians by Year of Graduation, 2010, continued

Country School	Total Physicians	Prior 1950	1950-1959	1960-1969	1970-1979	1980-1989	1990-1999	2000-Present
PR-Ponce Med Sch	1,520					324	543	653
" -San Juan Bautista Sch of Med	882					304	267	311
" -U Central Del Caribe	2,102					880	618	604
" -U Of Puerto Rico	5,121		191	399	943	1,405	1,070	1,113
RI-Brown U	2,674				292	702	796	884
SC-Med Coll Of So Carolina	6,466	106	348	579	1,182	1,471	1,303	1,477
" -U Of So Carolina	1,812					391	628	793
SD-U Of So Dakota	1,617				113	477	477	550
TN-East Tennessee State U	1,532					362	551	619
" -Meharry Med Coll	3,898	134	263	400	756	823	673	849
" -U Of Tennessee	9,095	302	930	1,339	1,711	1,668	1,495	1,650
" -Vanderbilt U	4,633	160	278	418	694	993	953	1,137
TX-Baylor Coll Of Med	7,488	129	401	676	1,343	1,544	1,605	1,790
" -Texas A&M U	1,549					325	472	752
" -Texas Tech U	3,266				179	766	978	1,343
" -U Of Tx (Dallas)	8,702	108	428	749	1,261	1,929	1,939	2,288
" -U Of Tx (Galveston)	9,282	192	668	983	1,607	1,860	1,851	2,121
" -U Of Tx (Houston)	5,935				346	1,557	1,848	2,184
" -U Of Tx (San Antonio)	6,679				855	1,716	1,944	2,164
UT-U Of Utah	4,567	86	243	417	794	985	969	1,073
VT-U Of Vermont	4,201	132	247	373	664	837	911	1,037
VA-Eastern Virginia Med Sch	2,995				153	793	934	1,115
" -Med Coll Of Va	7,849	289	537	650	1,275	1,596	1,605	1,897
" -U Of Virginia	6,301	199	403	590	1,000	1,304	1,323	1,482
WA-U Of Washington	7,248		389	666	1,104	1,664	1,565	1,860
WV-Marshall U	1,284					306	448	530
" -West Virginia U	3,627			322	717	821	784	983
WI-Med Coll Of Wisconsin	8,345	251	502	752	1,052	1,767	1,884	2,137
" -U Of Wisconsin	7,027	210	461	734	1,177	1,511	1,355	1,579
INA-Inactive Schools	601	215	7	29		305	31	14
CAN-Canadian Schools	11,857	402	1,205	1,745	2,497	2,568	2,429	1,011
IMG-Internat"L Schools	254,396	3,812	15,008	34,255	43,379	59,619	52,888	45,435

Table 1.18

Country and School of Graduation of Male Physicians by Year of Graduation, 2010

Country School	Total Physicians	Prior 1950	1950-1959	1960-1969	1970-1979	1980-1989	1990-1999	2000-Present
Total Physicians	688,468	19,468	49,158	87,755	129,516	154,028	127,962	120,581
US Active Schools	505,811	15,871	35,565	59,798	95,179	110,369	95,335	93,694
AL-U Of Alabama	5,126	27	245	562	974	1,197	1,061	1,060
" -U Of So Alabama	1,372				155	468	380	369
AZ-U Of Arizona	2,047				472	546	454	575
AR-U Of Arkansas	4,719	149	331	606	900	965	848	920
CA-Loma Linda U	5,359	247	497	652	1,038	981	972	972
" -Stanford U	2,993	175	352	373	632	486	506	469
" -U Of Cal (Davis)	2,028				463	539	539	487
" -U Of Cal (Irvine)	3,579			1,402	557	579	515	526
" -U Of Cal (LA)	4,814		115	497	1,131	1,180	997	894
" -U Of Cal (San Diego)	2,617				386	809	713	709
" -U Of Cal (SF)	4,823	227	432	786	1,009	871	771	727
" -U Of So Cal (LA)	4,876	125	358	533	830	1,124	942	964
CO-U Of Colorado	4,251	128	354	617	923	772	729	728
CT-U Of Connecticut	1,670				319	564	418	369
" -Yale U	3,681	178	400	606	722	659	579	537
DC-George Wash U	4,997	187	462	735	1,012	992	815	794
" -Georgetown U	6,714	236	542	829	1,335	1,524	1,282	966
" -Howard U	3,168	140	305	525	685	572	437	504
FL-Florida St U	155							155
" -U Of Florida	3,141			380	666	809	659	627
" -U Of Miami	4,762		101	521	1,126	1,298	908	808
" -U Of So Florida	2,041				240	607	597	597
GA-Emory U	4,047	165	379	547	806	826	673	651
" -Med Coll Of Georgia	6,076	126	386	694	1,154	1,372	1,170	1,174
" -Mercer U	636					50	255	331
" -Morehouse U	356					58	137	161
HI-U Of Hawaii	1,285				233	421	316	315
IL-Chgo Med School	5,196	112	418	563	822	1,058	1,050	1,173
" -Loyola U/Stritch	4,618	196	425	634	1,045	834	736	748
" -Northwestern U	6,631	365	816	1,085	1,296	1,152	944	973
" -Rush Med Coll	2,504	62			414	783	625	620
" -Southern Illinois U	1,418				194	438	391	395
" -U Of Chgo/Pritzker	3,798	161	379	526	731	782	636	583
" -U Of Illinois	10,846	530	871	1,447	2,057	2,283	1,881	1,777
IN-Indiana U	9,613	289	669	1,300	2,078	1,991	1,638	1,648
IA-U Of Iowa	5,996	227	552	873	1,240	1,156	1,035	913
KS-U Of Kansas	6,186	217	527	814	1,305	1,220	1,099	1,004
KY-U Of Kentucky	2,856			257	724	697	588	590
" -U Of Louisville	4,707	243	403	643	935	929	731	823
LA-Lsu (New Orleans)	6,101	195	502	857	1,183	1,256	1,072	1,036
" -Lsu (Shreveport)	2,286				274	725	653	634
" -Tulane U	5,952	323	661	969	1,171	1,024	885	919
MD-Johns Hopkins	4,324	215	400	640	878	830	683	678
" -U Of Maryland	5,528	331	521	793	1,182	1,164	822	715
" -Uniformed Services U	3,424					934	1,219	1,271
MA-Boston U	4,527	149	357	508	810	952	868	883
" -Harvard U	6,765	552	890	1,133	1,254	1,032	973	931

Table 1.18

Country and School of Graduation of Male by Year of Graduation, 2010, continued

Country School	Total Physicians	Prior 1950	1950-1959	1960-1969	1970-1979	1980-1989	1990-1999	2000-Present
" -Tufts U	5,764	296	617	886	1,104	973	863	1,025
" -U Of Massachusetts	1,807				198	598	506	505
MI-Michigan State U	1,990				409	570	526	485
" -U Of Michigan	8,143	342	929	1,437	1,743	1,538	1,166	988
" -Wayne State U	7,615	182	350	773	1,539	1,815	1,502	1,454
MN-Mayo Medical School	819				124	261	227	207
" -U Of Minnesota	8,478	419	721	1,120	1,936	1,798	1,273	1,211
MS-U Of Mississippi	3,763		72	480	851	1,021	673	666
MO-St Louis U	5,866	288	604	809	1,129	1,144	995	897
" -U Of Mo (Columbia)	3,340		56	556	816	783	600	529
" -U Of Mo (Kansas City)	1,430				156	475	406	393
" -Washington U	4,750	267	548	674	930	933	759	639
NE-Creighton U	4,249	153	375	542	842	872	788	677
" -U Of Nebraska	4,803	199	446	628	1,145	926	711	748
NV-U Of Nevada	923					317	302	304
NH-Dartmouth Med School	1,260				206	339	355	360
NJ-N Jersey Med Sch (Newark)	4,482			536	874	1,007	1,052	1,013
" -N Jersey Med Sch (Rutgers)	2,776				218	854	884	820
NM-U Of New Mexico	1,569			28	397	447	352	345
NY-Albany Med Coll	3,881	104	269	471	774	875	735	653
" -Albert Einstein Coll Of Med	4,843		37	713	1,136	1,094	926	937
" -Columbia U	5,854	378	659	921	1,052	1,033	910	901
" -Cornell U	4,012	246	499	690	788	699	560	530
" -Mt Sinai School Of Med	2,598				494	827	689	588
" -New York Med Coll	6,917	282	619	947	1,402	1,385	1,227	1,055
" -New York U	6,473	492	776	990	1,185	1,160	936	934
" -Suny (Brooklyn)	7,845	312	774	1,172	1,636	1,581	1,272	1,098
" -Suny (Buffalo)	4,743	208	398	664	999	913	836	725
" -Suny (Stony Brook)	1,791				100	473	621	597
" -Suny (Syracuse)	4,895	131	375	655	919	1,038	873	904
" -U Of Rochester	3,565	172	406	563	712	677	529	506
NC-Bowman Gray	3,492	85	269	397	639	758	681	663
" -Duke University	4,060	193	429	678	806	741	654	559
" -East Carolina U	1,093					327	378	388
" -U Of No Carolina	4,299		219	517	843	1,010	873	837
ND-U Of No Dakota	1,099				133	333	326	307
OH-Case Western Res	4,765	221	405	625	912	926	768	908
" -Northeastern Ohio U	1,595					453	559	583
" -Ohio State U	7,824	181	651	1,090	1,740	1,514	1,323	1,325
" -U Of Cincinnati	5,718	237	483	714	1,083	1,291	921	989
" -U of Toledo	2,855				377	796	784	898
" -Wright State U	1,434					561	444	429
OK-U Of Oklahoma	5,321	134	373	686	1,079	1,231	883	935
OR-U Of Oregon	3,763	181	359	578	835	730	519	561
PA-Jefferson Med Coll	10,050	446	927	1,291	1,634	1,647	1,498	2,607
" -Med Coll Of Penn	6,114	327	484	764	1,316	1,805	1,418	
" -Pennsylvania State U	2,332				500	634	552	646
" -Temple U	6,708	339	647	998	1,319	1,222	1,057	1,126
" -U Of Pennsylvania	6,262	439	755	1,100	1,196	1,018	881	873
" -U Of Pittsburgh	4,911	241	488	707	930	914	830	801

Table 1.18

Country and School of Graduation of Male by Year of Graduation, 2010, continued

Country School	Total Physicians	Prior 1950	1950-1959	1960-1969	1970-1979	1980-1989	1990-1999	2000-Present
PR-Ponce Med Sch	942					239	338	365
" -San Juan Bautista Sch of Med	482					192	162	128
" -U Central Del Caribe	1,311					623	373	315
" -U Of Puerto Rico	3,224		159	326	706	909	584	540
RI-Brown U	1,475				217	440	430	388
SC-Med Coll Of So Carolina	4,849	100	340	555	1,076	1,124	843	811
" -U Of So Carolina	1,148					287	414	447
SD-U Of So Dakota	1,042				93	357	285	307
TN-East Tennessee State U	921					249	339	333
" -Meharry Med Coll	2,575	113	246	361	596	530	341	388
" -U Of Tennessee	7,326	282	876	1,266	1,551	1,349	1,003	999
" -Vanderbilt U	3,512	154	262	396	624	771	646	659
TX-Baylor Coll Of Med	5,354	121	379	650	1,178	1,104	987	935
" -Texas A&M U	885					237	282	366
" -Texas Tech U	2,241				145	567	707	822
" -U Of Tx (Dallas)	6,453	94	400	713	1,113	1,498	1,277	1,358
" -U Of Tx (Galveston)	6,831	167	631	933	1,393	1,378	1,206	1,123
" -U Of Tx (Houston)	3,621				293	1,056	1,061	1,211
" -U Of Tx (San Antonio)	4,190				729	1,202	1,237	1,022
UT-U Of Utah	3,735	82	236	410	737	821	752	697
VT-U Of Vermont	2,777	121	225	354	582	574	476	445
VA-Eastern Virginia Med Sch	1,721				109	524	516	572
" -Med Coll Of Va	5,666	256	494	619	1,114	1,154	1,028	1,001
" -U Of Virginia	4,654	189	390	567	895	1,014	805	794
WA-U Of Washington	4,839		361	632	931	1,123	877	915
WV-Marshall U	818					217	293	308
" -West Virginia U	2,641			298	637	624	484	598
WI-Med Coll Of Wisconsin	6,099	231	476	725	949	1,273	1,183	1,262
" -U Of Wisconsin	4,931	189	421	686	994	1,087	801	753
INA-Inactive Schools	520	204	5	28		248	24	11
CAN-Canadian Schools	9,130	354	1,132	1,570	2,094	1,823	1,576	581
IMG-Internat"L Schools	173,007	3,039	12,456	26,359	32,243	41,588	31,027	26,295

Table 1.19

Country and School of Graduation of Female Physicians by Year of Graduation, 2010

Country School	Total Physicians	Prior 1950	1950-1959	1960-1969	1970-1979	1980-1989	1990-1999	2000-Present
Total Physicians	296,907	2,442	5,200	12,318	28,482	63,788	83,304	101,373
US Active Schools	212,710	1,610	2,573	4,246	16,943	44,955	60,583	81,800
AL-U Of Alabama	1,721	2	12	29	132	351	505	690
" -U Of So Alabama	699				29	135	227	308
AZ-U Of Arizona	1,377				125	272	428	552
AR-U Of Arkansas	1,444	7	23	32	110	276	426	570
CA-Loma Linda U	1,847	28	51	68	175	298	506	721
" -Stanford U	1,338	15	34	45	146	268	338	492
" -U Of Cal (Davis)	1,339				129	352	350	508
" -U Of Cal (Irvine)	1,273			80	92	276	364	461
" -U Of Cal (LA)	2,401		11	39	157	525	771	898
" -U Of Cal (San Diego)	1,416				90	298	451	577
" -U Of Cal (SF)	2,626	39	40	91	285	571	699	901
" -U Of So Cal (LA)	2,037	6	22	38	173	371	605	822
CO-U Of Colorado	1,934	17	36	48	174	443	522	694
CT-U Of Connecticut	1,187				76	258	382	471
" -Yale U	1,529	30	36	53	152	311	396	551
DC-George Wash U	2,352	33	28	56	200	462	670	903
" -Georgetown U	2,306	1	40	31	215	486	631	902
" -Howard U	1,859	23	55	95	224	451	449	562
FL-Florida St U	181							181
" -U Of Florida	1,553			25	111	305	465	647
" -U Of Miami	1,931		8	34	136	394	551	808
" -U Of So Florida	1,097				47	208	308	534
GA-Emory U	1,421	2	7	20	96	320	410	566
" -Med Coll Of Georgia	1,834	14	19	27	131	356	555	732
" -Mercer U	450					34	157	259
" -Morehouse U	511					60	165	286
HI-U Of Hawaii	797				54	200	223	320
IL-Chgo Med School	1,826	5	11	5	78	349	563	815
" -Loyola U/Stritch	1,806	14	19	26	183	362	514	688
" -Northwestern U	2,451	20	48	56	235	552	712	828
" -Rush Med Coll	1,723	9			99	403	539	673
" -Southern Illinois U	882				39	193	281	369
" -U Of Chgo/Pritzker	1,434	21	31	54	120	249	393	566
" -U Of Illinois	3,630	52	52	95	300	763	969	1,399
IN-Indiana U	3,325	21	32	77	302	766	879	1,248
IA-U Of Iowa	2,036	23	22	48	172	462	607	702
KS-U Of Kansas	2,135	19	23	27	215	469	586	796
KY-U Of Kentucky	1,139			24	128	265	289	433
" -U Of Louisville	1,765	12	25	32	143	365	495	693
LA-Lsu (New Orleans)	2,073	23	38	67	145	415	582	803
" -Lsu (Shreveport)	951				24	201	273	453
" -Tulane U	1,954	32	26	33	150	430	556	727
MD-Johns Hopkins	1,671	48	40	47	163	316	476	581
" -U Of Maryland	2,276	28	26	56	221	450	632	863
" -Uniformed Services U	1,086					240	362	484
MA-Boston U	2,166	22	38	74	216	485	584	747
" -Harvard U	2,521	5	50	78	301	527	682	878

Table 1.19

Country and School of Graduation of Female Physicians by Year of Graduation, 2010, continued

Country School	Total Physicians	Prior 1950	1950-1959	1960-1969	1970-1979	1980-1989	1990-1999	2000-Present
" -Tufts U	2,379	35	28	48	298	486	667	817
" -U Of Massachusetts	1,438				58	360	462	558
MI-Michigan State U	1,719				167	421	500	631
" -U Of Michigan	2,595	46	60	94	336	558	694	807
" -Wayne State U	3,185	18	20	58	251	656	973	1,209
MN-Mayo Medical School	534				31	115	162	226
" -U Of Minnesota	3,422	44	45	70	287	844	986	1,146
MS-U Of Mississippi	1,084		4	18	114	286	256	406
MO-St Louis U	1,595		10	33	119	305	407	721
" -U Of Mo (Columbia)	1,289		1	30	118	285	388	467
" -U Of Mo (Kansas City)	1,411				55	330	461	565
" -Washington U	1,643	20	36	44	180	320	421	622
NE-Creighton U	1,206	14	18	9	58	205	334	568
" -U Of Nebraska	1,590	16	20	27	144	374	465	544
NV-U Of Nevada	564					132	176	256
NH-Dartmouth Med School	909				66	223	282	338
NJ-N Jersey Med Sch (Newark)	2,028			44	138	458	605	783
" -N Jersey Med Sch (Rutgers)	1,748				76	337	545	790
NM-U Of New Mexico	1,109			3	93	247	333	433
NY-Albany Med Coll	1,852	15	14	30	140	366	553	734
" -Albert Einstein Coll Of Med	2,638		2	61	311	601	716	947
" -Columbia U	2,214	52	88	96	247	425	556	750
" -Cornell U	1,607	32	40	42	141	363	440	549
" -Mt Sinai School Of Med	1,816				140	422	608	646
" -New York Med Coll	2,694	51	62	73	244	545	671	1,048
" -New York U	2,426	68	82	122	275	514	537	828
" -Suny (Brooklyn)	2,882	22	68	134	305	573	754	1,026
" -Suny (Buffalo)	2,103	18	24	44	188	469	593	767
" -Suny (Stony Brook)	1,427				77	320	446	584
" -Suny (Syracuse)	2,023	18	27	49	147	425	593	764
" -U Of Rochester	1,437	19	29	32	110	291	427	529
NC-Bowman Gray	1,208	5	16	23	80	257	343	484
" -Duke University	1,422	13	26	28	174	340	362	479
" -East Carolina U	782					112	300	370
" -U Of No Carolina	2,138		8	17	147	502	651	813
ND-U Of No Dakota	622				18	108	198	298
OH-Case Western Res	2,158	16	45	67	203	529	636	662
" -Northeastern Ohio U	1,185					211	410	564
" -Ohio State U	2,521	14	24	75	248	572	730	858
" -U Of Cincinnati	1,954	27	21	27	129	526	556	668
" -U of Toledo	1,539				87	380	475	597
" -Wright State U	1,142					201	408	533
OK-U Of Oklahoma	1,654	10	18	35	118	384	473	616
OR-U Of Oregon	1,404	19	24	30	108	283	375	565
PA-Jefferson Med Coll	4,135			37	260	491	886	2,461
" -Med Coll Of Penn	3,737	162	297	391	715	1,064	1,108	
" -Pennsylvania State U	1,419				85	275	420	639
" -Temple U	2,391	36	58	99	210	506	628	854
" -U Of Pennsylvania	2,179	32	44	47	225	496	563	772
" -U Of Pittsburgh	1,809	18	18	43	173	361	463	733

Table 1.19

Country and School of Graduation of Female Physicians by Year of Graduation, 2010, continued

Country School	Total Physicians	Prior 1950	1950-1959	1960-1969	1970-1979	1980-1989	1990-1999	2000-Present
PR-Ponce Med Sch	578					85	205	288
" -San Juan Bautista Sch of Med	400					112	105	183
" -U Central Del Caribe	791					257	245	289
" -U Of Puerto Rico	1,897		32	73	237	496	486	573
RI-Brown U	1,199				75	262	366	496
SC-Med Coll Of So Carolina	1,617	6	8	24	106	347	460	666
" -U Of So Carolina	664					104	214	346
SD-U Of So Dakota	575				20	120	192	243
TN-East Tennessee State U	611					113	212	286
" -Meharry Med Coll	1,323	21	17	39	160	293	332	461
" -U Of Tennessee	1,769	20	54	73	160	319	492	651
" -Vanderbilt U	1,121	6	16	22	70	222	307	478
TX-Baylor Coll Of Med	2,134	8	22	26	165	440	618	855
" -Texas A&M U	664					88	190	386
" -Texas Tech U	1,025				34	199	271	521
" -U Of Tx (Dallas)	2,249	14	28	36	148	431	662	930
" -U Of Tx (Galveston)	2,451	25	37	50	214	482	645	998
" -U Of Tx (Houston)	2,314				53	501	787	973
" -U Of Tx (San Antonio)	2,489				126	514	707	1,142
UT-U Of Utah	832	4	7	7	57	164	217	376
VT-U Of Vermont	1,424	11	22	19	82	263	435	592
VA-Eastern Virginia Med Sch	1,274				44	269	418	543
" -Med Coll Of Va	2,183	33	43	31	161	442	577	896
" -U Of Virginia	1,647	10	13	23	105	290	518	688
WA-U Of Washington	2,409		28	34	173	541	688	945
WV-Marshall U	466					89	155	222
" -West Virginia U	986			24	80	197	300	385
WI-Med Coll Of Wisconsin	2,246	20	26	27	103	494	701	875
" -U Of Wisconsin	2,096	21	40	48	183	424	554	826
INA-Inactive Schools	81	11	2	1		57	7	3
CAN-Canadian Schools	2,727	48	73	175	403	745	853	430
IMG-Internat"L Schools	81,389	773	2,552	7,896	11,136	18,031	21,861	19,140

Table 1.20

Physicians by Race/Ethnicity, 2010

Specialty	Total Physicians	White	Black	Hispanic	Asian	Other	American Indian/ Alaskan Native	Unknown
Total Physicians	985,375	545,481	37,833	51,367	137,192	13,607	1,836	198,059
Aerospace Medicine	413	260	8	13	9	4	2	117
Allergy/Immunology	4,312	2,546	92	193	735	86	5	655
Anesthesiology	43,359	23,822	1,672	1,950	6,865	721	105	8,224
Cardiovascular Disease	22,888	12,078	624	1,124	4,230	539	39	4,254
Child Psychiatry	7,438	4,099	461	515	1,150	112	21	1,080
Colon/Rectal Surgery	1,491	988	53	110	182	18		140
Dermatology	11,316	7,998	343	472	984	106	21	1,392
Diagnostic Radiology	26,054	16,459	544	986	3,480	227	36	4,322
Emergency Medicine	33,278	22,085	1,380	1,576	2,651	341	110	5,135
Family Medicine	87,618	49,654	4,214	5,183	9,268	1,035	361	17,903
Forensic Pathology	670	476	31	28	54	3	2	76
Gastroenterology	13,210	7,112	431	717	2,538	305	8	2,099
General Practice	8,591	2,626	166	600	1,171	64	3	3,961
General Preventive Medicine	2,227	1,243	207	102	231	7	4	433
General Surgery	37,100	22,418	1,564	1,938	4,448	424	101	6,207
Internal Medicine	161,276	73,166	7,097	9,016	33,992	3,651	209	34,145
Medical Genetics	597	418	9	35	50	5		80
Neurological Surgery	5,781	3,746	204	249	655	75	13	839
Neurology	15,850	8,723	371	862	2,765	390	15	2,724
Nuclear Medicine	1,456	693	34	87	289	26	2	325
Obstetrics/Gynecology	42,797	25,035	3,297	2,435	3,950	502	85	7,493
Occupational Medicine	2,426	1,577	94	72	140	18	1	524
Ophthalmology	18,457	12,066	463	724	2,184	269	23	2,728
Orthopedic Surgery	25,241	17,875	720	742	1,588	182	57	4,077
Otolaryngology	10,326	7,052	239	394	1,166	85	12	1,378
Pathology-Anatomic/Clinical	19,027	10,609	403	896	2,983	258	24	3,854
Pediatric Cardiology	2,101	1,301	49	115	322	41	3	270
Pediatrics	76,401	40,764	3,953	5,229	11,454	1,330	159	13,512
Physical Medicine & Rehabilitation	9,045	4,642	476	591	1,896	150	23	1,267
Plastic Surgery	7,418	5,115	193	368	708	78	11	945
Psychiatry	39,738	21,741	1,533	2,134	5,783	673	75	7,799
Public Health & General Preventive Medicine	1,283	783	61	35	53	9	1	341
Pulmonary Diseases	11,126	6,009	296	689	2,041	238	13	1,840
Radiation Oncology	4,698	2,753	139	190	899	65	11	641
Radiology	9,386	5,365	169	421	1,229	73	11	2,118
Thoracic Surgery	4,605	2,874	154	193	500	63	7	814
Transplant Surgery	191	108	4	6	15	2		56
Urological Surgery	10,701	7,017	328	400	1,109	118	15	1,714
Vascular Medicine	30	22	1		2			5
Other Specialty	5,482	3,161	170	193	455	52	17	1,434
Unspecified	9,458	2,908	355	307	1,040	57	29	4,762
Inactive	125,928	80,216	1,558	3,707	9,535	784	22	30,106
Not Classified	64,153	25,877	3,673	5,769	12,392	421	180	15,841
Address Unknown	432	1		1	1			429

Table 1.21

Male Physicians by Race/Ethnicity, 2010

Specialty	Total Physicians	White	Black	Hispanic	Asian	Other	American Indian/ Alaskan Native	Unknown
Total Physicians	688,468	394,109	19,300	33,648	83,732	9,260	1,041	147,378
Aerospace Medicine	378	239	7	11	9	4	1	107
Allergy/Immunology	2,956	1,872	35	109	381	57	4	498
Anesthesiology	32,922	18,626	988	1,477	4,750	554	83	6,444
Cardiovascular Disease	20,294	10,755	490	980	3,609	490	30	3,940
Child Psychiatry	3,843	2,253	143	240	525	51	10	621
Colon/Rectal Surgery	1,245	831	40	84	147	16		127
Dermatology	6,385	4,625	120	221	382	58	10	969
Diagnostic Radiology	19,919	12,845	322	699	2,401	161	28	3,463
Emergency Medicine	24,978	16,706	770	1,147	1,816	258	71	4,210
Family Medicine	55,242	32,433	1,739	3,131	4,843	598	178	12,320
Forensic Pathology	440	307	22	23	33	2		53
Gastroenterology	11,359	6,279	316	563	2,017	270	8	1,906
General Practice	6,735	2,162	115	495	844	45	1	3,073
General Preventive Medicine	1,334	769	77	62	123	2	2	299
General Surgery	30,460	18,241	1,106	1,565	3,511	342	61	5,634
Internal Medicine	107,094	49,875	4,027	5,957	20,245	2,474	116	24,400
Medical Genetics	314	231	5	18	18	3		39
Neurological Surgery	5,351	3,479	180	230	580	69	12	801
Neurology	11,315	6,287	201	576	1,797	284	10	2,160
Nuclear Medicine	1,134	562	23	63	212	15	2	257
Obstetrics/Gynecology	21,977	12,856	1,031	1,354	1,524	256	22	4,934
Occupational Medicine	1,900	1,267	46	55	103	13	1	415
Ophthalmology	14,561	9,881	280	496	1,361	192	16	2,335
Orthopedic Surgery	23,804	16,824	649	688	1,469	169	49	3,956
Otolaryngology	8,779	6,066	175	312	884	65	8	1,269
Pathology-Anatomic/Clinical	12,014	6,941	176	513	1,574	142	14	2,654
Pediatric Cardiology	1,458	930	23	72	197	28	1	207
Pediatrics	33,322	18,256	1,102	2,250	4,349	632	52	6,681
Physical Medicine & Rehabilitation	6,036	3,215	270	396	1,195	94	16	850
Plastic Surgery	6,389	4,436	137	303	574	69	11	859
Psychiatry	25,474	14,008	759	1,351	3,416	431	45	5,464
Public Health & General Preventive Medicine	879	542	29	26	31	7	1	243
Pulmonary Diseases	9,248	5,015	229	549	1,608	216	9	1,622
Radiation Oncology	3,500	2,135	74	136	612	43	9	491
Radiology	7,819	4,519	131	325	1,000	63	9	1,772
Thoracic Surgery	4,384	2,731	142	187	468	62	7	787
Transplant Surgery	171	92	3	6	14	2		54
Urological Surgery	9,911	6,501	272	352	985	110	13	1,678
Vascular Medicine	23	16	1		1			5
Other Specialty	4,112	2,375	86	136	279	36	14	1,186
Unspecified	6,143	1,921	166	186	624	36	15	3,195
Inactive	107,072	70,067	1,157	3,107	6,834	617	15	25,275
Not Classified	35,498	14,138	1,636	3,197	6,387	224	87	9,829
Address Unknown	296							296

Table 1.22

Female Physicians by Race/Ethnicity, 2010

Specialty	Total Physicians	White	Black	Hispanic	Asian	Other	American Indian/ Alaskan Native	Unknown
Total Physicians	296,907	151,372	18,533	17,719	53,460	4,347	795	50,681
Aerospace Medicine	35	21	1	2			1	10
Allergy/Immunology	1,356	674	57	84	354	29	1	157
Anesthesiology	10,437	5,196	684	473	2,115	167	22	1,780
Cardiovascular Disease	2,594	1,323	134	144	621	49	9	314
Child Psychiatry	3,595	1,846	318	275	625	61	11	459
Colon/Rectal Surgery	246	157	13	26	35	2		13
Dermatology	4,931	3,373	223	251	602	48	11	423
Diagnostic Radiology	6,135	3,614	222	287	1,079	66	8	859
Emergency Medicine	8,300	5,379	610	429	835	83	39	925
Family Medicine	32,376	17,221	2,475	2,052	4,425	437	183	5,583
Forensic Pathology	230	169	9	5	21	1	2	23
Gastroenterology	1,851	833	115	154	521	35		193
General Practice	1,856	464	51	105	327	19	2	888
General Preventive Medicine	893	474	130	40	108	5	2	134
General Surgery	6,640	4,177	458	373	937	82	40	573
Internal Medicine	54,182	23,291	3,070	3,059	13,747	1,177	93	9,745
Medical Genetics	283	187	4	17	32	2		41
Neurological Surgery	430	267	24	19	75	6	1	38
Neurology	4,535	2,436	170	286	968	106	5	564
Nuclear Medicine	322	131	11	24	77	11		68
Obstetrics/Gynecology	20,820	12,179	2,266	1,081	2,426	246	63	2,559
Occupational Medicine	526	310	48	17	37	5		109
Ophthalmology	3,896	2,185	183	228	823	77	7	393
Orthopedic Surgery	1,437	1,051	71	54	119	13	8	121
Otolaryngology	1,547	986	64	82	282	20	4	109
Pathology-Anatomic/Clinical	7,013	3,668	227	383	1,409	116	10	1,200
Pediatric Cardiology	643	371	26	43	125	13	2	63
Pediatrics	43,079	22,508	2,851	2,979	7,105	698	107	6,831
Physical Medicine & Rehabilitation	3,009	1,427	206	195	701	56	7	417
Plastic Surgery	1,029	679	56	65	134	9		86
Psychiatry	14,264	7,733	774	783	2,367	242	30	2,335
Public Health & General Preventive Medicine	404	241	32	9	22	2		98
Pulmonary Diseases	1,878	994	67	140	433	22	4	218
Radiation Oncology	1,198	618	65	54	287	22	2	150
Radiology	1,567	846	38	96	229	10	2	346
Thoracic Surgery	221	143	12	6	32	1		27
Transplant Surgery	20	16	1		1			2
Urological Surgery	790	516	56	48	124	8	2	36
Vascular Medicine	7	6			1			
Other Specialty	1,370	786	84	57	176	16	3	248
Unspecified	3,315	987	189	121	416	21	14	1,567
Inactive	18,856	10,149	401	600	2,701	167	7	4,831
Not Classified	28,655	11,739	2,037	2,572	6,005	197	93	6,012
Address Unknown	136	1		1	1			133

Chapter 2

Physician Distribution

This chapter provides information on the geographic distribution of physicians in the US and Possessions. The tabulations consist of summary tables by state of location, age, and sex, and summary tables by state of location, Major Professional Activity, and sex. These tables provide this information for the physician population as a whole and for International Medical Graduates (IMGs).

State of Location, Age, and Activity by Sex

Total US Physicians

Table 2.1 demonstrates that of the total 2010 US physician population (985,375), more than half (55.0%) were located in 10 states, each having more than 25,000 physicians. These 10 leading states were California (118,110), New York (86,293), Texas (60,991), Florida (58,026), Pennsylvania (44,988), Illinois (41,724), Ohio (35,925), Massachusetts (35,334), New Jersey (30,976), and Michigan (29,331).

Physicians younger than 45 years comprised 30% or more of the total physicians in each of these states except Montana (23.6%), Wyoming (28.7%), Maine (29.1%), and Florida (29.9%). The state having the highest percentage of physicians in this age group was Massachusetts (44.4%).

Table 2.3 indicates that there were more female physicians in California in 2010 than in any other state (36,346, or 12.2% of total female physicians). New York followed with 29,467 female physicians and Texas with 17,982. These three states, in addition to Illinois (14,218), Pennsylvania (13,822), Florida (13,808), Massachusetts (12,920), and Ohio (10,859), accounted for more than half (50.3%) of all female physicians in 2010.

The distribution of physicians by age categories reveals a higher proportion of female physicians than male physicians younger than 35 years. Table C demonstrates the percentage distributions by age groups and sex.

Male physicians younger than 35 (Table 2.2) showed the highest concentrations in New York (9,242), California (8,056), Texas (5,892), Pennsylvania (5,007), and Illinois (4,463). Nearly two fifths (37.8%) of all male physicians younger than 35 years were located in these states. Table 2.3 reveals that female physicians younger than 35 years accounted for the highest counts in New York (8,800), California (8,368), Texas (5,302), Illinois (4,379), and

Table C

Percent Distribution of Physicians by Age and Sex, 2010

Sex	*Total*	*Under 35*	*35-44*	*45-54*	*55-64*	*65 and Over*
Both	100.0	16.8	21.8	22.4	19.2	19.8
Male	100.0	12.6	18.7	22.1	21.7	25.0
Female	100.0	26.6	29.0	23.2	13.7	7.6

Source: Tables 2.1, 2.2, and 2.3

Pennsylvania (4,331). Cumulatively, these five states accounted for 39.4% of all female physicians younger than 35 years.

State of Location and Activity

Tables 2.7 through 2.9 show the distribution of total physicians, male physicians, and female physicians among the states and major professional activity. Patient-Care physicians were in largest numbers in California (88,369), followed by New York (64,089), Texas (48,536), Florida (42,785), and Pennsylvania (33,568). Together, these states represented almost two fifths (36.9%) of all Patient-Care physicians. Residents/Fellows had the highest representation in New York, where they accounted nearly one fifth (21.3%) of Patient-Care physicians in that state.

For male physicians, Table 2.8 shows that Patient Care had the highest percentage representation in Alaska (80.3%), followed by North Dakota (80.1%), Alabama (79.7%), and Louisiana (79.6%). Lowest representation among male physicians in Patient Care was in Maryland (68.9), and the District of Columbia (68.9%).

Among female physicians (Table 2.9), Patient Care had the highest proportional representation in North Dakota (90.7%) and South Dakota (88.3%). Lowest was the District of Columbia (74.7%). Female Residents/Fellows were found in highest numbers in New York (6,375), California (4,924), and Texas (3,022).

International Medical Graduates (IMGs)

The states of New York (34,800), California (27,752), Florida (21,719), Texas (15,166), Illinois (14,166), and New Jersey (13,762) comprised half (50.1%) of all IMGs (Table 2.4). Of total IMGs, 37.5% were younger than 45 years. More than three fifths (57.5%) of IMGs in Nebraska were in the younger than 45-year age group, the highest proportion among the states.

The largest counts of male IMGs (Table 2.5) were found in New York (22,876), California (18,231), and Florida (16,247). Largest counts of female IMGs (Table 2.6) were found in New York (11,924), California (9,521), and Florida (5,472). The three highest-ranking states in each case accounted for approximately one third of the IMG population: 33.1% for male and 33.1% for female.

Table D indicates that the percentage distribution of female IMGs (Table 2.6) compared with the distribution of male IMGs (Table 2.5) varied widely in the younger and older age groups.

Of the five states with the largest counts of female IMGs New York, California, Florida, New Jersey, and Illinois proportionately the highest percentages of female IMGs younger than 35 years were found in New York (23.7%) and Illinois (22.5%).

More IMGs were in Office-Based practice in 2010 (55.1%) than in any other major professional activity (Table 2.10). Of the five states with the most IMGs (New York, California, Florida, Texas, and Illinois), California had the highest percentages of IMGs in Office-Based practice (63.9%), whereas New York had the lowest (46.3%).

New York (9,255), California (3,357), Pennsylvania (3,130), Florida (2,816), and Illinois (2,775) had the largest numbers of Hospital-Based IMGs. Of these states, Pennsylvania had the largest percentage of its IMG population (26.6%) as Hospital-Based.

Table D

Percent Distribution of International Medical Graduates by Age and Sex, 2010

Sex	*Total*	*Under 35*	*35-44*	*45-54*	*55-64*	*65 and Over*
Both	100.0	14.7	22.8	21.2	19.0	22.3
Male	100.0	12.0	19.8	21.3	20.7	26.2
Female	100.0	20.5	29.2	21.1	15.3	14.0

Source: Tables 2.4, 2.5, and 2.6

Table 2.1

Total Physicians by Age and State of Location, 2010

State	Total Physicians	< 35	35-44	45-54	55-64	≥ 65
Total Physicians	985,375	165,544	214,468	220,858	189,648	194,857
Alabama	11,613	1,932	2,450	2,904	2,328	1,999
Alaska	1,823	169	426	504	437	287
Arizona	16,944	2,213	4,004	3,889	3,184	3,654
Arkansas	6,771	1,097	1,451	1,560	1,399	1,264
California	118,110	16,424	25,723	23,724	24,247	27,992
Colorado	15,595	1,978	3,848	3,596	3,139	3,034
Connecticut	15,270	2,726	3,118	3,410	2,969	3,047
Delaware	2,550	392	582	589	459	528
District Of Columbia	5,776	1,834	1,147	837	879	1,079
Florida	58,026	6,231	11,129	13,865	11,537	15,264
Georgia	24,496	3,562	6,046	6,019	4,649	4,220
Hawaii	4,866	621	1,004	1,075	1,068	1,098
Idaho	3,215	240	771	869	665	670
Illinois	41,724	8,842	9,147	8,856	7,528	7,351
Indiana	15,898	2,358	3,578	4,041	3,251	2,670
Iowa	6,677	1,121	1,470	1,575	1,311	1,200
Kansas	7,558	1,229	1,609	1,711	1,483	1,526
Kentucky	11,417	1,911	2,575	2,722	2,281	1,928
Louisiana	13,587	2,641	3,034	2,871	2,629	2,412
Maine	4,426	394	892	1,071	1,024	1,045
Maryland	27,334	4,474	5,942	6,053	5,267	5,598
Massachusetts	35,334	7,522	8,161	7,386	6,231	6,034
Michigan	29,331	6,152	6,119	6,278	5,334	5,448
Minnesota	18,143	3,262	4,242	4,257	3,397	2,985
Mississippi	6,149	858	1,313	1,489	1,266	1,223
Missouri	16,802	3,697	3,627	3,762	2,991	2,725
Montana	2,658	144	482	698	655	679
Nebraska	5,150	1,033	1,145	1,173	944	855
Nevada	5,899	562	1,505	1,463	1,085	1,284
New Hampshire	4,563	579	1,007	1,136	931	910
New Jersey	30,976	4,233	6,403	7,504	6,467	6,369
New Mexico	5,759	726	1,182	1,226	1,417	1,208
New York	86,293	18,042	16,778	17,896	15,796	17,781
North Carolina	27,850	4,802	6,743	6,747	4,893	4,665
North Dakota	1,832	250	387	463	422	310
Ohio	35,925	7,416	7,969	7,975	6,227	6,338
Oklahoma	7,619	1,185	1,487	1,745	1,666	1,536
Oregon	13,007	1,593	3,078	2,874	2,747	2,715
Pennsylvania	44,988	9,338	8,603	9,868	8,612	8,567
Rhode Island	4,622	1,054	997	961	727	883
South Carolina	12,240	2,023	2,807	2,840	2,273	2,297
South Dakota	2,098	234	439	558	486	381
Tennessee	19,035	3,139	4,123	4,792	3,786	3,195
Texas	60,991	11,194	14,960	13,912	10,838	10,087
Utah	6,865	1,175	1,709	1,554	1,272	1,155
Vermont	2,752	374	526	673	556	623
Virginia	25,571	3,937	5,894	5,890	4,898	4,952
Washington	21,795	2,777	4,853	4,899	4,744	4,522
West Virginia	4,922	884	972	1,009	993	1,064
Wisconsin	17,220	2,766	3,875	4,361	3,245	2,973
Wyoming	1,242	88	268	292	319	275
Possessions	12,596	1,899	2,412	3,229	2,554	2,502
APO's and FPO's	1,040	215	451	207	97	70
Address Unknown	432	2	5		45	380

Table 2.2

Male Physicians by Age and State of Location, 2010

State	Total Physicians	< 35	35-44	45-54	55-64	≥ 65
Total Physicians	688,468	86,505	128,445	152,102	149,078	172,338
Alabama	8,846	1,140	1,675	2,208	1,956	1,867
Alaska	1,237	88	234	326	331	258
Arizona	12,335	1,185	2,526	2,720	2,566	3,338
Arkansas	5,167	636	970	1,223	1,159	1,179
California	81,764	8,056	14,783	15,547	18,697	24,681
Colorado	10,686	938	2,200	2,298	2,466	2,784
Connecticut	10,406	1,349	1,758	2,261	2,322	2,716
Delaware	1,726	178	333	414	345	456
District Of Columbia	3,420	840	588	503	619	870
Florida	44,218	3,361	7,273	10,321	9,541	13,722
Georgia	17,342	1,823	3,634	4,268	3,743	3,874
Hawaii	3,479	345	593	756	843	942
Idaho	2,562	128	551	668	572	643
Illinois	27,506	4,463	5,257	5,923	5,653	6,210
Indiana	11,590	1,272	2,298	2,926	2,659	2,435
Iowa	4,962	641	946	1,166	1,091	1,118
Kansas	5,483	653	1,003	1,227	1,202	1,398
Kentucky	8,392	1,084	1,721	1,977	1,873	1,737
Louisiana	9,938	1,480	1,985	2,138	2,164	2,171
Maine	3,179	200	529	691	812	947
Maryland	17,841	2,158	3,218	3,801	3,869	4,795
Massachusetts	22,414	3,684	4,407	4,508	4,540	5,275
Michigan	20,399	3,510	3,600	4,333	4,163	4,793
Minnesota	12,603	1,764	2,542	2,856	2,690	2,751
Mississippi	4,823	525	940	1,163	1,064	1,131
Missouri	11,844	2,003	2,266	2,674	2,440	2,461
Montana	2,029	64	295	502	529	639
Nebraska	3,777	591	719	866	783	818
Nevada	4,481	326	1,028	1,110	895	1,122
New Hampshire	3,233	311	580	742	775	825
New Jersey	20,738	2,183	3,539	4,954	4,819	5,243
New Mexico	3,839	382	644	732	1,019	1,062
New York	56,826	9,242	9,429	11,714	11,773	14,668
North Carolina	19,718	2,506	4,055	4,816	4,015	4,326
North Dakota	1,391	145	246	338	367	295
Ohio	25,066	4,063	4,915	5,630	4,911	5,547
Oklahoma	5,777	704	1,007	1,285	1,362	1,419
Oregon	9,032	764	1,793	1,853	2,131	2,491
Pennsylvania	31,166	5,007	5,109	6,858	6,737	7,455
Rhode Island	3,021	483	560	628	575	775
South Carolina	9,137	1,086	1,851	2,135	1,906	2,159
South Dakota	1,609	135	270	426	413	365
Tennessee	14,225	1,803	2,692	3,588	3,213	2,929
Texas	43,009	5,892	9,301	9,868	8,752	9,196
Utah	5,361	712	1,241	1,193	1,124	1,091
Vermont	1,841	182	285	409	410	555
Virginia	17,495	1,932	3,402	3,987	3,814	4,360
Washington	15,207	1,401	2,814	3,223	3,660	4,109
West Virginia	3,733	559	643	772	810	949
Wisconsin	12,278	1,476	2,351	3,070	2,651	2,730
Wyoming	965	51	178	214	260	262
Possessions	8,329	872	1,358	2,133	1,887	2,079
APO's and FPO's	727	128	308	160	71	60
Address Unknown	296	1	2		36	257

Table 2.3

Female Physicians by Age and State of Location, 2010

State	Total Physicians	< 35	35-44	45-54	55-64	≥ 65
Total Physicians	296,907	79,039	86,023	68,756	40,570	22,519
Alabama	2,767	792	775	696	372	132
Alaska	586	81	192	178	106	29
Arizona	4,609	1,028	1,478	1,169	618	316
Arkansas	1,604	461	481	337	240	85
California	36,346	8,368	10,940	8,177	5,550	3,311
Colorado	4,909	1,040	1,648	1,298	673	250
Connecticut	4,864	1,377	1,360	1,149	647	331
Delaware	824	214	249	175	114	72
District Of Columbia	2,356	994	559	334	260	209
Florida	13,808	2,870	3,856	3,544	1,996	1,542
Georgia	7,154	1,739	2,412	1,751	906	346
Hawaii	1,387	276	411	319	225	156
Idaho	653	112	220	201	93	27
Illinois	14,218	4,379	3,890	2,933	1,875	1,141
Indiana	4,308	1,086	1,280	1,115	592	235
Iowa	1,715	480	524	409	220	82
Kansas	2,075	576	606	484	281	128
Kentucky	3,025	827	854	745	408	191
Louisiana	3,649	1,161	1,049	733	465	241
Maine	1,247	194	363	380	212	98
Maryland	9,493	2,316	2,724	2,252	1,398	803
Massachusetts	12,920	3,838	3,754	2,878	1,691	759
Michigan	8,932	2,642	2,519	1,945	1,171	655
Minnesota	5,540	1,498	1,700	1,401	707	234
Mississippi	1,326	333	373	326	202	92
Missouri	4,958	1,694	1,361	1,088	551	264
Montana	629	80	187	196	126	40
Nebraska	1,373	442	426	307	161	37
Nevada	1,418	236	477	353	190	162
New Hampshire	1,330	268	427	394	156	85
New Jersey	10,238	2,050	2,864	2,550	1,648	1,126
New Mexico	1,920	344	538	494	398	146
New York	29,467	8,800	7,349	6,182	4,023	3,113
North Carolina	8,132	2,296	2,688	1,931	878	339
North Dakota	441	105	141	125	55	15
Ohio	10,859	3,353	3,054	2,345	1,316	791
Oklahoma	1,842	481	480	460	304	117
Oregon	3,975	829	1,285	1,021	616	224
Pennsylvania	13,822	4,331	3,494	3,010	1,875	1,112
Rhode Island	1,601	571	437	333	152	108
South Carolina	3,103	937	956	705	367	138
South Dakota	489	99	169	132	73	16
Tennessee	4,810	1,336	1,431	1,204	573	266
Texas	17,982	5,302	5,659	4,044	2,086	891
Utah	1,504	463	468	361	148	64
Vermont	911	192	241	264	146	68
Virginia	8,076	2,005	2,492	1,903	1,084	592
Washington	6,588	1,376	2,039	1,676	1,084	413
West Virginia	1,189	325	329	237	183	115
Wisconsin	4,942	1,290	1,524	1,291	594	243
Wyoming	277	37	90	78	59	13
Possessions	4,267	1,027	1,054	1,096	667	423
APO's and FPO's	313	87	143	47	26	10
Address Unknown	136	1	3		9	123

Table 2.4

IMGs by Age and State of Location, 2010

State	Total Physicians	< 35	35-44	45-54	55-64	≥ 65
Total Physicians	254,396	37,385	57,994	53,973	48,295	56,749
Alabama	1,884	324	503	482	324	251
Alaska	120	7	34	31	27	21
Arizona	3,954	549	1,194	898	629	684
Arkansas	1,086	260	359	242	139	86
California	27,752	1,857	5,773	6,204	6,920	6,998
Colorado	1,177	101	372	246	216	242
Connecticut	4,433	931	1,078	851	731	842
Delaware	790	78	230	150	110	222
District Of Columbia	1,175	313	277	175	168	242
Florida	21,719	1,738	4,048	5,252	4,483	6,198
Georgia	5,091	685	1,405	1,179	918	904
Hawaii	746	65	130	122	133	296
Idaho	146	8	47	33	30	28
Illinois	14,166	2,405	2,883	2,592	2,780	3,506
Indiana	3,384	395	900	794	653	642
Iowa	1,367	268	427	248	193	231
Kansas	1,482	258	388	280	239	317
Kentucky	2,422	344	711	568	394	405
Louisiana	2,710	641	705	519	481	364
Maine	649	100	198	96	106	149
Maryland	7,439	823	1,566	1,604	1,452	1,994
Massachusetts	7,850	1,392	2,223	1,665	1,181	1,389
Michigan	10,166	2,297	2,267	1,854	1,775	1,973
Minnesota	2,827	636	955	592	275	369
Mississippi	842	140	253	215	126	108
Missouri	3,820	795	1,042	661	576	746
Montana	122	6	22	27	35	32
Nebraska	755	211	223	146	88	87
Nevada	1,876	206	536	388	274	472
New Hampshire	734	125	207	132	99	171
New Jersey	13,762	1,737	2,603	3,119	3,150	3,153
New Mexico	1,013	149	268	210	206	180
New York	34,800	6,234	6,541	6,788	6,757	8,480
North Carolina	3,844	537	1,115	991	575	626
North Dakota	480	114	139	89	78	60
Ohio	10,362	1,956	2,530	1,834	1,637	2,405
Oklahoma	1,572	323	369	328	304	248
Oregon	1,214	157	379	269	155	254
Pennsylvania	11,760	2,542	2,508	2,293	2,092	2,325
Rhode Island	1,213	210	293	216	161	333
South Carolina	1,689	256	512	410	212	299
South Dakota	289	44	96	53	48	48
Tennessee	3,211	531	882	789	573	436
Texas	15,166	1,968	4,016	3,636	2,751	2,795
Utah	597	91	221	130	85	70
Vermont	260	67	52	46	33	62
Virginia	5,616	647	1,389	1,189	978	1,413
Washington	2,861	341	824	603	484	609
West Virginia	1,726	281	311	316	307	511
Wisconsin	3,219	526	937	738	427	591
Wyoming	144	25	54	24	25	16
Possessions	6,737	689	983	1,635	1,679	1,751
APO's and FPO's	91		12	21	22	36
Address Unknown	86	2	4		1	79

Table 2.5

Male IMGs by Age and State of Location, 2010

State	Total Physicians	< 35	35-44	45-54	55-64	≥ 65
Total Physicians	173,007	20,739	34,238	36,827	35,861	45,342
Alabama	1,382	200	351	371	251	209
Alaska	75	4	19	16	20	16
Arizona	2,832	331	775	659	508	559
Arkansas	777	161	243	189	110	74
California	18,231	856	3,022	3,810	5,038	5,505
Colorado	764	59	198	155	161	191
Connecticut	2,913	501	577	575	563	697
Delaware	542	35	143	104	79	181
District Of Columbia	701	164	141	110	108	178
Florida	16,247	952	2,715	3,881	3,534	5,165
Georgia	3,501	359	835	837	701	769
Hawaii	510	40	70	78	99	223
Idaho	109	3	30	25	27	24
Illinois	9,289	1,308	1,643	1,690	1,927	2,721
Indiana	2,395	213	562	583	501	536
Iowa998	164	297	191	147	199	
Kansas	1,040	148	248	203	183	258
Kentucky	1,747	205	490	429	307	316
Louisiana	1,903	388	460	385	371	299
Maine	463	56	131	60	80	136
Maryland	4,919	434	859	1,040	1,022	1,564
Massachusetts	4,962	769	1,227	1,044	851	1,071
Michigan	6,854	1,376	1,300	1,282	1,297	1,599
Minnesota	1,890	384	603	409	207	287
Mississippi	611	97	173	160	98	83
Missouri	2,658	493	659	467	427	612
Montana	95	2	17	21	28	27
Nebraska	535	132	153	106	69	75
Nevada	1,324	120	352	286	206	360
New Hampshire	499	72	124	86	74	143
New Jersey	8,699	865	1,280	2,002	2,201	2,351
New Mexico	710	90	174	133	165	148
New York	22,876	3,409	3,652	4,433	4,869	6,513
North Carolina	2,668	306	664	722	457	519
North Dakota	350	72	93	66	62	57
Ohio	7,257	1,141	1,604	1,335	1,243	1,934
Oklahoma	1,135	197	256	249	231	202
Oregon	813	89	233	177	118	196
Pennsylvania	7,957	1,432	1,480	1,593	1,600	1,852
Rhode Island	862	118	181	154	133	276
South Carolina	1,202	144	342	315	147	254
South Dakota	215	28	66	40	38	43
Tennessee	2,281	336	565	581	454	345
Texas	10,532	1,066	2,385	2,580	2,132	2,369
Utah	441	63	158	94	71	55
Vermont	188	41	33	35	26	53
Virginia	3,739	331	799	775	715	1,119
Washington	1,832	153	443	403	348	485
West Virginia	1,329	188	205	244	250	442
Wisconsin	2,223	302	589	514	327	491
Wyoming	96	16	33	15	20	12
Possessions	4,704	325	577	1,098	1,241	1,463
APO's and FPO's	70		7	17	18	28
Address Unknown	62	1	2		1	58

Table 2.6

Female IMGs by Age and State of Location, 2010

State	Total Physicians	< 35	35-44	45-54	55-64	≥ 65
Total Physicians	81,389	16,646	23,756	17,146	12,434	11,407
Alabama	502	124	152	111	73	42
Alaska	45	3	15	15	7	5
Arizona	1,122	218	419	239	121	125
Arkansas	309	99	116	53	29	12
California	9,521	1,001	2,751	2,394	1,882	1,493
Colorado	413	42	174	91	55	51
Connecticut	1,520	430	501	276	168	145
Delaware	248	43	87	46	31	41
District Of Columbia	474	149	136	65	60	64
Florida	5,472	786	1,333	1,371	949	1,033
Georgia	1,590	326	570	342	217	135
Hawaii	236	25	60	44	34	73
Idaho	37	5	17	8	3	4
Illinois	4,877	1,097	1,240	902	853	785
Indiana	989	182	338	211	152	106
Iowa	369	104	130	57	46	32
Kansas	442	110	140	77	56	59
Kentucky	675	139	221	139	87	89
Louisiana	807	253	245	134	110	65
Maine	186	44	67	36	26	13
Maryland	2,520	389	707	564	430	430
Massachusetts	2,888	623	996	621	330	318
Michigan	3,312	921	967	572	478	374
Minnesota	937	252	352	183	68	82
Mississippi	231	43	80	55	28	25
Missouri	1,162	302	383	194	149	134
Montana	27	4	5	6	7	5
Nebraska	220	79	70	40	19	12
Nevada	552	86	184	102	68	112
New Hampshire	235	53	83	46	25	28
New Jersey	5,063	872	1,323	1,117	949	802
New Mexico	303	59	94	77	41	32
New York	11,924	2,825	2,889	2,355	1,888	1,967
North Carolina	1,176	231	451	269	118	107
North Dakota	130	42	46	23	16	3
Ohio	3,105	815	926	499	394	471
Oklahoma	437	126	113	79	73	46
Oregon	401	68	146	92	37	58
Pennsylvania	3,803	1,110	1,028	700	492	473
Rhode Island	351	92	112	62	28	57
South Carolina	487	112	170	95	65	45
South Dakota	74	16	30	13	10	5
Tennessee	930	195	317	208	119	91
Texas	4,634	902	1,631	1,056	619	426
Utah	156	28	63	36	14	15
Vermont	72	26	19	11	7	9
Virginia	1,877	316	590	414	263	294
Washington	1,029	188	381	200	136	124
West Virginia	397	93	106	72	57	69
Wisconsin	996	224	348	224	100	100
Wyoming	48	9	21	9	5	4
Possessions	2,033	364	406	537	438	288
APO's and FPO's	21		5	4	4	8
Address Unknown	24	1	2			21

Table 2.7

Total Physicians by State of Location and Major Professional Activity, 2010

		Patient Care				Other Professional Activity			
				Hospital Based					
State	Total Physicians	Total Patient Care	Office Based	Resid./ Fellows	Phys. Staff	Admin.	Med. Teach.	Research	Other*
Total Physicians	985,375	752,572	565,024	108,142	79,406	14,009	9,909	13,755	194,698
Alabama	11,613	9,377	7,324	1,285	768	110	99	117	1,910
Alaska	1,823	1,502	1,188	44	270	31	10	14	266
Arizona	16,944	12,818	10,331	1,320	1,167	254	164	135	3,573
Arkansas	6,771	5,397	4,096	709	592	54	98	44	1,178
California	118,110	88,369	70,496	10,000	7,873	1,721	988	1,814	25,218
Colorado	15,595	11,932	9,692	1,130	1,110	261	146	222	3,034
Connecticut	15,270	11,447	8,276	1,978	1,193	277	189	295	3,062
Delaware	2,550	1,988	1,512	261	215	49	14	24	475
District Of Columbia	5,776	4,115	2,119	1,345	651	189	105	151	1,216
Florida	58,026	42,785	34,882	3,709	4,194	702	457	394	13,688
Georgia	24,496	19,195	15,387	2,013	1,795	354	266	320	4,361
Hawaii	4,866	3,668	2,850	349	469	76	50	45	1,027
Idaho	3,215	2,538	2,163	84	291	27	20	10	620
Illinois	41,724	32,274	23,508	5,763	3,003	553	396	435	8,066
Indiana	15,898	12,860	10,221	1,358	1,281	199	124	171	2,544
Iowa	6,677	5,118	3,803	709	606	58	94	115	1,292
Kansas	7,558	5,884	4,565	696	623	95	90	53	1,436
Kentucky	11,417	9,182	7,230	1,136	816	123	119	79	1,914
Louisiana	13,587	10,946	7,937	1,838	1,171	130	181	84	2,246
Maine	4,426	3,337	2,559	258	520	82	46	30	931
Maryland	27,334	19,430	13,717	2,894	2,819	699	306	1,182	5,717
Massachusetts	35,334	25,842	16,945	5,266	3,631	577	307	1,147	7,461
Michigan	29,331	22,764	16,112	4,478	2,174	404	329	322	5,512
Minnesota	18,143	14,377	10,901	2,205	1,271	242	157	251	3,116
Mississippi	6,149	4,900	3,753	525	622	66	55	23	1,105
Missouri	16,802	13,190	9,100	2,557	1,533	176	191	255	2,990
Montana	2,658	1,990	1,693	33	264	31	14	14	609
Nebraska	5,150	4,061	3,029	662	370	73	54	50	912
Nevada	5,899	4,558	3,952	236	370	68	33	20	1,220
New Hampshire	4,563	3,492	2,558	416	518	55	34	54	928
New Jersey	30,976	23,757	18,505	2,653	2,599	463	265	498	5,993
New Mexico	5,759	4,311	3,241	530	540	97	66	64	1,221
New York	86,293	64,089	42,410	13,649	8,030	1,406	970	1,403	18,425
North Carolina	27,850	21,593	16,576	2,922	2,095	365	308	438	5,146
North Dakota	1,832	1,514	1,145	123	246	25	18	6	269
Ohio	35,925	27,702	19,541	5,133	3,028	414	383	415	7,011
Oklahoma	7,619	6,030	4,697	751	582	94	98	43	1,354
Oregon	13,007	9,737	7,882	874	981	166	115	153	2,836
Pennsylvania	44,988	33,568	23,167	6,683	3,718	700	475	852	9,393
Rhode Island	4,622	3,515	2,318	779	418	72	46	67	922
South Carolina	12,240	9,851	7,681	1,206	964	119	158	89	2,023
South Dakota	2,098	1,691	1,391	90	210	23	22	8	354
Tennessee	19,035	15,143	11,775	2,122	1,246	250	175	218	3,249
Texas	60,991	48,536	37,367	6,838	4,331	711	715	579	10,450
Utah	6,865	5,334	4,062	766	506	84	68	109	1,270
Vermont	2,752	2,016	1,381	301	334	42	36	53	605
Virginia	25,571	19,819	14,961	2,404	2,454	398	248	227	4,879
Washington	21,795	16,274	12,934	1,683	1,657	330	204	404	4,583
West Virginia	4,922	3,819	2,796	580	443	57	80	24	942
Wisconsin	17,220	13,668	10,604	1,754	1,310	218	175	180	2,979
Wyoming	1,242	964	807	32	125	16	7	4	251
Possessions	12,596	9,491	7,443	986	1,062	196	138	47	2,724
APO's and FPO's	1,040	814	441	26	347	27	3	4	192

** Includes Other, Inactive and Not Classified Physicians*

Table 2.8

Male Physicians by State of Location and Major Professional Activity, 2010

		Patient Care				Other Professional Activity			
				Hospital Based					
State	Total Physicians	Total Patient Care	Office Based	Resid./ Fellows	Phys. Staff	Admin.	Med. Teach.	Research	Other*
Total Physicians	688,468	513,592	399,429	59,089	55,074	11,036	7,134	10,661	145,749
Alabama	8,846	7,054	5,706	806	542	92	83	99	1,518
Alaska	1,237	993	784	18	191	24	8	8	204
Arizona	12,335	9,038	7,458	723	857	213	112	102	2,870
Arkansas	5,167	4,052	3,207	414	431	41	73	38	963
California	81,764	59,276	48,774	5,076	5,426	1,364	736	1,415	18,973
Colorado	10,686	7,872	6,529	570	773	196	109	176	2,333
Connecticut	10,406	7,544	5,742	1,013	789	226	142	234	2,260
Delaware	1,726	1,311	1,054	120	137	35	11	18	351
District Of Columbia	3,420	2,356	1,299	639	418	142	75	111	736
Florida	44,218	31,661	26,478	2,115	3,068	576	330	318	11,333
Georgia	17,342	13,322	10,925	1,083	1,314	274	196	227	3,323
Hawaii	3,479	2,586	2,023	209	354	62	32	36	763
Idaho	2,562	1,973	1,716	36	221	24	13	7	545
Illinois	27,506	20,911	15,910	3,034	1,967	437	275	322	5,561
Indiana	11,590	9,201	7,538	760	903	165	98	135	1,991
Iowa	4,962	3,702	2,847	409	446	41	76	96	1,047
Kansas	5,483	4,153	3,331	389	433	79	68	45	1,138
Kentucky	8,392	6,665	5,393	687	585	105	87	64	1,471
Louisiana	9,938	7,914	5,984	1,067	863	109	131	70	1,714
Maine	3,179	2,304	1,800	128	376	69	34	20	752
Maryland	17,841	12,286	8,893	1,512	1,881	520	213	909	3,913
Massachusetts	22,414	15,769	10,739	2,709	2,321	462	220	864	5,099
Michigan	20,399	15,411	11,268	2,672	1,471	324	229	256	4,179
Minnesota	12,603	9,605	7,366	1,274	965	196	118	202	2,482
Mississippi	4,823	3,820	3,002	335	483	47	43	16	897
Missouri	11,844	9,134	6,555	1,480	1,099	143	139	210	2,218
Montana	2,029	1,465	1,270	12	183	24	7	13	520
Nebraska	3,777	2,886	2,238	389	259	60	41	41	749
Nevada	4,481	3,439	3,019	148	272	50	24	16	952
New Hampshire	3,233	2,404	1,789	242	373	46	26	44	713
New Jersey	20,738	15,725	12,665	1,457	1,603	351	166	375	4,121
New Mexico	3,839	2,785	2,138	291	356	69	40	46	899
New York	56,826	41,477	28,981	7,274	5,222	1,054	680	1,068	12,547
North Carolina	19,718	14,926	11,796	1,626	1,504	287	211	343	3,951
North Dakota	1,391	1,114	858	67	189	21	14	6	236
Ohio	25,066	18,896	13,907	2,886	2,103	338	278	314	5,240
Oklahoma	5,777	4,484	3,571	470	443	77	70	35	1,111
Oregon	9,032	6,444	5,322	432	690	131	94	121	2,242
Pennsylvania	31,166	22,770	16,553	3,676	2,541	544	329	665	6,858
Rhode Island	3,021	2,251	1,595	375	281	57	31	42	640
South Carolina	9,137	7,151	5,775	669	707	96	123	67	1,700
South Dakota	1,609	1,259	1,046	52	161	20	19	7	304
Tennessee	14,225	11,140	8,967	1,265	908	212	135	176	2,562
Texas	43,009	33,787	26,916	3,816	3,055	558	522	461	7,681
Utah	5,361	4,096	3,237	463	396	71	53	90	1,051
Vermont	1,841	1,269	888	155	226	33	24	43	472
Virginia	17,495	13,088	10,066	1,291	1,731	315	174	177	3,741
Washington	15,207	10,863	8,764	897	1,202	273	148	318	3,605
West Virginia	3,733	2,879	2,159	379	341	45	61	19	729
Wisconsin	12,278	9,448	7,539	960	949	183	115	138	2,394
Wyoming	965	721	606	15	100	14	5	3	222
Possessions	8,329	6,336	5,141	486	709	121	90	32	1,750
APO's and FPO's	727	576	302	18	256	20	3	3	125
Address Unknown	296								

** Includes Other, Inactive and Not Classified Physicians*

Table 2.9

Female Physicians by State of Location and Major Professional Activity, 2010

		Patient Care				Other Professional Activity			
				Hospital Based					
State	Total Physicians	Total Patient Care	Office Based	Resid./ Fellows	Phys. Staff	Admin.	Med. Teach.	Research	Other*
Total Physicians	296,907	238,980	165,595	49,053	24,332	2,973	2,775	3,094	48,949
Alabama	2,767	2,323	1,618	479	226	18	16	18	392
Alaska	586	509	404	26	79	7	2	6	62
Arizona	4,609	3,780	2,873	597	310	41	52	33	703
Arkansas	1,604	1,345	889	295	161	13	25	6	215
California	36,346	29,093	21,722	4,924	2,447	357	252	399	6,245
Colorado	4,909	4,060	3,163	560	337	65	37	46	701
Connecticut	4,864	3,903	2,534	965	404	51	47	61	802
Delaware	824	677	458	141	78	14	3	6	124
District Of Columbia	2,356	1,759	820	706	233	47	30	40	480
Florida	13,808	11,124	8,404	1,594	1,126	126	127	76	2,355
Georgia	7,154	5,873	4,462	930	481	80	70	93	1,038
Hawaii	1,387	1,082	827	140	115	14	18	9	264
Idaho	653	565	447	48	70	3	7	3	75
Illinois	14,218	11,363	7,598	2,729	1,036	116	121	113	2,505
Indiana	4,308	3,659	2,683	598	378	34	26	36	553
Iowa	1,715	1,416	956	300	160	17	18	19	245
Kansas	2,075	1,731	1,234	307	190	16	22	8	298
Kentucky	3,025	2,517	1,837	449	231	18	32	15	443
Louisiana	3,649	3,032	1,953	771	308	21	50	14	532
Maine	1,247	1,033	759	130	144	13	12	10	179
Maryland	9,493	7,144	4,824	1,382	938	179	93	273	1,804
Massachusetts	12,920	10,073	6,206	2,557	1,310	115	87	283	2,362
Michigan	8,932	7,353	4,844	1,806	703	80	100	66	1,333
Minnesota	5,540	4,772	3,535	931	306	46	39	49	634
Mississippi	1,326	1,080	751	190	139	19	12	7	208
Missouri	4,958	4,056	2,545	1,077	434	33	52	45	772
Montana	629	525	423	21	81	7	7	1	89
Nebraska	1,373	1,175	791	273	111	13	13	9	163
Nevada	1,418	1,119	933	88	98	18	9	4	268
New Hampshire	1,330	1,088	769	174	145	9	8	10	215
New Jersey	10,238	8,032	5,840	1,196	996	112	99	123	1,872
New Mexico	1,920	1,526	1,103	239	184	28	26	18	322
New York	29,467	22,612	13,429	6,375	2,808	352	290	335	5,878
North Carolina	8,132	6,667	4,780	1,296	591	78	97	95	1,195
North Dakota	441	400	287	56	57	4	4		33
Ohio	10,859	8,806	5,634	2,247	925	76	105	101	1,771
Oklahoma	1,842	1,546	1,126	281	139	17	28	8	243
Oregon	3,975	3,293	2,560	442	291	35	21	32	594
Pennsylvania	13,822	10,798	6,614	3,007	1,177	156	146	187	2,535
Rhode Island	1,601	1,264	723	404	137	15	15	25	282
South Carolina	3,103	2,700	1,906	537	257	23	35	22	323
South Dakota	489	432	345	38	49	3	3	1	50
Tennessee	4,810	4,003	2,808	857	338	38	40	42	687
Texas	17,982	14,749	10,451	3,022	1,276	153	193	118	2,769
Utah	1,504	1,238	825	303	110	13	15	19	219
Vermont	911	747	493	146	108	9	12	10	133
Virginia	8,076	6,731	4,895	1,113	723	83	74	50	1,138
Washington	6,588	5,411	4,170	786	455	57	56	86	978
West Virginia	1,189	940	637	201	102	12	19	5	213
Wisconsin	4,942	4,220	3,065	794	361	35	60	42	585
Wyoming	277	243	201	17	25	2	2	1	29
Possessions	4,267	3,155	2,302	500	353	75	48	15	974
APO's and FPO's	313	238	139	8	91	7		1	67
Address Unknown	136								

** Includes Other, Inactive and Not Classified Physicians*

Table 2.10

IMGs by State of Location and Major Professional Activity, 2010

		Patient Care				Other Professional Activity			
				Hospital Based					
State	Total Physicians	Total Patient Care	Office Based	Resid./ Fellows	Phys. Staff	Admin.	Med. Teach.	Research	Other*
Total Physicians	254,396	192,046	140,246	28,434	23,366	1,812	1,654	2,462	56,336
Alabama	1,884	1,537	1,094	255	188	7	9	18	313
Alaska	120	93	79	1	13	1	1	2	23
Arizona	3,954	3,091	2,475	318	298	18	33	21	791
Arkansas	1,086	883	543	209	131	2	7	10	184
California	27,752	21,094	17,737	1,207	2,150	215	164	303	5,976
Colorado	1,177	854	699	56	99	4	6	13	300
Connecticut	4,433	3,299	2,227	710	362	35	37	48	1,014
Delaware	790	598	455	71	72	9	1	4	178
District Of Columbia	1,175	798	394	274	130	14	17	23	323
Florida	21,719	16,007	13,201	1,164	1,642	143	116	129	5,324
Georgia	5,091	4,032	3,068	517	447	25	28	37	969
Hawaii	746	521	415	45	61	6	6	12	201
Idaho	146	111	84	3	24		3	1	31
Illinois	14,166	10,620	7,845	1,695	1,080	98	99	110	3,239
Indiana	3,384	2,766	2,158	279	329	16	14	16	572
Iowa	1,367	1,025	694	188	143	6	15	21	300
Kansas	1,482	1,164	764	208	192	11	10	16	281
Kentucky	2,422	1,955	1,447	273	235	8	17	14	428
Louisiana	2,710	2,175	1,306	591	278	20	29	19	467
Maine	649	502	351	68	83	4	2	3	138
Maryland	7,439	5,300	3,920	632	748	79	50	168	1,842
Massachusetts	7,850	5,583	3,643	1,039	901	54	33	165	2,015
Michigan	10,166	7,929	5,337	1,819	773	66	64	70	2,037
Minnesota	2,827	2,190	1,472	493	225	7	12	42	576
Mississippi	842	706	449	119	138	3	7	5	121
Missouri	3,820	2,893	1,866	645	382	16	35	32	844
Montana	122	93	71	3	19	1		1	27
Nebraska	755	602	363	176	63	5	3	6	139
Nevada	1,876	1,404	1,170	108	126	11	5	5	451
New Hampshire	734	567	404	67	96	1		8	158
New Jersey	13,762	10,647	7,943	1,309	1,395	121	70	141	2,783
New Mexico	1,013	812	583	131	98	8	4	7	182
New York	34,800	25,356	16,101	5,543	3,712	327	260	382	8,475
North Carolina	3,844	2,952	2,198	326	428	31	32	42	787
North Dakota	480	407	255	75	77	3	1		69
Ohio	10,362	7,624	5,101	1,544	979	50	67	86	2,535
Oklahoma	1,572	1,313	884	252	177	5	13	6	235
Oregon	1,214	849	684	69	96	9	8	14	334
Pennsylvania	11,760	8,877	5,747	2,001	1,129	89	76	139	2,579
Rhode Island	1,213	881	609	150	122	6	4	10	312
South Carolina	1,689	1,350	996	174	180	11	12	19	297
South Dakota	289	241	182	18	41	2		1	45
Tennessee	3,211	2,576	1,844	463	269	11	18	37	569
Texas	15,166	11,923	9,224	1,473	1,226	68	140	128	2,907
Utah	597	461	328	74	59	3	6	12	115
Vermont	260	170	86	57	27	3	3	5	79
Virginia	5,616	4,232	3,172	488	572	44	31	31	1,278
Washington	2,861	2,085	1,683	174	228	18	14	35	709
West Virginia	1,726	1,335	918	222	195	8	9	3	371
Wisconsin	3,219	2,581	1,913	404	264	8	26	20	584
Wyoming	144	123	91	19	13	1		1	19
Possessions	6,737	4,796	3,944	235	617	101	37	21	1,782
APO's and FPO's	91	63	29		34				28
Address Unknown	86								

** Includes Other, Inactive and Not Classified Physicians*

Table 2.11

Male IMGs by State of Location and Major Professional Activity, 2010

		Patient Care				Other Professional Activity			
				Hospital Based					
State	Total Physicians	Total Patient Care	Office Based	Resid./ Fellows	Phys. Staff	Admin.	Med. Teach.	Research	Other*
Total Physicians	173,007	129,866	97,654	16,303	15,909	1,325	1,179	1,902	38,673
Alabama	1,382	1,130	838	159	133	6	9	16	221
Alaska	75	57	53		4	1	1	1	15
Arizona	2,832	2,211	1,803	187	221	12	24	17	568
Arkansas	777	632	411	132	89	2	6	10	127
California	18,231	13,760	11,808	572	1,380	153	121	223	3,974
Colorado	764	534	438	26	70	4	4	10	212
Connecticut	2,913	2,110	1,488	391	231	22	31	42	708
Delaware	542	402	314	36	52	5	1	3	131
District Of Columbia	701	472	248	144	80	7	12	19	191
Florida	16,247	11,841	9,961	683	1,197	112	82	101	4,111
Georgia	3,501	2,756	2,161	282	313	15	22	29	679
Hawaii	510	364	293	29	42	5	2	10	129
Idaho	109	81	61	1	19		3	1	24
Illinois	9,289	6,906	5,244	956	706	78	71	81	2,153
Indiana	2,395	1,950	1,559	162	229	13	12	12	408
Iowa	998	738	519	109	110	4	11	15	230
Kansas	1,040	824	560	118	146	7	7	13	189
Kentucky	1,747	1,432	1,099	162	171	5	13	10	287
Louisiana	1,903	1,538	975	363	200	17	17	15	316
Maine	463	344	253	37	54	4	2	3	110
Maryland	4,919	3,466	2,622	347	497	52	33	125	1,243
Massachusetts	4,962	3,443	2,278	578	587	38	23	135	1,323
Michigan	6,854	5,295	3,687	1,098	510	47	50	57	1,405
Minnesota	1,890	1,424	957	299	168	6	9	32	419
Mississippi	611	526	340	80	106	1	6	4	74
Missouri	2,658	2,001	1,328	401	272	11	26	25	595
Montana	95	70	53	1	16	1		1	23
Nebraska	535	422	266	104	52	4	2	6	101
Nevada	1,324	1,010	850	69	91	8	2	4	300
New Hampshire	499	384	274	43	67	1		5	109
New Jersey	8,699	6,742	5,183	711	848	85	44	99	1,729
New Mexico	710	575	422	83	70	7	3	5	120
New York	22,876	16,544	11,015	3,107	2,422	248	175	292	5,617
North Carolina	2,668	2,043	1,550	191	302	24	23	36	542
North Dakota	350	294	197	41	56	3	1		52
Ohio	7,257	5,320	3,714	906	700	39	48	56	1,794
Oklahoma	1,135	942	643	158	141	3	10	6	174
Oregon	813	546	441	42	63	7	8	11	241
Pennsylvania	7,957	6,021	4,068	1,160	793	66	53	111	1,706
Rhode Island	862	630	452	87	91	5	2	7	218
South Carolina	1,202	941	718	102	121	9	8	13	231
South Dakota	215	181	137	11	33	1		1	32
Tennessee	2,281	1,832	1,354	289	189	11	15	29	394
Texas	10,532	8,311	6,566	888	857	52	93	100	1,976
Utah	441	331	237	48	46	2	5	12	91
Vermont	188	116	65	35	16	3	1	5	63
Virginia	3,739	2,733	2,083	262	388	33	24	25	924
Washington	1,832	1,309	1,062	90	157	13	11	31	468
West Virginia	1,329	1,031	734	144	153	6	7	3	282
Wisconsin	2,223	1,755	1,325	242	188	8	20	16	424
Wyoming	96	80	63	8	9	1		1	14
Possessions	4,704	3,418	2,861	129	428	58	26	18	1,184
APO's and FPO's	70	48	23		25				22
Address Unknown	62								

** Includes Other, Inactive and Not Classified Physicians*

Table 2.12

Female IMGs by State of Location and Major Professional Activity, 2010

		Patient Care				Other Professional Activity			
				Hospital Based					
State	Total Physicians	Total Patient Care	Office Based	Resid./ Fellows	Phys. Staff	Admin.	Med. Teach.	Research	Other*
Total Physicians	81,389	62,180	42,592	12,131	7,457	487	475	560	17,663
Alabama	502	407	256	96	55	1		2	92
Alaska	45	36	26	1	9			1	8
Arizona	1,122	880	672	131	77	6	9	4	223
Arkansas	309	251	132	77	42		1		57
California	9,521	7,334	5,929	635	770	62	43	80	2,002
Colorado	413	320	261	30	29		2	3	88
Connecticut	1,520	1,189	739	319	131	13	6	6	306
Delaware	248	196	141	35	20	4		1	47
District Of Columbia	474	326	146	130	50	7	5	4	132
Florida	5,472	4,166	3,240	481	445	31	34	28	1,213
Georgia	1,590	1,276	907	235	134	10	6	8	290
Hawaii	236	157	122	16	19	1	4	2	72
Idaho	37	30	23	2	5				7
Illinois	4,877	3,714	2,601	739	374	20	28	29	1,086
Indiana	989	816	599	117	100	3	2	4	164
Iowa	369	287	175	79	33	2	4	6	70
Kansas	442	340	204	90	46	4	3	3	92
Kentucky	675	523	348	111	64	3	4	4	141
Louisiana	807	637	331	228	78	3	12	4	151
Maine	186	158	98	31	29				28
Maryland	2,520	1,834	1,298	285	251	27	17	43	599
Massachusetts	2,888	2,140	1,365	461	314	16	10	30	692
Michigan	3,312	2,634	1,650	721	263	19	14	13	632
Minnesota	937	766	515	194	57	1	3	10	157
Mississippi	231	180	109	39	32	2	1	1	47
Missouri	1,162	892	538	244	110	5	9	7	249
Montana	27	23	18	2	3				4
Nebraska	220	180	97	72	11	1	1		38
Nevada	552	394	320	39	35	3	3	1	151
New Hampshire	235	183	130	24	29			3	49
New Jersey	5,063	3,905	2,760	598	547	36	26	42	1,054
New Mexico	303	237	161	48	28	1	1	2	62
New York	11,924	8,812	5,086	2,436	1,290	79	85	90	2,858
North Carolina	1,176	909	648	135	126	7	9	6	245
North Dakota	130	113	58	34	21				17
Ohio	3,105	2,304	1,387	638	279	11	19	30	741
Oklahoma	437	371	241	94	36	2	3		61
Oregon	401	303	243	27	33	2		3	93
Pennsylvania	3,803	2,856	1,679	841	336	23	23	28	873
Rhode Island	351	251	157	63	31	1	2	3	94
South Carolina	487	409	278	72	59	2	4	6	66
South Dakota	74	60	45	7	8	1			13
Tennessee	930	744	490	174	80		3	8	175
Texas	4,634	3,612	2,658	585	369	16	47	28	931
Utah	156	130	91	26	13	1	1		24
Vermont	72	54	21	22	11		2		16
Virginia	1,877	1,499	1,089	226	184	11	7	6	354
Washington	1,029	776	621	84	71	5	3	4	241
West Virginia	397	304	184	78	42	2	2		89
Wisconsin	996	826	588	162	76		6	4	160
Wyoming	48	43	28	11	4				5
Possessions	2,033	1,378	1,083	106	189	43	11	3	598
APO's and FPO's	21	15	6		9				6
Address Unknown	24								

** Includes Other, Inactive and Not Classified Physicians*

Chapter 3

Analysis of Professional Activity by Self-Designated Specialty and Geographic Region

This chapter includes detailed tables of physicians by specialty and major professional activity for census regions and divisions, metropolitan areas, states, and counties. These data are useful for determining health program options and strategies to complement policy-related research. It is recognized, however, that important influences not reflected in these data have an impact on the distribution patterns of physicians. These determinants of physician location include community of origin, medical education experience, hospital facilities, population size (as well as composition and change), urbanization, licensure requirements, and cultural, social, and environmental conditions.

Total US Physicians

Table 3.1

The geographic distribution for the 985,375 physicians in the US and Possessions is presented in Tables 3.1 through 3.12. Although no interpretation is presented or intended for the complex issue of physician diffusion, the data are useful to study the composition of the physician supply by specialty and major professional activity at the national, state, county, and metropolitan levels. In Table 3.1, total physician count includes the categories of Not Classified (64,153), Inactive (125,928), and Address Unknown (432).

In 2010, four fifths (76.4%) of the 985,375 physicians were in Patient Care (Table 3.1). Of the 752,572 physicians in Patient Care, 75.1% were in Office-Based practice, 14.4% were in residency/fellowship training, and 10.6% comprised full-time Hospital Staff. Of a total of 108,142 Residents/Fellows, more than half (52.9%) were specialists in the disciplines of Internal Medicine, Pediatrics, Family Medicine, General Surgery, and Anesthesiology. Percentages of total physicians in residency/fellowship training in these specialties are as follows: Internal Medicine, 22.4%; Pediatrics, 10.6%; Family Medicine, 7.5%; General Surgery, 7.4%; and Anesthesiology, 5.0%.

The five highest specialties ranked by size for total physicians included Internal Medicine, Family Medicine, Pediatrics, Obstetrics/Gynecology, and Anesthesiology. Table E illustrates the percentage distribution of physicians in these specialties by Patient Care, Office-Based practice, residency/fellowship training, full-time Hospital Staff, and other activities as of 2010.

International Medical Graduates (IMGs)

Tables 3.2 through 3.4

Nearly all (96.5%) IMGs who were not categorized as Inactive, Not Classified, or Address Unknown in 2010 were in Patient Care (Table 3.2). Internal Medicine comprised three fifths (62.1%) of all IMGs in the medical specialties, whereas 32.6% of all physicians in surgical specialties were in Obstetrics/Gynecology.

Of the 198,954 IMGs who were not categorized as Inactive, Not Classified, or Address Unknown, 60.4% were located in the South and Northeast census regions (Table 3.3). These regions consisted of nearly two thirds of all IMGs in Administration (62.3%) and in Research (64.7%). More than

Table E

Percent Distribution of Five Highest Ranking Self-Designated Specialties by Selected Major Professional Activity, 2010

Specialty	*Total*	*Patient Care**	*Office-Based*	*Residents/ Fellows*	*Hosp. Staff*	*Other Prof. Activity***
Internal Medicine	100.0	93.5	68.6	15.0	9.9	6.5
Family Medicine	100.0	96.2	79.8	9.3	7.2	3.8
Pediatrics	100.0	94.5	69.4	15.0	10.1	5.5
Obstetrics/Gynecology	100.0	96.9	79.6	10.6	6.8	3.1
Psychiatry	100.0	92.5	64.6	11.3	16.6	7.5

Source: Table 3.1
** Includes Office-Based practice, Residents/Fellows, and Hospital Staff*
*** Includes Medical Teaching, Administration, Research, and Other*

half (58.8%) of all IMGs in Medical Teaching were concentrated in the Middle Atlantic (406), South Atlantic (296), and East North Central (270) census divisions (Table 3.4). IMGs in Administration also represented the highest frequencies in these census divisions, or 62.9% of all IMGs in Administration.

US Physicians by Geographic Region

Tables 3.5 through 3.9

Regarding physicians in census regions, the South (33.1%) and the Northeast (23.3%) accounted for the largest percentages (Table 3.5). The North Central region had proportionately more physicians in Patient Care (78.2%) than any other region, whereas the Northeast had the greatest proportion of physicians in residency/fellowship training (14.0%).

Table 3.6 presents physician data by census division (see Appendix D). The South Atlantic census division had the highest number of physicians in 2010 with 188,765. The Middle Atlantic census division ranked second with 162,257, followed by the Pacific census division with 159,601 and the East North Central division with 140,098 physicians.

Population and physician/population ratios for the divisions are provided in Table F. These ratios are presented as general guidelines to compare the distribution of physicians among the divisions and not as definitive measures of physician supply. It is recognized that the quality and quantity of health care are predicated on a variety of factors such as medical need for services, demographic composition, geographical location, and socioeconomic variables, among others.

As Table F indicates, the New England and Middle Atlantic divisions had the largest numbers of physicians per 100,000 civilian population, with 463 and 396, respectively. The fewest numbers of physicians per 100,000 civilian population were located in the Mountain (260) and West South Central (244) divisions. The ratios for the divisions are illustrated in Figure 3.1.

Table 3.7 represents the distribution of physicians by state, specialty, and major professional activity. One third of all physicians (32.8%) were concentrated in California (12.0%), New York (8.8%), Texas (6.2%), and Florida (5.9%).

Table 3.9 reports the specialty and activity distributions of physicians by state and county. The top 10 counties with the largest numbers of physicians are Los Angeles, CA (32,420), Cook, IL (23,404), New York, NY (21,452), Harris, TX (13,347), San Diego, CA (11,602), Orange, CA (10,889), Maricopa, AZ (10,771), King, WA (10,518), Suffolk, MA (10,357), and Miami-Dade, FL (10,136). Taken together, these 10 counties make up 15.7% of the physicians in the US.

Table F

Physicians, Population, and Physician/Population Ratios by Census Division, 2010

Census Division	*Total Physicians*	*Population (000)***	*Physician Population/Ration*
Total*	**971,307**	**309,051**	**314**
New England	66,967	14,474	463
Middle Atlantic	162,257	40,943	396
East North Central	140,098	46,522	301
West North Central	58,260	20,451	285
South Atlantic	188,765	59,659	316
East South Central	48,214	18,368	262
West South Central	87,030	35,851	243
Mountain	58,177	22,379	260
Pacific	159,601	49,877	320

** Includes the 50 states and DC but excludes Possessions.*

*** Population estimates as of July 1, 2010.*

Source: Tables 3.6 and 3.8, US Census Bureau, Population Division, Table 1: Annual Estimates of the Population for the United States, Regions, and States and for Puerto Rico: April 1, 2000 to July 1, 2010

Figure 3.1

Physicians per 100,000 Civilian Population by Census Division, 2010*

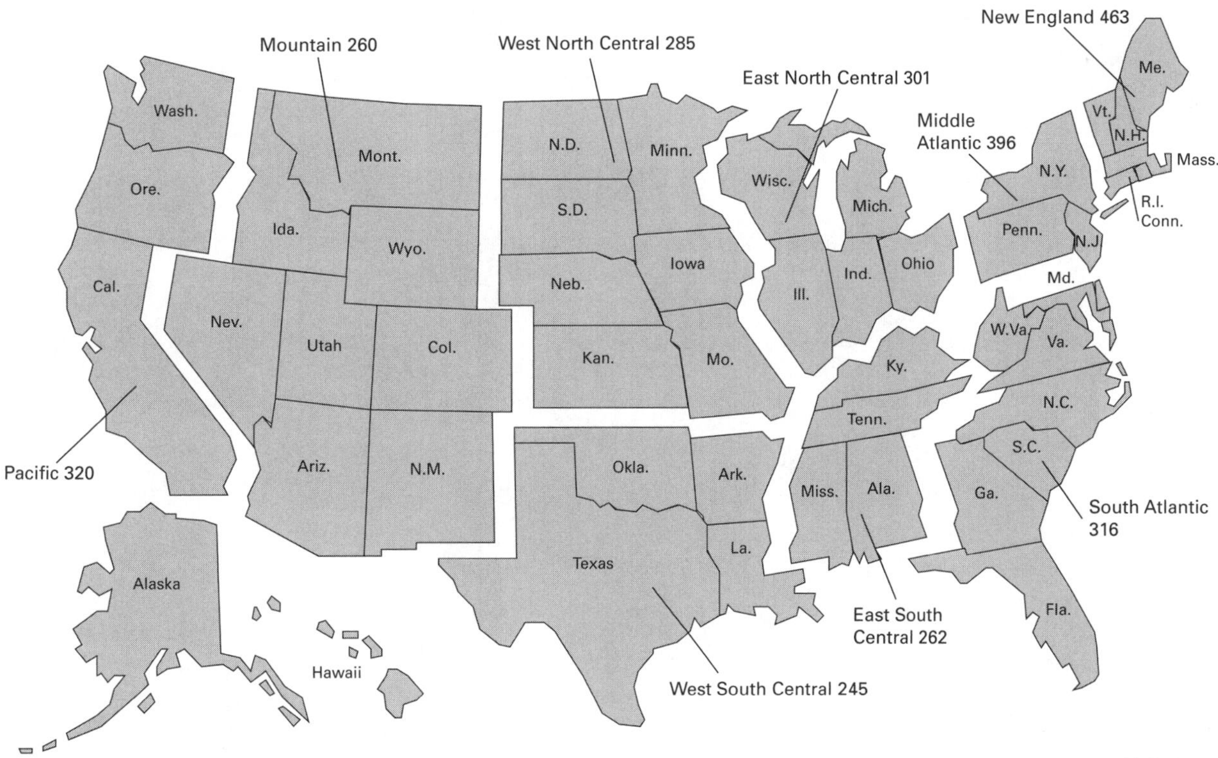

Source: Table F

**Physicians as of December 31, 2010, and population as of July 1, 2010, for 50 states and DC (excludes possessions)*

Metropolitan Data

Tables 3.10 through 3.12

In 2010, the 374 Metropolitan Statistical Areas listed in Table 3.10 contained 92.3% of the total physician population of 985,375. In those Metropolitan Statistical Areas, Office-Based medical specialties represented 28.7% of physicians in Patient Care, whereas Other Specialties were 20.2%, Surgical Specialties were 16.4%, and Family/General Practice were 9.1%.

Physicians in Metropolitan Statistical Areas comprised 95.0% of all physicians in Hospital-Based practice. This significant distribution reflects the clustering of interns, residents, fellows, and full-time staff in large metropolitan and university-affiliated teaching hospitals.

The 581 Micropolitan Statistical Areas listed in Table 3.11 contained only 5.5 % of the total physician population of 985,375, while the Non-Metropolitan physician population listed in Table 3.12 contained a mere 2.1% of MDs in the US.

The three states with the highest proportion of their population among Non-Metropolitan physicians were Maine (19.5%), Wyoming (17.6%), and Montana (16.5%). Five states — Connecticut, Delaware, Hawaii, New Jersey, and Rhode Island — and the District of Columbia had no physicians outside of a Metropolitan or Micropolitan Statistical Area.

Table 3.1

Total Physicians in the United States and Possessions by Self-Designated Specialty and Activity, 2010

		Patient Care				Other Professional Activity			
				Hospital Based					
Specialty	Total Physicians	Total Patient Care	Office Based	Resid./ Fellows	Phys. Staff	Admin.	Med. Teach.	Research	Other
Total Physicians	985,375	752,572	565,024	108,142	79,406	14,009	9,909	13,755	4,617
FM/GP	96,209	92,560	77,098	8,141	7,321	1,581	1,483	257	328
Family Medicine	87,618	84,317	69,896	8,141	6,280	1,389	1,453	214	245
General Practice	8,591	8,243	7,202		1,041	192	30	43	83
Medical Specialties	302,630	284,416	213,338	42,827	28,251	5,027	4,060	7,948	1,179
Allergy and Immunology	4,312	3,896	3,391	299	206	44	40	311	21
Cardiovascular Disease	22,888	21,640	17,454	2,502	1,684	236	301	639	72
Dermatology	11,316	11,069	9,272	1,285	512	45	78	102	22
Gastroenterology	13,210	12,603	10,466	1,338	799	110	157	311	29
Internal Medicine	161,276	150,721	110,612	24,178	15,931	3,113	2,107	4,650	685
Pediatric Cardiology	2,101	1,976	1,243	398	335	23	29	68	5
Pediatrics	76,401	72,223	53,054	11,444	7,725	1,267	1,146	1,451	314
Pulmonary Disease	11,126	10,288	7,846	1,383	1,059	189	202	416	31
Surgical Specialties	163,917	159,904	125,082	23,037	11,785	1,301	1,421	865	426
Colon and Rectal Surgery	1,491	1,462	1,275	78	109	6	14	5	4
General Surgery	37,100	36,001	24,327	8,019	3,655	407	363	220	109
Neurological Surgery	5,781	5,651	3,998	1,152	501	37	41	35	17
Obstetrics & Gynecology	42,797	41,491	34,083	4,516	2,892	444	518	250	94
Ophthalmology	18,457	18,078	15,723	1,493	862	83	123	140	33
Orthopedic Surgery	25,241	24,821	19,325	3,978	1,518	106	139	75	100
Otolaryngology	10,326	10,159	7,964	1,533	662	54	75	24	14
Plastic Surgery	7,418	7,313	6,180	798	335	27	40	19	19
Thoracic Surgery	4,605	4,441	3,601	274	566	61	40	55	8
Urology	10,701	10,487	8,606	1,196	685	76	68	42	28
Other Specialties	232,106	215,692	149,506	34,137	32,049	6,100	2,945	4,685	2,684
Aerospace Medicine	413	243	121		122	116	8	24	22
Anatomic/Clinical Pathology	19,027	16,415	10,688	2,804	2,923	659	382	715	856
Anesthesiology	43,359	42,329	31,819	5,397	5,113	271	472	208	79
Child & Adolescent Psychiatry	7,438	6,962	5,367	720	875	192	135	118	31
Diagnostic Radiology	26,054	25,305	17,503	4,840	2,962	137	232	113	267
Emergency Medicine	33,278	32,101	20,654	4,693	6,754	703	304	97	73
Forensic Pathology	670	473	373	39	61	33	8	7	149
General Preventive Medicine	2,227	1,754	1,224	245	285	214	40	151	68
Medical Genetics	597	450	260	84	106	17	25	95	10
Neurology	15,850	14,589	10,547	2,520	1,522	182	243	753	83
Nuclear Medicine	1,456	1,301	863	153	285	40	31	57	27
Occupational Medicine	2,426	1,755	1,438	1	316	455	35	78	103
Other Specialty	5,482	3,362	2,150	749	463	865	133	881	241
Physical Medicine and Rehabilitation	9,045	8,746	6,454	1,254	1,038	156	43	49	51
Psychiatry	39,738	36,770	25,690	4,487	6,593	1,297	562	833	276
Public Health and General Preventive Medicine	1,283	252	182	2	68	584	62	273	112
Radiation Oncology	4,698	4,600	3,379	610	611	35	22	33	8
Radiology	9,386	8,925	7,032	618	1,275	72	163	80	146
Transplant Surgery	191	175	133	1	41	3	5	7	1
Unspecified	9,458	9,156	3,606	4,920	630	69	40	112	81
Vascular Medicine	30	29	23		6			1	
Inactive	125,928								
Not Classified	64,153								
Address Unknown	432								

Subspecialties in this table are condensed into major specialties. See Appendix A.

Table 3.2

International Medical Graduates in the United States and Possessions by Self-Designated Specialty and Activity, 2010

		Patient Care				Other Professional Activity			
				Hospital Based					
Specialty	Total Physicians	Total Patient Care	Office Based	Resid./ Fellows	Phys. Staff	Admin.	Med. Teach.	Research	Other
Total Physicians	198,954	192,046	140,246	28,434	23,366	1,812	1,654	2,462	980
FM/GP	24,413	23,992	18,522	3,562	1,908	199	120	36	66
Family Medicine	20,105	19,806	14,988	3,562	1,256	126	111	27	35
General Practice	4,308	4,186	3,534		652	73	9	9	31
Medical Specialties	98,179	95,384	70,138	15,304	9,942	614	694	1,285	202
Allergy and Immunology	1,000	932	840	49	43	5	10	49	4
Cardiovascular Disease	7,089	6,869	5,407	943	519	21	61	125	13
Dermatology	605	581	490	46	45	3	8	12	1
Gastroenterology	3,675	3,551	2,854	437	260	21	34	65	4
Internal Medicine	60,935	59,386	42,611	10,423	6,352	368	349	710	122
Pediatric Cardiology	507	488	324	97	67	4	6	9	
Pediatrics	20,442	19,770	14,795	2,642	2,333	175	196	244	57
Pulmonary Disease	3,926	3,807	2,817	667	323	17	30	71	1
Surgical Specialties	21,426	20,848	16,284	2,522	2,042	147	189	177	65
Colon and Rectal Surgery	281	276	240	13	23		3	2	
General Surgery	6,580	6,400	4,403	1,180	817	52	62	42	24
Neurological Surgery	749	726	510	124	92	5	8	8	2
Obstetrics & Gynecology	6,981	6,803	5,522	752	529	59	56	49	14
Ophthalmology	1,343	1,306	1,132	88	86	4	10	20	3
Orthopedic Surgery	1,512	1,473	1,207	141	125	8	12	13	6
Otolaryngology	811	784	679	41	64	7	7	10	3
Plastic Surgery	804	786	681	60	45	2	2	8	6
Thoracic Surgery	953	921	730	71	120	2	9	20	1
Urology	1,412	1,373	1,180	52	141	8	20	5	6
Other Specialties	54,936	51,822	35,302	7,046	9,474	852	651	964	647
Aerospace Medicine	32	18	8		10	4	2	4	4
Anatomic/Clinical Pathology	6,157	5,403	3,349	883	1,171	146	128	204	276
Anesthesiology	11,423	11,142	8,581	742	1,819	45	145	66	25
Child & Adolescent Psychiatry	2,231	2,141	1,558	252	331	31	22	26	11
Diagnostic Radiology	2,871	2,742	1,845	391	506	14	41	25	49
Emergency Medicine	2,843	2,768	1,637	406	725	45	19	5	6
Forensic Pathology	144	93	74	7	12	6	3	2	40
General Preventive Medicine	320	282	206	49	27	13	4	14	7
Medical Genetics	154	131	71	32	28	2	4	16	1
Neurology	5,201	4,988	3,568	928	492	24	53	116	20
Nuclear Medicine	559	520	305	93	122	5	10	14	10
Occupational Medicine	349	295	248		47	35	4	4	11
Other Specialty	1,052	744	435	196	113	66	25	183	34
Physical Medicine and Rehabilitation	2,629	2,549	1,832	319	398	36	18	11	15
Psychiatry	12,591	12,024	7,703	1,484	2,837	265	94	166	42
Public Health and General Preventive Medicine	142	43	29	1	13	62	7	17	13
Radiation Oncology	727	707	549	19	139	6	5	9	
Radiology	1,679	1,549	1,045	164	340	14	40	34	42
Transplant Surgery	56	51	34	1	16		2	2	1
Unspecified	3,771	3,627	2,221	1,079	327	33	25	46	40
Vascular Medicine	5	5	4		1				

Note: Above excludes Inactive, Not Classified and Address Unknown Physicians.

Subspecialties in this table are condensed into major specialties. See Appendix A.

Table 3.3

International Medical Graduates by Census Region, Self-Designated Specialty, and Activity, 2010
Northeast

		Patient Care				Other Professional Activity			
				Hospital Based					
Specialty	Total Physicians	Total Patient Care	Office Based	Resid./ Fellows	Phys. Staff	Admin.	Med. Teach.	Research	Other
Total Physicians	58,212	55,882	37,111	10,944	7,827	640	485	901	304
FM/GP	4,126	4,038	2,922	777	339	44	21	11	12
Family Medicine	3,635	3,567	2,537	777	253	34	21	6	7
General Practice	491	471	385		86	10		5	5
Medical Specialties	29,805	28,833	19,051	6,543	3,239	228	215	451	78
Allergy and Immunology	274	248	220	14	14	3	2	20	1
Cardiovascular Disease	1,883	1,811	1,306	355	150	11	15	39	7
Dermatology	172	163	141	12	10	1	1	7	
Gastroenterology	1,011	966	721	174	71	9	10	23	3
Internal Medicine	19,023	18,465	11,740	4,707	2,018	144	106	254	54
Pediatric Cardiology	130	127	78	24	25		1	2	
Pediatrics	6,203	5,992	4,134	998	860	51	66	81	13
Pulmonary Disease	1,109	1,061	711	259	91	9	14	25	
Surgical Specialties	6,771	6,568	4,749	1,099	720	50	56	78	19
Colon and Rectal Surgery	74	72	68	4				2	
General Surgery	2,206	2,140	1,297	529	314	24	18	20	4
Neurological Surgery	182	174	119	30	25		2	6	
Obstetrics & Gynecology	2,348	2,288	1,688	398	202	15	18	19	8
Ophthalmology	386	372	325	23	24	2	2	8	2
Orthopedic Surgery	418	405	324	50	31	2	5	6	
Otolaryngology	246	232	204	7	21	3	5	5	1
Plastic Surgery	229	225	192	19	14			2	2
Thoracic Surgery	265	253	182	26	45	1	2	9	
Urology	417	407	350	13	44	3	4	1	2
Other Specialties	17,510	16,443	10,389	2,525	3,529	318	193	361	195
Aerospace Medicine	2	1	1						1
Anatomic/Clinical Pathology	2,042	1,801	1,000	323	478	50	42	65	84
Anesthesiology	3,792	3,700	2,770	315	615	24	36	23	9
Child & Adolescent Psychiatry	800	765	511	110	144	12	6	12	5
Diagnostic Radiology	916	879	565	163	151	6	8	10	13
Emergency Medicine	903	871	415	162	294	18	8	2	4
Forensic Pathology	42	24	21	1	2	3		2	13
General Preventive Medicine	76	71	47	13	11	1	1	1	2
Medical Genetics	33	25	14	5	6	1		7	
Neurology	1,524	1,448	956	313	179	8	16	43	9
Nuclear Medicine	177	163	85	34	44	2	3	5	4
Occupational Medicine	73	56	46		10	12	2	1	2
Other Specialty	305	196	110	51	35	18	7	77	7
Physical Medicine and Rehabilitation	985	943	664	127	152	21	9	2	10
Psychiatry	4,364	4,130	2,367	612	1,151	114	36	70	14
Public Health and General Preventive Medicine	32	8	6		2	15	3	3	3
Radiation Oncology	222	212	157	4	51	2	2	6	
Radiology	528	495	312	56	127	3	7	12	11
Transplant Surgery	19	19	13	1	5				
Unspecified	675	636	329	235	72	8	7	20	4

Note: Above excludes Inactive, Not Classified and Address Unknown Physicians.

Subspecialties in this table are condensed into major specialties. See Appendix A.

Table 3.3

International Medical Graduates by Census Region, Self-Designated Specialty, and Activity, 2010, continued
North Central

		Patient Care				Other Professional Activity			
				Hospital Based					
Specialty	Total Physicians	Total Patient Care	Office Based	Resid./ Fellows	Phys. Staff	Admin.	Med. Teach.	Research	Other
Total Physicians	41,290	40,042	27,950	7,544	4,548	288	346	420	194
FM/GP	5,468	5,393	3,836	1,160	397	32	25	5	13
Family Medicine	4,854	4,803	3,341	1,160	302	17	23	3	8
General Practice	614	590	495		95	15	2	2	5
Medical Specialties	20,250	19,773	13,936	3,850	1,987	82	146	224	25
Allergy and Immunology	223	217	189	15	13	2	1	3	
Cardiovascular Disease	1,574	1,537	1,220	205	112	1	7	28	1
Dermatology	124	122	92	19	11		2		
Gastroenterology	721	700	542	105	53	1	8	12	
Internal Medicine	13,000	12,725	8,806	2,628	1,291	56	78	127	14
Pediatric Cardiology	122	117	67	38	12	2	3		
Pediatrics	3,672	3,562	2,445	683	434	16	40	44	10
Pulmonary Disease	814	793	575	157	61	4	7	10	
Surgical Specialties	4,203	4,104	3,113	585	406	21	36	32	10
Colon and Rectal Surgery	75	74	61	4	9		1		
General Surgery	1,317	1,287	864	269	154	3	14	8	5
Neurological Surgery	199	194	139	33	22	2	1	1	1
Obstetrics & Gynecology	1,256	1,228	969	156	103	10	8	8	2
Ophthalmology	251	242	191	29	22	2	3	3	1
Orthopedic Surgery	275	270	214	30	26	1	1	3	
Otolaryngology	153	151	132	9	10			2	
Plastic Surgery	151	144	116	21	7		2	4	1
Thoracic Surgery	228	221	177	18	26	1	3	3	
Urology	298	293	250	16	27	2	3		
Other Specialties	11,369	10,772	7,065	1,949	1,758	153	139	159	146
Aerospace Medicine	3	2	1		1	1			
Anatomic/Clinical Pathology	1,438	1,263	795	232	236	30	35	39	71
Anesthesiology	2,351	2,298	1,694	244	360	5	33	10	5
Child & Adolescent Psychiatry	419	401	276	59	66	6	5	4	3
Diagnostic Radiology	672	647	421	125	101	1	8	3	13
Emergency Medicine	550	534	285	133	116	11	3	1	1
Forensic Pathology	29	20	15	1	4	1	2		6
General Preventive Medicine	50	46	36	8	2		1	3	
Medical Genetics	24	20	11	5	4		1	3	
Neurology	1,212	1,165	780	262	123	9	12	21	5
Nuclear Medicine	119	106	66	13	27		5	4	4
Occupational Medicine	78	69	61		8	5		2	2
Other Specialty	236	177	84	71	22	11	7	34	7
Physical Medicine and Rehabilitation	508	498	339	77	82	3	1	4	2
Psychiatry	2,308	2,219	1,470	314	435	51	13	19	6
Public Health and General Preventive Medicine	11	2	2			7			2
Radiation Oncology	195	191	154	3	34	3	1		
Radiology	392	362	249	41	72	5	10	4	11
Transplant Surgery	12	10	5		5		1	1	
Unspecified	759	739	318	361	60	4	1	7	8
Vascular Medicine	3	3	3						

Note: Above excludes Inactive, Not Classified and Address Unknown Physicians.

Subspecialties in this table are condensed into major specialties. See Appendix A.

Table 3.3

International Medical Graduates by Census Region, Self-Designated Specialty, and Activity, 2010, continued
South

		Patient Care				Other Professional Activity			
				Hospital Based					
Specialty	Total Physicians	Total Patient Care	Office Based	Resid./ Fellows	Phys. Staff	Admin.	Med. Teach.	Research	Other
Total Physicians	61,686	59,672	45,113	7,503	7,056	488	536	693	297
FM/GP	8,313	8,188	6,336	1,189	663	56	40	10	19
Family Medicine	7,111	7,012	5,359	1,189	464	42	37	10	10
General Practice	1,202	1,176	977		199	14	3		9
Medical Specialties	31,070	30,236	23,351	3,716	3,169	182	223	368	61
Allergy and Immunology	315	293	272	13	8		6	15	1
Cardiovascular Disease	2,549	2,480	1,993	320	167	7	26	33	3
Dermatology	176	171	149	8	14	1	2	1	1
Gastroenterology	1,273	1,243	1,034	122	87	3	11	16	
Internal Medicine	18,600	18,145	13,788	2,278	2,079	111	109	203	32
Pediatric Cardiology	177	171	125	27	19	2	1	3	
Pediatrics	6,631	6,416	4,975	764	677	56	62	74	23
Pulmonary Disease	1,349	1,317	1,015	184	118	2	6	23	1
Surgical Specialties	6,366	6,200	4,996	646	558	39	63	39	25
Colon and Rectal Surgery	91	89	76	4	9		2		
General Surgery	1,961	1,905	1,394	280	231	15	21	8	12
Neurological Surgery	241	233	156	47	30	3	4	1	
Obstetrics & Gynecology	1,870	1,828	1,542	171	115	14	18	9	1
Ophthalmology	435	423	373	30	20		5	7	
Orthopedic Surgery	504	492	403	49	40	3	3	3	3
Otolaryngology	252	245	206	16	23	1	1	3	2
Plastic Surgery	264	260	235	13	12	1		1	2
Thoracic Surgery	283	275	229	16	30		3	4	1
Urology	465	450	382	20	48	2	6	3	4
Other Specialties	15,937	15,048	10,430	1,952	2,666	211	210	276	192
Aerospace Medicine	16	8	4		4	2	1	3	2
Anatomic/Clinical Pathology	1,749	1,528	978	239	311	36	35	71	79
Anesthesiology	3,168	3,088	2,425	143	520	12	44	19	5
Child & Adolescent Psychiatry	627	604	469	56	79	8	7	6	2
Diagnostic Radiology	816	777	536	76	165	2	15	7	15
Emergency Medicine	886	873	592	78	203	6	5	1	1
Forensic Pathology	49	34	26	4	4	1			14
General Preventive Medicine	118	102	72	22	8	7	1	6	2
Medical Genetics	56	49	25	12	12		3	3	1
Neurology	1,703	1,644	1,233	284	127	5	19	30	5
Nuclear Medicine	160	153	91	29	33	2	2	2	1
Occupational Medicine	82	69	59		10	7	1		5
Other Specialty	305	225	128	58	39	22	8	38	12
Physical Medicine and Rehabilitation	726	710	512	94	104	6	4	4	2
Psychiatry	3,667	3,517	2,270	447	800	52	31	52	15
Public Health and General Preventive Medicine	60	17	13	1	3	26	3	11	3
Radiation Oncology	211	208	159	11	38	1	1	1	
Radiology	503	453	301	52	100	2	21	12	15
Transplant Surgery	17	15	9		6			1	1
Unspecified	1,017	973	527	346	100	14	9	9	12
Vascular Medicine	1	1	1						

Note: Above excludes Inactive, Not Classified and Address Unknown Physicians.

Subspecialties in this table are condensed into major specialties. See Appendix A.

Table 3.3

International Medical Graduates by Census Region, Self-Designated Specialty, and Activity, 2010, continued
West

		Patient Care				Other Professional Activity			
				Hospital Based					
Specialty	Total Physicians	Total Patient Care	Office Based	Resid./ Fellows	Phys. Staff	Admin.	Med. Teach.	Research	Other
Total Physicians	32,712	31,591	26,099	2,208	3,284	295	250	427	149
FM/GP	4,900	4,824	4,128	417	279	32	27	7	10
Family Medicine	4,082	4,017	3,397	417	203	23	27	7	8
General Practice	818	807	731		76	9			2
Medical Specialties	15,587	15,131	12,687	1,050	1,394	95	94	233	34
Allergy and Immunology	185	171	156	7	8		1	11	2
Cardiovascular Disease	1,008	972	822	61	89	2	10	23	1
Dermatology	125	117	103	7	7	1	3	4	
Gastroenterology	655	628	545	35	48	8	5	13	1
Internal Medicine	9,515	9,276	7,696	694	886	50	48	121	20
Pediatric Cardiology	74	69	51	8	10		1	4	
Pediatrics	3,406	3,296	2,822	177	297	32	23	45	10
Pulmonary Disease	619	602	492	61	49	2	3	12	
Surgical Specialties	3,592	3,496	3,034	176	286	30	28	28	10
Colon and Rectal Surgery	37	37	33	1	3				
General Surgery	958	935	744	102	89	9	5	6	3
Neurological Surgery	114	112	89	10	13		1		1
Obstetrics & Gynecology	1,270	1,228	1,131	16	81	15	12	13	2
Ophthalmology	251	249	225	6	18			2	
Orthopedic Surgery	291	285	247	11	27	1	1	1	3
Otolaryngology	137	133	117	9	7	3	1		
Plastic Surgery	154	151	133	7	11	1		1	1
Thoracic Surgery	173	168	139	11	18		1	4	
Urology	207	198	176	3	19	1	7	1	
Other Specialties	8,633	8,140	6,250	565	1,325	138	101	159	95
Aerospace Medicine	11	7	2		5	1	1	1	1
Anatomic/Clinical Pathology	878	771	549	82	140	28	14	29	36
Anesthesiology	2,028	1,973	1,632	36	305	4	32	13	6
Child & Adolescent Psychiatry	356	345	283	25	37	5	2	4	
Diagnostic Radiology	444	418	309	25	84	5	10	5	6
Emergency Medicine	405	399	299	18	82	3	2	1	
Forensic Pathology	21	12	9	1	2	1	1		7
General Preventive Medicine	63	52	41	6	5	4	1	4	2
Medical Genetics	40	36	20	10	6	1		3	
Neurology	722	693	570	67	56	2	5	22	
Nuclear Medicine	98	93	61	15	17	1		3	1
Occupational Medicine	85	75	62		13	6	1	1	2
Other Specialty	171	118	89	16	13	11	2	32	8
Physical Medicine and Rehabilitation	378	368	296	17	55	5	3	1	1
Psychiatry	2,045	1,959	1,445	102	412	44	14	22	6
Public Health and General Preventive Medicine	26	10	5		5	9	1	3	3
Radiation Oncology	93	91	76	1	14		1	1	
Radiology	240	223	170	15	38	4	2	6	5
Transplant Surgery	8	7	7				1		
Unspecified	520	489	325	129	35	4	8	8	11
Vascular Medicine	1	1			1				

Note: Above excludes Inactive, Not Classified and Address Unknown Physicians.

Subspecialties in this table are condensed into major specialties. See Appendix A.

Table 3.3

International Medical Graduates by Census Region, Self-Designated Specialty, and Activity, 2010, continued
Possessions

		Patient Care				Other Professional Activity			
				Hospital Based					
Specialty	Total Physicians	Total Patient Care	Office Based	Resid./ Fellows	Phys. Staff	Admin.	Med. Teach.	Research	Other
Total Physicians	5,054	4,859	3,973	235	651	101	37	21	36
FM/GP	1,606	1,549	1,300	19	230	35	7	3	12
Family Medicine	423	407	354	19	34	10	3	1	2
General Practice	1,183	1,142	946		196	25	4	2	10
Medical Specialties	1,467	1,411	1,113	145	153	27	16	9	4
Allergy and Immunology	3	3	3						
Cardiovascular Disease	75	69	66	2	1		3	2	1
Dermatology	8	8	5		3				
Gastroenterology	15	14	12	1	1			1	
Internal Medicine	797	775	581	116	78	7	8	5	2
Pediatric Cardiology	4	4	3		1				
Pediatrics	530	504	419	20	65	20	5		1
Pulmonary Disease	35	34	24	6	4			1	
Surgical Specialties	494	480	392	16	72	7	6		1
Colon and Rectal Surgery	4	4	2		2				
General Surgery	138	133	104		29	1	4		
Neurological Surgery	13	13	7	4	2				
Obstetrics & Gynecology	237	231	192	11	28	5			1
Ophthalmology	20	20	18		2				
Orthopedic Surgery	24	21	19	1	1	1	2		
Otolaryngology	23	23	20		3				
Plastic Surgery	6	6	5		1				
Thoracic Surgery	4	4	3		1				
Urology	25	25	22		3				
Other Specialties	1,487	1,419	1,168	55	196	32	8	9	19
Anatomic/Clinical Pathology	50	40	27	7	6	2	2		6
Anesthesiology	84	83	60	4	19			1	
Child & Adolescent Psychiatry	29	26	19	2	5		2		1
Diagnostic Radiology	23	21	14	2	5				2
Emergency Medicine	99	91	46	15	30	7	1		
Forensic Pathology	3	3	3						
General Preventive Medicine	13	11	10		1	1			1
Medical Genetics	1	1	1						
Neurology	40	38	29	2	7		1		1
Nuclear Medicine	5	5	2	2	1				
Occupational Medicine	31	26	20		6	5			
Other Specialty	35	28	24		4	4	1	2	
Physical Medicine and Rehabilitation	32	30	21	4	5	1	1		
Psychiatry	207	199	151	9	39	4		3	1
Public Health and General Preventive Medicine	13	6	3		3	5			2
Radiation Oncology	6	5	3		2			1	
Radiology	16	16	13		3				
Unspecified	800	790	722	8	60	3		2	5

Note: Above excludes Inactive, Not Classified and Address Unknown Physicians.

Subspecialties in this table are condensed into major specialties. See Appendix A.

Table 3.4

International Medical Graduates by Census Division, Self-Designated Specialty, and Activity, 2010
New England

		Patient Care				Other Professional Activity			
				Hospital Based					
Specialty	Total Physicians	Total Patient Care	Office Based	Resid./ Fellows	Phys. Staff	Admin.	Med. Teach.	Research	Other
Total Physicians	1,481	11,002	7,320	2,091	1,591	103	79	239	58
FM/GP	714	699	543	98	58	9	1	1	4
Family Medicine	626	613	468	98	47	8	1	1	3
General Practice	88	86	75		11	1			1
Medical Specialties	5,800	5,597	3,712	1,216	669	34	30	127	12
Allergy and Immunology	53	44	38	3	3		1	7	1
Cardiovascular Disease	385	370	240	91	39	2	3	9	1
Dermatology	46	41	32	5	4	1		4	
Gastroenterology	210	202	146	34	22			8	
Internal Medicine	4,009	3,894	2,512	918	464	20	15	70	10
Pediatric Cardiology	30	29	15	12	2		1		
Pediatrics	820	787	570	99	118	8	5	20	
Pulmonary Disease	247	230	159	54	17	3	5	9	
Surgical Specialties	1,192	1,153	834	183	136	7	8	19	5
Colon and Rectal Surgery	12	11	9	2				1	
General Surgery	379	366	204	106	56	3	4	5	1
Neurological Surgery	55	52	35	9	8		1	2	
Obstetrics & Gynecology	349	344	275	39	30		1	2	2
Ophthalmology	64	61	53	4	4	1		1	1
Orthopedic Surgery	78	74	59	7	8		1	3	
Otolaryngology	54	50	43	1	6	2		2	
Plastic Surgery	47	46	39	4	3				1
Thoracic Surgery	73	70	51	8	11			3	
Urology	81	79	66	3	10	1	1		
Other Specialties	3,775	3,553	2,231	594	728	53	40	92	37
Aerospace Medicine	1	1	1						
Anatomic/Clinical Pathology	511	454	270	87	97	7	10	20	20
Anesthesiology	835	812	565	104	143	3	12	5	3
Child & Adolescent Psychiatry	163	159	110	28	21	2	1	1	
Diagnostic Radiology	245	241	139	66	36			1	3
Emergency Medicine	172	166	87	20	59	5	1		
Forensic Pathology	4	2	2						2
General Preventive Medicine	35	34	24	6	4				1
Medical Genetics	14	9	5	3	1	1		4	
Neurology	363	346	210	78	58	1	2	13	1
Nuclear Medicine	31	28	15	7	6		1	2	
Occupational Medicine	18	13	11		2	4	1		
Other Specialty	65	40	22	12	6	5	3	17	
Physical Medicine and Rehabilitation	131	124	87	14	23	4	1		2
Psychiatry	787	744	447	92	205	17	5	17	4
Public Health and General Preventive Medicine	7	1	1			4	1	1	
Radiation Oncology	36	35	25		10			1	
Radiology	145	138	82	25	31		1	5	1
Transplant Surgery	4	4	4						
Unspecified	208	202	124	52	26		1	5	

Note: Above excludes Inactive, Not Classified and Address Unknown Physicians.

Subspecialties in this table are condensed into major specialties. See Appendix A.

Table 3.4

International Medical Graduates by Census Division, Self-Designated Specialty, and Activity, 2010, continued
Middle Atlantic

		Patient Care				Other Professional Activity			
				Hospital Based					
Specialty	Total Physicians	Total Patient Care	Office Based	Resid./ Fellows	Phys. Staff	Admin.	Med. Teach.	Research	Other
Total Physicians	46,731	44,880	29,791	8,853	6,236	537	406	662	246
FM/GP	3,412	3,339	2,379	679	281	35	20	10	8
Family Medicine	3,009	2,954	2,069	679	206	26	20	5	4
General Practice	403	385	310		75	9		5	4
Medical Specialties	24,005	23,236	15,339	5,327	2,570	194	185	324	66
Allergy and Immunology	221	204	182	11	11	3	1	13	
Cardiovascular Disease	1,498	1,441	1,066	264	111	9	12	30	6
Dermatology	126	122	109	7	6		1	3	
Gastroenterology	801	764	575	140	49	9	10	15	3
Internal Medicine	15,014	14,571	9,228	3,789	1,554	124	91	184	44
Pediatric Cardiology	100	98	63	12	23			2	
Pediatrics	5,383	5,205	3,564	899	742	43	61	61	13
Pulmonary Disease	862	831	552	205	74	6	9	16	
Surgical Specialties	5,579	5,415	3,915	916	584	43	48	59	14
Colon and Rectal Surgery	62	61	59	2				1	
General Surgery	1,827	1,774	1,093	423	258	21	14	15	3
Neurological Surgery	127	122	84	21	17		1	4	
Obstetrics & Gynecology	1,999	1,944	1,413	359	172	15	17	17	6
Ophthalmology	322	311	272	19	20	1	2	7	1
Orthopedic Surgery	340	331	265	43	23	2	4	3	
Otolaryngology	192	182	161	6	15	1	5	3	1
Plastic Surgery	182	179	153	15	11			2	1
Thoracic Surgery	192	183	131	18	34	1	2	6	
Urology	336	328	284	10	34	2	3	1	2
Other Specialties	13,735	12,890	8,158	1,931	2,801	265	153	269	158
Aerospace Medicine	1								1
Anatomic/Clinical Pathology	1,531	1,347	730	236	381	43	32	45	64
Anesthesiology	2,957	2,888	2,205	211	472	21	24	18	6
Child & Adolescent Psychiatry	637	606	401	82	123	10	5	11	5
Diagnostic Radiology	671	638	426	97	115	6	8	9	10
Emergency Medicine	731	705	328	142	235	13	7	2	4
Forensic Pathology	38	22	19	1	2	3		2	11
General Preventive Medicine	41	37	23	7	7	1	1	1	1
Medical Genetics	19	16	9	2	5			3	
Neurology	1,161	1,102	746	235	121	7	14	30	8
Nuclear Medicine	146	135	70	27	38	2	2	3	4
Occupational Medicine	55	43	35		8	8	1	1	2
Other Specialty	240	156	88	39	29	13	4	60	7
Physical Medicine and Rehabilitation	854	819	577	113	129	17	8	2	8
Psychiatry	3,577	3,386	1,920	520	946	97	31	53	10
Public Health and General Preventive Medicine	25	7	5		2	11	2	2	3
Radiation Oncology	186	177	132	4	41	2	2	5	
Radiology	383	357	230	31	96	3	6	7	10
Transplant Surgery	15	15	9	1	5				
Unspecified	467	434	205	183	46	8	6	15	4

Note: Above excludes Inactive, Not Classified and Address Unknown Physicians.

Subspecialties in this table are condensed into major specialties. See Appendix A.

Table 3.4

International Medical Graduates by Census Division, Self-Designated Specialty, and Activity, 2010, continued
East North Central

		Patient Care				Other Professional Activity			
				Hospital Based					
Specialty	Total Physicians	Total Patient Care	Office Based	Resid./ Fellows	Phys. Staff	Admin.	Med. Teach.	Research	Other
Total Physicians	32,495	31,520	22,354	5,741	3,425	238	270	302	165
FM/GP	4,343	4,282	3,102	882	298	24	21	4	12
Family Medicine	3,819	3,776	2,671	882	223	14	20	2	7
General Practice	524	506	431		75	10	1	2	5
Medical Specialties	16,102	15,737	11,214	3,028	1,495	70	112	161	22
Allergy and Immunology	172	169	149	9	11	1		2	
Cardiovascular Disease	1,201	1,176	953	144	79	1	3	20	1
Dermatology	103	101	79	14	8		2		
Gastroenterology	525	510	413	63	34	1	6	8	
Internal Medicine	10,333	10,124	7,076	2,088	960	49	60	87	13
Pediatric Cardiology	88	84	46	28	10	2	2		
Pediatrics	3,041	2,951	2,042	557	352	13	32	37	8
Pulmonary Disease	639	622	456	125	41	3	7	7	
Surgical Specialties	3,356	3,277	2,540	436	301	18	29	23	9
Colon and Rectal Surgery	63	62	50	3	9		1		
General Surgery	1,029	1,002	716	178	108	2	13	7	5
Neurological Surgery	153	149	103	27	19	2	1		1
Obstetrics & Gynecology	1,077	1,054	824	144	86	9	7	5	2
Ophthalmology	193	187	148	22	17	1	2	2	1
Orthopedic Surgery	196	192	159	16	17	1		3	
Otolaryngology	125	125	112	7	6				
Plastic Surgery	121	117	100	16	1		1	3	
Thoracic Surgery	176	169	139	11	19	1	3	3	
Urology	223	220	189	12	19	2	1		
Other Specialties	8,694	8,224	5,498	1,395	1,331	126	108	114	122
Aerospace Medicine	2	2	1		1				
Anatomic/Clinical Pathology	1,146	1,001	636	163	202	25	31	33	56
Anesthesiology	1,982	1,939	1,426	210	303	5	25	8	5
Child & Adolescent Psychiatry	289	277	195	41	41	4	4	2	2
Diagnostic Radiology	523	503	334	93	76	1	6	3	10
Emergency Medicine	461	448	239	121	88	10	2		1
Forensic Pathology	24	15	12	1	2	1	2		6
General Preventive Medicine	29	28	24	4				1	
Medical Genetics	16	14	7	4	3			2	
Neurology	860	830	574	174	82	6	8	12	4
Nuclear Medicine	89	78	52	7	19		4	3	4
Occupational Medicine	64	56	49		7	4		2	2
Other Specialty	170	128	56	55	17	9	6	23	4
Physical Medicine and Rehabilitation	382	373	255	57	61	3	1	3	2
Psychiatry	1,628	1,559	1,084	165	310	42	10	11	6
Public Health and General Preventive Medicine	10	2	2			6			2
Radiation Oncology	153	149	123	2	24	3	1		
Radiology	306	283	198	29	56	3	6	4	10
Transplant Surgery	8	6	4		2		1	1	
Unspecified	550	531	225	269	37	4	1	6	8
Vascular Medicine	2	2	2						

Note: Above excludes Inactive, Not Classified and Address Unknown Physicians.

Subspecialties in this table are condensed into major specialties. See Appendix A.

Table 3.4

International Medical Graduates by Census Division, Self-Designated Specialty, and Activity, 2010, continued
West North Central

		Patient Care				Other Professional Activity			
				Hospital Based					
Specialty	Total Physicians	Total Patient Care	Office Based	Resid./ Fellows	Phys. Staff	Admin.	Med. Teach.	Research	Other
Total Physicians	8,795	8,522	5,596	1,803	1,123	50	76	118	29
FM/GP	1,125	1,111	734	278	99	8	4	1	1
Family Medicine	1,035	1,027	670	278	79	3	3	1	1
General Practice	90	84	64		20	5	1		
Medical Specialties	4,148	4,036	2,722	822	492	12	34	63	3
Allergy and Immunology	51	48	40	6	2	1	1	1	
Cardiovascular Disease	373	361	267	61	33		4	8	
Dermatology	21	21	13	5	3				
Gastroenterology	196	190	129	42	19		2	4	
Internal Medicine	2,667	2,601	1,730	540	331	7	18	40	1
Pediatric Cardiology	34	33	21	10	2		1		
Pediatrics	631	611	403	126	82	3	8	7	2
Pulmonary Disease	175	171	119	32	20	1		3	
Surgical Specialties	847	827	573	149	105	3	7	9	1
Colon and Rectal Surgery	12	12	11	1					
General Surgery	288	285	148	91	46	1	1	1	
Neurological Surgery	46	45	36	6	3			1	
Obstetrics & Gynecology	179	174	145	12	17	1	1	3	
Ophthalmology	58	55	43	7	5	1	1	1	
Orthopedic Surgery	79	78	55	14	9		1		
Otolaryngology	28	26	20	2	4			2	
Plastic Surgery	30	27	16	5	6		1	1	1
Thoracic Surgery	52	52	38	7	7				
Urology	75	73	61	4	8		2		
Other Specialties	2,675	2,548	1,567	554	427	27	31	45	24
Aerospace Medicine	1					1			
Anatomic/Clinical Pathology	292	262	159	69	34	5	4	6	15
Anesthesiology	369	359	268	34	57		8	2	
Child & Adolescent Psychiatry	130	124	81	18	25	2	1	2	1
Diagnostic Radiology	149	144	87	32	25		2		3
Emergency Medicine	89	86	46	12	28	1	1	1	
Forensic Pathology	5	5	3		2				
General Preventive Medicine	21	18	12	4	2		1	2	
Medical Genetics	8	6	4	1	1		1	1	
Neurology	352	335	206	88	41	3	4	9	1
Nuclear Medicine	30	28	14	6	8		1	1	
Occupational Medicine	14	13	12		1	1			
Other Specialty	66	49	28	16	5	2	1	11	3
Physical Medicine and Rehabilitation	126	125	84	20	21			1	
Psychiatry	680	660	386	149	125	9	3	8	
Public Health and General Preventive Medicine	1					1			
Radiation Oncology	42	42	31	1	10				
Radiology	86	79	51	12	16	2	4		1
Transplant Surgery	4	4	1		3				
Unspecified	209	208	93	92	23			1	

Note: Above excludes Inactive, Not Classified and Address Unknown Physicians.

Subspecialties in this table are condensed into major specialties. See Appendix A.

Table 3.4

International Medical Graduates by Census Division, Self-Designated Specialty, and Activity, 2010, continued
South Atlantic

		Patient Care				Other Professional Activity			
				Hospital Based					
Specialty	Total Physicians	Total Patient Care	Office Based	Resid./ Fellows	Phys. Staff	Admin.	Med. Teach.	Research	Other
Total Physicians	37,933	36,604	28,322	3,868	4,414	364	296	456	213
FM/GP	4,842	4,761	3,855	512	394	42	19	5	15
Family Medicine	3,940	3,882	3,120	512	250	29	17	5	7
General Practice	902	879	735		144	13	2		8
Medical Specialties	19,021	18,481	14,560	1,946	1,975	137	125	232	46
Allergy and Immunology	185	168	157	6	5		4	12	1
Cardiovascular Disease	1,413	1,374	1,160	126	88	4	15	18	2
Dermatology	124	120	110	4	6		2	1	1
Gastroenterology	769	748	634	62	52	3	8	10	
Internal Medicine	11,638	11,339	8,773	1,255	1,311	84	62	131	22
Pediatric Cardiology	87	83	63	12	8	1	1	2	
Pediatrics	4,017	3,884	3,050	397	437	44	29	41	19
Pulmonary Disease	788	765	613	84	68	1	4	17	1
Surgical Specialties	4,107	4,005	3,270	371	364	26	34	26	16
Colon and Rectal Surgery	57	57	47	2	8				
General Surgery	1,264	1,231	913	167	151	10	8	7	8
Neurological Surgery	132	125	88	18	19	3	3	1	
Obstetrics & Gynecology	1,257	1,229	1,049	105	75	10	12	5	1
Ophthalmology	262	255	235	11	9		1	6	
Orthopedic Surgery	330	325	266	32	27	1	3	1	
Otolaryngology	163	158	133	12	13	1	1	2	1
Plastic Surgery	164	162	149	6	7			1	1
Thoracic Surgery	163	159	134	6	19		2	1	1
Urology	315	304	256	12	36	1	4	2	4
Other Specialties	9,963	9,357	6,637	1,039	1,681	159	118	193	136
Aerospace Medicine	6	3	1		2	1		2	
Anatomic/Clinical Pathology	1,023	876	572	110	194	25	14	48	60
Anesthesiology	1,984	1,935	1,531	89	315	7	25	14	3
Child & Adolescent Psychiatry	396	382	307	27	48	4	6	2	2
Diagnostic Radiology	504	478	342	39	97	2	6	7	11
Emergency Medicine	608	598	421	31	146	5	3	1	1
Forensic Pathology	35	25	19	2	4	1			9
General Preventive Medicine	91	76	59	14	3	7		6	2
Medical Genetics	29	24	11	7	6		1	3	1
Neurology	975	934	740	130	64	5	10	23	3
Nuclear Medicine	91	86	50	20	16	1	2	1	1
Occupational Medicine	46	35	28		7	7			4
Other Specialty	189	139	81	29	29	14	5	22	9
Physical Medicine and Rehabilitation	455	442	323	50	69	5	3	3	2
Psychiatry	2,386	2,278	1,501	244	533	38	24	37	9
Public Health and General Preventive Medicine	47	10	8		2	24	3	8	2
Radiation Oncology	117	116	94	8	14			1	
Radiology	328	294	200	33	61	1	12	9	12
Transplant Surgery	7	6	4		2			1	
Unspecified	645	619	344	206	69	12	4	5	5
Vascular Medicine	1	1	1						

Note: Above excludes Inactive, Not Classified and Address Unknown Physicians.

Subspecialties in this table are condensed into major specialties. See Appendix A.

Table 3.4

International Medical Graduates by Census Division, Self-Designated Specialty, and Activity, 2010, continued
East South Central

		Patient Care				Other Professional Activity			
				Hospital Based					
Specialty	Total Physicians	Total Patient Care	Office Based	Resid./ Fellows	Phys. Staff	Admin.	Med. Teach.	Research	Other
Total Physicians	6,960	6,774	4,834	1,110	830	29	51	74	32
FM/GP	954	944	662	196	86	4	3	2	1
Family Medicine	878	868	604	196	68	4	3	2	1
General Practice	76	76	58		18				
Medical Specialties	3,504	3,428	2,545	532	351	10	19	42	5
Allergy and Immunology	33	32	28	2	2			1	
Cardiovascular Disease	318	313	230	59	24		2	3	
Dermatology	8	8	6	1	1				
Gastroenterology	126	125	106	12	7			1	
Internal Medicine	2,165	2,120	1,560	328	232	7	11	23	4
Pediatric Cardiology	19	18	13	3	2			1	
Pediatrics	636	614	460	94	60	3	6	12	1
Pulmonary Disease	199	198	142	33	23			1	
Surgical Specialties	624	607	457	81	69	2	6	3	6
Colon and Rectal Surgery	9	9	7	1	1				
General Surgery	223	217	149	38	30	1	2		3
Neurological Surgery	26	25	15	7	3		1		
Obstetrics & Gynecology	142	139	110	14	15	1	1	1	
Ophthalmology	42	40	36	3	1		1	1	
Orthopedic Surgery	51	49	31	10	8				2
Otolaryngology	29	28	23	2	3				1
Plastic Surgery	27	27	24	1	2				
Thoracic Surgery	36	35	28	2	5			1	
Urology	39	38	34	3	1		1		
Other Specialties	1,878	1,795	1,170	301	324	13	23	27	20
Aerospace Medicine	2	1	1				1		
Anatomic/Clinical Pathology	194	175	103	38	34	2	5	7	5
Anesthesiology	342	335	257	12	66		4	3	
Child & Adolescent Psychiatry	56	55	39	8	8			1	
Diagnostic Radiology	78	75	50	9	16				3
Emergency Medicine	99	99	57	10	32				
Forensic Pathology	2	1	1						1
General Preventive Medicine	12	11	6	5			1		
Medical Genetics	5	3	3				2		
Neurology	263	255	189	49	17		3	4	1
Nuclear Medicine	28	27	15	7	5	1			
Occupational Medicine	6	6	5		1				
Other Specialty	37	25	15	6	4	4	1	5	2
Physical Medicine and Rehabilitation	68	68	50	10	8				
Psychiatry	484	468	270	93	105	4	2	6	4
Public Health and General Preventive Medicine	3	2	2			1			
Radiation Oncology	26	26	17	1	8				
Radiology	46	43	25	6	12	1	1		1
Transplant Surgery	2	2	1		1				
Unspecified	125	118	64	47	7		3	1	3

Note: Above excludes Inactive, Not Classified and Address Unknown Physicians.

Subspecialties in this table are condensed into major specialties. See Appendix A.

Table 3.4

International Medical Graduates by Census Division, Self-Designated Specialty, and Activity, 2010, continued
West South Central

		Patient Care				Other Professional Activity			
				Hospital Based					
Specialty	Total Physicians	Total Patient Care	Office Based	Resid./ Fellows	Phys. Staff	Admin.	Med. Teach.	Research	Other
Total Physicians	16,793	16,294	11,957	2,525	1,812	95	189	163	52
FM/GP	2,517	2,483	1,819	481	183	10	18	3	3
Family Medicine	2,293	2,262	1,635	481	146	9	17	3	2
General Practice	224	221	184		37	1	1		1
Medical Specialties	8,545	8,327	6,246	1,238	843	35	79	94	10
Allergy and Immunology	97	93	87	5	1		2	2	
Cardiovascular Disease	818	793	603	135	55	3	9	12	1
Dermatology	44	43	33	3	7	1			
Gastroenterology	378	370	294	48	28		3	5	
Internal Medicine	4,797	4,686	3,455	695	536	20	36	49	6
Pediatric Cardiology	71	70	49	12	9	1			
Pediatrics	1,978	1,918	1,465	273	180	9	27	21	3
Pulmonary Disease	362	354	260	67	27	1	2	5	
Surgical Specialties	1,635	1,588	1,269	194	125	11	23	10	3
Colon and Rectal Surgery	25	23	22	1			2		
General Surgery	474	457	332	75	50	4	11	1	1
Neurological Surgery	83	83	53	22	8				
Obstetrics & Gynecology	471	460	383	52	25	3	5	3	
Ophthalmology	131	128	102	16	10		3		
Orthopedic Surgery	123	118	106	7	5	2		2	1
Otolaryngology	60	59	50	2	7			1	
Plastic Surgery	73	71	62	6	3	1			1
Thoracic Surgery	84	81	67	8	6		1	2	
Urology	111	108	92	5	11	1	1	1	
Other Specialties	4,096	3,896	2,623	612	661	39	69	56	36
Aerospace Medicine	8	4	2		2	1		1	2
Anatomic/Clinical Pathology	532	477	303	91	83	9	16	16	14
Anesthesiology	842	818	637	42	139	5	15	2	2
Child & Adolescent Psychiatry	175	167	123	21	23	4	1	3	
Diagnostic Radiology	234	224	144	28	52		9		1
Emergency Medicine	179	176	114	37	25	1	2		
Forensic Pathology	12	8	6	2					4
General Preventive Medicine	15	15	7	3	5				
Medical Genetics	22	22	11	5	6				
Neurology	465	455	304	105	46		6	3	1
Nuclear Medicine	41	40	26	2	12			1	
Occupational Medicine	30	28	26		2		1		1
Other Specialty	79	61	32	23	6	4	2	11	1
Physical Medicine and Rehabilitation	203	200	139	34	27	1	1	1	
Psychiatry	797	771	499	110	162	10	5	9	2
Public Health and General Preventive Medicine	10	5	3	1	1	1		3	1
Radiation Oncology	68	66	48	2	16	1	1		
Radiology	129	116	76	13	27		8	3	2
Transplant Surgery	8	7	4		3				1
Unspecified	247	236	119	93	24	2	2	3	4

Note: Above excludes Inactive, Not Classified and Address Unknown Physicians.

Subspecialties in this table are condensed into major specialties. See Appendix A.

Table 3.4

International Medical Graduates by Census Division, Self-Designated Specialty, and Activity, 2010, continued
Mountain

		Patient Care				Other Professional Activity			
				Hospital Based					
Specialty	Total Physicians	Total Patient Care	Office Based	Resid./ Fellows	Phys. Staff	Admin.	Med. Teach.	Research	Other
Total Physicians	7,143	6,949	5,501	712	736	46	57	61	30
FM/GP	953	941	778	112	51	4	7		1
Family Medicine	868	858	706	112	40	2	7		1
General Practice	85	83	72		11	2			
Medical Specialties	3,759	3,686	2,961	377	348	16	20	33	4
Allergy and Immunology	47	47	45	2					
Cardiovascular Disease	250	245	198	25	22		1	4	
Dermatology	20	19	15	3	1			1	
Gastroenterology	187	182	151	16	15	2	1	2	
Internal Medicine	2,399	2,359	1,864	261	234	10	11	17	2
Pediatric Cardiology	14	13	12		1		1		
Pediatrics	672	654	539	51	64	3	5	8	2
Pulmonary Disease	170	167	137	19	11	1	1	1	
Surgical Specialties	628	609	486	63	60	6	7	5	1
Colon and Rectal Surgery	7	7	7						
General Surgery	210	206	142	39	25	1	2	1	
Neurological Surgery	24	24	16	7	1				
Obstetrics & Gynecology	197	189	170	6	13	3	1	3	1
Ophthalmology	36	35	28	3	4			1	
Orthopedic Surgery	48	48	34	6	8				
Otolaryngology	13	12	11		1		1		
Plastic Surgery	19	18	15		3	1			
Thoracic Surgery	35	34	30	2	2		1		
Urology	39	36	33		3	1	2		
Other Specialties	1,803	1,713	1,276	160	277	20	23	23	24
Aerospace Medicine	7	4	2		2	1	1		1
Anatomic/Clinical Pathology	167	145	99	21	25	2	3	5	12
Anesthesiology	421	410	353	6	51	1	7	1	2
Child & Adolescent Psychiatry	80	76	55	12	9	2	1	1	
Diagnostic Radiology	107	99	69	7	23	1	4	1	2
Emergency Medicine	113	112	84	5	23	1			
Forensic Pathology	7	6	5		1	1			
General Preventive Medicine	15	13	8	1	4	1		1	
Medical Genetics	9	9	5	1	3				
Neurology	194	190	135	34	21			4	
Nuclear Medicine	6	6	6						
Occupational Medicine	13	13	12		1				
Other Specialty	33	26	18	4	4	2		4	1
Physical Medicine and Rehabilitation	85	83	68		15	1			1
Psychiatry	394	382	267	43	72	5	4	2	1
Public Health and General Preventive Medicine	4	1			1	2		1	
Radiation Oncology	17	16	15		1		1		
Radiology	47	45	32	2	11			1	1
Transplant Surgery	2	2	2						
Unspecified	82	75	41	24	10		2	2	3

Note: Above excludes Inactive, Not Classified and Address Unknown Physicians.

Subspecialties in this table are condensed into major specialties. See Appendix A.

Table 3.4

International Medical Graduates by Census Division, Self-Designated Specialty, and Activity, 2010, continued
Pacific

		Patient Care				Other Professional Activity			
				Hospital Based					
Specialty	Total Physicians	Total Patient Care	Office Based	Resid./ Fellows	Phys. Staff	Admin.	Med. Teach.	Research	Other
Total Physicians	25,569	24,642	20,598	1,496	2,548	249	193	366	119
FM/GP	3,947	3,883	3,350	305	228	28	20	7	9
Family Medicine	3,214	3,159	2,691	305	163	21	20	7	7
General Practice	733	724	659		65	7			2
Medical Specialties	11,828	11,445	9,726	673	1,046	79	74	200	30
Allergy and Immunology	138	124	111	5	8		1	11	2
Cardiovascular Disease	758	727	624	36	67	2	9	19	1
Dermatology	105	98	88	4	6	1	3	3	
Gastroenterology	468	446	394	19	33	6	4	11	1
Internal Medicine	7,116	6,917	5,832	433	652	40	37	104	18
Pediatric Cardiology	60	56	39	8	9			4	
Pediatrics	2,734	2,642	2,283	126	233	29	18	37	8
Pulmonary Disease	449	435	355	42	38	1	2	11	
Surgical Specialties	2,964	2,887	2,548	113	226	24	21	23	9
Colon and Rectal Surgery	30	30	26	1	3				
General Surgery	748	729	602	63	64	8	3	5	3
Neurological Surgery	90	88	73	3	12		1		1
Obstetrics & Gynecology	1,073	1,039	961	10	68	12	11	10	1
Ophthalmology	215	214	197	3	14			1	
Orthopedic Surgery	243	237	213	5	19	1	1	1	3
Otolaryngology	124	121	106	9	6	3			
Plastic Surgery	135	133	118	7	8			1	1
Thoracic Surgery	138	134	109	9	16			4	
Urology	168	162	143	3	16		5	1	
Other Specialties	6,830	6,427	4,974	405	1,048	118	78	136	71
Aerospace Medicine	4	3			3			1	
Anatomic/Clinical Pathology	711	626	450	61	115	26	11	24	24
Anesthesiology	1,607	1,563	1,279	30	254	3	25	12	4
Child & Adolescent Psychiatry	276	269	228	13	28	3	1	3	
Diagnostic Radiology	337	319	240	18	61	4	6	4	4
Emergency Medicine	292	287	215	13	59	2	2	1	
Forensic Pathology	14	6	4	1	1		1		7
General Preventive Medicine	48	39	33	5	1	3	1	3	2
Medical Genetics	31	27	15	9	3	1		3	
Neurology	528	503	435	33	35	2	5	18	
Nuclear Medicine	92	87	55	15	17	1		3	1
Occupational Medicine	72	62	50		12	6	1	1	2
Other Specialty	138	92	71	12	9	9	2	28	7
Physical Medicine and Rehabilitation	293	285	228	17	40	4	3	1	
Psychiatry	1,651	1,577	1,178	59	340	39	10	20	5
Public Health and General Preventive Medicine	22	9	5		4	7	1	2	3
Radiation Oncology	76	75	61	1	13			1	
Radiology	193	178	138	13	27	4	2	5	4
Transplant Surgery	6	5	5				1		
Unspecified	438	414	284	105	25	4	6	6	8
Vascular Medicine	1	1			1				

Note: Above excludes Inactive, Not Classified and Address Unknown Physicians.

Subspecialties in this table are condensed into major specialties. See Appendix A.

Table 3.4

International Medical Graduates by Census Division, Self-Designated Specialty, and Activity, 2010, continued
Possessions

		Patient Care				Other Professional Activity			
				Hospital Based					
Specialty	Total Physicians	Total Patient Care	Office Based	Resid./ Fellows	Phys. Staff	Admin.	Med. Teach.	Research	Other
Total Physicians	5,054	4,859	3,973	235	651	101	37	21	36
FM/GP	1,606	1,549	1,300	19	230	35	7	3	12
Family Medicine	423	407	354	19	34	10	3	1	2
General Practice	1,183	1,142	946		196	25	4	2	10
Medical Specialties	1,467	1,411	1,113	145	153	27	16	9	4
Allergy and Immunology	3	3	3						
Cardiovascular Disease	75	69	66	2	1		3	2	1
Dermatology	8	8	5		3				
Gastroenterology	15	14	12	1	1			1	
Internal Medicine	797	775	581	116	78	7	8	5	2
Pediatric Cardiology	4	4	3		1				
Pediatrics	530	504	419	20	65	20	5		1
Pulmonary Disease	35	34	24	6	4			1	
Surgical Specialties	494	480	392	16	72	7	6		1
Colon and Rectal Surgery	4	4	2		2				
General Surgery	138	133	104		29	1	4		
Neurological Surgery	13	13	7	4	2				
Obstetrics & Gynecology	237	231	192	11	28	5			1
Ophthalmology	20	20	18		2				
Orthopedic Surgery	24	21	19	1	1	1	2		
Otolaryngology	23	23	20		3				
Plastic Surgery	6	6	5		1				
Thoracic Surgery	4	4	3		1				
Urology	25	25	22		3				
Other Specialties	1,487	1,419	1,168	55	196	32	8	9	19
Anatomic/Clinical Pathology	50	40	27	7	6	2	2		6
Anesthesiology	84	83	60	4	19			1	
Child & Adolescent Psychiatry	29	26	19	2	5		2		1
Diagnostic Radiology	23	21	14	2	5				2
Emergency Medicine	99	91	46	15	30	7	1		
Forensic Pathology	3	3	3						
General Preventive Medicine	13	11	10		1	1			1
Medical Genetics	1	1	1						
Neurology	40	38	29	2	7		1		1
Nuclear Medicine	5	5	2	2	1				
Occupational Medicine	31	26	20		6	5			
Other Specialty	35	28	24		4	4	1	2	
Physical Medicine and Rehabilitation	32	30	21	4	5	1	1		
Psychiatry	207	199	151	9	39	4		3	1
Public Health and General Preventive Medicine	13	6	3		3	5			2
Radiation Oncology	6	5	3		2			1	
Radiology	16	16	13		3				
Unspecified	800	790	722	8	60	3		2	5

Note: Above excludes Inactive, Not Classified and Address Unknown Physicians.

Subspecialties in this table are condensed into major specialties. See Appendix A.

Table 3.5

Physicians by Census Region, Self-Designated Specialty, and Activity, 2010
Northeast

		Patient Care				Other Professional Activity			
				Hospital Based					
Specialty	Total Physicians	Total Patient Care	Office Based	Resid./ Fellows	Phys. Staff	Admin.	Med. Teach.	Research	Other
Total Physicians	229,224	171,063	118,119	31,983	20,961	3,674	2,368	4,399	1,197
FM/GP	12,866	12,237	9,866	1,366	1,005	260	256	54	59
Family Medicine	11,950	11,381	9,130	1,366	885	231	253	38	47
General Practice	916	856	736		120	29	3	16	12
Medical Specialties	78,429	72,872	50,686	14,180	8,006	1,481	1,079	2,595	402
Allergy and Immunology	1,000	887	761	83	43	13	6	89	5
Cardiovascular Disease	6,134	5,736	4,347	867	522	88	74	202	34
Dermatology	2,573	2,494	2,053	342	99	15	18	41	5
Gastroenterology	3,451	3,271	2,588	450	233	35	43	91	11
Internal Medicine	43,779	40,368	27,073	8,774	4,521	967	586	1,602	256
Pediatric Cardiology	497	463	256	114	93	6	10	17	1
Pediatrics	18,204	17,105	11,805	3,099	2,201	304	284	429	82
Pulmonary Disease	2,791	2,548	1,803	451	294	53	58	124	8
Surgical Specialties	35,833	34,843	25,561	6,373	2,909	332	286	258	114
Colon and Rectal Surgery	392	385	339	19	27		3	3	1
General Surgery	8,497	8,205	4,908	2,354	943	120	74	66	32
Neurological Surgery	1,152	1,126	728	279	119	3	8	13	2
Obstetrics & Gynecology	9,245	8,924	6,831	1,303	790	115	109	71	26
Ophthalmology	4,272	4,190	3,630	373	187	13	24	34	11
Orthopedic Surgery	5,354	5,250	3,835	1,109	306	19	30	25	30
Otolaryngology	2,039	2,003	1,530	334	139	11	16	7	2
Plastic Surgery	1,515	1,498	1,225	206	67	6	4	3	4
Thoracic Surgery	999	944	698	82	164	22	8	24	1
Urology	2,368	2,318	1,837	314	167	23	10	12	5
Other Specialties	55,573	51,111	32,006	10,064	9,041	1,601	747	1,492	622
Aerospace Medicine	22	13	10		3	6		1	2
Anatomic/Clinical Pathology	4,490	3,818	2,064	811	943	188	90	208	186
Anesthesiology	9,690	9,421	6,498	1,607	1,316	73	107	70	19
Child & Adolescent Psychiatry	2,191	2,030	1,466	256	308	57	36	52	16
Diagnostic Radiology	6,029	5,829	3,622	1,511	696	39	52	51	58
Emergency Medicine	6,654	6,373	3,220	1,493	1,660	172	64	31	14
Forensic Pathology	122	75	63	6	6	13	1	3	30
General Preventive Medicine	378	310	209	65	36	32	10	16	10
Medical Genetics	118	90	44	23	23	3	2	21	2
Neurology	4,162	3,760	2,488	780	492	61	71	243	27
Nuclear Medicine	359	312	189	44	79	8	11	20	8
Occupational Medicine	415	267	205		62	97	9	19	23
Other Specialty	1,294	710	393	196	121	212	34	280	58
Physical Medicine and Rehabilitation	2,382	2,279	1,589	376	314	56	16	13	18
Psychiatry	12,004	10,954	7,129	1,532	2,293	440	187	344	79
Public Health and General Preventive Medicine	224	55	43		12	96	11	36	26
Radiation Oncology	1,033	1,004	651	180	173	7	6	13	3
Radiology	2,240	2,125	1,548	188	389	26	28	30	31
Transplant Surgery	52	48	37	1	10	2		2	
Unspecified	1,710	1,634	536	995	103	13	12	39	12
Vascular Medicine	4	4	2		2				
Inactive	27,538								
Not Classified	18,985								

Note: Above excludes Address Unknown.

Subspecialties in this table are contdensed into major specialties. See Appendix A.

Table 3.5

Physicians by Census Region, Self-Designated Specialty, and Activity, 2010, continued
North Central

		Patient Care				Other Professional Activity			
				Hospital Based					
Specialty	Total Physicians	Total Patient Care	Office Based	Resid./ Fellows	Phys. Staff	Admin.	Med. Teach.	Research	Other
Total Physicians	198,358	155,103	113,920	25,528	15,655	2,480	2,033	2,261	800
FM/GP	23,657	22,811	18,754	2,337	1,720	340	400	47	59
Family Medicine	22,388	21,600	17,707	2,337	1,556	307	393	43	45
General Practice	1,269	1,211	1,047		164	33	7	4	14
Medical Specialties	59,679	56,457	41,087	9,890	5,480	913	796	1,347	166
Allergy and Immunology	890	836	707	82	47	7	7	37	3
Cardiovascular Disease	4,581	4,344	3,490	542	312	35	60	132	10
Dermatology	2,095	2,067	1,632	329	106	4	13	9	2
Gastroenterology	2,413	2,297	1,848	297	152	15	31	66	4
Internal Medicine	31,910	30,051	21,696	5,418	2,937	599	431	731	98
Pediatric Cardiology	479	453	249	110	94	3	7	15	1
Pediatrics	15,198	14,448	9,988	2,819	1,641	209	210	289	42
Pulmonary Disease	2,113	1,961	1,477	293	191	41	37	68	6
Surgical Specialties	33,148	32,433	24,738	5,398	2,297	223	274	163	55
Colon and Rectal Surgery	329	323	280	18	25	3	3		
General Surgery	7,643	7,430	5,012	1,719	699	70	73	52	18
Neurological Surgery	1,273	1,251	838	298	115	8	6	5	3
Obstetrics & Gynecology	8,294	8,074	6,510	995	569	78	92	41	9
Ophthalmology	3,676	3,601	3,083	351	167	17	28	24	6
Orthopedic Surgery	5,297	5,230	3,917	1,004	309	16	26	16	9
Otolaryngology	2,131	2,100	1,562	406	132	8	14	6	3
Plastic Surgery	1,322	1,297	1,020	223	54	2	11	7	5
Thoracic Surgery	992	968	801	55	112	7	10	7	
Urology	2,191	2,159	1,715	329	115	14	11	5	2
Other Specialties	46,193	43,402	29,341	7,903	6,158	1,004	563	704	520
Aerospace Medicine	36	20	12		8	9	1	4	2
Anatomic/Clinical Pathology	4,221	3,679	2,461	635	583	143	81	129	189
Anesthesiology	8,711	8,537	6,137	1,340	1,060	43	85	34	12
Child & Adolescent Psychiatry	1,291	1,216	924	125	167	27	28	15	5
Diagnostic Radiology	5,714	5,571	3,772	1,180	619	23	49	9	62
Emergency Medicine	6,901	6,647	4,166	1,149	1,332	151	67	23	13
Forensic Pathology	124	90	71	7	12	5	2		27
General Preventive Medicine	262	216	166	29	21	19	2	18	7
Medical Genetics	115	91	55	14	22	1	5	16	2
Neurology	3,290	3,075	2,158	608	309	34	44	122	15
Nuclear Medicine	269	238	161	26	51	8	8	7	8
Occupational Medicine	590	464	373		91	85	4	16	21
Other Specialty	1,111	742	430	222	90	146	38	144	41
Physical Medicine and Rehabilitation	1,944	1,892	1,326	326	240	25	7	11	9
Psychiatry	6,592	6,164	4,344	787	1,033	193	93	102	40
Public Health and General Preventive Medicine	128	25	16		9	62	9	19	13
Radiation Oncology	1,046	1,032	736	157	139	7	2	4	1
Radiology	1,938	1,850	1,455	136	259	12	30	11	35
Transplant Surgery	49	43	31		12		2	4	
Unspecified	1,849	1,798	536	1,162	100	11	6	16	18
Vascular Medicine	12	12	11		1				
Inactive	23,459								
Not Classified	12,222								

Note: Above excludes Address Unknown.

Subspecialties in this table are condensed into major specialties. *See Appendix A.*

Table 3.5

Physicians by Census Region, Self-Designated Specialty, and Activity, 2010, continued
South

		Patient Care				Other Professional Activity			
				Hospital Based					
Specialty	Total Physicians	Total Patient Care	Office Based	Resid./ Fellows	Phys. Staff	Admin.	Med. Teach.	Research	Other
Total Physicians	325,947	252,106	193,810	32,538	25,758	4,470	3,482	4,036	1,460
FM/GP	33,680	32,439	27,120	2,711	2,608	533	519	81	108
Family Medicine	30,784	29,641	24,680	2,711	2,250	480	510	74	79
General Practice	2,896	2,798	2,440		358	53	9	7	29
Medical Specialties	98,964	93,385	72,155	12,172	9,058	1,523	1,416	2,283	357
Allergy and Immunology	1,494	1,345	1,186	96	63	11	20	111	7
Cardiovascular Disease	7,881	7,533	6,233	772	528	76	96	162	14
Dermatology	3,796	3,730	3,155	402	173	12	27	19	8
Gastroenterology	4,600	4,421	3,768	394	259	26	58	88	7
Internal Medicine	50,717	47,600	35,984	6,411	5,205	912	713	1,304	188
Pediatric Cardiology	708	665	452	114	99	9	7	24	3
Pediatrics	25,940	24,508	18,559	3,571	2,378	421	433	458	120
Pulmonary Disease	3,828	3,583	2,818	412	353	56	62	117	10
Surgical Specialties	58,078	56,683	45,162	7,519	4,002	436	559	246	154
Colon and Rectal Surgery	516	503	438	26	39	2	6	2	3
General Surgery	12,891	12,505	8,663	2,582	1,260	134	149	64	39
Neurological Surgery	2,098	2,050	1,508	366	176	19	15	8	6
Obstetrics & Gynecology	15,360	14,894	12,483	1,511	900	140	219	70	37
Ophthalmology	6,354	6,220	5,358	564	298	27	45	51	11
Orthopedic Surgery	8,768	8,639	6,857	1,255	527	38	49	16	26
Otolaryngology	3,839	3,781	3,023	520	238	19	24	7	8
Plastic Surgery	2,703	2,666	2,286	248	132	11	15	5	6
Thoracic Surgery	1,675	1,621	1,348	87	186	24	14	10	6
Urology	3,874	3,804	3,198	360	246	22	23	13	12
Other Specialties	74,832	69,599	49,373	10,136	10,090	1,978	988	1,426	841
Aerospace Medicine	229	130	64		66	69	5	15	10
Anatomic/Clinical Pathology	6,437	5,586	3,761	901	924	189	142	226	294
Anesthesiology	14,457	14,147	10,805	1,626	1,716	88	152	50	20
Child & Adolescent Psychiatry	2,267	2,124	1,669	206	249	62	47	28	6
Diagnostic Radiology	8,722	8,514	6,070	1,432	1,012	36	71	29	72
Emergency Medicine	10,918	10,571	7,226	1,234	2,111	195	99	25	28
Forensic Pathology	265	197	142	23	32	9	3	3	53
General Preventive Medicine	922	698	451	101	146	94	19	82	29
Medical Genetics	197	148	84	24	40	8	14	24	3
Neurology	5,155	4,794	3,623	731	440	49	80	214	18
Nuclear Medicine	445	400	258	54	88	15	8	18	4
Occupational Medicine	717	486	399	1	86	161	14	22	34
Other Specialty	1,745	1,119	735	228	156	256	38	263	69
Physical Medicine and Rehabilitation	2,650	2,567	1,940	341	286	44	13	15	11
Psychiatry	11,514	10,698	7,504	1,328	1,866	364	169	206	77
Public Health and General Preventive Medicine	595	98	68	2	28	282	26	153	36
Radiation Oncology	1,607	1,575	1,206	175	194	17	7	5	3
Radiology	3,138	2,982	2,402	176	404	12	68	21	55
Transplant Surgery	59	54	39		15	1	2	1	1
Unspecified	2,785	2,703	920	1,553	230	27	11	26	18
Vascular Medicine	8	8	7		1				
Inactive	41,734								
Not Classified	18,659								

Note: Above excludes Address Unknown.

Subspecialties in this table are condensed into major specialties. See Appendix A.

Table 3.5

Physicians by Census Region, Self-Designated Specialty, and Activity, 2010, continued
West

		Patient Care				Other Professional Activity			
				Hospital Based					
Specialty	Total Physicians	Total Patient Care	Office Based	Resid./ Fellows	Phys. Staff	Admin.	Med. Teach.	Research	Other
Total Physicians	217,778	163,995	131,291	17,081	15,623	3,162	1,885	3,008	1,098
FM/GP	23,631	22,791	19,490	1,690	1,611	395	287	71	87
Family Medicine	21,471	20,714	17,591	1,690	1,433	345	282	58	72
General Practice	2,160	2,077	1,899		178	50	5	13	15
Medical Specialties	62,099	58,414	46,944	6,184	5,286	1,038	703	1,701	243
Allergy and Immunology	912	813	726	36	51	12	7	74	6
Cardiovascular Disease	4,063	3,811	3,198	307	306	36	64	140	12
Dermatology	2,757	2,687	2,362	203	122	13	18	32	7
Gastroenterology	2,614	2,487	2,160	181	146	33	23	64	7
Internal Medicine	33,160	31,056	24,680	3,303	3,073	610	353	1,004	137
Pediatric Cardiology	403	381	276	60	45	5	5	12	
Pediatrics	15,895	15,072	11,866	1,875	1,331	291	194	271	67
Pulmonary Disease	2,295	2,107	1,676	219	212	38	39	104	7
Surgical Specialties	35,186	34,324	28,331	3,597	2,396	287	280	195	100
Colon and Rectal Surgery	245	242	214	14	14	1	2		
General Surgery	7,651	7,461	5,452	1,317	692	76	57	38	19
Neurological Surgery	1,225	1,193	906	198	89	7	10	9	6
Obstetrics & Gynecology	9,284	9,008	7,771	666	571	99	91	66	20
Ophthalmology	3,973	3,888	3,498	190	200	24	26	30	5
Orthopedic Surgery	5,659	5,543	4,592	588	363	32	31	18	35
Otolaryngology	2,230	2,189	1,783	265	141	15	21	4	1
Plastic Surgery	1,841	1,815	1,616	121	78	8	10	4	4
Thoracic Surgery	917	886	737	49	100	8	8	14	1
Urology	2,161	2,099	1,762	189	148	17	24	12	9
Other Specialties	52,232	48,466	36,526	5,610	6,330	1,442	615	1,041	668
Aerospace Medicine	111	68	31		37	30	2	4	7
Anatomic/Clinical Pathology	3,750	3,224	2,323	442	459	133	64	151	178
Anesthesiology	10,274	10,003	8,202	814	987	65	126	53	27
Child & Adolescent Psychiatry	1,604	1,512	1,250	127	135	45	21	23	3
Diagnostic Radiology	5,384	5,200	3,906	694	600	35	56	23	70
Emergency Medicine	8,568	8,286	5,924	777	1,585	174	72	18	18
Forensic Pathology	153	105	92	3	10	6	2	1	39
General Preventive Medicine	609	483	363	49	71	65	8	33	20
Medical Genetics	162	118	74	23	21	5	3	33	3
Neurology	3,097	2,821	2,177	380	264	38	45	171	22
Nuclear Medicine	347	318	231	24	63	7	3	12	7
Occupational Medicine	663	503	436		67	106	8	21	25
Other Specialty	1,274	749	558	102	89	240	21	191	73
Physical Medicine and Rehabilitation	1,847	1,789	1,431	179	179	29	6	10	13
Psychiatry	9,142	8,491	6,379	796	1,316	290	107	177	77
Public Health and General Preventive Medicine	313	67	52		15	135	16	63	32
Radiation Oncology	987	966	767	98	101	3	7	10	1
Radiology	1,999	1,900	1,569	118	213	21	36	17	25
Transplant Surgery	31	30	26		4		1		
Unspecified	1,911	1,828	732	984	112	15	11	29	28
Vascular Medicine	6	5	3		2			1	
Inactive	32,108								
Not Classified	12,522								

Note: Above excludes Address Unknown.

Subspecialties in this table are condensed into major specialties. See Appendix A.

Table 3.5

Physicians by Census Region, Self-Designated Specialty, and Activity, 2010, continued
Possessions

		Patient Care				Other Professional Activity			
				Hospital Based					
Specialty	Total Physicians	Total Patient Care	Office Based	Resid./ Fellows	Phys. Staff	Admin.	Med. Teach.	Research	Other
Total Physicians	13,636	10,305	7,884	1,012	1,409	223	141	51	62
FM/GP	2,375	2,282	1,868	37	377	53	21	4	15
Family Medicine	1,025	981	788	37	156	26	15	1	2
General Practice	1,350	1,301	1,080		221	27	6	3	13
Medical Specialties	3,459	3,288	2,466	401	421	72	66	22	11
Allergy and Immunology	16	15	11	2	2	1			
Cardiovascular Disease	229	216	186	14	16	1	7	3	2
Dermatology	95	91	70	9	12	1	2	1	
Gastroenterology	132	127	102	16	9	1	2	2	
Internal Medicine	1,710	1,646	1,179	272	195	25	24	9	6
Pediatric Cardiology	14	14	10		4				
Pediatrics	1,164	1,090	836	80	174	42	25	4	3
Pulmonary Disease	99	89	72	8	9	1	6	3	
Surgical Specialties	1,672	1,621	1,290	150	181	23	22	3	3
Colon and Rectal Surgery	9	9	4	1	4				
General Surgery	418	400	292	47	61	7	10		1
Neurological Surgery	33	31	18	11	2		2		
Obstetrics & Gynecology	614	591	488	41	62	12	7	2	2
Ophthalmology	182	179	154	15	10	2		1	
Orthopedic Surgery	163	159	124	22	13	1	3		
Otolaryngology	87	86	66	8	12	1			
Plastic Surgery	37	37	33		4				
Thoracic Surgery	22	22	17	1	4				
Urology	107	107	94	4	9				
Other Specialties	3,276	3,114	2,260	424	430	75	32	22	33
Aerospace Medicine	15	12	4		8	2			1
Anatomic/Clinical Pathology	129	108	79	15	14	6	5	1	9
Anesthesiology	227	221	177	10	34	2	2	1	1
Child & Adolescent Psychiatry	85	80	58	6	16	1	3		1
Diagnostic Radiology	205	191	133	23	35	4	4	1	5
Emergency Medicine	237	224	118	40	66	11	2		
Forensic Pathology	6	6	5		1				
General Preventive Medicine	56	47	35	1	11	4	1	2	2
Medical Genetics	5	3	3				1	1	
Neurology	146	139	101	21	17		3	3	1
Nuclear Medicine	36	33	24	5	4	2	1		
Occupational Medicine	41	35	25		10	6			
Other Specialty	58	42	34	1	7	11	2	3	
Physical Medicine and Rehabilitation	222	219	168	32	19	2	1		
Psychiatry	486	463	334	44	85	10	6	4	3
Public Health and General Preventive Medicine	23	7	3		4	9		2	5
Radiation Oncology	25	23	19		4	1		1	
Radiology	71	68	58		10	1	1	1	
Unspecified	1,203	1,193	882	226	85	3		2	5
Inactive	1,089								
Not Classified	1,765								

Note: Above excludes Address Unknown.

Subspecialties in this table are condensed into major specialties. See Appendix A.

Table 3.6

Physicians by Census Division, Self-Designated Specialty, and Activity, 2010
New England

		Patient Care				Other Professional Activity			
				Hospital Based					
Specialty	Total Physicians	Total Patient Care	Office Based	Resid./ Fellows	Phys. Staff	Admin.	Med. Teach.	Research	Other
Total Physicians	66,967	49,649	34,037	8,998	6,614	1,105	658	1,646	384
FM/GP	3,729	3,563	2,940	301	322	70	57	14	25
Family Medicine	3,525	3,377	2,772	301	304	62	55	10	21
General Practice	204	186	168		18	8	2	4	4
Medical Specialties	23,117	21,254	14,734	3,970	2,550	427	299	1,018	119
Allergy and Immunology	270	224	194	20	10	6	1	37	2
Cardiovascular Disease	1,684	1,563	1,112	275	176	20	22	68	11
Dermatology	744	714	566	107	41	8	2	19	1
Gastroenterology	939	877	679	120	78	9	14	39	
Internal Medicine	13,246	12,064	8,187	2,365	1,512	288	174	645	75
Pediatric Cardiology	152	149	80	47	22	1	2		
Pediatrics	5,249	4,920	3,410	906	604	78	68	156	27
Pulmonary Disease	833	743	506	130	107	17	16	54	3
Surgical Specialties	9,927	9,634	7,028	1,693	913	94	75	87	37
Colon and Rectal Surgery	86	83	71	7	5		2	1	
General Surgery	2,413	2,322	1,371	662	289	29	21	32	9
Neurological Surgery	338	332	218	78	36		2	4	
Obstetrics & Gynecology	2,526	2,442	1,887	326	229	33	27	17	7
Ophthalmology	1,105	1,086	924	90	72	2	4	9	4
Orthopedic Surgery	1,623	1,582	1,176	290	116	6	12	11	12
Otolaryngology	564	556	442	59	55	4	2	2	
Plastic Surgery	367	359	278	63	18	3	2		3
Thoracic Surgery	273	253	184	25	44	9	1	9	1
Urology	632	619	477	93	49	8	2	2	1
Other Specialties	16,669	15,198	9,335	3,034	2,829	514	227	527	203
Aerospace Medicine	10	5	5			4		1	
Anatomic/Clinical Pathology	1,517	1,293	686	307	300	59	27	82	56
Anesthesiology	2,654	2,567	1,700	503	364	20	43	20	4
Child & Adolescent Psychiatry	709	661	480	92	89	18	8	20	2
Diagnostic Radiology	1,831	1,772	1,077	475	220	13	16	14	16
Emergency Medicine	2,147	2,052	1,041	388	623	70	15	8	2
Forensic Pathology	23	11	10	1		1	1		10
General Preventive Medicine	136	113	70	27	16	10	2	7	4
Medical Genetics	54	39	19	10	10	3		11	1
Neurology	1,268	1,138	698	246	194	12	20	86	12
Nuclear Medicine	81	65	44	9	12		5	10	1
Occupational Medicine	146	95	76		19	26	3	9	13
Other Specialty	409	208	119	52	37	78	11	87	25
Physical Medicine and Rehabilitation	444	420	281	69	70	14	3	2	5
Psychiatry	3,665	3,322	2,194	464	664	141	56	117	29
Public Health and General Preventive Medicine	75	9	7		2	34	3	18	11
Radiation Oncology	302	291	185	47	59	3	2	6	
Radiology	658	621	436	73	112	6	7	16	8
Transplant Surgery	14	13	11		2	1			
Unspecified	525	502	196	271	35	1	5	13	4
Vascular Medicine	1	1			1				
Inactive	7,742								
Not Classified	5,783								

Note: Above excludes Address Unknown.

Subspecialties in this table are condensed into major specialties. See Appendix A.

Table 3.6

Physicians by Census Division, Self-Designated Specialty, and Activity, 2010, continued
Middle Atlantic

		Patient Care				Other Professional Activity			
				Hospital Based					
Specialty	Total Physicians	Total Patient Care	Office Based	Resid./ Fellows	Phys. Staff	Admin.	Med. Teach.	Research	Other
Total Physicians	162,257	121,414	84,082	22,985	14,347	2,569	1,710	2,753	813
FM/GP	9,137	8,674	6,926	1,065	683	190	199	40	34
Family Medicine	8,425	8,004	6,358	1,065	581	169	198	28	26
General Practice	712	670	568		102	21	1	12	8
Medical Specialties	55,312	51,618	35,952	10,210	5,456	1,054	780	1,577	283
Allergy and Immunology	730	663	567	63	33	7	5	52	3
Cardiovascular Disease	4,450	4,173	3,235	592	346	68	52	134	23
Dermatology	1,829	1,780	1,487	235	58	7	16	22	4
Gastroenterology	2,512	2,394	1,909	330	155	26	29	52	11
Internal Medicine	30,533	28,304	18,886	6,409	3,009	679	412	957	181
Pediatric Cardiology	345	314	176	67	71	5	8	17	1
Pediatrics	12,955	12,185	8,395	2,193	1,597	226	216	273	55
Pulmonary Disease	1,958	1,805	1,297	321	187	36	42	70	5
Surgical Specialties	25,906	25,209	18,533	4,680	1,996	238	211	171	77
Colon and Rectal Surgery	306	302	268	12	22		1	2	1
General Surgery	6,084	5,883	3,537	1,692	654	91	53	34	23
Neurological Surgery	814	794	510	201	83	3	6	9	2
Obstetrics & Gynecology	6,719	6,482	4,944	977	561	82	82	54	19
Ophthalmology	3,167	3,104	2,706	283	115	11	20	25	7
Orthopedic Surgery	3,731	3,668	2,659	819	190	13	18	14	18
Otolaryngology	1,475	1,447	1,088	275	84	7	14	5	2
Plastic Surgery	1,148	1,139	947	143	49	3	2	3	1
Thoracic Surgery	726	691	514	57	120	13	7	15	
Urology	1,736	1,699	1,360	221	118	15	8	10	4
Other Specialties	38,904	35,913	22,671	7,030	6,212	1,087	520	965	419
Aerospace Medicine	12	8	5		3	2			2
Anatomic/Clinical Pathology	2,973	2,525	1,378	504	643	129	63	126	130
Anesthesiology	7,036	6,854	4,798	1,104	952	53	64	50	15
Child & Adolescent Psychiatry	1,482	1,369	986	164	219	39	28	32	14
Diagnostic Radiology	4,198	4,057	2,545	1,036	476	26	36	37	42
Emergency Medicine	4,507	4,321	2,179	1,105	1,037	102	49	23	12
Forensic Pathology	99	64	53	5	6	12		3	20
General Preventive Medicine	242	197	139	38	20	22	8	9	6
Medical Genetics	64	51	25	13	13		2	10	1
Neurology	2,894	2,622	1,790	534	298	49	51	157	15
Nuclear Medicine	278	247	145	35	67	8	6	10	7
Occupational Medicine	269	172	129		43	71	6	10	10
Other Specialty	885	502	274	144	84	134	23	193	33
Physical Medicine and Rehabilitation	1,938	1,859	1,308	307	244	42	13	11	13
Psychiatry	8,339	7,632	4,935	1,068	1,629	299	131	227	50
Public Health and General Preventive Medicine	149	46	36		10	62	8	18	15
Radiation Oncology	731	713	466	133	114	4	4	7	3
Radiology	1,582	1,504	1,112	115	277	20	21	14	23
Transplant Surgery	38	35	26	1	8	1		2	
Unspecified	1,185	1,132	340	724	68	12	7	26	8
Vascular Medicine	3	3	2		1				
Inactive	19,796								
Not Classified	13,202								

Note: Above excludes Address Unknown.

Subspecialties in this table are condensed into major specialties. See Appendix A.

Table 3.6

Physicians by Census Division, Self-Designated Specialty, and Activity, 2010, continued
East North Central

		Patient Care				Other Professional Activity			
				Hospital Based					
Specialty	Total Physicians	Total Patient Care	Office Based	Resid./ Fellows	Phys. Staff	Admin.	Med. Teach.	Research	Other
Total Physicians	140,098	109,268	79,986	18,486	10,796	1,788	1,407	1,523	580
FM/GP	15,292	14,758	12,065	1,617	1,076	212	249	31	42
Family Medicine	14,355	13,859	11,280	1,617	962	191	245	28	32
General Practice	937	899	785		114	21	4	3	10
Medical Specialties	43,211	40,941	29,828	7,291	3,822	678	553	919	120
Allergy and Immunology	631	594	504	54	36	5	4	27	1
Cardiovascular Disease	3,180	3,026	2,441	379	206	26	38	83	7
Dermatology	1,469	1,448	1,140	230	78	4	9	6	2
Gastroenterology	1,671	1,594	1,289	199	106	10	22	42	3
Internal Medicine	23,401	22,086	16,033	4,012	2,041	448	299	495	73
Pediatric Cardiology	344	327	170	84	73	3	5	8	1
Pediatrics	11,031	10,489	7,207	2,124	1,158	151	152	211	28
Pulmonary Disease	1,484	1,377	1,044	209	124	31	24	47	5
Surgical Specialties	23,256	22,740	17,292	3,874	1,574	169	197	108	42
Colon and Rectal Surgery	229	224	190	12	22	2	3		
General Surgery	5,356	5,204	3,483	1,261	460	51	53	35	13
Neurological Surgery	888	871	580	208	83	7	5	3	2
Obstetrics & Gynecology	6,062	5,891	4,697	764	430	66	69	27	9
Ophthalmology	2,589	2,539	2,162	256	121	7	19	18	6
Orthopedic Surgery	3,542	3,495	2,629	678	188	12	20	11	4
Otolaryngology	1,415	1,396	1,057	257	82	6	9	1	3
Plastic Surgery	933	917	713	166	38	1	6	6	3
Thoracic Surgery	696	677	569	36	72	6	8	5	
Urology	1,546	1,526	1,212	236	78	11	5	2	2
Other Specialties	32,807	30,829	20,801	5,704	4,324	729	408	465	376
Aerospace Medicine	21	10	7		3	5	1	3	2
Anatomic/Clinical Pathology	2,920	2,539	1,666	427	446	105	62	85	129
Anesthesiology	6,355	6,228	4,436	995	797	31	61	24	11
Child & Adolescent Psychiatry	898	845	651	86	108	18	24	7	4
Diagnostic Radiology	3,900	3,806	2,550	828	428	15	33	6	40
Emergency Medicine	5,168	4,971	3,159	926	886	119	48	17	13
Forensic Pathology	83	59	50	4	5	4	2		18
General Preventive Medicine	162	136	106	20	10	11		9	6
Medical Genetics	79	66	42	9	15		2	11	
Neurology	2,238	2,097	1,486	397	214	19	33	75	14
Nuclear Medicine	191	172	117	18	37	4	5	4	6
Occupational Medicine	440	342	272		70	65	3	14	16
Other Specialty	764	515	288	166	61	93	28	100	28
Physical Medicine and Rehabilitation	1,438	1,397	971	252	174	19	5	8	9
Psychiatry	4,620	4,312	3,089	512	711	145	67	67	29
Public Health and General Preventive Medicine	92	14	9		5	51	6	11	10
Radiation Oncology	731	719	503	117	99	7	2	3	
Radiology	1,361	1,299	1,008	99	192	9	18	8	27
Transplant Surgery	33	28	21		7		2	3	
Unspecified	1,302	1,263	360	848	55	9	6	10	14
Vascular Medicine	11	11	10		1				
Inactive	16,432								
Not Classified	9,100								

Note: Above excludes Address Unknown.

Subspecialties in this table are condensed into major specialties. See Appendix A.

Table 3.6

Physicians by Census Division, Self-Designated Specialty, and Activity, 2010, continued
West North Central

		Patient Care				Other Professional Activity			
				Hospital Based					
Specialty	Total Physicians	Total Patient Care	Office Based	Resid./ Fellows	Phys. Staff	Admin.	Med. Teach.	Research	Other
Total Physicians	58,260	45,835	33,934	7,042	4,859	692	626	738	220
FM/GP	8,365	8,053	6,689	720	644	128	151	16	17
Family Medicine	8,033	7,741	6,427	720	594	116	148	15	13
General Practice	332	312	262		50	12	3	1	4
Medical Specialties	16,468	15,516	11,259	2,599	1,658	235	243	428	46
Allergy and Immunology	259	242	203	28	11	2	3	10	2
Cardiovascular Disease	1,401	1,318	1,049	163	106	9	22	49	3
Dermatology	626	619	492	99	28		4	3	
Gastroenterology	742	703	559	98	46	5	9	24	1
Internal Medicine	8,509	7,965	5,663	1,406	896	151	132	236	25
Pediatric Cardiology	135	126	79	26	21		2	7	
Pediatrics	4,167	3,959	2,781	695	483	58	58	78	14
Pulmonary Disease	629	584	433	84	67	10	13	21	1
Surgical Specialties	9,892	9,693	7,446	1,524	723	54	77	55	13
Colon and Rectal Surgery	100	99	90	6	3	1			
General Surgery	2,287	2,226	1,529	458	239	19	20	17	5
Neurological Surgery	385	380	258	90	32	1	1	2	1
Obstetrics & Gynecology	2,232	2,183	1,813	231	139	12	23	14	
Ophthalmology	1,087	1,062	921	95	46	10	9	6	
Orthopedic Surgery	1,755	1,735	1,288	326	121	4	6	5	5
Otolaryngology	716	704	505	149	50	2	5	5	
Plastic Surgery	389	380	307	57	16	1	5	1	2
Thoracic Surgery	296	291	232	19	40	1	2	2	
Urology	645	633	503	93	37	3	6	3	
Other Specialties	13,386	12,573	8,540	2,199	1,834	275	155	239	144
Aerospace Medicine	15	10	5		5	4		1	
Anatomic/Clinical Pathology	1,301	1,140	795	208	137	38	19	44	60
Anesthesiology	2,356	2,309	1,701	345	263	12	24	10	1
Child & Adolescent Psychiatry	393	371	273	39	59	9	4	8	1
Diagnostic Radiology	1,814	1,765	1,222	352	191	8	16	3	22
Emergency Medicine	1,733	1,676	1,007	223	446	32	19	6	
Forensic Pathology	41	31	21	3	7	1			9
General Preventive Medicine	100	80	60	9	11	8	2	9	1
Medical Genetics	36	25	13	5	7	1	3	5	2
Neurology	1,052	978	672	211	95	15	11	47	1
Nuclear Medicine	78	66	44	8	14	4	3	3	2
Occupational Medicine	150	122	101		21	20	1	2	5
Other Specialty	347	227	142	56	29	53	10	44	13
Physical Medicine and Rehabilitation	506	495	355	74	66	6	2	3	
Psychiatry	1,972	1,852	1,255	275	322	48	26	35	11
Public Health and General Preventive Medicine	36	11	7		4	11	3	8	3
Radiation Oncology	315	313	233	40	40			1	1
Radiology	577	551	447	37	67	3	12	3	8
Transplant Surgery	16	15	10		5			1	
Unspecified	547	535	176	314	45	2		6	4
Vascular Medicine	1	1	1						
Inactive	7,027								
Not Classified	3,122								

Note: Above excludes Address Unknown.

Subspecialties in this table are condensed into major specialties. See Appendix A.

Table 3.6

Physicians by Census Division, Self-Designated Specialty, and Activity, 2010, continued
South Atlantic

		Patient Care				Other Professional Activity			
				Hospital Based					
Specialty	Total Physicians	Total Patient Care	Office Based	Resid./ Fellows	Phys. Staff	Admin.	Med. Teach.	Research	Other
Total Physicians	188,765	142,595	109,631	17,334	15,630	2,932	1,942	2,849	987
FM/GP	17,685	16,953	14,115	1,313	1,525	329	276	56	71
Family Medicine	16,026	15,366	12,758	1,313	1,295	289	269	51	51
General Practice	1,659	1,587	1,357		230	40	7	5	20
Medical Specialties	58,033	54,375	42,235	6,588	5,552	1,018	797	1,564	279
Allergy and Immunology	830	722	632	50	40	9	13	81	5
Cardiovascular Disease	4,555	4,339	3,636	392	311	50	55	100	11
Dermatology	2,231	2,186	1,894	194	98	11	13	14	7
Gastroenterology	2,731	2,623	2,247	214	162	15	30	56	7
Internal Medicine	30,418	28,332	21,487	3,635	3,210	610	414	918	144
Pediatric Cardiology	403	374	252	68	54	6	7	14	2
Pediatrics	14,668	13,756	10,465	1,808	1,483	284	233	298	97
Pulmonary Disease	2,197	2,043	1,622	227	194	33	32	83	6
Surgical Specialties	32,195	31,381	24,961	3,939	2,481	256	278	176	104
Colon and Rectal Surgery	275	269	231	12	26	1		2	3
General Surgery	7,100	6,863	4,715	1,371	777	87	78	46	26
Neurological Surgery	1,141	1,108	794	204	110	11	9	7	6
Obstetrics & Gynecology	8,551	8,287	6,962	760	565	82	111	42	29
Ophthalmology	3,667	3,580	3,099	304	177	14	21	44	8
Orthopedic Surgery	4,804	4,737	3,743	659	335	19	27	11	10
Otolaryngology	2,060	2,033	1,614	274	145	9	9	5	4
Plastic Surgery	1,560	1,538	1,337	118	83	8	6	5	3
Thoracic Surgery	894	868	696	59	113	12	5	4	5
Urology	2,143	2,098	1,770	178	150	13	12	10	10
Other Specialties	43,392	39,886	28,320	5,494	6,072	1,329	591	1,053	533
Aerospace Medicine	115	67	27		40	39	1	5	3
Anatomic/Clinical Pathology	3,494	2,956	1,987	444	525	114	84	154	186
Anesthesiology	7,784	7,602	5,808	785	1,009	51	83	34	14
Child & Adolescent Psychiatry	1,369	1,280	1,028	113	139	43	30	14	2
Diagnostic Radiology	4,812	4,687	3,397	716	574	25	40	21	39
Emergency Medicine	6,559	6,332	4,319	724	1,289	131	59	18	19
Forensic Pathology	151	115	82	15	18	5	3	2	26
General Preventive Medicine	698	509	321	76	112	72	16	77	24
Medical Genetics	110	81	44	14	23	3	8	17	1
Neurology	3,037	2,787	2,118	405	264	38	39	159	14
Nuclear Medicine	261	232	145	33	54	9	5	11	4
Occupational Medicine	381	238	185		53	92	8	16	27
Other Specialty	1,079	640	400	139	101	172	21	196	50
Physical Medicine and Rehabilitation	1,508	1,458	1,092	192	174	26	8	12	4
Psychiatry	7,140	6,579	4,672	745	1,162	247	118	146	50
Public Health and General Preventive Medicine	465	61	42		19	222	20	132	30
Radiation Oncology	930	909	703	96	110	10	4	4	3
Radiology	1,809	1,719	1,371	115	233	8	38	16	28
Transplant Surgery	26	23	14		9	1	1	1	
Unspecified	1,661	1,608	563	882	163	21	5	18	9
Vascular Medicine	3	3	2		1				
Inactive	26,736								
Not Classified	10,724								

Note: Above excludes Address Unknown.

Subspecialties in this table are condensed into major specialties. See Appendix A.

Table 3.6

Physicians by Census Division, Self-Designated Specialty, and Activity, 2010, continued
East South Central

		Patient Care				Other Professional Activity			
				Hospital Based					
Specialty	Total Physicians	Total Patient Care	Office Based	Resid./ Fellows	Phys. Staff	Admin.	Med. Teach.	Research	Other
Total Physicians	48,214	38,602	30,082	5,068	3,452	549	448	437	192
FM/GP	5,505	5,328	4,531	410	387	83	74	8	12
Family Medicine	5,085	4,916	4,160	410	346	77	74	8	10
General Practice	420	412	371		41	6			2
Medical Specialties	14,688	14,023	10,954	1,907	1,162	184	175	274	32
Allergy and Immunology	219	208	185	17	6	1	2	7	1
Cardiovascular Disease	1,194	1,150	946	138	66	7	13	23	1
Dermatology	493	489	433	42	14		2	2	
Gastroenterology	647	621	538	53	30	3	10	13	
Internal Medicine	7,499	7,141	5,461	962	718	110	87	140	21
Pediatric Cardiology	92	85	61	13	11			7	
Pediatrics	3,870	3,689	2,824	607	258	55	54	64	8
Pulmonary Disease	674	640	506	75	59	8	7	18	1
Surgical Specialties	9,265	9,072	7,325	1,219	528	66	82	24	21
Colon and Rectal Surgery	63	61	51	4	6		2		
General Surgery	2,258	2,204	1,552	470	182	16	26	6	6
Neurological Surgery	340	337	254	59	24		3		
Obstetrics & Gynecology	2,321	2,253	1,913	224	116	24	28	13	3
Ophthalmology	895	883	790	69	24	4	4	3	1
Orthopedic Surgery	1,470	1,451	1,153	225	73	8	3	1	7
Otolaryngology	635	627	522	74	31		6		2
Plastic Surgery	366	363	314	35	14		3		
Thoracic Surgery	298	284	242	8	34	9	3	1	1
Urology	619	609	534	51	24	5	4		1
Other Specialties	10,770	10,179	7,272	1,532	1,375	216	117	131	127
Aerospace Medicine	22	14	9		5	4	2	2	
Anatomic/Clinical Pathology	1,021	897	609	150	138	28	18	29	49
Anesthesiology	2,116	2,066	1,572	265	229	16	26	7	1
Child & Adolescent Psychiatry	274	261	210	24	27	1	7	4	1
Diagnostic Radiology	1,420	1,392	1,007	251	134	5	5	4	14
Emergency Medicine	1,510	1,475	1,008	157	310	21	7	4	3
Forensic Pathology	47	30	21	2	7	2			15
General Preventive Medicine	78	68	45	12	11	5	2	1	2
Medical Genetics	25	16	11		5	2	2	3	2
Neurology	766	721	556	110	55	5	15	23	2
Nuclear Medicine	61	56	41	9	6	1		4	
Occupational Medicine	107	78	69		9	21	2	3	3
Other Specialty	248	185	131	29	25	35	3	20	5
Physical Medicine and Rehabilitation	329	318	253	31	34	7			4
Psychiatry	1,531	1,461	1,012	189	260	29	15	17	9
Public Health and General Preventive Medicine	53	17	15		2	25	2	7	2
Radiation Oncology	249	244	180	28	36	4		1	
Radiology	478	458	382	16	60	2	7		11
Transplant Surgery	8	8	6		2				
Unspecified	425	412	133	259	20	3	4	2	4
Vascular Medicine	2	2	2						
Inactive	5,591								
Not Classified	2,395								

Note: Above excludes Address Unknown.

Subspecialties in this table are condensed into major specialties. See Appendix A.

Table 3.6

Physicians by Census Division, Self-Designated Specialty, and Activity, 2010, continued
West South Central

		Patient Care				Other Professional Activity			
				Hospital Based					
Specialty	Total Physicians	Total Patient Care	Office Based	Resid./ Fellows	Phys. Staff	Admin.	Med. Teach.	Research	Other
Total Physicians	88,968	70,909	54,097	10,136	6,676	989	1,092	750	281
FM/GP	10,490	10,158	8,474	988	696	121	169	17	25
Family Medicine	9,673	9,359	7,762	988	609	114	167	15	18
General Practice	817	799	712		87	7	2	2	7
Medical Specialties	26,243	24,987	18,966	3,677	2,344	321	444	445	46
Allergy and Immunology	445	415	369	29	17	1	5	23	1
Cardiovascular Disease	2,132	2,044	1,651	242	151	19	28	39	2
Dermatology	1,072	1,055	828	166	61	1	12	3	1
Gastroenterology	1,222	1,177	983	127	67	8	18	19	
Internal Medicine	12,800	12,127	9,036	1,814	1,277	192	212	246	23
Pediatric Cardiology	213	206	139	33	34	3		3	1
Pediatrics	7,402	7,063	5,270	1,156	637	82	146	96	15
Pulmonary Disease	957	900	690	110	100	15	23	16	3
Surgical Specialties	16,618	16,230	12,876	2,361	993	114	199	46	29
Colon and Rectal Surgery	178	173	156	10	7	1	4		
General Surgery	3,533	3,438	2,396	741	301	31	45	12	7
Neurological Surgery	617	605	460	103	42	8	3	1	
Obstetrics & Gynecology	4,488	4,354	3,608	527	219	34	80	15	5
Ophthalmology	1,792	1,757	1,469	191	97	9	20	4	2
Orthopedic Surgery	2,494	2,451	1,961	371	119	11	19	4	9
Otolaryngology	1,144	1,121	887	172	62	10	9	2	2
Plastic Surgery	777	765	635	95	35	3	6		3
Thoracic Surgery	483	469	410	20	39	3	6	5	
Urology	1,112	1,097	894	131	72	4	7	3	1
Other Specialties	20,670	19,534	13,781	3,110	2,643	433	280	242	181
Aerospace Medicine	92	49	28		21	26	2	8	7
Anatomic/Clinical Pathology	1,922	1,733	1,165	307	261	47	40	43	59
Anesthesiology	4,557	4,479	3,425	576	478	21	43	9	5
Child & Adolescent Psychiatry	624	583	431	69	83	18	10	10	3
Diagnostic Radiology	2,490	2,435	1,666	465	304	6	26	4	19
Emergency Medicine	2,849	2,764	1,899	353	512	43	33	3	6
Forensic Pathology	67	52	39	6	7	2		1	12
General Preventive Medicine	146	121	85	13	23	17	1	4	3
Medical Genetics	62	51	29	10	12	3	4	4	
Neurology	1,352	1,286	949	216	121	6	26	32	2
Nuclear Medicine	123	112	72	12	28	5	3	3	
Occupational Medicine	229	170	145	1	24	48	4	3	4
Other Specialty	418	294	204	60	30	49	14	47	14
Physical Medicine and Rehabilitation	813	791	595	118	78	11	5	3	3
Psychiatry	2,843	2,658	1,820	394	444	88	36	43	18
Public Health and General Preventive Medicine	77	20	11	2	7	35	4	14	4
Radiation Oncology	428	422	323	51	48	3	3		
Radiology	851	805	649	45	111	2	23	5	16
Transplant Surgery	25	23	19		4		1		1
Unspecified	699	683	224	412	47	3	2	6	5
Vascular Medicine	3	3	3						
Inactive	9,407								
Not Classified	5,540								

Note: Above excludes Address Unknown.

Subspecialties in this table are condensed into major specialties. See Appendix A.

Table 3.6

Physicians by Census Division, Self-Designated Specialty, and Activity, 2010, continued
Mountain

		Patient Care				Other Professional Activity			
				Hospital Based					
Specialty	Total Physicians	Total Patient Care	Office Based	Resid./ Fellows	Phys. Staff	Admin.	Med. Teach.	Research	Other
Total Physicians	58,177	44,445	35,941	4,131	4,373	838	518	578	256
FM/GP	7,051	6,798	5,731	500	567	112	102	18	21
Family Medicine	6,664	6,434	5,406	500	528	95	101	15	19
General Practice	387	364	325		39	17	1	3	2
Medical Specialties	15,731	14,892	11,871	1,553	1,468	273	202	316	48
Allergy and Immunology	229	213	193	9	11	3	1	11	1
Cardiovascular Disease	1,097	1,043	897	67	79	6	16	28	4
Dermatology	666	646	581	42	23	3	5	10	2
Gastroenterology	711	689	600	50	39	7	6	8	1
Internal Medicine	8,145	7,687	5,970	839	878	164	105	164	25
Pediatric Cardiology	115	108	83	17	8	2	3	2	
Pediatrics	4,077	3,872	3,032	474	366	76	58	57	14
Pulmonary Disease	691	634	515	55	64	12	8	36	1
Surgical Specialties	9,778	9,565	8,090	851	624	71	68	45	29
Colon and Rectal Surgery	65	65	62	2	1				
General Surgery	2,192	2,147	1,635	305	207	18	12	9	6
Neurological Surgery	369	363	284	62	17	2	1	3	
Obstetrics & Gynecology	2,572	2,497	2,159	193	145	26	22	20	7
Ophthalmology	982	967	885	37	45	6	3	4	2
Orthopedic Surgery	1,679	1,649	1,418	135	96	5	11	6	8
Otolaryngology	572	556	471	46	39	4	11	1	
Plastic Surgery	451	446	410	17	19	3	1		1
Thoracic Surgery	258	251	217	10	24	3	2	1	1
Urology	638	624	549	44	31	4	5	1	4
Other Specialties	14,075	13,190	10,249	1,227	1,714	382	146	199	158
Aerospace Medicine	46	26	10		16	15	2	1	2
Anatomic/Clinical Pathology	1,000	883	663	110	110	24	14	33	46
Anesthesiology	2,994	2,933	2,548	151	234	13	30	10	8
Child & Adolescent Psychiatry	434	405	329	30	46	16	5	8	
Diagnostic Radiology	1,568	1,522	1,183	143	196	11	15	2	18
Emergency Medicine	2,575	2,500	1,820	226	454	50	15	4	6
Forensic Pathology	41	36	33		3	2			3
General Preventive Medicine	143	114	85	11	18	17		10	2
Medical Genetics	35	28	14	6	8	1	1	4	1
Neurology	859	798	604	122	72	10	13	35	3
Nuclear Medicine	48	45	34		11	1		1	1
Occupational Medicine	185	144	126		18	29	3	2	7
Other Specialty	328	209	148	33	28	70	1	30	18
Physical Medicine and Rehabilitation	533	516	442	35	39	7	1	3	6
Psychiatry	2,025	1,876	1,371	159	346	71	28	29	21
Public Health and General Preventive Medicine	74	15	12		3	34	1	20	4
Radiation Oncology	263	259	217	19	23	1	2		1
Radiology	615	583	490	30	63	8	12	4	8
Transplant Surgery	6	6	5		1				
Unspecified	302	291	115	152	24	2	3	3	3
Vascular Medicine	1	1			1				
Inactive	8,794								
Not Classified	2,748								

Note: Above excludes Address Unknown.

Subspecialties in this table are condensed into major specialties. See Appendix A.

Table 3.6

Physicians by Census Division, Self-Designated Specialty, and Activity, 2010, continued
Pacific

		Patient Care				Other Professional Activity			
				Hospital Based					
Specialty	Total Physicians	Total Patient Care	Office Based	Resid./ Fellows	Phys. Staff	Admin.	Med. Teach.	Research	Other
Total Physicians	159,601	119,550	95,350	12,950	11,250	2,324	1,367	2,430	842
FM/GP	16,580	15,993	13,759	1,190	1,044	283	185	53	66
Family Medicine	14,807	14,280	12,185	1,190	905	250	181	43	53
General Practice	1,773	1,713	1,574		139	33	4	10	13
Medical Specialties	46,368	43,522	35,073	4,631	3,818	765	501	1,385	195
Allergy and Immunology	683	600	533	27	40	9	6	63	5
Cardiovascular Disease	2,966	2,768	2,301	240	227	30	48	112	8
Dermatology	2,091	2,041	1,781	161	99	10	13	22	5
Gastroenterology	1,903	1,798	1,560	131	107	26	17	56	6
Internal Medicine	25,015	23,369	18,710	2,464	2,195	446	248	840	112
Pediatric Cardiology	288	273	193	43	37	3	2	10	
Pediatrics	11,818	11,200	8,834	1,401	965	215	136	214	53
Pulmonary Disease	1,604	1,473	1,161	164	148	26	31	68	6
Surgical Specialties	25,408	24,759	20,241	2,746	1,772	216	212	150	71
Colon and Rectal Surgery	180	177	152	12	13	1	2		
General Surgery	5,459	5,314	3,817	1,012	485	58	45	29	13
Neurological Surgery	856	830	622	136	72	5	9	6	6
Obstetrics & Gynecology	6,712	6,511	5,612	473	426	73	69	46	13
Ophthalmology	2,991	2,921	2,613	153	155	18	23	26	3
Orthopedic Surgery	3,980	3,894	3,174	453	267	27	20	12	27
Otolaryngology	1,658	1,633	1,312	219	102	11	10	3	1
Plastic Surgery	1,390	1,369	1,206	104	59	5	9	4	3
Thoracic Surgery	659	635	520	39	76	5	6	13	
Urology	1,523	1,475	1,213	145	117	13	19	11	5
Other Specialties	38,157	35,276	26,277	4,383	4,616	1,060	469	842	510
Aerospace Medicine	65	42	21		21	15		3	5
Anatomic/Clinical Pathology	2,750	2,341	1,660	332	349	109	50	118	132
Anesthesiology	7,280	7,070	5,654	663	753	52	96	43	19
Child & Adolescent Psychiatry	1,170	1,107	921	97	89	29	16	15	3
Diagnostic Radiology	3,816	3,678	2,723	551	404	24	41	21	52
Emergency Medicine	5,993	5,786	4,104	551	1,131	124	57	14	12
Forensic Pathology	112	69	59	3	7	4	2	1	36
General Preventive Medicine	466	369	278	38	53	48	8	23	18
Medical Genetics	127	90	60	17	13	4	2	29	2
Neurology	2,238	2,023	1,573	258	192	28	32	136	19
Nuclear Medicine	299	273	197	24	52	6	3	11	6
Occupational Medicine	478	359	310		49	77	5	19	18
Other Specialty	946	540	410	69	61	170	20	161	55
Physical Medicine and Rehabilitation	1,314	1,273	989	144	140	22	5	7	7
Psychiatry	7,117	6,615	5,008	637	970	219	79	148	56
Public Health and General Preventive Medicine	239	52	40		12	101	15	43	28
Radiation Oncology	724	707	550	79	78	2	5	10	
Radiology	1,384	1,317	1,079	88	150	13	24	13	17
Transplant Surgery	25	24	21		3		1		
Unspecified	1,609	1,537	617	832	88	13	8	26	25
Vascular Medicine	5	4	3		1			1	
Inactive	23,314								
Not Classified	9,774								

Note: Above excludes Address Unknown.

Subspecialties in this table are condensed into major specialties. See Appendix A.

Table 3.6

Physicians by Census Division, Self-Designated Specialty, and Activity, 2010, continued
Possessions

		Patient Care				Other Professional Activity			
				Hospital Based					
Specialty	Total Physicians	Total Patient Care	Office Based	Resid./ Fellows	Phys. Staff	Admin.	Med. Teach.	Research	Other
Total Physicians	13,636	10,305	7,884	1,012	1,409	223	141	51	62
FM/GP	2,375	2,282	1,868	37	377	53	21	4	15
Family Medicine	1,025	981	788	37	156	26	15	1	2
General Practice	1,350	1,301	1,080		221	27	6	3	13
Medical Specialties	3,459	3,288	2,466	401	421	72	66	22	11
Allergy and Immunology	16	15	11	2	2	1			
Cardiovascular Disease	229	216	186	14	16	1	7	3	2
Dermatology	95	91	70	9	12	1	2	1	
Gastroenterology	132	127	102	16	9	1	2	2	
Internal Medicine	1,710	1,646	1,179	272	195	25	24	9	6
Pediatric Cardiology	14	14	10		4				
Pediatrics	1,164	1,090	836	80	174	42	25	4	3
Pulmonary Disease	99	89	72	8	9	1	6	3	
Surgical Specialties	1,672	1,621	1,290	150	181	23	22	3	3
Colon and Rectal Surgery	9	9	4	1	4				
General Surgery	418	400	292	47	61	7	10		1
Neurological Surgery	33	31	18	11	2		2		
Obstetrics & Gynecology	614	591	488	41	62	12	7	2	2
Ophthalmology	182	179	154	15	10	2		1	
Orthopedic Surgery	163	159	124	22	13	1	3		
Otolaryngology	87	86	66	8	12	1			
Plastic Surgery	37	37	33		4				
Thoracic Surgery	22	22	17	1	4				
Urology	107	107	94	4	9				
Other Specialties	3,276	3,114	2,260	424	430	75	32	22	33
Aerospace Medicine	15	12	4		8	2			1
Anatomic/Clinical Pathology	129	108	79	15	14	6	5	1	9
Anesthesiology	227	221	177	10	34	2	2	1	1
Child & Adolescent Psychiatry	85	80	58	6	16	1	3		1
Diagnostic Radiology	205	191	133	23	35	4	4	1	5
Emergency Medicine	237	224	118	40	66	11	2		
Forensic Pathology	6	6	5		1				
General Preventive Medicine	56	47	35	1	11	4	1	2	2
Medical Genetics	5	3	3				1	1	
Neurology	146	139	101	21	17		3	3	1
Nuclear Medicine	36	33	24	5	4	2	1		
Occupational Medicine	41	35	25		10	6			
Other Specialty	58	42	34	1	7	11	2	3	
Physical Medicine and Rehabilitation	222	219	168	32	19	2	1		
Psychiatry	486	463	334	44	85	10	6	4	3
Public Health and General Preventive Medicine	23	7	3		4	9		2	5
Radiation Oncology	25	23	19		4	1		1	
Radiology	71	68	58		10	1	1	1	
Unspecified	1,203	1,193	882	226	85	3		2	5
Inactive	1,089								
Not Classified	1,765								

Note: Above excludes Address Unknown.

Subspecialties in this table are condensed into major specialties. See Appendix A.

Table 3.7

Physicians by State, Self-Designated Specialty, and Activity, 2010
Alabama

		Patient Care				Other Professional Activity			
				Hospital Based					
Specialty	Total Physicians	Total Patient Care	Office Based	Resid./ Fellows	Phys. Staff	Admin.	Med. Teach.	Research	Other
Total Physicians	11,613	9,377	7,324	1,285	768	110	99	117	42
FM/GP	1,366	1,338	1,113	128	97	13	12	1	2
Family Medicine	1,273	1,246	1,030	128	88	12	12	1	2
General Practice	93	92	83		9	1			
Medical Specialties	3,521	3,362	2,665	461	236	39	41	72	7
Allergy and Immunology	39	34	31	2	1		1	4	
Cardiovascular Disease	283	270	233	19	18		2	11	
Dermatology	126	126	113	12	1				
Gastroenterology	161	155	134	12	9		3	3	
Internal Medicine	1,873	1,778	1,372	254	152	27	22	40	6
Pediatric Cardiology	14	14	11	1	2				
Pediatrics	875	842	650	143	49	9	11	12	1
Pulmonary Disease	150	143	121	18	4	3	2	2	
Surgical Specialties	2,298	2,258	1,884	269	105	10	18	5	7
Colon and Rectal Surgery	19	19	17	2					
General Surgery	534	523	383	103	37	3	4		4
Neurological Surgery	83	83	62	16	5				
Obstetrics & Gynecology	569	548	480	44	24	5	11	4	1
Ophthalmology	222	220	202	15	3			1	1
Orthopedic Surgery	394	393	315	62	16				1
Otolaryngology	186	185	166	14	5		1		
Plastic Surgery	77	76	66	4	6		1		
Thoracic Surgery	66	64	58		6	1	1		
Urology	148	147	135	9	3	1			
Other Specialties	2,560	2,419	1,662	427	330	48	28	39	26
Aerospace Medicine	9	4	2		2	2	1	2	
Anatomic/Clinical Pathology	239	217	140	50	27	5	4	7	6
Anesthesiology	508	496	356	76	64	7	3	2	
Child & Adolescent Psychiatry	70	68	55	4	9		1	1	
Diagnostic Radiology	339	334	225	77	32			2	3
Emergency Medicine	299	290	188	32	70	5	2	2	
Forensic Pathology	13	5	4		1	1			7
General Preventive Medicine	20	19	14	1	4			1	
Medical Genetics	6	1	1				2	2	1
Neurology	208	197	150	36	11	1	4	5	1
Nuclear Medicine	11	10	6	3	1			1	
Occupational Medicine	25	18	15		3	5	2		
Other Specialty	64	49	33	7	9	6	2	6	1
Physical Medicine and Rehabilitation	82	80	61	11	8	2			
Psychiatry	352	338	236	38	64	6	2	5	1
Public Health and General Preventive Medicine	11	1	1			7		2	1
Radiation Oncology	65	64	49	8	7			1	
Radiology	110	100	83	6	11	1	4		5
Transplant Surgery	2	2	2						
Unspecified	126	125	40	78	7		1		
Vascular Medicine	1	1	1						
Inactive	1,302								
Not Classified	566								

Note: Excludes Address Unknown.

Subspecialties in this table are condensed into major specialties. See Appendix A.

Table 3.7

Physicians by State, Self-Designated Specialty, and Activity, 2010, continued
Alaska

		Patient Care				Other Professional Activity			
				Hospital Based					
Specialty	Total Physicians	Total Patient Care	Office Based	Resid./ Fellows	Phys. Staff	Admin.	Med. Teach.	Research	Other
Total Physicians	1,823	1,502	1,188	44	270	31	10	14	11
FM/GP	422	411	310	31	70	7	3	1	
Family Medicine	398	387	290	31	66	7	3	1	
General Practice	24	24	20		4				
Medical Specialties	363	351	289	5	57	7	1	4	
Allergy and Immunology	6	6	2	1	3				
Cardiovascular Disease	28	28	24		4				
Dermatology	11	11	10		1				
Gastroenterology	12	12	10		2				
Internal Medicine	170	163	134	2	27	3	1	3	
Pediatric Cardiology	2	2	2						
Pediatrics	122	117	97	2	18	4		1	
Pulmonary Disease	12	12	10		2				
Surgical Specialties	345	339	275	2	62	2	1	2	1
Colon and Rectal Surgery	3	3	3						
General Surgery	77	74	54	1	19	1	1		1
Neurological Surgery	10	10	10						
Obstetrics & Gynecology	85	85	76		9				
Ophthalmology	30	30	24		6				
Orthopedic Surgery	75	74	59		15			1	
Otolaryngology	31	31	21		10				
Plastic Surgery	9	8	7		1			1	
Thoracic Surgery	5	5	4		1				
Urology	20	19	17	1	1	1			
Other Specialties	438	401	314	6	81	15	5	7	10
Aerospace Medicine	6	3	1		2	2			1
Anatomic/Clinical Pathology	22	17	13		4		1	1	3
Anesthesiology	83	81	71	1	9		2		
Child & Adolescent Psychiatry	10	9	8		1			1	
Diagnostic Radiology	48	46	37	1	8				2
Emergency Medicine	105	101	71		30	4			
Forensic Pathology	3	3	3						
General Preventive Medicine	12	8	4	2	2	1		2	1
Neurology	18	18	15		3				
Occupational Medicine	4	2	2			1		1	
Other Specialty	6	4	4			2			
Physical Medicine and Rehabilitation	12	12	11		1				
Psychiatry	79	72	53	1	18	3	1	1	2
Public Health and General Preventive Medicine	5	1	1			2		1	1
Radiation Oncology	7	7	5		2				
Radiology	12	11	10		1		1		
Unspecified	6	6	5	1					
Inactive	206								
Not Classified	49								

Note: Excludes Address Unknown.

Subspecialties in this table are condensed into major specialties. See Appendix A.

Table 3.7

Physicians by State, Self-Designated Specialty, and Activity, 2010, continued
Arizona

		Patient Care				Other Professional Activity			
				Hospital Based					
Specialty	Total Physicians	Total Patient Care	Office Based	Resid./ Fellows	Phys. Staff	Admin.	Med. Teach.	Research	Other
Total Physicians	16,944	12,818	10,331	1,320	1,167	254	164	135	79
FM/GP	1,586	1,512	1,300	102	110	35	27	7	5
Family Medicine	1,459	1,395	1,196	102	97	28	27	5	4
General Practice	127	117	104		13	7		2	1
Medical Specialties	4,959	4,735	3,780	502	453	81	66	65	12
Allergy and Immunology	58	58	56		2				
Cardiovascular Disease	374	363	312	29	22	2	3	3	3
Dermatology	210	206	187	12	7		2	2	
Gastroenterology	235	229	195	21	13	2	2	2	
Internal Medicine	2,599	2,470	1,925	274	271	46	33	45	5
Pediatric Cardiology	37	36	32		4		1		
Pediatrics	1,216	1,159	892	148	119	24	22	8	3
Pulmonary Disease	230	214	181	18	15	7	3	5	1
Surgical Specialties	2,765	2,695	2,242	301	152	19	21	19	11
Colon and Rectal Surgery	28	28	26	1	1				
General Surgery	670	654	474	128	52	3	5	4	4
Neurological Surgery	105	104	69	29	6			1	
Obstetrics & Gynecology	736	705	602	69	34	11	7	10	3
Ophthalmology	280	276	253	12	11	2	1	1	
Orthopedic Surgery	399	390	340	29	21	2	2	3	2
Otolaryngology	133	130	113	10	7	1	2		
Plastic Surgery	144	144	133	4	7				
Thoracic Surgery	82	80	71	3	6		2		
Urology	188	184	161	16	7		2		2
Other Specialties	4,140	3,876	3,009	415	452	119	50	44	51
Aerospace Medicine	7	5	3		2	1		1	
Anatomic/Clinical Pathology	274	240	188	23	29	8	4	5	17
Anesthesiology	956	939	817	54	68	3	11	1	2
Child & Adolescent Psychiatry	109	102	86	6	10	4	1	2	
Diagnostic Radiology	469	453	343	60	50	4	6	1	5
Emergency Medicine	692	670	463	95	112	11	7	1	3
Forensic Pathology	14	13	11		2				1
General Preventive Medicine	28	21	19		2	4		3	
Medical Genetics	6	5	4		1			1	
Neurology	305	287	199	58	30	2	6	9	1
Nuclear Medicine	23	21	16		5	1			1
Occupational Medicine	41	31	29		2	9		1	
Other Specialty	117	73	53	11	9	29	1	7	7
Physical Medicine and Rehabilitation	122	119	108	4	7	1			2
Psychiatry	569	524	387	49	88	25	9	5	6
Public Health and General Preventive Medicine	21	3	3			10	1	6	1
Radiation Oncology	86	86	75	6	5				
Radiology	214	200	166	12	22	6	3		5
Transplant Surgery	1	1	1						
Unspecified	85	82	38	37	7	1	1	1	
Vascular Medicine	1	1			1				
Inactive	2,653								
Not Classified	841								

Note: Excludes Address Unknown.

Subspecialties in this table are condensed into major specialties. *See Appendix A.*

Table 3.7

Physicians by State, Self-Designated Specialty, and Activity, 2010, continued
Arkansas

		Patient Care				Other Professional Activity			
				Hospital Based					
Specialty	Total Physicians	Total Patient Care	Office Based	Resid./ Fellows	Phys. Staff	Admin.	Med. Teach.	Research	Other
Total Physicians	6,771	5,397	4,096	709	592	54	98	44	24
FM/GP	1,302	1,262	1,025	148	89	6	29	1	4
Family Medicine	1,209	1,171	943	148	80	6	29	1	2
General Practice	93	91	82		9				2
Medical Specialties	1,713	1,629	1,193	239	197	18	36	26	4
Allergy and Immunology	27	25	25				1	1	
Cardiovascular Disease	161	153	116	16	21	2	2	4	
Dermatology	75	74	61	12	1			1	
Gastroenterology	87	84	72	9	3		2	1	
Internal Medicine	745	713	531	86	96	7	13	10	2
Pediatric Cardiology	17	17	6	6	5				
Pediatrics	535	502	333	103	66	7	16	8	2
Pulmonary Disease	66	61	49	7	5	2	2	1	
Surgical Specialties	1,157	1,137	935	118	84	6	11	1	2
Colon and Rectal Surgery	7	7	7						
General Surgery	262	256	184	44	28	3	2	1	
Neurological Surgery	49	49	40	5	4				
Obstetrics & Gynecology	281	276	244	16	16	1	4		
Ophthalmology	132	129	107	10	12	1	2		
Orthopedic Surgery	181	179	152	21	6	1	1		
Otolaryngology	94	92	69	16	7		1		1
Plastic Surgery	33	32	31		1				1
Thoracic Surgery	39	38	32		6		1		
Urology	79	79	69	6	4				
Other Specialties	1,445	1,369	943	204	222	24	22	16	14
Aerospace Medicine	2					1	1		
Anatomic/Clinical Pathology	136	123	88	20	15	3	1	2	7
Anesthesiology	279	276	201	43	32	1	1	1	
Child & Adolescent Psychiatry	38	36	26	2	8		1	1	
Diagnostic Radiology	182	176	126	31	19		5		1
Emergency Medicine	203	200	122	24	54		2		1
Forensic Pathology	4	4	3		1				
General Preventive Medicine	7	7	4	1	2				
Medical Genetics	2	1			1	1			
Neurology	98	94	68	17	9		2	2	
Nuclear Medicine	15	15	9	2	4				
Occupational Medicine	8	8	6		2				
Other Specialty	39	25	19	3	3	7	2	3	2
Physical Medicine and Rehabilitation	60	57	37	11	9	1	1	1	
Psychiatry	232	215	139	30	46	6	4	5	2
Public Health and General Preventive Medicine	4					4			
Radiation Oncology	22	22	21		1				
Radiology	80	77	62	6	9		2		1
Unspecified	34	33	12	14	7			1	
Inactive	863								
Not Classified	291								

Note: Excludes Address Unknown.

Subspecialties in this table are condensed into major specialties. See Appendix A.

Table 3.7

Physicians by State, Self-Designated Specialty, and Activity, 2010, continued
California

		Patient Care				Other Professional Activity			
				Hospital Based					
Specialty	Total Physicians	Total Patient Care	Office Based	Resid./ Fellows	Phys. Staff	Admin.	Med. Teach.	Research	Other
Total Physicians	118,110	88,369	70,496	10,000	7,873	1,721	988	1,814	598
FM/GP	11,121	10,760	9,295	826	639	172	109	34	46
Family Medicine	9,682	9,370	8,015	826	529	147	106	25	34
General Practice	1,439	1,390	1,280		110	25	3	9	12
Medical Specialties	35,346	33,174	26,818	3,679	2,677	591	384	1,048	149
Allergy and Immunology	541	471	422	24	25	7	5	54	4
Cardiovascular Disease	2,326	2,162	1,805	196	161	24	39	93	8
Dermatology	1,630	1,594	1,378	138	78	8	8	16	4
Gastroenterology	1,428	1,343	1,148	114	81	21	16	44	4
Internal Medicine	18,847	17,599	14,206	1,884	1,509	339	188	637	84
Pediatric Cardiology	228	215	150	35	30	3	2	8	
Pediatrics	9,120	8,658	6,813	1,154	691	172	105	145	40
Pulmonary Disease	1,226	1,132	896	134	102	17	21	51	5
Surgical Specialties	18,778	18,298	15,007	2,070	1,221	164	157	107	52
Colon and Rectal Surgery	136	134	113	9	12	1	1		
General Surgery	3,939	3,837	2,789	719	329	37	32	21	12
Neurological Surgery	610	595	437	104	54	4	5	3	3
Obstetrics & Gynecology	5,041	4,889	4,198	378	313	64	48	31	9
Ophthalmology	2,245	2,189	1,954	118	117	13	18	22	3
Orthopedic Surgery	2,872	2,812	2,307	352	153	18	16	8	18
Otolaryngology	1,188	1,167	943	165	59	10	8	2	1
Plastic Surgery	1,136	1,119	986	87	46	5	7	3	2
Thoracic Surgery	507	487	402	31	54	4	6	10	
Urology	1,104	1,069	878	107	84	8	16	7	4
Other Specialties	28,245	26,137	19,376	3,425	3,336	794	338	625	351
Aerospace Medicine	35	22	11		11	8		2	3
Anatomic/Clinical Pathology	2,050	1,746	1,220	255	271	91	39	91	83
Anesthesiology	5,365	5,212	4,138	498	576	40	64	32	17
Child & Adolescent Psychiatry	889	842	702	76	64	24	11	11	1
Diagnostic Radiology	2,711	2,609	1,915	408	286	18	31	16	37
Emergency Medicine	4,268	4,127	2,897	474	756	84	40	9	8
Forensic Pathology	83	54	46	2	6	2	1		26
General Preventive Medicine	318	258	199	28	31	32	5	10	13
Medical Genetics	94	69	46	13	10	3		21	1
Neurology	1,676	1,503	1,175	196	132	24	25	114	10
Nuclear Medicine	226	207	149	15	43	5	2	7	5
Occupational Medicine	338	258	224		34	54	4	12	10
Other Specialty	670	377	278	56	43	121	15	114	43
Physical Medicine and Rehabilitation	946	921	709	108	104	14	3	5	3
Psychiatry	5,534	5,146	3,942	489	715	178	56	115	39
Public Health and General Preventive Medicine	161	32	23		9	74	10	25	20
Radiation Oncology	529	517	399	63	55	1	3	8	
Radiology	1,033	978	799	59	120	11	21	8	15
Transplant Surgery	20	19	17		2		1		
Unspecified	1,295	1,237	485	685	67	10	7	24	17
Vascular Medicine	4	3	2		1			1	
Inactive	16,904								
Not Classified	7,716								

Note: Excludes Address Unknown.

Subspecialties in this table are condensed into major specialties. See Appendix A.

Table 3.7

Physicians by State, Self-Designated Specialty, and Activity, 2010, continued
Colorado

		Patient Care				Other Professional Activity			
				Hospital Based					
Specialty	Total Physicians	Total Patient Care	Office Based	Resid./ Fellows	Phys. Staff	Admin.	Med. Teach.	Research	Other
Total Physicians	15,595	11,932	9,692	1,130	1,110	261	146	222	59
FM/GP	1,938	1,863	1,579	140	144	37	28	4	6
Family Medicine	1,868	1,795	1,516	140	139	35	28	4	6
General Practice	70	68	63		5	2			
Medical Specialties	4,249	3,966	3,177	447	342	82	55	132	14
Allergy and Immunology	97	84	69	8	7	3	1	8	1
Cardiovascular Disease	246	231	201	14	16	2	4	9	
Dermatology	181	175	152	16	7	2		3	1
Gastroenterology	168	166	144	9	13			2	
Internal Medicine	2,166	2,014	1,605	224	185	47	30	66	9
Pediatric Cardiology	36	32	20	10	2	1	2	1	
Pediatrics	1,152	1,082	838	148	96	26	14	27	3
Pulmonary Disease	203	182	148	18	16	1	4	16	
Surgical Specialties	2,588	2,526	2,125	234	167	21	23	12	6
Colon and Rectal Surgery	12	12	12						
General Surgery	561	552	423	83	46	6	3		
Neurological Surgery	99	96	76	12	8	1	1	1	
Obstetrics & Gynecology	715	697	585	66	46	5	4	6	3
Ophthalmology	262	257	232	10	15	2	1	2	
Orthopedic Surgery	455	443	383	36	24	2	6	2	2
Otolaryngology	162	156	128	15	13		6		
Plastic Surgery	108	107	103	1	3	1			
Thoracic Surgery	54	50	42	3	5	3		1	
Urology	160	156	141	8	7	1	2		1
Other Specialties	3,845	3,577	2,811	309	457	121	40	74	33
Aerospace Medicine	19	8	3		5	9	2		
Anatomic/Clinical Pathology	272	243	178	33	32	5	5	11	8
Anesthesiology	774	757	662	28	67	4	10	2	1
Child & Adolescent Psychiatry	152	142	119	9	14	5	2	3	
Diagnostic Radiology	372	363	275	31	57	4	2	1	2
Emergency Medicine	725	699	526	46	127	18	4	3	1
Forensic Pathology	8	7	7			1			
General Preventive Medicine	53	39	30	5	4	9		5	
Medical Genetics	13	11	5	4	2			2	
Neurology	192	175	140	23	12	3	3	10	1
Nuclear Medicine	12	12	8		4				
Occupational Medicine	74	60	54		6	8	1	1	4
Other Specialty	81	45	35	6	4	18		13	5
Physical Medicine and Rehabilitation	174	165	137	16	12	3	1	2	3
Psychiatry	599	556	436	39	81	21	4	12	6
Public Health and General Preventive Medicine	23	4	3		1	12		6	1
Radiation Oncology	59	56	45	6	5	1	2		
Radiology	145	139	114	10	15		3	2	1
Transplant Surgery	1	1	1						
Unspecified	97	95	33	53	9		1	1	
Inactive	2,270								
Not Classified	705								

Note: Excludes Address Unknown.

Subspecialties in this table are condensed into major specialties. See Appendix A.

Table 3.7

Physicians by State, Self-Designated Specialty, and Activity, 2010, continued
Connecticut

		Patient Care				Other Professional Activity			
				Hospital Based					
Specialty	Total Physicians	Total Patient Care	Office Based	Resid./ Fellows	Phys. Staff	Admin.	Med. Teach.	Research	Other
Total Physicians	15,270	11,447	8,276	1,978	1,193	277	189	295	90
FM/GP	610	578	487	52	39	14	11	2	5
Family Medicine	574	543	454	52	37	13	11	2	5
General Practice	36	35	33		2	1			
Medical Specialties	5,475	5,089	3,668	950	471	106	94	164	22
Allergy and Immunology	70	60	56	4		1		7	2
Cardiovascular Disease	403	387	306	53	28	5	4	6	1
Dermatology	191	185	160	17	8			5	1
Gastroenterology	247	232	192	27	13	3	7	5	
Internal Medicine	3,172	2,921	1,987	637	297	77	55	106	13
Pediatric Cardiology	26	24	18	6		1	1		
Pediatrics	1,156	1,093	809	174	110	16	19	24	4
Pulmonary Disease	210	187	140	32	15	3	8	11	1
Surgical Specialties	2,515	2,440	1,911	396	133	27	24	16	8
Colon and Rectal Surgery	33	32	29	3				1	
General Surgery	546	524	324	150	50	6	10	4	2
Neurological Surgery	85	84	62	16	6		1		
Obstetrics & Gynecology	708	685	537	106	42	11	6	5	1
Ophthalmology	303	295	267	19	9	1	1	3	3
Orthopedic Surgery	379	370	316	45	9	3	4	1	1
Otolaryngology	150	148	120	21	7	1		1	
Plastic Surgery	101	100	84	14	2	1			
Thoracic Surgery	61	57	49	4	4	3	1		
Urology	149	145	123	18	4	1	1	1	1
Other Specialties	3,698	3,340	2,210	580	550	130	60	113	55
Aerospace Medicine	4	3	3			1			
Anatomic/Clinical Pathology	326	270	148	50	72	18	8	15	15
Anesthesiology	593	574	441	78	55	5	11	1	2
Child & Adolescent Psychiatry	183	170	122	25	23	5	2	6	
Diagnostic Radiology	458	442	299	114	29	4	5	1	6
Emergency Medicine	451	425	198	85	142	20	4	2	
Forensic Pathology	4	1	1			1			2
General Preventive Medicine	34	29	23	2	4	2	1	1	1
Medical Genetics	13	7	4	2	1	2		3	1
Neurology	223	203	147	36	20	2	2	14	2
Nuclear Medicine	26	21	15	5	1		2	3	
Occupational Medicine	44	26	19		7	8	3	3	4
Other Specialty	86	38	23	8	7	17	2	18	11
Physical Medicine and Rehabilitation	90	83	73	2	8	4	1		2
Psychiatry	865	776	530	90	156	35	14	35	5
Public Health and General Preventive Medicine	10	2	2			3		3	2
Radiation Oncology	63	59	42	10	7	1		3	
Radiology	125	116	95	7	14	1	4	2	2
Transplant Surgery	3	3	3						
Unspecified	97	92	22	66	4	1	1	3	
Inactive	1,891								
Not Classified	1,081								

Note: Excludes Address Unknown.

Subspecialties in this table are condensed into major specialties. See Appendix A.

Table 3.7

Physicians by State, Self-Designated Specialty, and Activity, 2010, continued
Delaware

		Patient Care				Other Professional Activity			
				Hospital Based					
Specialty	Total Physicians	Total Patient Care	Office Based	Resid./ Fellows	Phys. Staff	Admin.	Med. Teach.	Research	Other
Total Physicians	2,550	1,988	1,512	261	215	49	14	24	9
FM/GP	260	248	196	31	21	7	4	1	
Family Medicine	246	235	184	31	20	7	3	1	
General Practice	14	13	12		1		1		
Medical Specialties	786	748	587	83	78	17	3	14	4
Allergy and Immunology	11	10	8	2				1	
Cardiovascular Disease	65	63	50	9	4	1	1		
Dermatology	17	17	17						
Gastroenterology	35	33	30		3			2	
Internal Medicine	362	343	280	29	34	12		6	1
Pediatric Cardiology	9	8	7	1				1	
Pediatrics	259	248	172	41	35	3	2	3	3
Pulmonary Disease	28	26	23	1	2	1		1	
Surgical Specialties	414	404	336	39	29	8	2		
Colon and Rectal Surgery	4	4	4						
General Surgery	102	98	71	21	6	4			
Neurological Surgery	14	13	11		2	1			
Obstetrics & Gynecology	98	95	74	14	7	1	2		
Ophthalmology	49	48	47		1	1			
Orthopedic Surgery	61	61	56	2	3				
Otolaryngology	21	21	18		3				
Plastic Surgery	23	23	22		1				
Thoracic Surgery	16	15	10	1	4	1			
Urology	26	26	23	1	2				
Other Specialties	624	588	393	108	87	17	5	9	5
Aerospace Medicine	1	1			1				
Anatomic/Clinical Pathology	38	34	22	2	10	1	1		2
Anesthesiology	90	87	73	1	13	2	1		
Child & Adolescent Psychiatry	22	21	17		4	1			
Diagnostic Radiology	79	77	51	22	4	1			1
Emergency Medicine	115	111	62	35	14	4			
Forensic Pathology	5	4	3		1		1		
General Preventive Medicine	2	2			2				
Medical Genetics	1	1			1				
Neurology	31	31	29		2				
Nuclear Medicine	2	2	1		1				
Occupational Medicine	9	6	4		2	3			
Other Specialty	39	30	8	21	1	1		6	2
Physical Medicine and Rehabilitation	33	33	30	1	2				
Psychiatry	96	93	61	15	17	1	1	1	
Public Health and General Preventive Medicine	4					3		1	
Radiation Oncology	14	14	9	1	4				
Radiology	25	24	19		5		1		
Unspecified	18	17	4	10	3			1	
Inactive	329								
Not Classified	137								

Note: Excludes Address Unknown.

Subspecialties in this table are condensed into major specialties. See Appendix A.

Table 3.7

Physicians by State, Self-Designated Specialty, and Activity, 2010, continued
District of Columbia

		Patient Care				Other Professional Activity			
				Hospital Based					
Specialty	Total Physicians	Total Patient Care	Office Based	Resid./ Fellows	Phys. Staff	Admin.	Med. Teach.	Research	Other
Total Physicians	5,776	4,115	2,119	1,345	651	189	105	151	49
FM/GP	219	196	131	25	40	12	8	2	1
Family Medicine	195	173	115	25	33	11	8	2	1
General Practice	24	23	16		7	1			
Medical Specialties	2,015	1,799	898	616	285	68	40	89	19
Allergy and Immunology	23	13	10	1	2	2	1	7	
Cardiovascular Disease	110	90	55	20	15	7	5	8	
Dermatology	65	61	46	13	2	1	1		2
Gastroenterology	78	74	47	19	8		2	2	
Internal Medicine	1,081	967	471	341	155	38	16	49	11
Pediatric Cardiology	23	19	11	6	2	3			1
Pediatrics	559	506	231	188	87	17	12	19	5
Pulmonary Disease	76	69	27	28	14		3	4	
Surgical Specialties	953	908	462	346	100	13	20	8	4
Colon and Rectal Surgery	9	9	6	2	1				
General Surgery	282	262	88	135	39	7	9	3	1
Neurological Surgery	42	41	15	20	6		1		
Obstetrics & Gynecology	215	204	138	48	18	3	4	2	2
Ophthalmology	114	109	67	36	6	1	2	2	
Orthopedic Surgery	98	96	54	33	9		2		
Otolaryngology	66	65	26	32	7	1			
Plastic Surgery	44	42	16	20	6		2		
Thoracic Surgery	26	24	17	2	5	1			1
Urology	57	56	35	18	3			1	
Other Specialties	1,422	1,212	628	358	226	96	37	52	25
Aerospace Medicine	6	5	2		3	1			
Anatomic/Clinical Pathology	103	73	34	11	28	9	5	9	7
Anesthesiology	189	179	90	48	41	3	7		
Child & Adolescent Psychiatry	60	54	38	12	4	3	2	1	
Diagnostic Radiology	122	118	59	40	19		2	2	
Emergency Medicine	178	170	72	65	33	5	2	1	
Forensic Pathology	2	1	1						1
General Preventive Medicine	24	12	8	1	3	6		3	3
Medical Genetics	6	3			3		1	2	
Neurology	125	111	43	47	21	2	2	8	2
Nuclear Medicine	15	11	5	1	5	2	1		1
Occupational Medicine	20	5	4		1	9	1	2	3
Other Specialty	52	25	15	3	7	15	3	7	2
Physical Medicine and Rehabilitation	26	25	13	3	9	1			
Psychiatry	343	303	190	81	32	20	8	8	4
Public Health and General Preventive Medicine	30	1	1			18	2	7	2
Radiation Oncology	19	19	10	4	5				
Radiology	55	54	34	13	7		1		
Transplant Surgery	2	2	1		1				
Unspecified	45	41	8	29	4	2		2	
Inactive	501								
Not Classified	666								

Note: Excludes Address Unknown.

Subspecialties in this table are condensed into major specialties. See Appendix A.

Table 3.7

Physicians by State, Self-Designated Specialty, and Activity, 2010, continued
Florida

		Patient Care				Other Professional Activity			
				Hospital Based					
Specialty	Total Physicians	Total Patient Care	Office Based	Resid./ Fellows	Phys. Staff	Admin.	Med. Teach.	Research	Other
Total Physicians	58,026	42,785	34,882	3,709	4,194	702	457	394	276
FM/GP	5,126	4,935	4,201	306	428	98	61	8	24
Family Medicine	4,297	4,135	3,496	306	333	81	60	7	14
General Practice	829	800	705		95	17	1	1	10
Medical Specialties	17,359	16,656	13,825	1,411	1,420	238	188	223	54
Allergy and Immunology	213	206	189	8	9	2	2	3	
Cardiovascular Disease	1,644	1,590	1,420	85	85	17	13	19	5
Dermatology	788	779	696	57	26	2	2	4	1
Gastroenterology	903	878	784	48	46	5	11	9	
Internal Medicine	9,001	8,613	7,023	770	820	129	103	125	31
Pediatric Cardiology	119	115	88	13	14	1	2	1	
Pediatrics	3,990	3,810	3,060	389	361	72	51	43	14
Pulmonary Disease	701	665	565	41	59	10	4	19	3
Surgical Specialties	9,604	9,401	7,933	831	637	61	72	36	34
Colon and Rectal Surgery	109	106	89	6	11	1		1	1
General Surgery	1,951	1,902	1,424	274	204	16	14	8	11
Neurological Surgery	362	353	266	56	31	3	4	1	1
Obstetrics & Gynecology	2,308	2,240	1,961	151	128	19	35	8	6
Ophthalmology	1,217	1,200	1,080	74	46	2	4	8	3
Orthopedic Surgery	1,437	1,416	1,167	145	104	6	7	4	4
Otolaryngology	587	579	498	44	37	2	4	1	1
Plastic Surgery	615	609	561	31	17	2	1	1	2
Thoracic Surgery	311	301	266	9	26	7		2	1
Urology	707	695	621	41	33	3	3	2	4
Other Specialties	12,525	11,793	8,923	1,161	1,709	305	136	127	164
Aerospace Medicine	35	21	8		13	9	1	3	1
Anatomic/Clinical Pathology	1,003	860	633	85	142	31	18	26	68
Anesthesiology	2,691	2,640	2,128	203	309	19	20	9	3
Child & Adolescent Psychiatry	294	277	236	18	23	10	5	1	1
Diagnostic Radiology	1,526	1,491	1,110	187	194	7	11	2	15
Emergency Medicine	1,855	1,787	1,247	167	373	46	15	2	5
Forensic Pathology	63	48	36	7	5	3			12
General Preventive Medicine	127	103	64	17	22	15	2	4	3
Medical Genetics	21	13	9	1	3		4	4	
Neurology	959	918	740	115	63	9	11	17	4
Nuclear Medicine	72	68	42	8	18		1	1	2
Occupational Medicine	82	63	50		13	12	1	1	5
Other Specialty	237	149	113	8	28	45	9	19	15
Physical Medicine and Rehabilitation	406	395	331	24	40	9			2
Psychiatry	1,738	1,630	1,216	105	309	47	25	24	12
Public Health and General Preventive Medicine	50	10	9		1	31	2	6	1
Radiation Oncology	329	323	255	28	40	3	2	1	
Radiology	564	540	452	20	68	1	7	4	12
Transplant Surgery	8	6	2		4		1	1	
Unspecified	464	450	241	168	41	8	1	2	3
Vascular Medicine	1	1	1						
Inactive	10,775								
Not Classified	2,637								

Note: Excludes Address Unknown.

Subspecialties in this table are condensed into major specialties. See Appendix A.

Table 3.7

Physicians by State, Self-Designated Specialty, and Activity, 2010, continued
Georgia

		Patient Care				Other Professional Activity			
				Hospital Based					
Specialty	Total Physicians	Total Patient Care	Office Based	Resid./ Fellows	Phys. Staff	Admin.	Med. Teach.	Research	Other
Total Physicians	24,496	19,195	15,387	2,013	1,795	354	266	320	151
FM/GP	2,454	2,363	1,962	197	204	38	42	4	7
Family Medicine	2,286	2,203	1,831	197	175	33	41	4	5
General Practice	168	160	131		29	5	1		2
Medical Specialties	7,711	7,298	5,913	740	645	122	111	139	41
Allergy and Immunology	90	84	77	5	2		3	3	
Cardiovascular Disease	553	537	434	62	41	1	8	7	
Dermatology	290	286	251	26	9	2	1	1	
Gastroenterology	339	333	297	20	16	1	2	2	1
Internal Medicine	4,056	3,813	3,031	398	384	77	66	81	19
Pediatric Cardiology	55	52	37	10	5			3	
Pediatrics	2,066	1,948	1,582	198	168	38	25	35	20
Pulmonary Disease	262	245	204	21	20	3	6	7	1
Surgical Specialties	4,526	4,432	3,725	451	256	37	30	12	15
Colon and Rectal Surgery	42	42	38	2	2				
General Surgery	1,043	1,008	758	175	75	12	13	5	5
Neurological Surgery	139	136	103	18	15	1			2
Obstetrics & Gynecology	1,359	1,324	1,175	89	60	17	10	4	4
Ophthalmology	419	411	357	33	21	4	1	2	1
Orthopedic Surgery	653	648	539	73	36	2	2		1
Otolaryngology	306	303	262	28	13		1	1	1
Plastic Surgery	190	189	175	4	10		1		
Thoracic Surgery	112	110	90	12	8	1			1
Urology	263	261	228	17	16		2		
Other Specialties	5,595	5,102	3,787	625	690	157	83	165	88
Aerospace Medicine	13	6	3		3	6		1	
Anatomic/Clinical Pathology	460	393	277	65	51	13	9	13	32
Anesthesiology	999	982	800	87	95	7	8		2
Child & Adolescent Psychiatry	142	135	111	12	12	1	6		
Diagnostic Radiology	603	592	444	80	68	1	5	1	4
Emergency Medicine	861	830	603	76	151	17	8	4	2
Forensic Pathology	23	17	13	2	2	1			5
General Preventive Medicine	151	107	62	10	35	9	4	25	6
Medical Genetics	12	9	6		3		2	1	
Neurology	353	326	273	29	24	5	2	19	1
Nuclear Medicine	22	18	11	3	4		2	1	1
Occupational Medicine	65	45	36		9	11	1	3	5
Other Specialty	114	72	45	11	16	16	4	11	11
Physical Medicine and Rehabilitation	180	174	131	23	20	1	3	2	
Psychiatry	879	826	616	72	138	23	14	13	3
Public Health and General Preventive Medicine	140	17	7		10	42	7	64	10
Radiation Oncology	120	118	100	14	4		1	1	
Radiology	259	242	200	9	33	1	7	3	6
Transplant Surgery	1	1	1						
Unspecified	197	191	48	132	11	3		3	
Vascular Medicine	1	1			1				
Inactive	2,888								
Not Classified	1,322								

Note: Excludes Address Unknown.

Subspecialties in this table are condensed into major specialties. See Appendix A.

Table 3.7

Physicians by State, Self-Designated Specialty, and Activity, 2010, continued
Hawaii

		Patient Care				Other Professional Activity			
				Hospital Based					
Specialty	Total Physicians	Total Patient Care	Office Based	Resid./ Fellows	Phys. Staff	Admin.	Med. Teach.	Research	Other
Total Physicians	4,866	3,668	2,850	349	469	76	50	45	35
FM/GP	440	421	347	22	52	8	5	2	4
Family Medicine	365	350	282	22	46	6	4	2	3
General Practice	75	71	65		6	2	1		1
Medical Specialties	1,434	1,362	1,087	99	176	27	16	20	9
Allergy and Immunology	19	17	14		3		1	1	
Cardiovascular Disease	69	68	54	3	11			1	
Dermatology	54	52	45	1	6	1		1	
Gastroenterology	46	45	43		2		1		
Internal Medicine	809	771	614	66	91	15	10	8	5
Pediatric Cardiology	5	4	3		1			1	
Pediatrics	393	371	287	28	56	9	4	6	3
Pulmonary Disease	39	34	27	1	6	2		2	1
Surgical Specialties	804	778	601	108	69	7	12	3	4
Colon and Rectal Surgery	4	4	4						
General Surgery	178	171	106	46	19	4	2	1	
Neurological Surgery	15	13	11	1	1			1	1
Obstetrics & Gynecology	240	227	183	27	17		10	1	2
Ophthalmology	102	101	98		3	1			
Orthopedic Surgery	124	122	85	23	14	1			1
Otolaryngology	45	45	33	6	6				
Plastic Surgery	30	30	28		2				
Thoracic Surgery	18	18	16		2				
Urology	48	47	37	5	5	1			
Other Specialties	1,196	1,107	815	120	172	34	17	20	18
Aerospace Medicine	6	4	2		2	2			
Anatomic/Clinical Pathology	83	72	52	12	8	3		2	6
Anesthesiology	156	154	134	2	18	1	1		
Child & Adolescent Psychiatry	65	62	52	4	6	1	2		
Diagnostic Radiology	120	118	88	12	18			1	1
Emergency Medicine	199	190	151	1	38	8	1		
Forensic Pathology	3					1			2
General Preventive Medicine	30	23	16		7	2		3	2
Medical Genetics	1	1			1				
Neurology	51	50	35	3	12			1	
Nuclear Medicine	15	13	10		3		1	1	
Occupational Medicine	18	14	12		2	3			1
Other Specialty	40	26	16	6	4	5	1	7	1
Physical Medicine and Rehabilitation	40	38	33	2	3	1			1
Psychiatry	249	232	156	39	37	6	7	1	3
Public Health and General Preventive Medicine	10	3	2		1		3	3	1
Radiation Oncology	16	16	13		3				
Radiology	43	41	33		8		1	1	
Unspecified	51	50	10	39	1	1			
Inactive	759								
Not Classified	233								

Note: Excludes Address Unknown.

Subspecialties in this table are condensed into major specialties. See Appendix A.

Table 3.7

Physicians by State, Self-Designated Specialty, and Activity, 2010, continued
Idaho

		Patient Care				Other Professional Activity			
				Hospital Based					
Specialty	Total Physicians	Total Patient Care	Office Based	Resid./ Fellows	Phys. Staff	Admin.	Med. Teach.	Research	Other
Total Physicians	3,215	2,538	2,163	84	291	27	20	10	7
FM/GP	608	595	498	48	49	2	11		
Family Medicine	576	563	469	48	46	2	11		
General Practice	32	32	29		3				
Medical Specialties	639	613	512	26	75	11	6	6	3
Allergy and Immunology	13	13	13						
Cardiovascular Disease	49	48	43		5			1	
Dermatology	35	35	34		1				
Gastroenterology	38	35	34		1	1		1	1
Internal Medicine	323	310	240	23	47	7	3	2	1
Pediatric Cardiology	4	4	3		1				
Pediatrics	141	134	119	3	12	3	3		1
Pulmonary Disease	36	34	26		8			2	
Surgical Specialties	617	612	565	1	46	2	1	1	1
Colon and Rectal Surgery	4	4	4						
General Surgery	142	141	122	1	18	1			
Neurological Surgery	28	28	28						
Obstetrics & Gynecology	145	143	131		12	1		1	
Ophthalmology	59	59	57		2				
Orthopedic Surgery	126	125	116		9				1
Otolaryngology	40	39	39				1		
Plastic Surgery	21	21	21						
Thoracic Surgery	9	9	8		1				
Urology	43	43	39		4				
Other Specialties	738	718	588	9	121	12	2	3	3
Aerospace Medicine	3	1			1	2			
Anatomic/Clinical Pathology	41	39	32		7	1		1	
Anesthesiology	108	108	96	2	10				
Child & Adolescent Psychiatry	17	17	15		2				
Diagnostic Radiology	156	154	129		25		1		1
Emergency Medicine	166	165	125	1	39	1			
Forensic Pathology	2	2	2						
General Preventive Medicine	4	3	2		1	1			
Neurology	34	32	30		2			1	1
Nuclear Medicine	1	1	1						
Occupational Medicine	9	6	4		2	2			1
Other Specialty	12	10	8	2		2			
Physical Medicine and Rehabilitation	31	31	29		2				
Psychiatry	75	70	47		23	3	1	1	
Public Health and General Preventive Medicine	1	1	1						
Radiation Oncology	17	17	16		1				
Radiology	46	46	41		5				
Unspecified	15	15	10	4	1				
Inactive	526								
Not Classified	87								

Note: Excludes Address Unknown.

Subspecialties in this table are condensed into major specialties. See Appendix A.

Table 3.7

Physicians by State, Self-Designated Specialty, and Activity, 2010, continued
Illinois

		Patient Care				Other Professional Activity			
				Hospital Based					
Specialty	Total Physicians	Total Patient Care	Office Based	Resid./ Fellows	Phys. Staff	Admin.	Med. Teach.	Research	Other
Total Physicians	41,724	32,274	23,508	5,763	3,003	553	396	435	188
FM/GP	4,023	3,893	3,104	511	278	51	55	9	15
Family Medicine	3,691	3,578	2,832	511	235	42	54	6	11
General Practice	332	315	272		43	9	1	3	4
Medical Specialties	13,604	12,915	9,482	2,417	1,016	237	153	255	44
Allergy and Immunology	208	194	168	16	10	4	1	9	
Cardiovascular Disease	973	922	742	127	53	13	8	29	1
Dermatology	464	455	361	72	22	2	4	2	1
Gastroenterology	528	503	413	60	30	4	9	10	2
Internal Medicine	7,691	7,275	5,222	1,459	594	158	84	146	28
Pediatric Cardiology	90	85	58	18	9	1	1	2	1
Pediatrics	3,207	3,066	2,200	600	266	44	39	48	10
Pulmonary Disease	443	415	318	65	32	11	7	9	1
Surgical Specialties	6,555	6,405	4,910	1,074	421	45	53	34	18
Colon and Rectal Surgery	55	53	40	4	9	1	1		
General Surgery	1,407	1,362	917	323	122	14	15	10	6
Neurological Surgery	258	254	162	64	28	2	1		1
Obstetrics & Gynecology	1,826	1,779	1,443	218	118	16	15	12	4
Ophthalmology	743	728	632	62	34	1	7	5	2
Orthopedic Surgery	971	957	726	194	37	1	8	3	2
Otolaryngology	393	389	288	79	22	2	1		1
Plastic Surgery	275	269	209	47	13		2	2	2
Thoracic Surgery	180	175	149	13	13	1	2	2	
Urology	447	439	344	70	25	7	1		
Other Specialties	9,664	9,061	6,012	1,761	1,288	220	135	137	111
Aerospace Medicine	3					3			
Anatomic/Clinical Pathology	874	759	501	129	129	28	26	27	34
Anesthesiology	1,900	1,863	1,292	338	233	6	22	5	4
Child & Adolescent Psychiatry	238	223	176	29	18	6	5	2	2
Diagnostic Radiology	1,043	1,016	675	216	125	5	9	2	11
Emergency Medicine	1,465	1,406	836	269	301	36	15	6	2
Forensic Pathology	25	19	17	1	1		2		4
General Preventive Medicine	55	47	37	7	3	2		3	3
Medical Genetics	17	16	9	3	4			1	
Neurology	665	625	433	121	71	7	9	22	2
Nuclear Medicine	48	44	26	5	13		1		3
Occupational Medicine	111	84	71		13	15	2	1	9
Other Specialty	225	141	89	36	16	35	10	30	9
Physical Medicine and Rehabilitation	470	453	280	105	68	9	2	3	3
Psychiatry	1,467	1,369	1,017	158	194	46	23	20	9
Public Health and General Preventive Medicine	28	5	4		1	14	1	5	3
Radiation Oncology	196	193	145	27	21		1	2	
Radiology	370	349	264	25	60	4	5	4	8
Transplant Surgery	7	6	4		2			1	
Unspecified	454	440	134	292	14	4	2	3	5
Vascular Medicine	3	3	2		1				
Inactive	4,630								
Not Classified	3,248								

Note: Excludes Address Unknown.

Subspecialties in this table are condensed into major specialties. See Appendix A.

Table 3.7

Physicians by State, Self-Designated Specialty, and Activity, 2010, continued
Indiana

		Patient Care				Other Professional Activity			
				Hospital Based					
Specialty	Total Physicians	Total Patient Care	Office Based	Resid./ Fellows	Phys. Staff	Admin.	Med. Teach.	Research	Other
Total Physicians	15,898	12,860	10,221	1,358	1,281	199	124	171	85
FM/GP	2,436	2,359	1,924	214	221	37	32	1	7
Family Medicine	2,306	2,234	1,814	214	206	34	32	1	5
General Practice	130	125	110		15	3			2
Medical Specialties	4,471	4,235	3,297	483	455	58	40	121	17
Allergy and Immunology	52	49	48		1	1		2	
Cardiovascular Disease	406	390	342	25	23	1	4	8	3
Dermatology	152	151	126	17	8		1		
Gastroenterology	192	187	164	14	9	1		4	
Internal Medicine	2,241	2,089	1,633	230	226	37	25	80	10
Pediatric Cardiology	29	29	17	6	6				
Pediatrics	1,209	1,160	822	176	162	16	7	23	3
Pulmonary Disease	190	180	145	15	20	2	3	4	1
Surgical Specialties	2,687	2,637	2,245	249	143	18	20	8	4
Colon and Rectal Surgery	33	32	31	1			1		
General Surgery	585	573	447	87	39	2	5	4	1
Neurological Surgery	98	98	76	16	6				
Obstetrics & Gynecology	700	673	568	54	51	14	10	1	2
Ophthalmology	273	272	248	21	3	1			
Orthopedic Surgery	450	447	394	33	20		1	2	
Otolaryngology	177	175	151	18	6		1		1
Plastic Surgery	102	102	93	4	5				
Thoracic Surgery	97	94	85	1	8	1	1	1	
Urology	172	171	152	14	5		1		
Other Specialties	3,845	3,629	2,755	412	462	86	32	41	57
Aerospace Medicine	3	2	2						1
Anatomic/Clinical Pathology	336	283	195	38	50	18	5	10	20
Anesthesiology	996	982	794	81	107	5	5	2	2
Child & Adolescent Psychiatry	88	83	64	6	13	1	2	1	1
Diagnostic Radiology	459	449	354	70	25	2	2	1	5
Emergency Medicine	575	553	405	51	97	17	4		1
Forensic Pathology	7	5	4		1				2
General Preventive Medicine	9	8	7		1			1	
Medical Genetics	6	6	4	2					
Neurology	269	253	209	27	17	3	5	5	3
Nuclear Medicine	17	14	13	1		1			2
Occupational Medicine	56	44	33		11	10			2
Other Specialty	91	68	34	28	6	7	3	9	4
Physical Medicine and Rehabilitation	130	127	101	12	14	1		1	1
Psychiatry	433	397	290	18	89	13	4	10	9
Public Health and General Preventive Medicine	5					5			
Radiation Oncology	99	98	78	8	12			1	
Radiology	171	167	142	11	14	1	1		2
Transplant Surgery	5	5	5						
Unspecified	89	84	20	59	5	2	1		2
Vascular Medicine	1	1	1						
Inactive	1,884								
Not Classified	575								

Note: Excludes Address Unknown.

Subspecialties in this table are condensed into major specialties. See Appendix A.

Table 3.7

Physicians by State, Self-Designated Specialty, and Activity, 2010, continued
Iowa

		Patient Care				Other Professional Activity			
				Hospital Based					
Specialty	Total Physicians	Total Patient Care	Office Based	Resid./ Fellows	Phys. Staff	Admin.	Med. Teach.	Research	Other
Total Physicians	6,677	5,118	3,803	709	606	58	94	115	19
FM/GP	1,172	1,128	911	118	99	12	27	2	3
Family Medicine	1,126	1,086	871	118	97	9	27	2	2
General Practice	46	42	40		2	3			1
Medical Specialties	1,599	1,477	1,084	220	173	18	30	71	3
Allergy and Immunology	28	25	20	3	2	1		2	
Cardiovascular Disease	141	129	107	15	7	1	2	9	
Dermatology	78	78	58	13	7				
Gastroenterology	80	75	59	9	7		1	4	
Internal Medicine	786	719	523	111	85	11	15	40	1
Pediatric Cardiology	20	18	9	5	4		1	1	
Pediatrics	391	366	262	55	49	5	8	10	2
Pulmonary Disease	75	67	46	9	12		3	5	
Surgical Specialties	1,147	1,120	871	136	113	4	13	8	2
Colon and Rectal Surgery	4	4	4						
General Surgery	274	266	201	26	39	1	4	1	2
Neurological Surgery	37	37	18	13	6				
Obstetrics & Gynecology	223	214	170	18	26	2	5	2	
Ophthalmology	156	149	124	18	7	1	3	3	
Orthopedic Surgery	191	189	157	18	14			2	
Otolaryngology	104	104	71	25	8				
Plastic Surgery	32	31	29		2		1		
Thoracic Surgery	40	40	31	3	6				
Urology	86	86	66	15	5				
Other Specialties	1,486	1,393	937	235	221	24	24	34	11
Aerospace Medicine	1	1	1						
Anatomic/Clinical Pathology	169	149	113	23	13	3	3	8	6
Anesthesiology	310	301	214	51	36		7	2	
Child & Adolescent Psychiatry	41	39	31	5	3	1	1		
Diagnostic Radiology	174	170	132	17	21	1	1		2
Emergency Medicine	141	138	74	17	47	3			
Forensic Pathology	6	6	4		2				
General Preventive Medicine	16	13	9	3	1	1		2	
Medical Genetics	3	3	1	1	1				
Neurology	116	109	67	24	18	1	1	4	1
Nuclear Medicine	16	14	11		3	1	1		
Occupational Medicine	20	19	14		5			1	
Other Specialty	50	39	20	14	5	8	1	1	1
Physical Medicine and Rehabilitation	40	39	31	3	5	1			
Psychiatry	199	178	121	12	45	4	6	11	
Public Health and General Preventive Medicine	5	1	1				1	2	1
Radiation Oncology	43	43	31	7	5				
Radiology	56	54	43	4	7		2		
Unspecified	80	77	19	54	4			3	
Inactive	907								
Not Classified	366								

Note: Excludes Address Unknown.

Subspecialties in this table are condensed into major specialties. See Appendix A.

Table 3.7

Physicians by State, Self-Designated Specialty, and Activity, 2010, continued
Kansas

		Patient Care				Other Professional Activity			
				Hospital Based					
Specialty	Total Physicians	Total Patient Care	Office Based	Resid./ Fellows	Phys. Staff	Admin.	Med. Teach.	Research	Other
Total Physicians	7,558	5,884	4,565	696	623	95	90	53	28
FM/GP	1,179	1,119	925	98	96	24	31	3	2
Family Medicine	1,117	1,060	882	98	80	21	31	3	2
General Practice	62	59	43		16	3			
Medical Specialties	1,882	1,798	1,391	194	213	24	31	21	8
Allergy and Immunology	33	32	25	2	5			1	
Cardiovascular Disease	179	171	148	9	14		6	2	
Dermatology	69	68	54	10	4		1		
Gastroenterology	76	75	64	10	1				1
Internal Medicine	941	892	680	103	109	14	18	15	2
Pediatric Cardiology	9	9	7		2				
Pediatrics	490	469	348	49	72	7	6	3	5
Pulmonary Disease	85	82	65	11	6	3			
Surgical Specialties	1,322	1,299	1,046	165	88	6	8	6	3
Colon and Rectal Surgery	11	11	10		1				
General Surgery	303	294	210	52	32	3	3	2	1
Neurological Surgery	40	39	34	4	1	1			
Obstetrics & Gynecology	299	296	249	29	18		2	1	
Ophthalmology	141	137	129	2	6	2	1	1	
Orthopedic Surgery	239	238	184	40	14				1
Otolaryngology	92	91	69	18	4			1	
Plastic Surgery	64	62	53	7	2		1		1
Thoracic Surgery	41	40	37		3			1	
Urology	92	91	71	13	7		1		
Other Specialties	1,767	1,668	1,203	239	226	41	20	23	15
Aerospace Medicine	4	2	1		1	2			
Anatomic/Clinical Pathology	156	140	103	14	23	5	2	4	5
Anesthesiology	341	335	270	43	22	1	4		1
Child & Adolescent Psychiatry	60	58	43	5	10	2			
Diagnostic Radiology	254	247	186	40	21	1	2		4
Emergency Medicine	192	190	135	8	47	1	1		
Forensic Pathology	4	3	3						1
General Preventive Medicine	7	5	4		1			2	
Medical Genetics	2	1			1				1
Neurology	118	114	79	13	22	2	1	1	
Nuclear Medicine	4	4	1		3				
Occupational Medicine	17	15	11		4				2
Other Specialty	45	28	20	4	4	8	1	8	
Physical Medicine and Rehabilitation	64	64	49	8	7				
Psychiatry	301	273	185	45	43	14	7	6	1
Public Health and General Preventive Medicine	2					2			
Radiation Oncology	40	39	30	4	5			1	
Radiology	69	66	55	2	9	1	2		
Unspecified	87	84	28	53	3	2		1	
Inactive	1,053								
Not Classified	355								

Note: Excludes Address Unknown.

Subspecialties in this table are condensed into major specialties. See Appendix A.

Table 3.7

Physicians by State, Self-Designated Specialty, and Activity, 2010, continued
Kentucky

		Patient Care				Other Professional Activity			
				Hospital Based					
Specialty	Total Physicians	Total Patient Care	Office Based	Resid./ Fellows	Phys. Staff	Admin.	Med. Teach.	Research	Other
Total Physicians	11,417	9,182	7,230	1,136	816	123	119	79	44
FM/GP	1,357	1,309	1,121	88	100	23	19	3	3
Family Medicine	1,252	1,204	1,024	88	92	23	19	3	3
General Practice	105	105	97		8				
Medical Specialties	3,375	3,245	2,569	410	266	32	47	44	7
Allergy and Immunology	68	68	64	1	3				
Cardiovascular Disease	283	275	215	43	17	1	5	2	
Dermatology	136	136	125	10	1				
Gastroenterology	142	135	114	17	4		3	4	
Internal Medicine	1,637	1,569	1,226	189	154	19	20	25	4
Pediatric Cardiology	21	19	15		4			2	
Pediatrics	934	897	699	132	66	11	17	6	3
Pulmonary Disease	154	146	111	18	17	1	2	5	
Surgical Specialties	2,079	2,031	1,655	245	131	15	19	8	6
Colon and Rectal Surgery	22	21	17	1	3		1		
General Surgery	547	531	382	102	47	3	9	4	
Neurological Surgery	68	66	52	9	5		2		
Obstetrics & Gynecology	510	496	418	48	30	9	3	2	
Ophthalmology	195	193	174	14	5	1		1	
Orthopedic Surgery	324	318	253	46	19		1		5
Otolaryngology	122	121	106	9	6		1		
Plastic Surgery	95	93	79	12	2		2		
Thoracic Surgery	74	71	61	2	8	1		1	1
Urology	122	121	113	2	6	1			
Other Specialties	2,736	2,597	1,885	393	319	53	34	24	28
Aerospace Medicine	6	4	3		1	2			
Anatomic/Clinical Pathology	224	191	124	27	40	7	8	5	13
Anesthesiology	559	545	421	65	59	4	10		
Child & Adolescent Psychiatry	78	73	62	8	3		3	1	1
Diagnostic Radiology	340	335	260	39	36	1	2		2
Emergency Medicine	437	432	310	44	78	3	1	1	
Forensic Pathology	16	10	6	2	2				6
General Preventive Medicine	11	10	5	3	2	1			
Medical Genetics	6	5	5			1			
Neurology	163	152	114	24	14	3	2	6	
Nuclear Medicine	12	11	9		2			1	
Occupational Medicine	27	22	21		1	3		2	
Other Specialty	61	46	33	10	3	12	1	2	
Physical Medicine and Rehabilitation	102	100	75	18	7	2			
Psychiatry	387	368	273	50	45	8	3	5	3
Public Health and General Preventive Medicine	8	3	2		1	2	1	1	1
Radiation Oncology	66	64	45	12	7	2			
Radiology	84	80	66		14		2		2
Transplant Surgery	2	2	2						
Unspecified	147	144	49	91	4	2	1		
Inactive	1,284								
Not Classified	586								

Note: Excludes Address Unknown.

Subspecialties in this table are condensed into major specialties. See Appendix A.

Table 3.7

Physicians by State, Self-Designated Specialty, and Activity, 2010, continued
Louisiana

		Patient Care				Other Professional Activity			
				Hospital Based					
Specialty	Total Physicians	Total Patient Care	Office Based	Resid./ Fellows	Phys. Staff	Admin.	Med. Teach.	Research	Other
Total Physicians	13,587	10,946	7,937	1,838	1,171	130	181	84	32
FM/GP	1,400	1,363	1,074	162	127	9	23	4	1
Family Medicine	1,252	1,217	949	162	106	8	23	4	
General Practice	148	146	125		21	1			1
Medical Specialties	4,185	3,994	2,846	724	424	50	84	53	4
Allergy and Immunology	66	64	54	10			2		
Cardiovascular Disease	373	360	265	72	23	2	6	5	
Dermatology	179	176	142	28	6		3		
Gastroenterology	180	178	147	25	6	1		1	
Internal Medicine	2,054	1,949	1,302	403	244	30	42	31	2
Pediatric Cardiology	28	26	19	2	5	2			
Pediatrics	1,123	1,076	799	162	115	14	20	12	1
Pulmonary Disease	182	165	118	22	25	1	11	4	1
Surgical Specialties	2,830	2,765	2,118	457	190	17	37	7	4
Colon and Rectal Surgery	31	29	23	3	3		2		
General Surgery	615	597	391	157	49	6	8	2	2
Neurological Surgery	109	106	75	23	8	1	1	1	
Obstetrics & Gynecology	737	717	567	97	53	7	11	2	
Ophthalmology	316	307	249	38	20	1	6	2	
Orthopedic Surgery	419	413	319	71	23		5		1
Otolaryngology	238	236	180	43	13	1	1		
Plastic Surgery	93	91	81	8	2		2		
Thoracic Surgery	74	74	68	1	5				
Urology	198	195	165	16	14	1	1		1
Other Specialties	2,958	2,824	1,899	495	430	54	37	20	23
Aerospace Medicine	1					1			
Anatomic/Clinical Pathology	256	225	152	32	41	9	9	3	10
Anesthesiology	541	536	365	80	91	2	2	1	
Child & Adolescent Psychiatry	76	69	48	14	7	3	2	2	
Diagnostic Radiology	360	351	235	63	53	1	5		3
Emergency Medicine	548	534	327	103	104	9	4		1
Forensic Pathology	8	6	4		2			1	1
General Preventive Medicine	22	22	17	3	2				
Medical Genetics	7	6	6				1		
Neurology	203	196	139	38	19		4	3	
Nuclear Medicine	14	12	7	1	4	2			
Occupational Medicine	34	30	25		5	3	1		
Other Specialty	74	61	31	26	4	4	3	4	2
Physical Medicine and Rehabilitation	124	122	92	19	11	1	1		
Psychiatry	449	428	294	77	57	14	5	1	1
Public Health and General Preventive Medicine	10	2			2	4		4	
Radiation Oncology	52	52	46		6				
Radiology	101	95	78		17			1	5
Transplant Surgery	4	4	4						
Unspecified	74	73	29	39	5	1			
Inactive	1,396								
Not Classified	818								

Note: Excludes Address Unknown.

Subspecialties in this table are condensed into major specialties. See Appendix A.

Table 3.7

Physicians by State, Self-Designated Specialty, and Activity, 2010, continued
Maine

		Patient Care				Other Professional Activity			
				Hospital Based					
Specialty	Total Physicians	Total Patient Care	Office Based	Resid./ Fellows	Phys. Staff	Admin.	Med. Teach.	Research	Other
Total Physicians	4,426	3,337	2,559	258	520	82	46	30	37
FM/GP	645	611	488	59	64	14	14	3	3
Family Medicine	625	592	471	59	62	13	14	3	3
General Practice	20	19	17		2	1			
Medical Specialties	1,154	1,089	872	74	143	22	15	13	15
Allergy and Immunology	10	9	8		1			1	
Cardiovascular Disease	90	85	73	6	6		3	1	1
Dermatology	23	23	22		1				
Gastroenterology	44	42	37	1	4	1		1	
Internal Medicine	644	608	480	38	90	13	7	6	10
Pediatric Cardiology	10	10	6	2	2				
Pediatrics	272	257	202	26	29	6	2	3	4
Pulmonary Disease	61	55	44	1	10	2	3	1	
Surgical Specialties	706	688	550	38	100	7	7	3	1
Colon and Rectal Surgery	3	3	3						
General Surgery	199	197	139	22	36	1	1		
Neurological Surgery	22	21	18		3			1	
Obstetrics & Gynecology	164	158	122	14	22	2	4		
Ophthalmology	72	70	65		5		2		
Orthopedic Surgery	126	123	104	1	18	1		1	1
Otolaryngology	34	34	29		5				
Plastic Surgery	16	16	16						
Thoracic Surgery	25	22	17		5	2		1	
Urology	45	44	37	1	6	1			
Other Specialties	1,027	949	649	87	213	39	10	11	18
Anatomic/Clinical Pathology	57	50	45		5		1	3	3
Anesthesiology	180	176	135	17	24	2	1	1	
Child & Adolescent Psychiatry	50	44	34	4	6	2	1	3	
Diagnostic Radiology	104	102	65	18	19				2
Emergency Medicine	198	188	92	25	71	8	1		1
Forensic Pathology	2								2
General Preventive Medicine	8	6	3		3	2			
Medical Genetics	2	1			1			1	
Neurology	59	53	44		9	2	1		3
Nuclear Medicine	1	1	1						
Occupational Medicine	15	14	12		2				1
Other Specialty	24	11	9		2	9		2	2
Physical Medicine and Rehabilitation	35	30	19	2	9	2	2		1
Psychiatry	213	200	130	18	52	9	1	1	2
Public Health and General Preventive Medicine	6	1	1			3	1		1
Radiation Oncology	13	13	10		3				
Radiology	37	36	31	1	4		1		
Unspecified	23	23	18	2	3				
Inactive	741								
Not Classified	153								

Note: Excludes Address Unknown.

Subspecialties in this table are condensed into major specialties. See Appendix A.

Table 3.7

Physicians by State, Self-Designated Specialty, and Activity, 2010, continued
Maryland

		Patient Care				Other Professional Activity			
				Hospital Based					
Specialty	Total Physicians	Total Patient Care	Office Based	Resid./ Fellows	Phys. Staff	Admin.	Med. Teach.	Research	Other
Total Physicians	27,334	19,430	13,717	2,894	2,819	699	306	1,182	202
FM/GP	1,356	1,272	1,062	69	141	41	19	15	9
Family Medicine	1,218	1,143	953	69	121	38	19	12	6
General Practice	138	129	109		20	3		3	3
Medical Specialties	9,363	8,204	5,903	1,231	1,070	277	149	649	84
Allergy and Immunology	202	141	112	13	16	4	3	52	2
Cardiovascular Disease	619	560	451	59	50	11	11	34	3
Dermatology	291	276	224	26	26	2	4	6	3
Gastroenterology	362	339	275	37	27	4	3	15	1
Internal Medicine	5,270	4,573	3,192	790	591	176	82	396	43
Pediatric Cardiology	39	35	16	9	10	1	1	2	
Pediatrics	2,253	1,987	1,427	252	308	74	38	123	31
Pulmonary Disease	327	293	206	45	42	5	7	21	1
Surgical Specialties	4,276	4,089	2,955	651	483	59	41	65	22
Colon and Rectal Surgery	29	27	26		1			1	1
General Surgery	945	892	519	240	133	14	16	18	5
Neurological Surgery	166	159	100	40	19	2	1	3	1
Obstetrics & Gynecology	1,175	1,117	870	120	127	23	14	12	9
Ophthalmology	538	509	414	45	50	4	2	21	2
Orthopedic Surgery	627	616	447	113	56	7	2	2	
Otolaryngology	252	248	174	39	35	1	1	1	1
Plastic Surgery	191	185	153	19	13	3		2	1
Thoracic Surgery	105	98	66	10	22	1	3	2	1
Urology	248	238	186	25	27	4	2	3	1
Other Specialties	6,824	5,865	3,797	943	1,125	322	97	453	87
Aerospace Medicine	22	13	8		5	8			1
Anatomic/Clinical Pathology	602	479	259	93	127	21	12	68	22
Anesthesiology	1,096	1,059	753	100	206	7	12	17	1
Child & Adolescent Psychiatry	261	243	196	15	32	12	3	3	
Diagnostic Radiology	607	583	392	100	91	7	5	7	5
Emergency Medicine	721	686	465	59	162	18	8	5	4
Forensic Pathology	21	16	10	1	5			1	4
General Preventive Medicine	208	141	87	34	20	24	7	29	7
Medical Genetics	34	21	9	9	3	2		10	1
Neurology	498	398	267	62	69	13	8	76	3
Nuclear Medicine	64	54	29	15	10	5		5	
Occupational Medicine	69	29	19		10	23	1	8	8
Other Specialty	259	102	47	28	27	39	2	109	7
Physical Medicine and Rehabilitation	236	223	143	42	38	4	2	6	1
Psychiatry	1,297	1,140	808	121	211	69	22	51	15
Public Health and General Preventive Medicine	124	12	10		2	60	4	43	5
Radiation Oncology	122	113	75	15	23	4	1	2	2
Radiology	221	203	136	25	42	2	9	6	1
Transplant Surgery	4	3	2		1	1			
Unspecified	358	347	82	224	41	3	1	7	
Inactive	3,170								
Not Classified	2,345								

Note: Excludes Address Unknown.

Subspecialties in this table are condensed into major specialties. See Appendix A.

Table 3.7

Physicians by State, Self-Designated Specialty, and Activity, 2010, continued
Massachusetts

		Patient Care				Other Professional Activity			
				Hospital Based					
Specialty	Total Physicians	Total Patient Care	Office Based	Resid./ Fellows	Phys. Staff	Admin.	Med. Teach.	Research	Other
Total Physicians	35,334	25,842	16,945	5,266	3,631	577	307	1,147	205
FM/GP	1,403	1,337	1,123	118	96	29	22	4	11
Family Medicine	1,298	1,245	1,042	118	85	23	21	1	8
General Practice	105	92	81		11	6	1	3	3
Medical Specialties	12,702	11,511	7,726	2,305	1,480	245	138	738	70
Allergy and Immunology	158	125	101	16	8	4	1	28	
Cardiovascular Disease	918	826	545	170	111	14	14	55	9
Dermatology	395	377	293	57	27	5	1	12	
Gastroenterology	501	459	336	77	46	3	6	33	
Internal Medicine	7,306	6,547	4,371	1,315	861	166	85	464	44
Pediatric Cardiology	101	100	47	38	15		1		
Pediatrics	2,901	2,705	1,797	557	351	43	27	111	15
Pulmonary Disease	422	372	236	75	61	10	3	35	2
Surgical Specialties	4,753	4,595	3,169	928	498	46	31	58	23
Colon and Rectal Surgery	39	37	29	3	5		2		
General Surgery	1,178	1,124	602	377	145	17	8	24	5
Neurological Surgery	165	162	100	41	21			3	
Obstetrics & Gynecology	1,139	1,099	845	144	110	15	11	9	5
Ophthalmology	555	546	438	65	43	1	1	6	1
Orthopedic Surgery	745	722	503	159	60	2	5	7	9
Otolaryngology	279	274	208	28	38	2	2	1	
Plastic Surgery	191	186	136	36	14	1	2		2
Thoracic Surgery	149	138	88	20	30	3		7	1
Urology	313	307	220	55	32	5		1	
Other Specialties	9,220	8,399	4,927	1,915	1,557	257	116	347	101
Aerospace Medicine	5	2	2			2		1	
Anatomic/Clinical Pathology	870	746	394	202	150	31	12	53	28
Anesthesiology	1,455	1,399	832	355	212	10	27	17	2
Child & Adolescent Psychiatry	368	345	257	42	46	8	3	11	1
Diagnostic Radiology	947	917	515	271	131	4	9	12	5
Emergency Medicine	1,088	1,042	534	226	282	33	8	5	
Forensic Pathology	9	5	5				1		3
General Preventive Medicine	54	44	30	10	4	2		5	3
Medical Genetics	36	28	14	8	6	1		7	
Neurology	797	705	386	174	145	6	11	69	6
Nuclear Medicine	48	37	24	3	10		3	7	1
Occupational Medicine	64	38	33		5	13		6	7
Other Specialty	204	102	58	24	20	36	5	51	10
Physical Medicine and Rehabilitation	262	254	154	58	42	5		2	1
Psychiatry	2,034	1,845	1,209	276	360	75	30	65	19
Public Health and General Preventive Medicine	49	5	3		2	23	2	13	6
Radiation Oncology	185	178	102	36	40	2	2	3	
Radiology	396	373	237	58	78	5	1	12	5
Transplant Surgery	8	7	6		1	1			
Unspecified	340	326	132	172	22		2	8	4
Vascular Medicine	1	1			1				
Inactive	3,459								
Not Classified	3,797								

Note: Excludes Address Unknown.

Subspecialties in this table are condensed into major specialties. See Appendix A.

Table 3.7

Physicians by State, Self-Designated Specialty, and Activity, 2010, continued
Michigan

		Patient Care				Other Professional Activity			
				Hospital Based					
Specialty	Total Physicians	Total Patient Care	Office Based	Resid./ Fellows	Phys. Staff	Admin.	Med. Teach.	Research	Other
Total Physicians	29,331	22,764	16,112	4,478	2,174	404	329	322	102
FM/GP	2,886	2,775	2,226	356	193	47	52	7	5
Family Medicine	2,716	2,613	2,078	356	179	41	50	7	5
General Practice	170	162	148		14	6	2		
Medical Specialties	9,103	8,614	6,192	1,637	785	139	142	194	14
Allergy and Immunology	144	140	118	12	10		2	2	
Cardiovascular Disease	629	601	472	101	28	3	5	19	1
Dermatology	303	300	234	50	16	1		2	
Gastroenterology	314	293	216	54	23	1	4	15	1
Internal Medicine	5,101	4,806	3,438	934	434	98	80	112	5
Pediatric Cardiology	76	73	32	24	17	2		1	
Pediatrics	2,246	2,134	1,473	422	239	26	46	34	6
Pulmonary Disease	290	267	209	40	18	8	5	9	1
Surgical Specialties	4,974	4,857	3,532	985	340	46	44	21	6
Colon and Rectal Surgery	58	56	50	2	4	1	1		
General Surgery	1,216	1,186	744	334	108	12	10	6	2
Neurological Surgery	167	165	119	34	12	1	1		
Obstetrics & Gynecology	1,363	1,314	981	215	118	20	21	7	1
Ophthalmology	592	582	480	76	26	1	4	3	2
Orthopedic Surgery	664	651	454	174	23	8	5		
Otolaryngology	264	263	190	57	16	1			
Plastic Surgery	215	209	161	41	7	1	1	3	1
Thoracic Surgery	129	127	111	5	11	1		1	
Urology	306	304	242	47	15		1	1	
Other Specialties	6,958	6,518	4,162	1,500	856	172	91	100	77
Aerospace Medicine	3	1	1			1		1	
Anatomic/Clinical Pathology	606	530	328	99	103	22	12	15	27
Anesthesiology	1,047	1,026	714	199	113	4	10	4	3
Child & Adolescent Psychiatry	202	184	134	18	32	7	8	3	
Diagnostic Radiology	913	891	524	271	96	2	11	2	7
Emergency Medicine	1,259	1,219	711	328	180	25	11	1	3
Forensic Pathology	18	11	9	1	1	2			5
General Preventive Medicine	30	22	18	4		6		1	1
Medical Genetics	20	16	12	1	3		1	3	
Neurology	443	409	288	80	41	2	10	18	4
Nuclear Medicine	55	47	30	6	11	2	3	3	
Occupational Medicine	96	76	66		10	15		4	1
Other Specialty	137	93	50	28	15	18	3	18	5
Physical Medicine and Rehabilitation	314	304	229	51	24	4	2	1	3
Psychiatry	1,007	932	664	115	153	36	15	17	7
Public Health and General Preventive Medicine	30	4	3		1	20		4	2
Radiation Oncology	162	157	95	37	25	5			
Radiology	285	269	204	25	40	1	5	2	8
Transplant Surgery	7	6	6					1	
Unspecified	323	320	75	237	8			2	1
Vascular Medicine	1	1	1						
Inactive	3,494								
Not Classified	1,916								

Note: Excludes Address Unknown.

Subspecialties in this table are condensed into major specialties. See Appendix A.

Table 3.7

Physicians by State, Self-Designated Specialty, and Activity, 2010, continued
Minnesota

		Patient Care				Other Professional Activity			
				Hospital Based					
Specialty	Total Physicians	Total Patient Care	Office Based	Resid./ Fellows	Phys. Staff	Admin.	Med. Teach.	Research	Other
Total Physicians	18,143	14,377	10,901	2,205	1,271	242	157	251	67
FM/GP	2,913	2,819	2,426	213	180	38	43	6	7
Family Medicine	2,854	2,764	2,379	213	172	35	42	6	7
General Practice	59	55	47		8	3	1		
Medical Specialties	5,166	4,858	3,636	810	412	83	55	156	14
Allergy and Immunology	75	70	65	5		1	1	3	
Cardiovascular Disease	436	411	317	56	38	2	4	18	1
Dermatology	212	209	163	39	7		2	1	
Gastroenterology	249	232	184	33	15	2	4	11	
Internal Medicine	2,708	2,522	1,834	440	248	60	30	86	10
Pediatric Cardiology	50	46	33	11	2			4	
Pediatrics	1,263	1,207	915	201	91	14	14	25	3
Pulmonary Disease	173	161	125	25	11	4		8	
Surgical Specialties	2,806	2,756	2,082	495	179	14	18	17	1
Colon and Rectal Surgery	48	48	43	4	1				
General Surgery	631	618	400	161	57	4	3	5	1
Neurological Surgery	101	99	61	29	9		1	1	
Obstetrics & Gynecology	636	626	550	49	27	1	6	3	
Ophthalmology	300	295	256	23	16	3	1	1	
Orthopedic Surgery	550	544	383	130	31	3	1	2	
Otolaryngology	190	186	130	42	14	1	2	1	
Plastic Surgery	96	95	79	11	5	1			
Thoracic Surgery	76	74	52	11	11		1	1	
Urology	178	171	128	35	8	1	3	3	
Other Specialties	4,209	3,944	2,757	687	500	107	41	72	45
Aerospace Medicine	2	2			2				
Anatomic/Clinical Pathology	392	347	233	68	46	13	5	11	16
Anesthesiology	606	594	448	89	57	3	4	5	
Child & Adolescent Psychiatry	107	101	81	9	11	3	1	2	
Diagnostic Radiology	611	596	433	105	58	3	3	1	8
Emergency Medicine	600	574	353	93	128	17	8	1	
Forensic Pathology	14	9	4	2	3	1			4
General Preventive Medicine	44	38	31	6	1	3		3	
Medical Genetics	13	9	6	1	2			3	1
Neurology	355	329	244	63	22	5	5	16	
Nuclear Medicine	11	11	9		2				
Occupational Medicine	61	43	39		4	15	1		2
Other Specialty	122	82	48	28	6	19	3	15	3
Physical Medicine and Rehabilitation	190	183	122	42	19	3	1	3	
Psychiatry	587	556	388	82	86	16	5	6	4
Public Health and General Preventive Medicine	20	7	6		1	5	2	6	
Radiation Oncology	87	87	64	14	9				
Radiology	195	187	163	7	17	1	3		4
Transplant Surgery	8	8	5		3				
Unspecified	183	180	79	78	23				3
Vascular Medicine	1	1	1						
Inactive	2,193								
Not Classified	856								

Note: Excludes Address Unknown.

Subspecialties in this table are condensed into major specialties. See Appendix A.

Table 3.7

Physicians by State, Self-Designated Specialty, and Activity, 2010, continued
Mississippi

		Patient Care				Other Professional Activity			
				Hospital Based					
Specialty	Total Physicians	Total Patient Care	Office Based	Resid./ Fellows	Phys. Staff	Admin.	Med. Teach.	Research	Other
Total Physicians	6,149	4,900	3,753	525	622	66	55	23	37
FM/GP	806	781	651	49	81	11	10	1	3
Family Medicine	729	706	585	49	72	10	10	1	2
General Practice	77	75	66		9	1			1
Medical Specialties	1,684	1,628	1,256	176	196	22	18	14	2
Allergy and Immunology	25	23	19	2	2		1		1
Cardiovascular Disease	144	138	113	13	12	2	3	1	
Dermatology	46	45	43		2		1		
Gastroenterology	98	95	83	5	7		2	1	
Internal Medicine	869	841	610	104	127	13	4	10	1
Pediatric Cardiology	3	3	3						
Pediatrics	418	402	329	45	28	7	7	2	
Pulmonary Disease	81	81	56	7	18				
Surgical Specialties	1,258	1,229	970	147	112	14	11	2	2
Colon and Rectal Surgery	2	2	1		1				
General Surgery	271	264	183	42	39	3	2	1	1
Neurological Surgery	57	56	39	7	10		1		
Obstetrics & Gynecology	324	317	268	29	20	2	4	1	
Ophthalmology	131	128	116	9	3	1	2		
Orthopedic Surgery	180	177	132	28	17	3			
Otolaryngology	109	108	81	17	10				1
Plastic Surgery	50	50	44	6					
Thoracic Surgery	46	42	36		6	4			
Urology	88	85	70	9	6	1	2		
Other Specialties	1,333	1,262	876	153	233	19	16	6	30
Aerospace Medicine	3	2	1		1		1		
Anatomic/Clinical Pathology	130	111	70	15	26	3	1	2	13
Anesthesiology	259	253	189	29	35	1	5		
Child & Adolescent Psychiatry	33	33	24	3	6				
Diagnostic Radiology	162	158	119	25	14				4
Emergency Medicine	220	210	132	27	51	4	3	1	2
Forensic Pathology	1	1			1				
General Preventive Medicine	15	11	8		3	1	1		2
Medical Genetics	6	4	2		2	1			1
Neurology	103	98	74	13	11		3	1	1
Nuclear Medicine	8	7	5		2	1			
Occupational Medicine	4	4	3		1				
Other Specialty	22	18	13	1	4	2		1	1
Physical Medicine and Rehabilitation	34	32	23	1	8	1			1
Psychiatry	195	191	116	21	54	1	2		1
Public Health and General Preventive Medicine	9	5	4		1	3		1	
Radiation Oncology	28	27	23		4	1			
Radiology	66	64	57	1	6				2
Transplant Surgery	1	1			1				
Unspecified	34	32	13	17	2				2
Inactive	828								
Not Classified	240								

Note: Excludes Address Unknown.

Subspecialties in this table are condensed into major specialties. *See Appendix A.*

Table 3.7

Physicians by State, Self-Designated Specialty, and Activity, 2010, continued
Missouri

		Patient Care				Other Professional Activity			
				Hospital Based					
Specialty	Total Physicians	Total Patient Care	Office Based	Resid./ Fellows	Phys. Staff	Admin.	Med. Teach.	Research	Other
Total Physicians	16,802	13,190	9,100	2,557	1,533	176	191	255	60
FM/GP	1,413	1,366	1,128	114	124	23	17	5	2
Family Medicine	1,326	1,283	1,060	114	109	22	16	4	1
General Practice	87	83	68		15	1	1	1	1
Medical Specialties	5,515	5,195	3,510	1,079	606	66	96	148	10
Allergy and Immunology	87	80	61	15	4		2	3	2
Cardiovascular Disease	445	410	318	58	34	4	10	19	2
Dermatology	194	191	150	36	5		1	2	
Gastroenterology	256	244	186	40	18	1	2	9	
Internal Medicine	2,814	2,648	1,799	548	301	37	50	75	4
Pediatric Cardiology	43	40	22	10	8		1	2	
Pediatrics	1,469	1,386	840	342	204	22	26	33	2
Pulmonary Disease	207	196	134	30	32	2	4	5	
Surgical Specialties	2,985	2,916	2,125	572	219	18	28	17	6
Colon and Rectal Surgery	26	26	23	2	1				
General Surgery	657	639	417	152	70	5	6	6	1
Neurological Surgery	136	135	90	36	9			1	
Obstetrics & Gynecology	730	709	561	103	45	9	6	6	
Ophthalmology	326	321	262	45	14	2	3		
Orthopedic Surgery	482	473	316	115	42		5		4
Otolaryngology	207	201	134	55	12		3	3	
Plastic Surgery	138	134	94	35	5		2	1	1
Thoracic Surgery	95	93	74	4	15	1	1		
Urology	188	185	154	25	6	1	2		
Other Specialties	3,959	3,713	2,337	792	584	69	50	85	42
Aerospace Medicine	4	2	2			1		1	
Anatomic/Clinical Pathology	371	319	209	76	34	11	6	15	20
Anesthesiology	732	716	490	126	100	5	8	3	
Child & Adolescent Psychiatry	109	101	71	13	17	2	1	5	
Diagnostic Radiology	522	507	290	157	60	2	7	2	4
Emergency Medicine	558	540	300	84	156	9	7	2	
Forensic Pathology	14	11	8	1	2				3
General Preventive Medicine	23	16	11		5	3	2	1	1
Medical Genetics	11	6	3	1	2	1	2	2	
Neurology	337	305	181	98	26	6	2	24	
Nuclear Medicine	32	24	14	6	4	3	2	3	
Occupational Medicine	38	33	29		4	4		1	
Other Specialty	83	52	36	8	8	10	3	12	6
Physical Medicine and Rehabilitation	140	138	98	20	20	1	1		
Psychiatry	584	559	369	91	99	7	4	9	5
Public Health and General Preventive Medicine	6	2			2	3			1
Radiation Oncology	94	94	67	13	14				
Radiology	182	172	127	20	25	1	5	3	1
Transplant Surgery	3	3	2		1				
Unspecified	116	113	30	78	5			2	1
Inactive	1,731								
Not Classified	1,199								

Note: Excludes Address Unknown.

Subspecialties in this table are condensed into major specialties. See Appendix A.

Table 3.7

Physicians by State, Self-Designated Specialty, and Activity, 2010, continued
Montana

		Patient Care				Other Professional Activity			
				Hospital Based					
Specialty	Total Physicians	Total Patient Care	Office Based	Resid./ Fellows	Phys. Staff	Admin.	Med. Teach.	Research	Other
Total Physicians	2,658	1,990	1,693	33	264	31	14	14	7
FM/GP	457	445	377	20	48	8	4		
Family Medicine	439	428	361	20	47	7	4		
General Practice	18	17	16		1	1			
Medical Specialties	554	532	452	2	78	9	3	7	3
Allergy and Immunology	12	11	10		1			1	
Cardiovascular Disease	46	45	40		5			1	
Dermatology	30	30	28		2				
Gastroenterology	27	27	25		2				
Internal Medicine	297	284	229	2	53	6	2	3	2
Pediatric Cardiology	1	1	1						
Pediatrics	116	111	100		11	2	1	1	1
Pulmonary Disease	25	23	19		4	1		1	
Surgical Specialties	473	464	418	2	44	4	3		2
Colon and Rectal Surgery	1	1	1						
General Surgery	100	98	81	1	16	1			1
Neurological Surgery	24	24	22		2				
Obstetrics & Gynecology	100	97	87		10	2	1		
Ophthalmology	46	45	43		2	1			
Orthopedic Surgery	108	105	99		6		2		1
Otolaryngology	29	29	26	1	2				
Plastic Surgery	15	15	15						
Thoracic Surgery	18	18	13		5				
Urology	32	32	31		1				
Other Specialties	572	549	446	9	94	10	4	7	2
Anatomic/Clinical Pathology	45	41	32		9		1	2	1
Anesthesiology	128	126	117		9	1	1		
Child & Adolescent Psychiatry	16	15	12		3	1			
Diagnostic Radiology	73	71	62		9	1	1		
Emergency Medicine	108	105	76	2	27	3			
Forensic Pathology	2	1	1						1
General Preventive Medicine	6	6	4		2				
Medical Genetics	3	3			3				
Neurology	32	32	30		2				
Nuclear Medicine	1	1	1						
Occupational Medicine	6	6	5		1				
Other Specialty	14	9	7		2	2		3	
Physical Medicine and Rehabilitation	19	19	16		3				
Psychiatry	73	69	54	1	14	2	1	1	
Public Health and General Preventive Medicine	1	1			1				
Radiation Oncology	12	12	8		4				
Radiology	24	23	19		4			1	
Unspecified	9	9	2	6	1				
Inactive	550								
Not Classified	52								

Note: Excludes Address Unknown.

Subspecialties in this table are condensed into major specialties. See Appendix A.

Table 3.7

Physicians by State, Self-Designated Specialty, and Activity, 2010, continued
Nebraska

		Patient Care				Other Professional Activity			
				Hospital Based					
Specialty	Total Physicians	Total Patient Care	Office Based	Resid./ Fellows	Phys. Staff	Admin.	Med. Teach.	Research	Other
Total Physicians	5,150	4,061	3,029	662	370	73	54	50	22
FM/GP	875	840	695	88	57	15	17		3
Family Medicine	846	815	673	88	54	14	16		1
General Practice	29	25	22		3	1	1		2
Medical Specialties	1,347	1,274	910	252	112	25	18	23	7
Allergy and Immunology	22	21	18	3				1	
Cardiovascular Disease	131	130	98	25	7	1			
Dermatology	32	32	31		1				
Gastroenterology	49	47	38	6	3	2			
Internal Medicine	692	649	430	163	56	14	10	15	4
Pediatric Cardiology	7	7	4		3				
Pediatrics	359	340	254	46	40	8	3	6	2
Pulmonary Disease	55	48	37	9	2		5	1	1
Surgical Specialties	918	897	713	136	48	10	6	5	
Colon and Rectal Surgery	7	6	6			1			
General Surgery	223	214	146	50	18	5	1	3	
Neurological Surgery	41	41	31	8	2				
Obstetrics & Gynecology	209	203	160	31	12		4	2	
Ophthalmology	95	92	83	7	2	2	1		
Orthopedic Surgery	170	170	142	22	6				
Otolaryngology	70	69	59	8	2	1			
Plastic Surgery	33	33	28	4	1				
Thoracic Surgery	16	16	14	1	1				
Urology	54	53	44	5	4	1			
Other Specialties	1,120	1,050	711	186	153	23	13	22	12
Aerospace Medicine	2	1			1	1			
Anatomic/Clinical Pathology	127	110	78	20	12	4	1	6	6
Anesthesiology	238	235	173	34	28	2	1		
Child & Adolescent Psychiatry	39	38	25	5	8			1	
Diagnostic Radiology	150	146	100	32	14		3		1
Emergency Medicine	134	130	74	21	35	1	2	1	
Forensic Pathology	1	1	1						
General Preventive Medicine	5	3	3			1		1	
Medical Genetics	4	4	1	2	1				
Neurology	72	67	53	12	2	1	2	2	
Nuclear Medicine	9	8	5	2	1				1
Occupational Medicine	6	5	2		3	1			
Other Specialty	34	16	11	2	3	6	2	8	2
Physical Medicine and Rehabilitation	31	31	23	1	7				
Psychiatry	159	149	104	22	23	5	2	2	1
Public Health and General Preventive Medicine	1					1			
Radiation Oncology	25	25	18	2	5				
Radiology	42	41	31	4	6				1
Transplant Surgery	4	3	2		1			1	
Unspecified	37	37	7	27	3				
Inactive	628								
Not Classified	262								

Note: Excludes Address Unknown.

Subspecialties in this table are condensed into major specialties. See Appendix A.

Table 3.7

Physicians by State, Self-Designated Specialty, and Activity, 2010, continued
Nevada

		Patient Care				Other Professional Activity			
				Hospital Based					
Specialty	Total Physicians	Total Patient Care	Office Based	Resid./ Fellows	Phys. Staff	Admin.	Med. Teach.	Research	Other
Total Physicians	5,899	4,558	3,952	236	370	68	33	20	27
FM/GP	583	568	497	28	43	6	5		4
Family Medicine	536	524	457	28	39	3	5		4
General Practice	47	44	40		4	3			
Medical Specialties	1,744	1,688	1,431	111	146	27	16	9	4
Allergy and Immunology	18	17	16		1			1	
Cardiovascular Disease	142	138	127	1	10	1	1	2	
Dermatology	51	51	50		1				
Gastroenterology	73	72	72				1		
Internal Medicine	1,019	977	798	77	102	22	12	5	3
Pediatric Cardiology	12	12	12						
Pediatrics	378	371	309	33	29	3	2	1	1
Pulmonary Disease	51	50	47		3	1			
Surgical Specialties	968	954	861	41	52	5	4	2	3
Colon and Rectal Surgery	6	6	6						
General Surgery	215	214	169	22	23	1			
Neurological Surgery	29	29	29						
Obstetrics & Gynecology	280	275	258	9	8	2	3		
Ophthalmology	97	96	87	1	8				1
Orthopedic Surgery	145	144	138	3	3	1			
Otolaryngology	46	44	40		4		1	1	
Plastic Surgery	54	53	45	6	2				1
Thoracic Surgery	32	32	30		2				
Urology	64	61	59		2	1		1	1
Other Specialties	1,411	1,348	1,163	56	129	30	8	9	16
Aerospace Medicine	3	3	1		2				
Anatomic/Clinical Pathology	83	77	72		5	3			3
Anesthesiology	370	366	352		14	2	1	1	
Child & Adolescent Psychiatry	32	30	24	3	3		1	1	
Diagnostic Radiology	169	165	150	1	14				4
Emergency Medicine	251	249	198	19	32	2			
Forensic Pathology	6	4	4			1			1
General Preventive Medicine	13	10	7		3	2			1
Medical Genetics	3	1	1			1		1	
Neurology	75	70	65	1	4	1	2	2	
Nuclear Medicine	3	3	3						
Occupational Medicine	12	8	6		2	3			1
Other Specialty	24	19	14	1	4	5			
Physical Medicine and Rehabilitation	63	60	57		3	3			
Psychiatry	182	171	116	19	36	5	3		3
Public Health and General Preventive Medicine	6	2	2			1		3	
Radiation Oncology	31	30	29		1				1
Radiology	65	60	55		5	1	1	1	2
Transplant Surgery	1	1			1				
Unspecified	19	19	7	12					
Inactive	896								
Not Classified	297								

Note: Excludes Address Unknown.

Subspecialties in this table are condensed into major specialties. See Appendix A.

Table 3.7

Physicians by State, Self-Designated Specialty, and Activity, 2010, continued
New Hampshire

		Patient Care				Other Professional Activity			
				Hospital Based					
Specialty	Total Physicians	Total Patient Care	Office Based	Resid./ Fellows	Phys. Staff	Admin.	Med. Teach.	Research	Other
Total Physicians	4,563	3,492	2,558	416	518	55	34	54	21
FM/GP	499	484	407	14	63	6	2	2	5
Family Medicine	482	468	393	14	61	6	2	2	4
General Practice	17	16	14		2				1
Medical Specialties	1,324	1,264	928	142	194	16	13	27	4
Allergy and Immunology	13	13	12		1				
Cardiovascular Disease	105	104	77	14	13			1	
Dermatology	43	43	37	5	1				
Gastroenterology	57	56	42	10	4		1		
Internal Medicine	746	704	493	84	127	12	7	21	2
Pediatric Cardiology	5	5	4		1				
Pediatrics	306	291	231	24	36	3	5	5	2
Pulmonary Disease	49	48	32	5	11	1			
Surgical Specialties	801	786	588	111	87	4	3	6	2
Colon and Rectal Surgery	3	3	2	1					
General Surgery	202	195	122	41	32	2	1	2	2
Neurological Surgery	27	27	18	7	2				
Obstetrics & Gynecology	201	198	159	16	23		2	1	
Ophthalmology	69	69	62	2	5				
Orthopedic Surgery	153	151	109	26	16			2	
Otolaryngology	41	41	36	4	1				
Plastic Surgery	28	27	20	5	2	1			
Thoracic Surgery	22	20	17		3	1		1	
Urology	55	55	43	9	3				
Other Specialties	1,032	958	635	149	174	29	16	19	10
Aerospace Medicine	1					1			
Anatomic/Clinical Pathology	91	81	44	18	19	2	1	3	4
Anesthesiology	200	196	131	32	33	1	3		
Child & Adolescent Psychiatry	33	32	25	5	2		1		
Diagnostic Radiology	123	119	88	19	12	2			2
Emergency Medicine	163	159	98	3	58	3			1
Forensic Pathology	2	1		1					1
General Preventive Medicine	22	20	5	14	1	2			
Neurology	68	66	48	9	9	1		1	
Nuclear Medicine	1	1			1				
Occupational Medicine	10	5	4		1	4			1
Other Specialty	30	14	7	1	6	7	3	5	1
Physical Medicine and Rehabilitation	26	25	20	4	1	1			
Psychiatry	182	166	116	31	19	3	7	6	
Public Health and General Preventive Medicine	3					2		1	
Radiation Oncology	14	14	8		6				
Radiology	39	37	30	2	5		1	1	
Transplant Surgery	1	1	1						
Unspecified	23	21	10	10	1			2	
Inactive	686								
Not Classified	221								

Note: Excludes Address Unknown.

Subspecialties in this table are condensed into major specialties. See Appendix A.

Table 3.7

Physicians by State, Self-Designated Specialty, and Activity, 2010, continued
New Jersey

		Patient Care				Other Professional Activity			
				Hospital Based					
Specialty	Total Physicians	Total Patient Care	Office Based	Resid./ Fellows	Phys. Staff	Admin.	Med. Teach.	Research	Other
Total Physicians	30,976	23,757	18,505	2,653	2,599	463	265	498	194
FM/GP	1,552	1,466	1,205	152	109	27	36	14	9
Family Medicine	1,385	1,312	1,087	152	73	21	36	10	6
General Practice	167	154	118		36	6		4	3
Medical Specialties	11,530	10,830	8,445	1,250	1,135	201	137	290	72
Allergy and Immunology	175	164	151	7	6	2	1	6	2
Cardiovascular Disease	973	915	784	60	71	13	9	29	7
Dermatology	320	312	294	10	8	2		5	1
Gastroenterology	514	496	445	35	16	3	3	9	3
Internal Medicine	6,193	5,761	4,329	844	588	129	69	182	52
Pediatric Cardiology	59	53	39	1	13		3	3	
Pediatrics	2,908	2,768	2,103	258	407	40	43	50	7
Pulmonary Disease	388	361	300	35	26	12	9	6	
Surgical Specialties	5,103	4,977	4,145	509	323	47	31	33	15
Colon and Rectal Surgery	66	65	61		4			1	
General Surgery	1,132	1,104	764	214	126	15	4	5	4
Neurological Surgery	117	115	87	17	11		1	1	
Obstetrics & Gynecology	1,468	1,415	1,197	119	99	19	17	13	4
Ophthalmology	603	593	562	20	11	1	3	4	2
Orthopedic Surgery	721	711	616	80	15	3	1	2	4
Otolaryngology	259	254	230	15	9	3	2		
Plastic Surgery	228	225	199	19	7	2	1		
Thoracic Surgery	136	128	98	3	27	2		6	
Urology	373	367	331	22	14	2	2	1	1
Other Specialties	6,992	6,484	4,710	742	1,032	188	61	161	98
Aerospace Medicine	2	2	1		1				
Anatomic/Clinical Pathology	505	427	280	55	92	25	7	19	27
Anesthesiology	1,533	1,503	1,184	97	222	10	6	10	4
Child & Adolescent Psychiatry	257	239	184	19	36	4	3	7	4
Diagnostic Radiology	755	727	552	122	53	3	4	9	12
Emergency Medicine	733	706	447	97	162	18	5	3	1
Forensic Pathology	16	8	7		1	4		2	2
General Preventive Medicine	34	25	18	3	4	2	2	3	2
Medical Genetics	9	6	3	1	2		1	1	1
Neurology	516	468	367	62	39	9	8	25	6
Nuclear Medicine	47	38	29	1	8	1	1	3	4
Occupational Medicine	66	44	34		10	15	2	2	3
Other Specialty	164	81	58	6	17	31	4	42	6
Physical Medicine and Rehabilitation	385	369	283	39	47	10		3	3
Psychiatry	1,325	1,237	846	116	275	44	12	23	9
Public Health and General Preventive Medicine	17	4	4			8	2	1	2
Radiation Oncology	135	132	110	7	15			2	1
Radiology	306	293	252	7	34	3	1	2	7
Transplant Surgery	8	7	6		1			1	
Unspecified	179	168	45	110	13	1	3	3	4
Inactive	3,825								
Not Classified	1,974								

Note: Excludes Address Unknown.

Subspecialties in this table are condensed into major specialties. See Appendix A.

Table 3.7

Physicians by State, Self-Designated Specialty, and Activity, 2010, continued
New Mexico

		Patient Care				Other Professional Activity			
				Hospital Based					
Specialty	Total Physicians	Total Patient Care	Office Based	Resid./ Fellows	Phys. Staff	Admin.	Med. Teach.	Research	Other
Total Physicians	5,759	4,311	3,241	530	540	97	66	64	44
FM/GP	827	796	634	75	87	12	12	4	3
Family Medicine	776	747	593	75	79	11	12	3	3
General Practice	51	49	41		8	1		1	
Medical Specialties	1,544	1,444	1,091	168	185	32	29	30	9
Allergy and Immunology	12	12	12						
Cardiovascular Disease	101	95	79	7	9		3	2	1
Dermatology	50	46	41	5			2	1	1
Gastroenterology	77	71	52	12	7	2	2	2	
Internal Medicine	841	783	579	94	110	22	13	19	4
Pediatric Cardiology	5	5	5						
Pediatrics	406	381	282	44	55	8	9	5	3
Pulmonary Disease	52	51	41	6	4			1	
Surgical Specialties	840	819	631	107	81	7	9	2	3
Colon and Rectal Surgery	3	3	3						
General Surgery	203	196	140	28	28	2	3	1	1
Neurological Surgery	26	25	17	7	1	1			
Obstetrics & Gynecology	229	224	186	23	15	1	3	1	
Ophthalmology	76	75	73		2				1
Orthopedic Surgery	153	152	103	34	15				1
Otolaryngology	48	46	32	6	8	1	1		
Plastic Surgery	27	25	19		6	1	1		
Thoracic Surgery	22	22	21		1				
Urology	53	51	37	9	5	1	1		
Other Specialties	1,371	1,252	885	180	187	46	16	28	29
Aerospace Medicine	10	6	2		4	2			2
Anatomic/Clinical Pathology	124	103	69	24	10	3	1	8	9
Anesthesiology	224	221	171	29	21		1	1	1
Child & Adolescent Psychiatry	55	50	33	8	9	3	1	1	
Diagnostic Radiology	123	116	76	25	15	2	1		4
Emergency Medicine	256	246	162	35	49	8	2		
Forensic Pathology	8	8	7		1				
General Preventive Medicine	18	15	10		5	1		1	1
Medical Genetics	2	1	1						1
Neurology	84	78	52	17	9	1	1	4	
Nuclear Medicine	5	5	3		2				
Occupational Medicine	19	16	13		3	3			
Other Specialty	35	21	15	2	4	7		3	4
Physical Medicine and Rehabilitation	29	29	26	1	2				
Psychiatry	274	249	175	30	44	8	6	7	4
Public Health and General Preventive Medicine	14	3	2		1	7		2	2
Radiation Oncology	20	20	18		2				
Radiology	48	45	37	3	5		3		
Unspecified	23	20	13	6	1	1		1	1
Inactive	841								
Not Classified	336								

Note: Excludes Address Unknown.

Subspecialties in this table are condensed into major specialties. See Appendix A.

Table 3.7

Physicians by State, Self-Designated Specialty, and Activity, 2010, continued
New York

		Patient Care				Other Professional Activity			
				Hospital Based					
Specialty	Total Physicians	Total Patient Care	Office Based	Resid./ Fellows	Phys. Staff	Admin.	Med. Teach.	Research	Other
Total Physicians	86,293	64,089	42,410	13,649	8,030	1,406	970	1,403	375
FM/GP	3,770	3,613	2,876	428	309	72	64	13	8
Family Medicine	3,446	3,306	2,606	428	272	64	63	9	4
General Practice	324	307	270		37	8	1	4	4
Medical Specialties	29,819	27,820	18,505	6,269	3,046	607	460	797	135
Allergy and Immunology	372	330	275	37	18	5	3	34	
Cardiovascular Disease	2,198	2,058	1,522	346	190	38	32	63	7
Dermatology	1,020	994	822	143	29	4	13	7	2
Gastroenterology	1,320	1,251	964	205	82	16	18	30	5
Internal Medicine	16,768	15,553	9,872	3,956	1,725	401	247	482	85
Pediatric Cardiology	179	163	90	34	39	3	5	8	
Pediatrics	6,981	6,573	4,364	1,357	852	127	114	135	32
Pulmonary Disease	981	898	596	191	111	13	28	38	4
Surgical Specialties	13,469	13,114	9,320	2,659	1,135	112	118	89	36
Colon and Rectal Surgery	147	146	126	8	12		1		
General Surgery	3,077	2,975	1,707	924	344	43	33	19	7
Neurological Surgery	416	405	254	107	44		4	6	1
Obstetrics & Gynecology	3,553	3,436	2,549	564	323	38	41	28	10
Ophthalmology	1,704	1,671	1,434	165	72	6	11	12	4
Orthopedic Surgery	1,896	1,861	1,256	477	128	6	11	8	10
Otolaryngology	787	774	550	165	59	2	7	3	1
Plastic Surgery	637	632	534	70	28	1	1	2	1
Thoracic Surgery	345	329	243	33	53	6	4	6	
Urology	907	885	667	146	72	10	5	5	2
Other Specialties	21,185	19,542	11,709	4,293	3,540	615	328	504	196
Aerospace Medicine	5	2			2	1			2
Anatomic/Clinical Pathology	1,543	1,307	684	282	341	71	39	66	60
Anesthesiology	3,680	3,585	2,396	699	490	28	37	20	10
Child & Adolescent Psychiatry	873	804	559	105	140	25	21	16	7
Diagnostic Radiology	2,127	2,051	1,198	585	268	18	17	17	24
Emergency Medicine	2,335	2,246	1,050	680	516	49	30	8	2
Forensic Pathology	57	38	31	3	4	7		1	11
General Preventive Medicine	153	128	86	35	7	16	5	2	2
Medical Genetics	32	24	13	5	6		1	7	
Neurology	1,618	1,460	940	335	185	29	37	87	5
Nuclear Medicine	155	141	75	24	42	6	3	3	2
Occupational Medicine	111	66	51		15	34	2	6	3
Other Specialty	446	273	133	91	49	61	12	88	12
Physical Medicine and Rehabilitation	1,018	970	654	180	136	22	13	5	8
Psychiatry	5,120	4,680	2,872	743	1,065	192	90	131	27
Public Health and General Preventive Medicine	99	36	27		9	37	5	15	6
Radiation Oncology	358	348	212	78	58	2	3	4	1
Radiology	810	768	542	56	170	13	9	10	10
Transplant Surgery	18	18	14		4				
Unspecified	626	596	172	392	32	4	4	18	4
Vascular Medicine	1	1			1				
Inactive	10,115								
Not Classified	7,935								

Note: Excludes Address Unknown.

Subspecialties in this table are condensed into major specialties. *See Appendix A.*

Table 3.7

Physicians by State, Self-Designated Specialty, and Activity, 2010, continued
North Carolina

		Patient Care				Other Professional Activity			
				Hospital Based					
Specialty	Total Physicians	Total Patient Care	Office Based	Resid./ Fellows	Phys. Staff	Admin.	Med. Teach.	Research	Other
Total Physicians	27,850	21,593	16,576	2,922	2,095	365	308	438	102
FM/GP	3,051	2,942	2,481	222	239	45	45	9	10
Family Medicine	2,928	2,825	2,381	222	222	42	44	9	8
General Practice	123	117	100		17	3	1		2
Medical Specialties	8,523	7,974	6,118	1,073	783	134	122	271	22
Allergy and Immunology	91	80	66	9	5	1	1	8	1
Cardiovascular Disease	666	634	519	77	38	5	5	22	
Dermatology	349	344	298	33	13	1	1	3	
Gastroenterology	426	402	343	40	19	3	7	12	2
Internal Medicine	4,378	4,071	3,028	553	490	86	57	154	10
Pediatric Cardiology	60	55	34	13	8		2	3	
Pediatrics	2,221	2,087	1,595	302	190	35	45	46	8
Pulmonary Disease	332	301	235	46	20	3	4	23	1
Surgical Specialties	4,866	4,751	3,752	679	320	35	43	28	9
Colon and Rectal Surgery	18	18	15	1	2				
General Surgery	1,100	1,069	760	212	97	16	8	6	1
Neurological Surgery	165	158	119	29	10	1	3	2	1
Obstetrics & Gynecology	1,317	1,281	1,071	141	69	9	17	8	2
Ophthalmology	496	486	426	41	19	1	4	5	
Orthopedic Surgery	785	771	594	134	43	2	6	3	3
Otolaryngology	335	332	260	51	21	1		2	
Plastic Surgery	181	179	149	19	11	2			
Thoracic Surgery	121	118	83	15	20		2		1
Urology	348	339	275	36	28	3	3	2	1
Other Specialties	6,366	5,926	4,225	948	753	151	98	130	61
Aerospace Medicine	2	1	1			1			
Anatomic/Clinical Pathology	475	407	284	76	47	13	11	22	22
Anesthesiology	1,037	1,010	706	177	127	6	14	5	2
Child & Adolescent Psychiatry	230	208	165	23	20	7	9	5	1
Diagnostic Radiology	744	721	543	123	55	5	9	4	5
Emergency Medicine	1,107	1,076	743	145	188	14	13	2	2
Forensic Pathology	11	9	6	2	1		1	1	
General Preventive Medicine	79	63	48	7	8	4		11	1
Medical Genetics	13	11	4	2	5	1	1		
Neurology	444	415	320	66	29	3	6	18	2
Nuclear Medicine	33	32	23	2	7			1	
Occupational Medicine	46	31	26		5	11	1		3
Other Specialty	142	88	56	26	6	24	1	23	6
Physical Medicine and Rehabilitation	246	236	168	43	25	6	3	1	
Psychiatry	1,099	1,011	729	126	156	36	20	26	6
Public Health and General Preventive Medicine	31	5	4		1	14	2	7	3
Radiation Oncology	150	147	111	17	19	2			1
Radiology	298	285	224	31	30	1	6	1	5
Transplant Surgery	5	5	4		1				
Unspecified	173	164	59	82	23	3	1	3	2
Vascular Medicine	1	1	1						
Inactive	3,425								
Not Classified	1,619								

Note: Excludes Address Unknown.

Subspecialties in this table are condensed into major specialties. See Appendix A.

Table 3.7

Physicians by State, Self-Designated Specialty, and Activity, 2010, continued
North Dakota

		Patient Care				Other Professional Activity			
				Hospital Based					
Specialty	Total Physicians	Total Patient Care	Office Based	Resid./ Fellows	Phys. Staff	Admin.	Med. Teach.	Research	Other
Total Physicians	1,832	1,514	1,145	123	246	25	18	6	12
FM/GP	391	376	273	55	48	9	6		
Family Medicine	370	355	256	55	44	9	6		
General Practice	21	21	17		4				
Medical Specialties	449	434	338	24	72	8	3	3	1
Allergy and Immunology	8	8	8						
Cardiovascular Disease	26	26	23		3				
Dermatology	17	17	16		1				
Gastroenterology	11	11	11						
Internal Medicine	276	265	190	23	52	5	3	2	1
Pediatric Cardiology	2	2	2						
Pediatrics	94	92	78	1	13	2			
Pulmonary Disease	15	13	10		3	1		1	
Surgical Specialties	327	320	265	17	38	1	4	1	1
Colon and Rectal Surgery	2	2	2						
General Surgery	102	98	69	15	14	1	3		
Neurological Surgery	10	9	5		4				1
Obstetrics & Gynecology	59	59	55	1	3				
Ophthalmology	32	32	32						
Orthopedic Surgery	50	49	42		7			1	
Otolaryngology	24	24	20	1	3				
Plastic Surgery	14	13	12		1		1		
Thoracic Surgery	15	15	12		3				
Urology	19	19	16		3				
Other Specialties	408	384	269	27	88	7	5	2	10
Aerospace Medicine	2	2	1		1				
Anatomic/Clinical Pathology	42	35	29		6	1	2		4
Anesthesiology	60	60	41	2	17				
Child & Adolescent Psychiatry	20	18	11		7	1			1
Diagnostic Radiology	45	42	34		8	1			2
Emergency Medicine	54	52	32		20		1	1	
Forensic Pathology	2	1	1						1
General Preventive Medicine	2	2	1		1				
Medical Genetics	1						1		
Neurology	21	21	16	1	4				
Occupational Medicine	1	1	1						
Other Specialty	5	4	4			1			
Physical Medicine and Rehabilitation	17	16	13		3	1			
Psychiatry	82	78	54	12	12	2	1	1	
Public Health and General Preventive Medicine	2	1			1				1
Radiation Oncology	12	12	12						
Radiology	16	15	13		2				1
Unspecified	24	24	6	12	6				
Inactive	216								
Not Classified	41								

Note: Excludes Address Unknown.

Subspecialties in this table are condensed into major specialties. See Appendix A.

Table 3.7

Physicians by State, Self-Designated Specialty, and Activity, 2010, continued
Ohio

		Patient Care				Other Professional Activity			
				Hospital Based					
Specialty	Total Physicians	Total Patient Care	Office Based	Resid./ Fellows	Phys. Staff	Admin.	Med. Teach.	Research	Other
Total Physicians	35,925	27,702	19,541	5,133	3,028	414	383	415	128
FM/GP	3,464	3,341	2,763	354	224	41	70	7	5
Family Medicine	3,243	3,126	2,581	354	191	38	69	7	3
General Practice	221	215	182		33	3	1		2
Medical Specialties	11,235	10,639	7,341	2,123	1,175	155	157	252	32
Allergy and Immunology	129	120	95	15	10		1	7	1
Cardiovascular Disease	836	790	620	92	78	7	16	21	2
Dermatology	356	349	268	62	19	1	3	2	1
Gastroenterology	439	415	333	48	34	4	8	12	
Internal Medicine	5,836	5,536	3,889	1,093	554	99	80	102	19
Pediatric Cardiology	108	101	44	25	32		3	4	
Pediatrics	3,146	2,967	1,840	719	408	43	43	85	8
Pulmonary Disease	385	361	252	69	40	1	3	19	1
Surgical Specialties	6,170	6,045	4,361	1,208	476	39	56	25	5
Colon and Rectal Surgery	62	62	52	3	7				
General Surgery	1,504	1,464	912	402	150	13	18	9	
Neurological Surgery	246	237	138	73	26	3	3	3	
Obstetrics & Gynecology	1,506	1,472	1,157	218	97	10	16	6	2
Ophthalmology	642	632	522	72	38	2	5	3	
Orthopedic Surgery	955	945	648	225	72	2	4	3	1
Otolaryngology	375	368	266	74	28	3	4		
Plastic Surgery	240	238	183	47	8		2		
Thoracic Surgery	212	206	166	12	28	3	2	1	
Urology	428	421	317	82	22	3	2		2
Other Specialties	8,173	7,677	5,076	1,448	1,153	179	100	131	86
Aerospace Medicine	12	7	4		3	1	1	2	1
Anatomic/Clinical Pathology	746	652	417	121	114	23	15	24	32
Anesthesiology	1,550	1,523	1,051	248	224	7	12	6	2
Child & Adolescent Psychiatry	242	230	176	23	31	3	7	1	1
Diagnostic Radiology	920	895	614	166	115	5	7	1	12
Emergency Medicine	1,300	1,242	818	229	195	28	17	7	6
Forensic Pathology	22	18	14	2	2	1			3
General Preventive Medicine	53	46	35	8	3	3		3	1
Medical Genetics	26	20	10	2	8			6	
Neurology	584	548	349	133	66	6	8	19	3
Nuclear Medicine	41	39	25	1	13	1		1	
Occupational Medicine	128	93	68		25	23		8	4
Other Specialty	220	157	81	59	17	21	5	30	7
Physical Medicine and Rehabilitation	322	317	222	59	36	3	1	1	
Psychiatry	1,124	1,055	710	156	189	39	14	14	2
Public Health and General Preventive Medicine	17	4	2		2	8	3	1	1
Radiation Oncology	178	176	120	28	28	1	1		
Radiology	350	332	251	24	57	3	5	2	8
Transplant Surgery	9	6	3		3		2	1	
Unspecified	324	312	101	189	22	3	2	4	3
Vascular Medicine	5	5	5						
Inactive	4,190								
Not Classified	2,693								

Note: Excludes Address Unknown.

Subspecialties in this table are condensed into major specialties. See Appendix A.

Table 3.7

Physicians by State, Self-Designated Specialty, and Activity, 2010, continued
Oklahoma

		Patient Care				Other Professional Activity			
				Hospital Based					
Specialty	Total Physicians	Total Patient Care	Office Based	Resid./ Fellows	Phys. Staff	Admin.	Med. Teach.	Research	Other
Total Physicians	7,619	6,030	4,697	751	582	94	98	43	34
FM/GP	1,111	1,080	863	126	91	12	14	1	4
Family Medicine	1,027	999	793	126	80	11	14	1	2
General Practice	84	81	70		11	1			2
Medical Specialties	2,050	1,939	1,514	234	191	40	39	28	4
Allergy and Immunology	24	23	23					1	
Cardiovascular Disease	190	183	156	12	15	3	2	2	
Dermatology	71	70	59	10	1		1		
Gastroenterology	109	107	93	8	6		2		
Internal Medicine	1,061	996	752	125	119	28	18	16	3
Pediatric Cardiology	11	11	11						
Pediatrics	506	475	360	69	46	7	14	9	1
Pulmonary Disease	78	74	60	10	4	2	2		
Surgical Specialties	1,395	1,366	1,122	162	82	10	15	2	2
Colon and Rectal Surgery	15	14	13		1	1			
General Surgery	307	298	219	48	31	2	6		1
Neurological Surgery	68	67	54	9	4	1			
Obstetrics & Gynecology	336	323	266	35	22	3	7	2	1
Ophthalmology	148	147	130	14	3		1		
Orthopedic Surgery	235	234	199	28	7	1			
Otolaryngology	90	89	70	12	7	1			
Plastic Surgery	50	50	48	2					
Thoracic Surgery	35	35	32		3				
Urology	111	109	91	14	4	1	1		
Other Specialties	1,743	1,645	1,198	229	218	32	30	12	24
Aerospace Medicine	10	5	3		2	2		2	1
Anatomic/Clinical Pathology	142	125	98	14	13	4	6	1	6
Anesthesiology	378	372	304	32	36		5		1
Child & Adolescent Psychiatry	44	40	24	2	14	2	1	1	
Diagnostic Radiology	230	223	163	43	17		2		5
Emergency Medicine	214	207	146	19	42	2	4	1	
Forensic Pathology	3	1	1						2
General Preventive Medicine	10	9	6		3	1			
Medical Genetics	3	3	3						
Neurology	105	99	69	17	13	1	4	1	
Nuclear Medicine	12	11	6	2	3	1			
Occupational Medicine	33	25	21		4	6			2
Other Specialty	34	27	23	3	1	3		3	1
Physical Medicine and Rehabilitation	42	42	38	2	2				
Psychiatry	296	280	183	45	52	7	6	3	
Public Health and General Preventive Medicine	7	2	1	1		2	2		1
Radiation Oncology	45	44	38	4	2	1			
Radiology	60	57	51		6				3
Transplant Surgery	4	3	2		1				1
Unspecified	69	68	16	45	7				1
Vascular Medicine	2	2	2						
Inactive	1,044								
Not Classified	276								

Note: Excludes Address Unknown.

Subspecialties in this table are condensed into major specialties. See Appendix A.

Table 3.7

Physicians by State, Self-Designated Specialty, and Activity, 2010, continued
Oregon

		Patient Care				Other Professional Activity			
				Hospital Based					
Specialty	Total Physicians	Total Patient Care	Office Based	Resid./ Fellows	Phys. Staff	Admin.	Med. Teach.	Research	Other
Total Physicians	13,007	9,737	7,882	874	981	166	115	153	72
FM/GP	1,492	1,437	1,252	89	96	28	17	4	6
Family Medicine	1,411	1,361	1,183	89	89	24	17	3	6
General Practice	81	76	69		7	4		1	
Medical Specialties	3,553	3,370	2,709	342	319	49	40	82	12
Allergy and Immunology	40	37	37			1		2	
Cardiovascular Disease	197	189	151	21	17	2	2	4	
Dermatology	149	145	126	13	6		1	3	
Gastroenterology	156	150	132	8	10	3		3	
Internal Medicine	2,112	1,994	1,543	229	222	33	23	52	10
Pediatric Cardiology	18	18	11	3	4				
Pediatrics	765	732	621	59	52	8	11	12	2
Pulmonary Disease	116	105	88	9	8	2	3	6	
Surgical Specialties	2,176	2,130	1,771	210	149	15	11	13	7
Colon and Rectal Surgery	18	18	15	3					
General Surgery	509	499	361	94	44	5	2	3	
Neurological Surgery	103	101	82	11	8		2		
Obstetrics & Gynecology	546	534	473	31	30	3	3	5	1
Ophthalmology	252	245	219	17	9	2	2	3	
Orthopedic Surgery	335	324	276	14	34	4	1		6
Otolaryngology	150	148	123	17	8	1		1	
Plastic Surgery	75	75	62	7	6				
Thoracic Surgery	50	49	46	2	1			1	
Urology	138	137	114	14	9		1		
Other Specialties	3,022	2,800	2,150	233	417	74	47	54	47
Aerospace Medicine	2	1	1			1			
Anatomic/Clinical Pathology	204	166	123	14	29	6	3	9	20
Anesthesiology	608	593	504	38	51	3	10	2	
Child & Adolescent Psychiatry	85	82	70	6	6	1		1	1
Diagnostic Radiology	311	302	237	28	37	3	2	1	3
Emergency Medicine	613	592	414	37	141	9	10	2	
Forensic Pathology	9	4	4				1	1	3
General Preventive Medicine	33	22	15	3	4	7	1	2	1
Medical Genetics	8	5	4	1				3	
Neurology	186	165	130	18	17	1	5	12	3
Nuclear Medicine	11	11	9	1	1				
Occupational Medicine	28	20	19		1	5	1	1	1
Other Specialty	88	54	42	3	9	15	2	11	6
Physical Medicine and Rehabilitation	91	88	79	2	7	3			
Psychiatry	471	440	318	33	89	13	10	3	5
Public Health and General Preventive Medicine	22	9	7		2	7		4	2
Radiation Oncology	65	64	52	5	7		1		
Radiology	99	97	83	4	10			1	1
Transplant Surgery	1	1			1				
Unspecified	86	83	38	40	5		1	1	1
Vascular Medicine	1	1	1						
Inactive	2,082								
Not Classified	682								

Note: Excludes Address Unknown.

Subspecialties in this table are condensed into major specialties. See Appendix A.

Table 3.7

Physicians by State, Self-Designated Specialty, and Activity, 2010, continued
Pennsylvania

		Patient Care				Other Professional Activity			
				Hospital Based					
Specialty	Total Physicians	Total Patient Care	Office Based	Resid./ Fellows	Phys. Staff	Admin.	Med. Teach.	Research	Other
Total Physicians	44,988	33,568	23,167	6,683	3,718	700	475	852	244
FM/GP	3,815	3,595	2,845	485	265	91	99	13	17
Family Medicine	3,594	3,386	2,665	485	236	84	99	9	16
General Practice	221	209	180		29	7		4	1
Medical Specialties	13,963	12,968	9,002	2,691	1,275	246	183	490	76
Allergy and Immunology	183	169	141	19	9		1	12	1
Cardiovascular Disease	1,279	1,200	929	186	85	17	11	42	9
Dermatology	489	474	371	82	21	1	3	10	1
Gastroenterology	678	647	500	90	57	7	8	13	3
Internal Medicine	7,572	6,990	4,685	1,609	696	149	96	293	44
Pediatric Cardiology	107	98	47	32	19	2		6	1
Pediatrics	3,066	2,844	1,928	578	338	59	59	88	16
Pulmonary Disease	589	546	401	95	50	11	5	26	1
Surgical Specialties	7,334	7,118	5,068	1,512	538	79	62	49	26
Colon and Rectal Surgery	93	91	81	4	6			1	1
General Surgery	1,875	1,804	1,066	554	184	33	16	10	12
Neurological Surgery	281	274	169	77	28	3	1	2	1
Obstetrics & Gynecology	1,698	1,631	1,198	294	139	25	24	13	5
Ophthalmology	860	840	710	98	32	4	6	9	1
Orthopedic Surgery	1,114	1,096	787	262	47	4	6	4	4
Otolaryngology	429	419	308	95	16	2	5	2	1
Plastic Surgery	283	282	214	54	14			1	
Thoracic Surgery	245	234	173	21	40	5	3	3	
Urology	456	447	362	53	32	3	1	4	1
Other Specialties	10,727	9,887	6,252	1,995	1,640	284	131	300	125
Aerospace Medicine	5	4	4			1			
Anatomic/Clinical Pathology	925	791	414	167	210	33	17	41	43
Anesthesiology	1,823	1,766	1,218	308	240	15	21	20	1
Child & Adolescent Psychiatry	352	326	243	40	43	10	4	9	3
Diagnostic Radiology	1,316	1,279	795	329	155	5	15	11	6
Emergency Medicine	1,439	1,369	682	328	359	35	14	12	9
Forensic Pathology	26	18	15	2	1	1			7
General Preventive Medicine	55	44	35		9	4	1	4	2
Medical Genetics	23	21	9	7	5			2	
Neurology	760	694	483	137	74	11	6	45	4
Nuclear Medicine	76	68	41	10	17	1	2	4	1
Occupational Medicine	92	62	44		18	22	2	2	4
Other Specialty	275	148	83	47	18	42	7	63	15
Physical Medicine and Rehabilitation	535	520	371	88	61	10		3	2
Psychiatry	1,894	1,715	1,217	209	289	63	29	73	14
Public Health and General Preventive Medicine	33	6	5		1	17	1	2	7
Radiation Oncology	238	233	144	48	41	2	1	1	1
Radiology	466	443	318	52	73	4	11	2	6
Transplant Surgery	12	10	6	1	3	1		1	
Unspecified	380	368	123	222	23	7		5	
Vascular Medicine	2	2	2						
Inactive	5,856								
Not Classified	3,293								

Note: Excludes Address Unknown.

Subspecialties in this table are condensed into major specialties. See Appendix A.

Table 3.7

Physicians by State, Self-Designated Specialty, and Activity, 2010, continued
Puerto Rico

		Patient Care				Other Professional Activity			
				Hospital Based					
Specialty	Total Physicians	Total Patient Care	Office Based	Resid./ Fellows	Phys. Staff	Admin.	Med. Teach.	Research	Other
Total Physicians	12,154	9,133	7,166	981	986	191	137	47	54
FM/GP	2,078	1,993	1,684	29	280	47	20	4	14
Family Medicine	749	712	619	29	64	20	14	1	2
General Practice	1,329	1,281	1,065		216	27	6	3	12
Medical Specialties	3,142	2,985	2,283	397	305	62	64	20	11
Allergy and Immunology	11	11	9	2					
Cardiovascular Disease	220	207	180	14	13	1	7	3	2
Dermatology	83	80	65	9	6		2	1	
Gastroenterology	126	121	98	16	7	1	2	2	
Internal Medicine	1,561	1,501	1,079	270	152	23	24	7	6
Pediatric Cardiology	11	11	10		1				
Pediatrics	1,035	968	771	78	119	37	23	4	3
Pulmonary Disease	95	86	71	8	7		6	3	
Surgical Specialties	1,435	1,389	1,127	148	114	18	22	3	3
Colon and Rectal Surgery	6	6	4	1	1				
General Surgery	352	335	244	47	44	6	10		1
Neurological Surgery	30	28	15	11	2		2		
Obstetrics & Gynecology	531	511	426	40	45	9	7	2	2
Ophthalmology	165	163	141	15	7	1		1	
Orthopedic Surgery	128	124	102	21	1	1	3		
Otolaryngology	71	70	59	8	3	1			
Plastic Surgery	33	33	30		3				
Thoracic Surgery	21	21	17	1	3				
Urology	98	98	89	4	5				
Other Specialties	2,907	2,766	2,072	407	287	64	31	20	26
Aerospace Medicine	1	1	1						
Anatomic/Clinical Pathology	112	94	73	15	6	5	5	1	7
Anesthesiology	193	188	161	9	18	1	2	1	1
Child & Adolescent Psychiatry	70	65	52	6	7	1	3		1
Diagnostic Radiology	171	158	117	19	22	3	4	1	5
Emergency Medicine	173	160	82	38	40	11	2		
Forensic Pathology	3	3	3						
General Preventive Medicine	21	16	14		2	2	1	1	1
Medical Genetics	5	3	3				1	1	
Neurology	134	127	93	21	13		3	3	1
Nuclear Medicine	35	32	24	5	3	2	1		
Occupational Medicine	35	30	23		7	5			
Other Specialty	55	41	34	1	6	10	2	2	
Physical Medicine and Rehabilitation	214	212	163	32	17	1	1		
Psychiatry	423	401	298	43	60	10	5	4	3
Public Health and General Preventive Medicine	18	6	3		3	8		2	2
Radiation Oncology	23	21	18		3	1		1	
Radiology	66	63	55		8	1	1	1	
Unspecified	1,155	1,145	855	218	72	3		2	5
Inactive	997								
Not Classified	1,595								

Note: Excludes Address Unknown.

Subspecialties in this table are condensed into major specialties. See Appendix A.

Table 3.7

Physicians by State, Self-Designated Specialty, and Activity, 2010, continued
Rhode Island

		Patient Care				Other Professional Activity			
				Hospital Based					
Specialty	Total Physicians	Total Patient Care	Office Based	Resid./ Fellows	Phys. Staff	Admin.	Med. Teach.	Research	Other
Total Physicians	4,622	3,515	2,318	779	418	72	46	67	19
FM/GP	235	224	163	38	23	5	5	1	
Family Medicine	222	211	150	38	23	5	5	1	
General Practice	13	13	13						
Medical Specialties	1,698	1,604	1,063	382	159	24	25	40	5
Allergy and Immunology	11	11	11						
Cardiovascular Disease	117	116	87	21	8			1	
Dermatology	69	64	37	23	4	3	1	1	
Gastroenterology	63	62	51	3	8	1			
Internal Medicine	951	896	594	224	78	15	10	27	3
Pediatric Cardiology	7	7	5	1	1				
Pediatrics	421	393	238	100	55	5	12	9	2
Pulmonary Disease	59	55	40	10	5		2	2	
Surgical Specialties	744	724	521	157	46	8	7	4	1
Colon and Rectal Surgery	7	7	7						
General Surgery	178	174	112	49	13	2		2	
Neurological Surgery	26	25	15	7	3		1		
Obstetrics & Gynecology	208	199	149	34	16	4	3	2	
Ophthalmology	67	67	56	4	7				
Orthopedic Surgery	140	137	91	43	3		2		1
Otolaryngology	33	32	30	1	1	1			
Plastic Surgery	22	22	14	8					
Thoracic Surgery	12	12	9	1	2				
Urology	51	49	38	10	1	1	1		
Other Specialties	1,042	963	571	202	190	35	9	22	13
Anatomic/Clinical Pathology	97	79	24	17	38	5	2	5	6
Anesthesiology	120	118	95	4	19	1		1	
Child & Adolescent Psychiatry	49	44	25	12	7	3	1		1
Diagnostic Radiology	128	125	81	29	15	1		1	1
Emergency Medicine	175	169	91	49	29	5		1	
Forensic Pathology	4	2	2						2
General Preventive Medicine	7	7	5	1	1				
Medical Genetics	1	1			1				
Neurology	76	71	52	14	5	1	4		
Nuclear Medicine	5	5	4	1					
Occupational Medicine	10	10	6		4				
Other Specialty	46	36	17	18	1	3		6	1
Physical Medicine and Rehabilitation	14	12	7		5	1			1
Psychiatry	220	198	111	37	50	13	2	6	1
Public Health and General Preventive Medicine	4	1	1			2		1	
Radiation Oncology	18	18	14	1	3				
Radiology	37	36	26	3	7			1	
Transplant Surgery	2	2	1		1				
Unspecified	29	29	9	16	4				
Inactive	524								
Not Classified	379								

Note: Excludes Address Unknown.

Subspecialties in this table are condensed into major specialties. See Appendix A.

Table 3.7

Physicians by State, Self-Designated Specialty, and Activity, 2010, continued
South Carolina

		Patient Care				Other Professional Activity			
				Hospital Based					
Specialty	Total Physicians	Total Patient Care	Office Based	Resid./ Fellows	Phys. Staff	Admin.	Med. Teach.	Research	Other
Total Physicians	12,240	9,851	7,681	1,206	964	119	158	89	34
FM/GP	1,687	1,622	1,315	180	127	21	34	6	4
Family Medicine	1,592	1,535	1,235	180	120	16	34	5	2
General Practice	95	87	80		7	5		1	2
Medical Specialties	3,430	3,278	2,558	403	317	32	69	46	5
Allergy and Immunology	53	52	49	1	2		1		
Cardiovascular Disease	278	268	235	19	14	3	7		
Dermatology	130	126	110	11	5	2	2		
Gastroenterology	176	171	148	12	11		2	3	
Internal Medicine	1,685	1,609	1,229	195	185	14	27	33	2
Pediatric Cardiology	35	34	20	10	4			1	
Pediatrics	946	899	666	139	94	9	27	8	3
Pulmonary Disease	127	119	101	16	2	4	3	1	
Surgical Specialties	2,304	2,251	1,819	282	150	14	24	10	5
Colon and Rectal Surgery	16	16	14		2				
General Surgery	535	518	360	105	53	8	6	2	1
Neurological Surgery	71	69	59	8	2	1		1	
Obstetrics & Gynecology	616	602	506	55	41		11	1	2
Ophthalmology	255	251	222	24	5			4	
Orthopedic Surgery	368	361	289	53	19		4	2	1
Otolaryngology	139	136	112	19	5	1	2		
Plastic Surgery	90	89	78	5	6	1			
Thoracic Surgery	67	66	54	4	8	1			
Urology	147	143	125	9	9	2	1		1
Other Specialties	2,830	2,700	1,989	341	370	52	31	27	20
Aerospace Medicine	5	5	2		3				
Anatomic/Clinical Pathology	234	210	154	33	23	6	8	3	7
Anesthesiology	507	497	411	43	43	4	3	2	1
Child & Adolescent Psychiatry	134	128	100	15	13	1	2	3	
Diagnostic Radiology	310	303	223	40	40	1	1	1	4
Emergency Medicine	526	516	354	50	112	5	4	1	
Forensic Pathology	10	9	6	1	2		1		
General Preventive Medicine	18	14	8	4	2	2	1	1	
Medical Genetics	12	12	11	1					
Neurology	150	144	116	19	9	2	1	3	
Nuclear Medicine	13	12	8	2	2			1	
Occupational Medicine	26	24	16		8	2			
Other Specialty	56	44	31	9	4	6		5	1
Physical Medicine and Rehabilitation	79	78	71	1	6				1
Psychiatry	472	444	288	71	85	9	9	6	4
Public Health and General Preventive Medicine	20	3	3			14	1		2
Radiation Oncology	51	51	46	5					
Radiology	105	104	95	1	8			1	
Transplant Surgery	3	3	2		1				
Unspecified	99	99	44	46	9				
Inactive	1,579								
Not Classified	410								

Note: Excludes Address Unknown.

Subspecialties in this table are condensed into major specialties. See Appendix A.

Table 3.7

Physicians by State, Self-Designated Specialty, and Activity, 2010, continued
South Dakota

		Patient Care				Other Professional Activity			
				Hospital Based					
Specialty	Total Physicians	Total Patient Care	Office Based	Resid./ Fellows	Phys. Staff	Admin.	Med. Teach.	Research	Other
Total Physicians	2,098	1,691	1,391	90	210	23	22	8	12
FM/GP	422	405	331	34	40	7	10		
Family Medicine	394	378	306	34	38	6	10		
General Practice	28	27	25		2	1			
Medical Specialties	510	480	390	20	70	11	10	6	3
Allergy and Immunology	6	6	6						
Cardiovascular Disease	43	41	38		3	1		1	
Dermatology	24	24	20	1	3				
Gastroenterology	21	19	17		2		2		
Internal Medicine	292	270	207	18	45	10	6	3	3
Pediatric Cardiology	4	4	2		2				
Pediatrics	101	99	84	1	14		1	1	
Pulmonary Disease	19	17	16		1		1	1	
Surgical Specialties	387	385	344	3	38	1		1	
Colon and Rectal Surgery	2	2	2						
General Surgery	97	97	86	2	9				
Neurological Surgery	20	20	19		1				
Obstetrics & Gynecology	76	76	68		8				
Ophthalmology	37	36	35		1			1	
Orthopedic Surgery	73	72	64	1	7	1			
Otolaryngology	29	29	22		7				
Plastic Surgery	12	12	12						
Thoracic Surgery	13	13	12		1				
Urology	28	28	24		4				
Other Specialties	437	421	326	33	62	4	2	1	9
Anatomic/Clinical Pathology	44	40	30	7	3	1			3
Anesthesiology	69	68	65		3	1			
Child & Adolescent Psychiatry	17	16	11	2	3		1		
Diagnostic Radiology	58	57	47	1	9				1
Emergency Medicine	54	52	39		13	1		1	
General Preventive Medicine	3	3	1		2				
Medical Genetics	2	2	2						
Neurology	33	33	32		1				
Nuclear Medicine	6	5	4		1				1
Occupational Medicine	7	6	5		1				1
Other Specialty	8	6	3		3	1			1
Physical Medicine and Rehabilitation	24	24	19		5				
Psychiatry	60	59	34	11	14		1		
Radiation Oncology	14	13	11		2				1
Radiology	17	16	15		1				1
Transplant Surgery	1	1	1						
Unspecified	20	20	7	12	1				
Inactive	299								
Not Classified	43								

Note: Excludes Address Unknown.

Subspecialties in this table are condensed into major specialties. See Appendix A.

Table 3.7

Physicians by State, Self-Designated Specialty, and Activity, 2010, continued
Tennessee

		Patient Care				Other Professional Activity			
				Hospital Based					
Specialty	Total Physicians	Total Patient Care	Office Based	Resid./ Fellows	Phys. Staff	Admin.	Med. Teach.	Research	Other
Total Physicians	19,035	15,143	11,775	2,122	1,246	250	175	218	69
FM/GP	1,976	1,900	1,646	145	109	36	33	3	4
Family Medicine	1,831	1,760	1,521	145	94	32	33	3	3
General Practice	145	140	125		15	4			1
Medical Specialties	6,108	5,788	4,464	860	464	91	69	144	16
Allergy and Immunology	87	83	71	12		1		3	
Cardiovascular Disease	484	467	385	63	19	4	3	9	1
Dermatology	185	182	152	20	10		1	2	
Gastroenterology	246	236	207	19	10	3	2	5	
Internal Medicine	3,120	2,953	2,253	415	285	51	41	65	10
Pediatric Cardiology	54	49	32	12	5			5	
Pediatrics	1,643	1,548	1,146	287	115	28	19	44	4
Pulmonary Disease	289	270	218	32	20	4	3	11	1
Surgical Specialties	3,630	3,554	2,816	558	180	27	34	9	6
Colon and Rectal Surgery	20	19	16	1	2		1		
General Surgery	906	886	604	223	59	7	11	1	1
Neurological Surgery	132	132	101	27	4				
Obstetrics & Gynecology	918	892	747	103	42	8	10	6	2
Ophthalmology	347	342	298	31	13	2	2	1	
Orthopedic Surgery	572	563	453	89	21	5	2	1	1
Otolaryngology	218	213	169	34	10		4		1
Plastic Surgery	144	144	125	13	6				
Thoracic Surgery	112	107	87	6	14	3	2		
Urology	261	256	216	31	9	2	2		1
Other Specialties	4,141	3,901	2,849	559	493	96	39	62	43
Aerospace Medicine	4	4	3		1				
Anatomic/Clinical Pathology	428	378	275	58	45	13	5	15	17
Anesthesiology	790	772	606	95	71	4	8	5	1
Child & Adolescent Psychiatry	93	87	69	9	9	1	3	2	
Diagnostic Radiology	579	565	403	110	52	4	3	2	5
Emergency Medicine	554	543	378	54	111	9	1		1
Forensic Pathology	17	14	11		3	1			2
General Preventive Medicine	32	28	18	8	2	3	1		
Medical Genetics	7	6	3		3			1	
Neurology	292	274	218	37	19	1	6	11	
Nuclear Medicine	30	28	21	6	1			2	
Occupational Medicine	51	34	30		4	13		1	3
Other Specialty	101	72	52	11	9	15		11	3
Physical Medicine and Rehabilitation	111	106	94	1	11	2			3
Psychiatry	597	564	387	80	97	14	8	7	4
Public Health and General Preventive Medicine	25	8	8			13	1	3	
Radiation Oncology	90	89	63	8	18	1			
Radiology	218	214	176	9	29	1	1		2
Transplant Surgery	3	3	2		1				
Unspecified	118	111	31	73	7	1	2	2	2
Vascular Medicine	1	1	1						
Inactive	2,177								
Not Classified	1,003								

Note: Excludes Address Unknown.

Subspecialties in this table are condensed into major specialties. See Appendix A.

Table 3.7

Physicians by State, Self-Designated Specialty, and Activity, 2010, continued
Texas

Specialty	Total Physicians	Patient Care				Other Professional Activity			
				Hospital Based					
		Total Patient Care	Office Based	Resid./ Fellows	Phys. Staff	Admin.	Med. Teach.	Research	Other
Total Physicians	60,991	48,536	37,367	6,838	4,331	711	715	579	191
FM/GP	6,677	6,453	5,512	552	389	94	103	11	16
Family Medicine	6,185	5,972	5,077	552	343	89	101	9	14
General Practice	492	481	435		46	5	2	2	2
Medical Specialties	18,295	17,425	13,413	2,480	1,532	213	285	338	34
Allergy and Immunology	328	303	267	19	17	1	2	21	1
Cardiovascular Disease	1,408	1,348	1,114	142	92	12	18	28	2
Dermatology	747	735	566	116	53	1	8	2	1
Gastroenterology	846	808	671	85	52	7	14	17	
Internal Medicine	8,940	8,469	6,451	1,200	818	127	139	189	16
Pediatric Cardiology	157	152	103	25	24	1		3	1
Pediatrics	5,238	5,010	3,778	822	410	54	96	67	11
Pulmonary Disease	631	600	463	71	66	10	8	11	2
Surgical Specialties	11,236	10,962	8,701	1,624	637	81	136	36	21
Colon and Rectal Surgery	125	123	113	7	3		2		
General Surgery	2,349	2,287	1,602	492	193	20	29	9	4
Neurological Surgery	391	383	291	66	26	6	2		
Obstetrics & Gynecology	3,134	3,038	2,531	379	128	23	58	11	4
Ophthalmology	1,196	1,174	983	129	62	7	11	2	2
Orthopedic Surgery	1,659	1,625	1,291	251	83	9	13	4	8
Otolaryngology	722	704	568	101	35	8	7	2	1
Plastic Surgery	601	592	475	85	32	3	4		2
Thoracic Surgery	335	322	278	19	25	3	5	5	
Urology	724	714	569	95	50	2	5	3	
Other Specialties	14,524	13,696	9,741	2,182	1,773	323	191	194	120
Aerospace Medicine	79	44	25		19	22	1	6	6
Anatomic/Clinical Pathology	1,388	1,260	827	241	192	31	24	37	36
Anesthesiology	3,359	3,295	2,555	421	319	18	35	7	4
Child & Adolescent Psychiatry	466	438	333	51	54	13	6	6	3
Diagnostic Radiology	1,718	1,685	1,142	328	215	5	14	4	10
Emergency Medicine	1,884	1,823	1,304	207	312	32	23	2	4
Forensic Pathology	52	41	31	6	4	2			9
General Preventive Medicine	107	83	58	9	16	16	1	4	3
Medical Genetics	50	41	20	10	11	2	3	4	
Neurology	946	897	673	144	80	5	16	26	2
Nuclear Medicine	82	74	50	7	17	2	3	3	
Occupational Medicine	154	107	93	1	13	39	3	3	2
Other Specialty	271	181	131	28	22	35	9	37	9
Physical Medicine and Rehabilitation	587	570	428	86	56	9	3	2	3
Psychiatry	1,866	1,735	1,204	242	289	61	21	34	15
Public Health and General Preventive Medicine	56	16	10	1	5	25	2	10	3
Radiation Oncology	309	304	218	47	39	2	3		
Radiology	610	576	458	39	79	2	21	4	7
Transplant Surgery	17	16	13		3		1		
Unspecified	522	509	167	314	28	2	2	5	4
Vascular Medicine	1	1	1						
Inactive	6,104								
Not Classified	4,155								

Note: Excludes Address Unknown.

Subspecialties in this table are condensed into major specialties. *See Appendix A.*

Table 3.7

Physicians by State, Self-Designated Specialty, and Activity, 2010, continued
Utah

		Patient Care				Other Professional Activity			
				Hospital Based					
Specialty	Total Physicians	Total Patient Care	Office Based	Resid./ Fellows	Phys. Staff	Admin.	Med. Teach.	Research	Other
Total Physicians	6,865	5,334	4,062	766	506	84	68	109	28
FM/GP	795	769	648	64	57	10	11	3	2
Family Medicine	766	744	627	64	53	7	11	3	1
General Practice	29	25	21		4	3			1
Medical Specialties	1,812	1,690	1,242	292	156	26	27	66	3
Allergy and Immunology	16	15	14	1				1	
Cardiovascular Disease	126	111	84	16	11	1	5	9	
Dermatology	99	93	80	9	4	1	1	4	
Gastroenterology	83	79	70	8	1	2	1	1	
Internal Medicine	769	722	496	140	86	10	12	24	1
Pediatric Cardiology	20	18	10	7	1	1		1	
Pediatrics	613	580	443	98	39	9	7	15	2
Pulmonary Disease	86	72	45	13	14	2	1	11	
Surgical Specialties	1,281	1,253	1,019	165	69	12	5	9	2
Colon and Rectal Surgery	11	11	10	1					
General Surgery	242	233	170	42	21	4	1	4	
Neurological Surgery	49	48	34	14				1	
Obstetrics & Gynecology	304	295	250	26	19	3	3	2	1
Ophthalmology	145	143	124	14	5	1		1	
Orthopedic Surgery	232	230	185	33	12		1	1	
Otolaryngology	100	98	81	14	3	2			
Plastic Surgery	79	78	71	6	1	1			
Thoracic Surgery	37	36	28	4	4				1
Urology	82	81	66	11	4	1			
Other Specialties	1,735	1,622	1,153	245	224	36	25	31	21
Aerospace Medicine	3	2	1		1	1			
Anatomic/Clinical Pathology	137	119	74	30	15	3	3	5	7
Anesthesiology	379	362	283	38	41	3	6	4	4
Child & Adolescent Psychiatry	48	44	36	4	4	3		1	
Diagnostic Radiology	175	169	123	25	21		4		2
Emergency Medicine	319	311	232	28	51	5	2		1
Forensic Pathology	1	1	1						
General Preventive Medicine	19	19	12	6	1				
Medical Genetics	8	7	3	2	2		1		
Neurology	124	112	78	23	11	2	1	9	
Nuclear Medicine	3	2	2					1	
Occupational Medicine	22	16	14		2	4	1		1
Other Specialty	40	28	12	11	5	6		4	2
Physical Medicine and Rehabilitation	87	86	63	14	9			1	
Psychiatry	209	196	129	21	46	4	4	3	2
Public Health and General Preventive Medicine	8	1	1			4		3	
Radiation Oncology	33	33	22	7	4				
Radiology	67	64	53	4	7	1	2		
Transplant Surgery	3	3	3						
Unspecified	50	47	11	32	4		1		2
Inactive	835								
Not Classified	407								

Note: Excludes Address Unknown.

Subspecialties in this table are condensed into major specialties. See Appendix A.

Table 3.7

Physicians by State, Self-Designated Specialty, and Activity, 2010, continued
Vermont

		Patient Care				Other Professional Activity			
				Hospital Based					
Specialty	Total Physicians	Total Patient Care	Office Based	Resid./ Fellows	Phys. Staff	Admin.	Med. Teach.	Research	Other
Total Physicians	2,752	2,016	1,381	301	334	42	36	53	12
FM/GP	337	329	272	20	37	2	3	2	1
Family Medicine	324	318	262	20	36	2	2	1	1
General Practice	13	11	10		1		1	1	
Medical Specialties	764	697	477	117	103	14	14	36	3
Allergy and Immunology	8	6	6			1		1	
Cardiovascular Disease	51	45	24	11	10	1	1	4	
Dermatology	23	22	17	5				1	
Gastroenterology	27	26	21	2	3	1			
Internal Medicine	427	388	262	67	59	5	10	21	3
Pediatric Cardiology	3	3			3				
Pediatrics	193	181	133	25	23	5	3	4	
Pulmonary Disease	32	26	14	7	5	1		5	
Surgical Specialties	408	401	289	63	49	2	3		2
Colon and Rectal Surgery	1	1	1						
General Surgery	110	108	72	23	13	1	1		
Neurological Surgery	13	13	5	7	1				
Obstetrics & Gynecology	106	103	75	12	16	1	1		1
Ophthalmology	39	39	36		3				
Orthopedic Surgery	80	79	53	16	10		1		
Otolaryngology	27	27	19	5	3				
Plastic Surgery	9	8	8						1
Thoracic Surgery	4	4	4						
Urology	19	19	16		3				
Other Specialties	650	589	343	101	145	24	16	15	6
Anatomic/Clinical Pathology	76	67	31	20	16	3	3	3	
Anesthesiology	106	104	66	17	21	1	1		
Child & Adolescent Psychiatry	26	26	17	4	5				
Diagnostic Radiology	71	67	29	24	14	2	2		
Emergency Medicine	72	69	28		41	1	2		
Forensic Pathology	2	2	2						
General Preventive Medicine	11	7	4		3	2	1	1	
Medical Genetics	2	2	1		1				
Neurology	45	40	21	13	6		2	2	1
Occupational Medicine	3	2	2			1			
Other Specialty	19	7	5	1	1	6	1	5	
Physical Medicine and Rehabilitation	17	16	8	3	5	1			
Psychiatry	151	137	98	12	27	6	2	4	2
Public Health and General Preventive Medicine	3					1			2
Radiation Oncology	9	9	9						
Radiology	24	23	17	2	4				1
Unspecified	13	11	5	5	1		2		
Inactive	441								
Not Classified	152								

Note: Excludes Address Unknown.

Subspecialties in this table are condensed into major specialties. See Appendix A.

Table 3.7

Physicians by State, Self-Designated Specialty, and Activity, 2010, continued
Virginia

		Patient Care				Other Professional Activity			
				Hospital Based					
Specialty	Total Physicians	Total Patient Care	Office Based	Resid./ Fellows	Phys. Staff	Admin.	Med. Teach.	Research	Other
Total Physicians	25,571	19,819	14,961	2,404	2,454	398	248	227	142
FM/GP	2,864	2,740	2,258	204	278	58	43	10	13
Family Medicine	2,665	2,551	2,113	204	234	52	40	10	12
General Practice	199	189	145		44	6	3		1
Medical Specialties	7,507	7,141	5,498	821	822	113	85	122	46
Allergy and Immunology	131	120	105	11	4		2	7	2
Cardiovascular Disease	493	476	382	39	55	4	3	8	2
Dermatology	268	266	225	25	16	1			1
Gastroenterology	357	340	279	33	28	2	2	10	3
Internal Medicine	3,880	3,670	2,760	452	458	67	47	71	25
Pediatric Cardiology	54	49	32	6	11	1	1	2	1
Pediatrics	2,048	1,957	1,500	237	220	34	26	19	12
Pulmonary Disease	276	263	215	18	30	4	4	5	
Surgical Specialties	4,336	4,247	3,311	517	419	24	36	16	13
Colon and Rectal Surgery	43	42	34	1	7				1
General Surgery	898	876	578	159	139	8	8	4	2
Neurological Surgery	143	141	93	28	20	1			1
Obstetrics & Gynecology	1,261	1,230	1,021	114	95	8	13	6	4
Ophthalmology	474	463	399	38	26	1	8	2	
Orthopedic Surgery	645	639	505	78	56	2	3		1
Otolaryngology	288	283	215	47	21	3	1		1
Plastic Surgery	198	194	159	20	15		2	2	
Thoracic Surgery	99	99	78	5	16				
Urology	287	280	229	27	24	1	1	2	3
Other Specialties	6,127	5,691	3,894	862	935	203	84	79	70
Aerospace Medicine	30	14	3		11	14		1	1
Anatomic/Clinical Pathology	456	391	263	69	59	16	19	11	19
Anesthesiology	1,015	991	732	105	154	3	16	1	4
Child & Adolescent Psychiatry	203	192	149	14	29	7	3	1	
Diagnostic Radiology	675	659	468	108	83	3	4	4	5
Emergency Medicine	1,008	979	657	109	213	16	6	1	6
Forensic Pathology	16	11	7	2	2	1			4
General Preventive Medicine	82	61	42		19	12	2	3	4
Medical Genetics	10	10	4	1	5				
Neurology	395	365	270	54	41	4	7	17	2
Nuclear Medicine	38	34	25	2	7	2		2	
Occupational Medicine	51	27	22		5	18	3		3
Other Specialty	144	98	69	20	9	23	2	16	5
Physical Medicine and Rehabilitation	272	265	180	55	30	4		3	
Psychiatry	1,047	974	669	119	186	39	13	16	5
Public Health and General Preventive Medicine	59	13	8		5	37	1	2	6
Radiation Oncology	108	107	82	12	13	1			
Radiology	235	225	174	15	36	1	6	1	2
Transplant Surgery	3	3	2		1				
Unspecified	280	272	68	177	27	2	2		4
Inactive	3,460								
Not Classified	1,277								

Note: Excludes Address Unknown.

Subspecialties in this table are condensed into major specialties. See Appendix A.

Table 3.7

Physicians by State, Self-Designated Specialty, and Activity, 2010, continued
Virgin Islands

		Patient Care				Other Professional Activity			
				Hospital Based					
Specialty	Total Physicians	Total Patient Care	Office Based	Resid./ Fellows	Phys. Staff	Admin.	Med. Teach.	Research	Other
Total Physicians	209	171	135	1	35	2			
FM/GP	24	24	21		3				
Family Medicine	20	20	18		2				
General Practice	4	4	3		1				
Medical Specialties	54	54	42	1	11				
Allergy and Immunology	1	1	1						
Cardiovascular Disease	4	4	3		1				
Dermatology	2	2	2						
Gastroenterology	2	2	2						
Internal Medicine	29	29	24	1	4				
Pediatrics	16	16	10		6				
Surgical Specialties	54	53	47		6	1			
General Surgery	12	12	11		1				
Obstetrics & Gynecology	23	22	19		3	1			
Ophthalmology	6	6	6						
Orthopedic Surgery	6	6	6						
Otolaryngology	2	2	2						
Plastic Surgery	2	2	2						
Urology	3	3	1		2				
Other Specialties	41	40	25		15	1			
Anesthesiology	8	8	4		4				
Diagnostic Radiology	3	3	2		1				
Emergency Medicine	7	7	4		3				
Forensic Pathology	1	1	1						
General Preventive Medicine	1	1	1						
Neurology	3	3	3						
Nuclear Medicine	1	1			1				
Occupational Medicine	1	1	1						
Physical Medicine and Rehabilitation	3	2	1		1	1			
Psychiatry	5	5	2		3				
Public Health and General Preventive Medicine	1	1			1				
Radiation Oncology	1	1			1				
Radiology	2	2	2						
Unspecified	4	4	4						
Inactive	25								
Not Classified	11								

Note: Excludes Address Unknown.

Subspecialties in this table are condensed into major specialties. See Appendix A.

Table 3.7

Physicians by State, Self-Designated Specialty, and Activity, 2010, continued
Washington

		Patient Care				Other Professional Activity			
				Hospital Based					
Specialty	Total Physicians	Total Patient Care	Office Based	Resid./ Fellows	Phys. Staff	Admin.	Med. Teach.	Research	Other
Total Physicians	21,795	16,274	12,934	1,683	1,657	330	204	404	126
FM/GP	3,105	2,964	2,555	222	187	68	51	12	10
Family Medicine	2,951	2,812	2,415	222	175	66	51	12	10
General Practice	154	152	140		12	2			
Medical Specialties	5,672	5,265	4,170	506	589	91	60	231	25
Allergy and Immunology	77	69	58	2	9	1		6	1
Cardiovascular Disease	346	321	267	20	34	4	7	14	
Dermatology	247	239	222	9	8	1	4	2	1
Gastroenterology	261	248	227	9	12	2		9	2
Internal Medicine	3,077	2,842	2,213	283	346	56	26	140	13
Pediatric Cardiology	35	34	27	5	2			1	
Pediatrics	1,418	1,322	1,016	158	148	22	16	50	8
Pulmonary Disease	211	190	140	20	30	5	7	9	
Surgical Specialties	3,305	3,214	2,587	356	271	28	31	25	7
Colon and Rectal Surgery	19	18	17		1		1		
General Surgery	756	733	507	152	74	11	8	4	
Neurological Surgery	118	111	82	20	9	1	2	2	2
Obstetrics & Gynecology	800	776	682	37	57	6	8	9	1
Ophthalmology	362	356	318	18	20	2	3	1	
Orthopedic Surgery	574	562	447	64	51	4	3	3	2
Otolaryngology	244	242	192	31	19		2		
Plastic Surgery	140	137	123	10	4		2		1
Thoracic Surgery	79	76	52	6	18	1		2	
Urology	213	203	167	18	18	3	2	4	1
Other Specialties	5,256	4,831	3,622	599	610	143	62	136	84
Aerospace Medicine	16	12	6		6	2		1	1
Anatomic/Clinical Pathology	391	340	252	51	37	9	7	15	20
Anesthesiology	1,068	1,030	807	124	99	8	19	9	2
Child & Adolescent Psychiatry	121	112	89	11	12	3	3	2	1
Diagnostic Radiology	626	603	446	102	55	3	8	3	9
Emergency Medicine	808	776	571	39	166	19	6	3	4
Forensic Pathology	14	8	6	1	1	1			5
General Preventive Medicine	73	58	44	5	9	6	2	6	1
Medical Genetics	24	15	10	3	2	1	2	5	1
Neurology	307	287	218	41	28	3	2	9	6
Nuclear Medicine	47	42	29	8	5	1		3	1
Occupational Medicine	90	65	53		12	14		5	6
Other Specialty	142	79	70	4	5	27	2	29	5
Physical Medicine and Rehabilitation	225	214	157	32	25	4	2	2	3
Psychiatry	784	725	539	75	111	19	5	28	7
Public Health and General Preventive Medicine	41	7	7			18	2	10	4
Radiation Oncology	107	103	81	11	11	1	1	2	
Radiology	197	190	154	25	11	2	1	3	1
Transplant Surgery	4	4	4						
Unspecified	171	161	79	67	15	2		1	7
Inactive	3,363								
Not Classified	1,094								

Note: Excludes Address Unknown.

Subspecialties in this table are condensed into major specialties. See Appendix A.

Table 3.7

Physicians by State, Self-Designated Specialty, and Activity, 2010, continued
West Virginia

		Patient Care				Other Professional Activity			
				Hospital Based					
Specialty	Total Physicians	Total Patient Care	Office Based	Resid./ Fellows	Phys. Staff	Admin.	Med. Teach.	Research	Other
Total Physicians	4,922	3,819	2,796	580	443	57	80	24	22
FM/GP	668	635	509	79	47	9	20	1	3
Family Medicine	599	566	450	79	37	9	20	1	3
General Practice	69	69	59		10				
Medical Specialties	1,339	1,277	935	210	132	17	30	11	4
Allergy and Immunology	16	16	16						
Cardiovascular Disease	127	121	90	22	9	1	2	2	1
Dermatology	33	31	27	3	1		2		
Gastroenterology	55	53	44	5	4		1	1	
Internal Medicine	705	673	473	107	93	11	16	3	2
Pediatric Cardiology	9	7	7				1	1	
Pediatrics	326	314	232	62	20	2	7	2	1
Pulmonary Disease	68	62	46	11	5	3	1	2	
Surgical Specialties	916	898	668	143	87	5	10	1	2
Colon and Rectal Surgery	5	5	5						
General Surgery	244	238	157	50	31	2	4		
Neurological Surgery	39	38	28	5	5	1			
Obstetrics & Gynecology	202	194	146	28	20	2	5	1	
Ophthalmology	105	103	87	13	3				2
Orthopedic Surgery	130	129	92	28	9		1		
Otolaryngology	66	66	49	14	3				
Plastic Surgery	28	28	24		4				
Thoracic Surgery	37	37	32	1	4				
Urology	60	60	48	4	8				
Other Specialties	1,079	1,009	684	148	177	26	20	11	13
Aerospace Medicine	1	1			1				
Anatomic/Clinical Pathology	123	109	61	10	38	4	1	2	7
Anesthesiology	160	157	115	21	21		2		1
Child & Adolescent Psychiatry	23	22	16	4	2	1			
Diagnostic Radiology	146	143	107	16	20		3		
Emergency Medicine	188	177	116	18	43	6	3	2	
General Preventive Medicine	7	6	2	3	1			1	
Medical Genetics	1	1	1						
Neurology	82	79	60	13	6		2	1	
Nuclear Medicine	2	1	1				1		
Occupational Medicine	13	8	8			3		2	
Other Specialty	36	32	16	13	3	3			1
Physical Medicine and Rehabilitation	30	29	25		4	1			
Psychiatry	169	158	95	35	28	3	6	1	1
Public Health and General Preventive Medicine	7					3	1	2	1
Radiation Oncology	17	17	15		2				
Radiology	47	42	37	1	4	2	1		2
Unspecified	27	27	9	14	4				
Inactive	609								
Not Classified	311								

Note: Excludes Address Unknown.

Subspecialties in this table are condensed into major specialties. See Appendix A.

Table 3.7

Physicians by State, Self-Designated Specialty, and Activity, 2010, continued
Wisconsin

		Patient Care				Other Professional Activity			
				Hospital Based					
Specialty	Total Physicians	Total Patient Care	Office Based	Resid./ Fellows	Phys. Staff	Admin.	Med. Teach.	Research	Other
Total Physicians	17,220	13,668	10,604	1,754	1,310	218	175	180	77
FM/GP	2,483	2,390	2,048	182	160	36	40	7	10
Family Medicine	2,399	2,308	1,975	182	151	36	40	7	8
General Practice	84	82	73		9				2
Medical Specialties	4,798	4,538	3,516	631	391	89	61	97	13
Allergy and Immunology	98	91	75	11	5			7	
Cardiovascular Disease	336	323	265	34	24	2	5	6	
Dermatology	194	193	151	29	13		1		
Gastroenterology	198	196	163	23	10		1	1	
Internal Medicine	2,532	2,380	1,851	296	233	56	30	55	11
Pediatric Cardiology	41	39	19	11	9		1	1	
Pediatrics	1,223	1,162	872	207	83	22	17	21	1
Pulmonary Disease	176	154	120	20	14	9	6	6	1
Surgical Specialties	2,870	2,796	2,244	358	194	21	24	20	9
Colon and Rectal Surgery	21	21	17	2	2				
General Surgery	644	619	463	115	41	10	5	6	4
Neurological Surgery	119	117	85	21	11	1			1
Obstetrics & Gynecology	667	653	548	59	46	6	7	1	
Ophthalmology	339	325	280	25	20	2	3	7	2
Orthopedic Surgery	502	495	407	52	36	1	2	3	1
Otolaryngology	206	201	162	29	10		3	1	1
Plastic Surgery	101	99	67	27	5		1	1	
Thoracic Surgery	78	75	58	5	12		3		
Urology	193	191	157	23	11	1		1	
Other Specialties	4,167	3,944	2,796	583	565	72	50	56	45
Anatomic/Clinical Pathology	358	315	225	40	50	14	4	9	16
Anesthesiology	862	834	585	129	120	9	12	7	
Child & Adolescent Psychiatry	128	125	101	10	14	1	2		
Diagnostic Radiology	565	555	383	105	67	1	4		5
Emergency Medicine	569	551	389	49	113	13	1	3	1
Forensic Pathology	11	6	6			1			4
General Preventive Medicine	15	13	9	1	3			1	1
Medical Genetics	10	8	7	1			1	1	
Neurology	277	262	207	36	19	1	1	11	2
Nuclear Medicine	30	28	23	5			1		1
Occupational Medicine	49	45	34		11	2	1	1	
Other Specialty	91	56	34	15	7	12	7	13	3
Physical Medicine and Rehabilitation	202	196	139	25	32	2		2	2
Psychiatry	589	559	408	65	86	11	11	6	2
Public Health and General Preventive Medicine	12	1			1	4	2	1	4
Radiation Oncology	96	95	65	17	13	1			
Radiology	185	182	147	14	21		2		1
Transplant Surgery	5	5	3		2				
Unspecified	112	107	30	71	6		1	1	3
Vascular Medicine	1	1	1						
Inactive	2,234								
Not Classified	668								

Note: Excludes Address Unknown.

Subspecialties in this table are condensed into major specialties. See Appendix A.

Table 3.7

Physicians by State, Self-Designated Specialty, and Activity, 2010, continued
Wyoming

		Patient Care				Other Professional Activity			
				Hospital Based					
Specialty	Total Physicians	Total Patient Care	Office Based	Resid./ Fellows	Phys. Staff	Admin.	Med. Teach.	Research	Other
Total Physicians	1,242	964	807	32	125	16	7	4	5
FM/GP	257	250	198	23	29	2	4		1
Family Medicine	244	238	187	23	28	2	3		1
General Practice	13	12	11		1		1		
Medical Specialties	230	224	186	5	33	5		1	
Allergy and Immunology	3	3	3						
Cardiovascular Disease	13	12	11		1			1	
Dermatology	10	10	9		1				
Gastroenterology	10	10	8		2				
Internal Medicine	131	127	98	5	24	4			
Pediatrics	55	54	49		5	1			
Pulmonary Disease	8	8	8						
Surgical Specialties	246	242	229		13	1	2		1
General Surgery	59	59	56		3				
Neurological Surgery	9	9	9						
Obstetrics & Gynecology	63	61	60		1	1	1		
Ophthalmology	17	16	16				1		
Orthopedic Surgery	61	60	54		6				1
Otolaryngology	14	14	12		2				
Plastic Surgery	3	3	3						
Thoracic Surgery	4	4	4						
Urology	16	16	15		1				
Other Specialties	263	248	194	4	50	8	1	3	3
Aerospace Medicine	1	1			1				
Anatomic/Clinical Pathology	24	21	18		3	1		1	1
Anesthesiology	55	54	50		4			1	
Child & Adolescent Psychiatry	5	5	4		1				
Diagnostic Radiology	31	31	25	1	5				
Emergency Medicine	58	55	38		17	2			1
General Preventive Medicine	2	1	1					1	
Neurology	13	12	10		2	1			
Occupational Medicine	2	1	1				1		
Other Specialty	5	4	4			1			
Physical Medicine and Rehabilitation	8	7	6		1				1
Psychiatry	44	41	27		14	3			
Radiation Oncology	5	5	4		1				
Radiology	6	6	5	1					
Unspecified	4	4	1	2	1				
Inactive	223								
Not Classified	23								

Note: Excludes Address Unknown.

Subspecialties in this table are condensed into major specialties. See Appendix A.

Table 3.7

Physicians by State, Self-Designated Specialty, and Activity, 2010, continued
Pacific Islands

		Patient Care				Other Professional Activity			
				Hospital Based					
Specialty	Total Physicians	Total Patient Care	Office Based	Resid./ Fellows	Phys. Staff	Admin.	Med. Teach.	Research	Other
Total Physicians	233	187	142	4	41	3	1		3
FM/GP	48	48	44		4				
Family Medicine	40	40	37		3				
General Practice	8	8	7		1				
Medical Specialties	64	63	52	1	10		1		
Dermatology	2	2	2						
Internal Medicine	36	36	31	1	4				
Pediatrics	26	25	19		6		1		
Surgical Specialties	36	35	27	1	7	1			
General Surgery	10	10	9		1				
Obstetrics & Gynecology	14	14	11		3				
Ophthalmology	4	3	2		1	1			
Orthopedic Surgery	3	3	2	1					
Otolaryngology	2	2	1		1				
Plastic Surgery	1	1	1						
Urology	2	2	1		1				
Other Specialties	46	41	19	2	20	2			3
Aerospace Medicine	1	1			1				
Anatomic/Clinical Pathology	3	2	1		1				1
Anesthesiology	8	8	4		4				
Diagnostic Radiology	6	6	3		3				
Emergency Medicine	10	10	3		7				
General Preventive Medicine	2	2	1	1					
Neurology	2	2	1		1				
Other Specialty	2	1			1	1			
Psychiatry	7	7	5		2				
Public Health and General Preventive Medicine	3					1			2
Radiation Oncology	1	1	1						
Unspecified	1	1		1					
Inactive	22								
Not Classified	17								

Note: Excludes Address Unknown.

Subspecialties in this table are condensed into major specialties. See Appendix A.

Table 3.8

Female Physicians by State, Self-Designated Specialty, and Activity, 2010
Alabama

		Patient Care				Other Professional Activity			
				Hospital Based					
Specialty	Total Physicians	Total Patient Care	Office Based	Resid./ Fellows	Phys. Staff	Admin.	Med. Teach.	Research	Other
Total Physicians	2,767	2,323	1,618	479	226	18	16	18	14
FM/GP	381	374	286	54	34	2	2	1	2
Family Medicine	369	362	276	54	32	2	2	1	2
General Practice	12	12	10		2				
Medical Specialties	1,073	1,045	761	206	78	5	9	12	2
Allergy and Immunology	14	14	12	1	1				
Cardiovascular Disease	26	24	20	4			1	1	
Dermatology	56	56	48	7	1				
Gastroenterology	16	15	10	4	1			1	
Internal Medicine	481	467	323	96	48	2	6	5	1
Pediatric Cardiology	3	3	3						
Pediatrics	456	447	332	88	27	2	2	4	1
Pulmonary Disease	21	19	13	6		1		1	
Surgical Specialties	327	323	228	79	16		2		2
Colon and Rectal Surgery	1	1	1						
General Surgery	70	69	33	31	5				1
Neurological Surgery	6	6	1	4	1				
Obstetrics & Gynecology	188	186	145	31	10		2		
Ophthalmology	20	20	18	2					
Orthopedic Surgery	13	12	8	4					1
Otolaryngology	16	16	11	5					
Plastic Surgery	2	2	2						
Thoracic Surgery	1	1	1						
Urology	10	10	8	2					
Other Specialties	608	581	343	140	98	11	3	5	8
Anatomic/Clinical Pathology	86	79	41	28	10	2	1	1	3
Anesthesiology	87	86	53	16	17	1			
Child & Adolescent Psychiatry	36	35	30	2	3			1	
Diagnostic Radiology	57	55	35	15	5			1	1
Emergency Medicine	59	59	36	6	17				
Forensic Pathology	2	1	1						1
General Preventive Medicine	7	7	6		1				
Medical Genetics	1								1
Neurology	46	45	25	16	4				1
Nuclear Medicine	3	3	1	1	1				
Occupational Medicine	2	2	1		1				
Other Specialty	19	18	8	5	5	1			
Physical Medicine and Rehabilitation	25	23	15	3	5	2			
Psychiatry	108	104	66	15	23	2	1	1	
Public Health and General Preventive Medicine	4	1	1			3			
Radiation Oncology	14	13	8	2	3			1	
Radiology	13	11	10	1			1		1
Unspecified	39	39	6	30	3				
Inactive	152								
Not Classified	226								

Note: Excludes Address Unknown.

Subspecialties in this table are condensed into major specialties. See Appendix A.

Table 3.8

Female Physicians by State, Self-Designated Specialty, and Activity, 2010, continued
Alaska

		Patient Care				Other Professional Activity			
				Hospital Based					
Specialty	Total Physicians	Total Patient Care	Office Based	Resid./ Fellows	Phys. Staff	Admin.	Med. Teach.	Research	Other
Total Physicians	586	509	404	26	79	7	2	6	6
FM/GP	194	190	143	20	27	3		1	
Family Medicine	190	186	139	20	27	3		1	
General Practice	4	4	4						
Medical Specialties	144	141	112	4	25	1		2	
Allergy and Immunology	3	3		1	2				
Cardiovascular Disease	1	1	1						
Dermatology	4	4	4						
Internal Medicine	64	63	52	1	10			1	
Pediatric Cardiology	1	1	1						
Pediatrics	68	66	51	2	13	1		1	
Pulmonary Disease	3	3	3						
Surgical Specialties	71	70	64		6				1
Colon and Rectal Surgery	1	1	1						
General Surgery	14	13	12		1				1
Neurological Surgery	1	1	1						
Obstetrics & Gynecology	41	41	40		1				
Ophthalmology	4	4	3		1				
Orthopedic Surgery	4	4	2		2				
Otolaryngology	4	4	3		1				
Plastic Surgery	2	2	2						
Other Specialties	121	108	85	2	21	3	2	3	5
Aerospace Medicine	1	1			1				
Anatomic/Clinical Pathology	8	4	3		1		1	1	2
Anesthesiology	17	16	15		1		1		
Child & Adolescent Psychiatry	5	5	5						
Diagnostic Radiology	10	9	7	1	1				1
Emergency Medicine	35	33	24		9	2			
Forensic Pathology	1	1	1						
General Preventive Medicine	3	3	2		1				
Neurology	5	5	5						
Occupational Medicine	1							1	
Physical Medicine and Rehabilitation	5	5	5						
Psychiatry	26	24	17		7			1	1
Public Health and General Preventive Medicine	2					1			1
Radiation Oncology	1	1	1						
Unspecified	1	1		1					
Inactive	37								
Not Classified	19								

Note: Excludes Address Unknown.

Subspecialties in this table are condensed into major specialties. See Appendix A.

Table 3.8

Female Physicians by State, Self-Designated Specialty, and Activity, 2010, continued
Arizona

		Patient Care				Other Professional Activity			
				Hospital Based					
Specialty	Total Physicians	Total Patient Care	Office Based	Resid./ Fellows	Phys. Staff	Admin.	Med. Teach.	Research	Other
Total Physicians	4,609	3,780	2,873	597	310	41	52	33	18
FM/GP	571	552	453	61	38	9	6	1	3
Family Medicine	549	532	437	61	34	7	6	1	3
General Practice	22	20	16		4	2			
Medical Specialties	1,640	1,577	1,193	246	138	15	31	13	4
Allergy and Immunology	12	12	12						
Cardiovascular Disease	36	35	27	7	1			1	
Dermatology	83	81	72	6	3		1	1	
Gastroenterology	34	34	22	10	2				
Internal Medicine	793	762	574	115	73	7	14	8	2
Pediatric Cardiology	3	2	2				1		
Pediatrics	643	617	459	100	58	8	14	2	2
Pulmonary Disease	36	34	25	8	1		1	1	
Surgical Specialties	625	612	464	121	27	1	4	5	3
Colon and Rectal Surgery	9	9	9						
General Surgery	131	130	82	39	9				1
Neurological Surgery	7	7	3	4					
Obstetrics & Gynecology	358	347	279	58	10	1	4	4	2
Ophthalmology	51	50	38	8	4			1	
Orthopedic Surgery	19	19	16	3					
Otolaryngology	8	8	5	2	1				
Plastic Surgery	20	20	16	2	2				
Thoracic Surgery	6	6	5		1				
Urology	16	16	11	5					
Other Specialties	1,088	1,039	763	169	107	16	11	14	8
Aerospace Medicine	1							1	
Anatomic/Clinical Pathology	105	97	76	12	9	1	2	2	3
Anesthesiology	191	183	151	18	14	2	5		1
Child & Adolescent Psychiatry	58	53	46	2	5	2	1	2	
Diagnostic Radiology	99	98	71	19	8				1
Emergency Medicine	180	178	111	37	30	1	1		
Forensic Pathology	3	3	3						
General Preventive Medicine	14	12	12					2	
Neurology	88	86	52	30	4		1		1
Nuclear Medicine	3	3	3						
Occupational Medicine	7	5	5			2			
Other Specialty	29	25	16	6	3	2		1	1
Physical Medicine and Rehabilitation	27	26	25	1					1
Psychiatry	205	197	142	24	31	5	1	2	
Public Health and General Preventive Medicine	7	2	2			1		4	
Radiation Oncology	20	20	18	1	1				
Radiology	25	25	24	1					
Unspecified	26	26	6	18	2				
Inactive	338								
Not Classified	347								

Note: Excludes Address Unknown.

Subspecialties in this table are condensed into major specialties. See Appendix A.

Table 3.8

Female Physicians by State, Self-Designated Specialty, and Activity, 2010, continued
Arkansas

		Patient Care				Other Professional Activity			
				Hospital Based					
Specialty	Total Physicians	Total Patient Care	Office Based	Resid./ Fellows	Phys. Staff	Admin.	Med. Teach.	Research	Other
Total Physicians	1,604	1,345	889	295	161	13	25	6	7
FM/GP	299	288	217	54	17	1	7	1	2
Family Medicine	289	279	208	54	17	1	7	1	1
General Practice	10	9	9						1
Medical Specialties	520	498	319	108	71	5	12	5	
Allergy and Immunology	11	11	11						
Cardiovascular Disease	12	11	9	2				1	
Dermatology	20	19	11	8				1	
Gastroenterology	6	5	4		1		1		
Internal Medicine	185	178	112	35	31	1	5	1	
Pediatric Cardiology	5	5	2	1	2				
Pediatrics	268	257	162	61	34	4	5	2	
Pulmonary Disease	13	12	8	1	3		1		
Surgical Specialties	190	186	130	43	13	1	3		
Colon and Rectal Surgery	1	1	1						
General Surgery	37	36	17	17	2	1			
Neurological Surgery	1	1	1						
Obstetrics & Gynecology	98	96	78	12	6		2		
Ophthalmology	25	25	16	6	3				
Orthopedic Surgery	6	6	4	2					
Otolaryngology	14	14	8	5	1				
Plastic Surgery	3	3	3						
Thoracic Surgery	2	1	1				1		
Urology	3	3	1	1	1				
Other Specialties	387	373	223	90	60	6	3		5
Aerospace Medicine	1					1			
Anatomic/Clinical Pathology	49	46	30	11	5				3
Anesthesiology	71	71	42	21	8				
Child & Adolescent Psychiatry	13	13	9	1	3				
Diagnostic Radiology	34	33	18	11	4		1		
Emergency Medicine	38	38	25	4	9				
General Preventive Medicine	2	2	1		1				
Neurology	28	28	16	8	4				
Nuclear Medicine	7	7	3	1	3				
Occupational Medicine	1	1	1						
Other Specialty	9	5	2	3		3	1		
Physical Medicine and Rehabilitation	21	21	14	4	3				
Psychiatry	82	79	42	19	18	1	1		1
Public Health and General Preventive Medicine	1					1			
Radiation Oncology	5	5	4		1				
Radiology	12	11	10	1					1
Unspecified	13	13	6	6	1				
Inactive	86								
Not Classified	122								

Note: Excludes Address Unknown.

Subspecialties in this table are condensed into major specialties. See Appendix A.

Table 3.8

Female Physicians by State, Self-Designated Specialty, and Activity, 2010, continued
California

		Patient Care				Other Professional Activity			
				Hospital Based					
Specialty	Total Physicians	Total Patient Care	Office Based	Resid./ Fellows	Phys. Staff	Admin.	Med. Teach.	Research	Other
Total Physicians	36,346	29,093	21,722	4,924	2,447	357	252	399	179
FM/GP	4,108	4,007	3,303	487	217	33	39	14	15
Family Medicine	3,816	3,723	3,050	487	186	30	37	13	13
General Practice	292	284	253		31	3	2	1	2
Medical Specialties	13,484	12,934	9,853	2,046	1,035	139	109	250	52
Allergy and Immunology	157	143	114	18	11		1	11	2
Cardiovascular Disease	284	259	189	45	25	5	5	14	1
Dermatology	700	687	573	82	32		3	8	2
Gastroenterology	218	212	154	43	15		1	5	
Internal Medicine	6,613	6,324	4,807	971	546	69	49	143	28
Pediatric Cardiology	67	63	42	14	7		1	3	
Pediatrics	5,248	5,059	3,848	825	386	65	46	59	19
Pulmonary Disease	197	187	126	48	13		3	7	
Surgical Specialties	4,532	4,466	3,304	847	315	22	22	12	10
Colon and Rectal Surgery	29	29	24	4	1				
General Surgery	764	757	408	287	62	1		4	2
Neurological Surgery	50	50	29	16	5				
Obstetrics & Gynecology	2,519	2,476	1,977	333	166	19	15	4	5
Ophthalmology	498	491	412	48	31	1	2	3	1
Orthopedic Surgery	168	165	111	40	14		1		2
Otolaryngology	217	216	147	54	15		1		
Plastic Surgery	146	145	113	24	8		1		
Thoracic Surgery	38	37	20	9	8		1		
Urology	103	100	63	32	5	1	1	1	
Other Specialties	8,156	7,686	5,262	1,544	880	163	82	123	102
Aerospace Medicine	2	2	1		1				
Anatomic/Clinical Pathology	756	675	445	154	76	30	9	17	25
Anesthesiology	1,307	1,274	911	215	148	8	13	8	4
Child & Adolescent Psychiatry	427	413	338	44	31	6	4	4	
Diagnostic Radiology	666	642	452	126	64		9	4	11
Emergency Medicine	1,028	1,005	659	214	132	10	9	2	2
Forensic Pathology	17	13	11	1	1	1			3
General Preventive Medicine	142	112	86	11	15	11	3	5	11
Medical Genetics	46	38	26	8	4	1		6	1
Neurology	482	451	314	101	36	6	3	19	3
Nuclear Medicine	52	47	30	6	11			2	3
Occupational Medicine	83	59	55		4	12	3	4	5
Other Specialty	168	119	74	30	15	16	2	18	13
Physical Medicine and Rehabilitation	303	296	216	33	47	6			1
Psychiatry	1,840	1,765	1,268	266	231	33	16	21	5
Public Health and General Preventive Medicine	47	8	5		3	19	4	6	10
Radiation Oncology	134	131	100	18	13			3	
Radiology	175	165	127	16	22	2	5	1	2
Transplant Surgery	2	2	2						
Unspecified	479	469	142	301	26	2	2	3	3
Inactive	2,517								
Not Classified	3,549								

Note: Excludes Address Unknown.

Subspecialties in this table are condensed into major specialties. See Appendix A.

Table 3.8

Female Physicians by State, Self-Designated Specialty, and Activity, 2010, continued
Colorado

		Patient Care				Other Professional Activity			
				Hospital Based					
Specialty	Total Physicians	Total Patient Care	Office Based	Resid./ Fellows	Phys. Staff	Admin.	Med. Teach.	Research	Other
Total Physicians	4,909	4,060	3,163	560	337	65	37	46	18
FM/GP	792	767	627	89	51	14	8		3
Family Medicine	782	758	618	89	51	13	8		3
General Practice	10	9	9			1			
Medical Specialties	1,674	1,612	1,256	231	125	20	12	26	4
Allergy and Immunology	27	24	21	2	1	1	1		1
Cardiovascular Disease	31	31	27	2	2				
Dermatology	85	83	68	11	4	1		1	
Gastroenterology	27	27	22	2	3				
Internal Medicine	790	761	597	105	59	8	6	14	1
Pediatric Cardiology	9	9	5	3	1				
Pediatrics	668	644	488	101	55	10	5	7	2
Pulmonary Disease	37	33	28	5				4	
Surgical Specialties	681	669	521	104	44	3	3	4	2
Colon and Rectal Surgery	4	4	4						
General Surgery	109	108	68	32	8	1			
Neurological Surgery	7	7	3	1	3				
Obstetrics & Gynecology	417	409	329	55	25	1	2	3	2
Ophthalmology	51	51	45	4	2				
Orthopedic Surgery	36	35	29	5	1			1	
Otolaryngology	28	27	21	4	2		1		
Plastic Surgery	11	10	10			1			
Thoracic Surgery	1	1			1				
Urology	17	17	12	3	2				
Other Specialties	1,079	1,012	759	136	117	28	14	16	9
Anatomic/Clinical Pathology	85	80	56	14	10	2	1	2	
Anesthesiology	178	170	150	12	8	1	5	1	1
Child & Adolescent Psychiatry	65	60	52	4	4	3	2		
Diagnostic Radiology	71	69	48	7	14	1	1		
Emergency Medicine	189	184	132	25	27	4	1		
Forensic Pathology	3	2	2			1			
General Preventive Medicine	23	14	12	1	1	6		3	
Medical Genetics	7	7	3	3	1				
Neurology	71	67	49	10	8	1		3	
Occupational Medicine	13	11	10		1		1		1
Other Specialty	16	14	8	5	1			1	1
Physical Medicine and Rehabilitation	53	50	38	6	6				3
Psychiatry	218	207	154	23	30	4	2	3	2
Public Health and General Preventive Medicine	10	2	2			5		2	1
Radiation Oncology	19	19	13	5	1				
Radiology	23	21	18		3		1	1	
Unspecified	35	35	12	21	2				
Inactive	320								
Not Classified	363								

Note: Excludes Address Unknown.

tSubspecialties in this table are condensed into major specialties. See Appendix A.

Table 3.8

Female Physicians by State, Self-Designated Specialty, and Activity, 2010, continued
Connecticut

		Patient Care				Other Professional Activity			
				Hospital Based					
Specialty	Total Physicians	Total Patient Care	Office Based	Resid./ Fellows	Phys. Staff	Admin.	Med. Teach.	Research	Other
Total Physicians	4,864	3,903	2,534	965	404	51	47	61	25
FM/GP	230	224	184	27	13	1	3		2
Family Medicine	220	214	175	27	12	1	3		2
General Practice	10	10	9		1				
Medical Specialties	2,056	1,949	1,270	487	192	31	26	40	10
Allergy and Immunology	18	16	13	3				1	1
Cardiovascular Disease	48	48	34	12	2				
Dermatology	84	83	67	11	5			1	
Gastroenterology	54	49	31	14	4	1	4		
Internal Medicine	1,130	1,063	632	310	121	24	12	24	7
Pediatric Cardiology	11	10	7	3			1		
Pediatrics	662	637	456	123	58	4	8	11	2
Pulmonary Disease	49	43	30	11	2	2	1	3	
Surgical Specialties	654	648	432	185	31		3	1	2
Colon and Rectal Surgery	10	10	8	2					
General Surgery	122	119	47	65	7		1	1	1
Neurological Surgery	7	7	4	3					
Obstetrics & Gynecology	380	377	278	80	19		2		1
Ophthalmology	64	64	52	9	3				
Orthopedic Surgery	20	20	11	8	1				
Otolaryngology	20	20	11	9					
Plastic Surgery	17	17	13	3	1				
Urology	14	14	8	6					
Other Specialties	1,147	1,082	648	266	168	19	15	20	11
Aerospace Medicine	1	1	1						
Anatomic/Clinical Pathology	125	114	55	30	29	5	1	2	3
Anesthesiology	174	171	110	41	20	1	2		
Child & Adolescent Psychiatry	81	77	53	16	8	1	1	2	
Diagnostic Radiology	131	129	79	38	12		1		1
Emergency Medicine	113	108	46	31	31	2	2	1	
Forensic Pathology	2	1	1						1
General Preventive Medicine	15	11	9	1	1	1	1	1	1
Medical Genetics	7	5	3	1	1			1	1
Neurology	72	68	41	20	7	1		3	
Nuclear Medicine	9	9	6	3					
Occupational Medicine	9	6	3		3		2	1	
Other Specialty	23	14	7	4	3	3	1	3	2
Physical Medicine and Rehabilitation	24	23	20	1	2				1
Psychiatry	290	277	183	48	46	4	3	5	1
Public Health and General Preventive Medicine	3	2	2			1			
Radiation Oncology	16	15	10	3	2			1	
Radiology	18	17	14	2	1		1		
Transplant Surgery	1	1	1						
Unspecified	33	33	4	27	2				
Inactive	269								
Not Classified	508								

Note: Excludes Address Unknown.

Subspecialties in this table are condensed into major specialties. See Appendix A.

Table 3.8

Female Physicians by State, Self-Designated Specialty, and Activity, 2010, continued
Delaware

		Patient Care				Other Professional Activity			
				Hospital Based					
Specialty	Total Physicians	Total Patient Care	Office Based	Resid./ Fellows	Phys. Staff	Admin.	Med. Teach.	Research	Other
Total Physicians	824	677	458	141	78	14	3	6	2
FM/GP	129	123	89	22	12	4	1	1	
Family Medicine	127	121	87	22	12	4	1	1	
General Practice	2	2	2						
Medical Specialties	281	267	190	48	29	8	1	3	2
Allergy and Immunology	1	1		1					
Cardiovascular Disease	7	6	3	3		1			
Dermatology	6	6	6						
Gastroenterology	3	3	3						
Internal Medicine	110	103	82	10	11	6		1	
Pediatric Cardiology	1	1		1					
Pediatrics	148	142	93	33	16	1	1	2	2
Pulmonary Disease	5	5	3		2				
Surgical Specialties	96	96	67	25	4				
Colon and Rectal Surgery	1	1	1						
General Surgery	23	23	13	10					
Obstetrics & Gynecology	54	54	37	14	3				
Ophthalmology	8	8	7		1				
Orthopedic Surgery	3	3	2	1					
Otolaryngology	2	2	2						
Plastic Surgery	3	3	3						
Urology	2	2	2						
Other Specialties	196	191	112	46	33	2	1	2	
Anatomic/Clinical Pathology	13	13	8	1	4				
Anesthesiology	23	23	21		2				
Child & Adolescent Psychiatry	8	8	6		2				
Diagnostic Radiology	24	23	13	7	3	1			
Emergency Medicine	43	43	22	17	4				
Forensic Pathology	1	1			1				
General Preventive Medicine	1	1			1				
Medical Genetics	1	1			1				
Neurology	3	3	3						
Nuclear Medicine	1	1			1				
Other Specialty	15	14	3	10	1			1	
Physical Medicine and Rehabilitation	6	6	5		1				
Psychiatry	40	39	23	8	8		1		
Public Health and General Preventive Medicine	1					1			
Radiation Oncology	3	3	3						
Radiology	5	5	3		2				
Unspecified	8	7	2	3	2			1	
Inactive	57								
Not Classified	65								

Note: Excludes Address Unknown.

Subspecialties in this table are condensed into major specialties. See Appendix A.

Table 3.8

Female Physicians by State, Self-Designated Specialty, and Activity, 2010, continued
District of Columbia

		Patient Care				Other Professional Activity			
				Hospital Based					
Specialty	Total Physicians	Total Patient Care	Office Based	Resid./ Fellows	Phys. Staff	Admin.	Med. Teach.	Research	Other
Total Physicians	2,356	1,759	820	706	233	47	30	40	19
FM/GP	93	84	58	18	8	5	3		1
Family Medicine	90	82	56	18	8	4	3		1
General Practice	3	2	2			1			
Medical Specialties	961	892	401	369	122	21	13	26	9
Allergy and Immunology	7	4	3	1		1		2	
Cardiovascular Disease	33	30	14	10	6	2		1	
Dermatology	39	38	29	7	2				1
Gastroenterology	16	16	6	7	3				
Internal Medicine	450	418	178	180	60	9	6	12	5
Pediatric Cardiology	13	12	6	5	1	1			
Pediatrics	382	354	160	149	45	8	7	10	3
Pulmonary Disease	21	20	5	10	5			1	
Surgical Specialties	318	311	137	144	30	1	1	3	2
Colon and Rectal Surgery	7	7	4	2	1				
General Surgery	92	90	22	54	14			1	1
Neurological Surgery	4	4	1	2	1				
Obstetrics & Gynecology	122	119	76	36	7	1	1		1
Ophthalmology	49	47	23	20	4			2	
Orthopedic Surgery	10	10	1	7	2				
Otolaryngology	21	21	6	15					
Plastic Surgery	6	6	2	4					
Thoracic Surgery	3	3	1	1	1				
Urology	4	4	1	3					
Other Specialties	523	472	224	175	73	20	13	11	7
Anatomic/Clinical Pathology	42	29	14	8	7	6	1	2	4
Anesthesiology	65	61	30	16	15		4		
Child & Adolescent Psychiatry	35	31	21	8	2	1	2	1	
Diagnostic Radiology	37	36	22	8	6		1		
Emergency Medicine	81	79	29	38	12		2		
Forensic Pathology	2	1	1						1
General Preventive Medicine	10	5	4		1	1		2	2
Medical Genetics	1							1	
Neurology	43	40	14	21	5		1	2	
Nuclear Medicine	4	4	1	1	2				
Occupational Medicine	3	1	1			2			
Other Specialty	14	12	9	1	2	1		1	
Physical Medicine and Rehabilitation	10	9	4	1	4	1			
Psychiatry	129	125	62	50	13	2	2		
Public Health and General Preventive Medicine	7					6		1	
Radiation Oncology	6	6	2	3	1				
Radiology	17	17	8	7	2				
Unspecified	17	16	2	13	1			1	
Inactive	126								
Not Classified	335								

Note: Excludes Address Unknown.

Subspecialties in this table are condensed into major specialties. See Appendix A.

Table 3.8

Female Physicians by State, Self-Designated Specialty, and Activity, 2010, continued
Florida

		Patient Care				Other Professional Activity			
				Hospital Based					
Specialty	Total Physicians	Total Patient Care	Office Based	Resid./ Fellows	Phys. Staff	Admin.	Med. Teach.	Research	Other
Total Physicians	13,808	11,124	8,404	1,594	1,126	126	127	76	73
FM/GP	1,620	1,570	1,311	152	107	15	22	4	9
Family Medicine	1,446	1,402	1,164	152	86	13	22	3	6
General Practice	174	168	147		21	2		1	3
Medical Specialties	5,254	5,071	3,886	702	483	57	62	45	19
Allergy and Immunology	64	62	56	4	2	1		1	
Cardiovascular Disease	133	127	99	19	9	2	1	1	2
Dermatology	269	268	233	29	6	1			
Gastroenterology	87	83	60	16	7	1	2	1	
Internal Medicine	2,473	2,385	1,789	327	269	24	28	27	9
Pediatric Cardiology	36	35	25	6	4		1		
Pediatrics	2,117	2,040	1,573	286	181	28	28	13	8
Pulmonary Disease	75	71	51	15	5		2	2	
Surgical Specialties	1,590	1,571	1,187	262	122	2	9	4	4
Colon and Rectal Surgery	19	17	14	3		1		1	
General Surgery	253	250	135	82	33			1	2
Neurological Surgery	21	20	13	2	5		1		
Obstetrics & Gynecology	868	860	699	112	49		6	1	1
Ophthalmology	209	207	164	28	15		2		
Orthopedic Surgery	54	54	37	8	9				
Otolaryngology	64	63	54	8	1			1	
Plastic Surgery	66	65	51	10	4				1
Thoracic Surgery	15	14	7	3	4	1			
Urology	21	21	13	6	2				
Other Specialties	3,062	2,912	2,020	478	414	52	34	23	41
Aerospace Medicine	3	2	1		1	1			
Anatomic/Clinical Pathology	333	293	202	46	45	7	7	7	19
Anesthesiology	547	536	398	76	62	1	9	1	
Child & Adolescent Psychiatry	133	131	104	16	11		2		
Diagnostic Radiology	327	319	233	47	39	1	3		4
Emergency Medicine	418	410	262	74	74	5	1		2
Forensic Pathology	23	19	13	4	2				4
General Preventive Medicine	41	33	18	10	5	4	1	1	2
Medical Genetics	10	8	6		2		1	1	
Neurology	207	201	141	47	13	2	1	3	
Nuclear Medicine	10	10	6	2	2				
Occupational Medicine	21	16	11		5	2		1	2
Other Specialty	29	23	15	3	5	5			1
Physical Medicine and Rehabilitation	112	106	81	9	16	5			1
Psychiatry	523	501	352	54	95	11	6	5	
Public Health and General Preventive Medicine	14	4	4			7	1	1	1
Radiation Oncology	68	67	50	8	9		1		
Radiology	82	78	59	4	15		1	1	2
Transplant Surgery	1	1			1				
Unspecified	160	154	64	78	12	1		2	3
Inactive	1,297								
Not Classified	985								

Note: Excludes Address Unknown.

Subspecialties in this table are condensed into major specialties. See Appendix A.

Table 3.8

Female Physicians by State, Self-Designated Specialty, and Activity, 2010, continued
Georgia

		Patient Care				Other Professional Activity			
				Hospital Based					
Specialty	Total Physicians	Total Patient Care	Office Based	Resid./ Fellows	Phys. Staff	Admin.	Med. Teach.	Research	Other
Total Physicians	7,154	5,873	4,462	930	481	80	70	93	55
FM/GP	869	843	687	102	54	9	13	1	3
Family Medicine	836	814	665	102	47	7	12	1	2
General Practice	33	29	22		7	2	1		1
Medical Specialties	2,822	2,699	2,092	372	235	35	33	34	21
Allergy and Immunology	26	24	21	3			1	1	
Cardiovascular Disease	57	55	41	12	2		1	1	
Dermatology	129	128	107	19	2		1		
Gastroenterology	51	51	43	8					
Internal Medicine	1,340	1,282	949	186	147	19	15	17	7
Pediatric Cardiology	9	9	8	1					
Pediatrics	1,170	1,113	891	139	83	16	14	13	14
Pulmonary Disease	40	37	32	4	1		1	2	
Surgical Specialties	925	913	712	166	35	7	3	1	1
Colon and Rectal Surgery	7	7	5	2					
General Surgery	128	125	65	53	7		2	1	
Neurological Surgery	11	11	4	5	2				
Obstetrics & Gynecology	612	606	510	75	21	4	1		1
Ophthalmology	62	60	45	13	2	2			
Orthopedic Surgery	23	22	17	5		1			
Otolaryngology	41	41	30	9	2				
Plastic Surgery	23	23	23						
Thoracic Surgery	3	3	2	1					
Urology	15	15	11	3	1				
Other Specialties	1,555	1,418	971	290	157	29	21	57	30
Aerospace Medicine	2	1			1	1			
Anatomic/Clinical Pathology	156	136	96	29	11	1	1	5	13
Anesthesiology	224	221	161	38	22	2	1		
Child & Adolescent Psychiatry	71	68	57	8	3		3		
Diagnostic Radiology	124	121	88	21	12		1		2
Emergency Medicine	222	215	148	35	32		3	3	1
Forensic Pathology	8	7	4	1	2				1
General Preventive Medicine	65	46	28	7	11	2	2	10	5
Medical Genetics	4	3	3					1	
Neurology	81	76	53	17	6	1		4	
Nuclear Medicine	4	4	2	1	1				
Occupational Medicine	16	10	10			3	1	1	1
Other Specialty	26	16	10	5	1	1	1	5	3
Physical Medicine and Rehabilitation	53	51	36	10	5	1		1	
Psychiatry	313	298	211	49	38	4	6	4	1
Public Health and General Preventive Medicine	40	5	1		4	11	1	20	3
Radiation Oncology	28	28	21	6	1				
Radiology	37	35	28	2	5		1	1	
Unspecified	81	77	14	61	2	2		2	
Inactive	353								
Not Classified	630								

Note: Excludes Address Unknown.

Subspecialties in this table are condensed into major specialties. See Appendix A.

Table 3.8

Female Physicians by State, Self-Designated Specialty, and Activity, 2010, continued
Hawaii

		Patient Care				Other Professional Activity			
				Hospital Based					
Specialty	Total Physicians	Total Patient Care	Office Based	Resid./ Fellows	Phys. Staff	Admin.	Med. Teach.	Research	Other
Total Physicians	1,387	1,082	827	140	115	14	18	9	10
FM/GP	161	155	128	14	13	2	3	1	
Family Medicine	150	144	118	14	12	2	3	1	
General Practice	11	11	10		1				
Medical Specialties	488	463	372	39	52	7	9	5	4
Allergy and Immunology	3	3	3						
Cardiovascular Disease	8	7	6	1				1	
Dermatology	18	16	14	1	1	1		1	
Gastroenterology	3	3	2		1				
Internal Medicine	252	239	192	21	26	4	6		3
Pediatrics	197	189	149	16	24	1	3	3	1
Pulmonary Disease	7	6	6			1			
Surgical Specialties	200	195	137	44	14	1	3	1	
Colon and Rectal Surgery	1	1	1						
General Surgery	40	39	17	18	4	1			
Obstetrics & Gynecology	121	117	90	21	6		3	1	
Ophthalmology	16	16	15		1				
Orthopedic Surgery	9	9	5	2	2				
Otolaryngology	7	7	3	3	1				
Urology	6	6	6						
Other Specialties	284	269	190	43	36	4	3	2	6
Aerospace Medicine	1	1			1				
Anatomic/Clinical Pathology	28	25	16	6	3				3
Anesthesiology	29	29	25		4				
Child & Adolescent Psychiatry	19	19	16	1	2				
Diagnostic Radiology	17	17	9	3	5				
Emergency Medicine	34	32	26		6	2			
Forensic Pathology	1								1
General Preventive Medicine	7	5	4		1			1	1
Neurology	11	10	5	2	3			1	
Nuclear Medicine	1	1	1						
Occupational Medicine	4	3	3			1			
Other Specialty	9	9	4	5					
Physical Medicine and Rehabilitation	10	9	9						1
Psychiatry	80	78	55	15	8	1	1		
Public Health and General Preventive Medicine	3	2	1		1		1		
Radiation Oncology	3	3	2		1				
Radiology	12	11	10		1		1		
Unspecified	15	15	4	11					
Inactive	147								
Not Classified	107								

Note: Excludes Address Unknown.

Subspecialties in this table are condensed into major specialties. See Appendix A.

Table 3.8

Female Physicians by State, Self-Designated Specialty, and Activity, 2010, continued
Idaho

		Patient Care				Other Professional Activity			
				Hospital Based					
Specialty	Total Physicians	Total Patient Care	Office Based	Resid./ Fellows	Phys. Staff	Admin.	Med. Teach.	Research	Other
Total Physicians	653	565	447	48	70	3	7	3	1
FM/GP	176	172	131	31	10	1	3		
Family Medicine	174	170	129	31	10	1	3		
General Practice	2	2	2						
Medical Specialties	190	183	141	14	28	2	3	1	1
Cardiovascular Disease	4	4	4						
Dermatology	6	6	5		1				
Gastroenterology	4	4	4						
Internal Medicine	111	109	79	11	19	1	1		
Pediatric Cardiology	2	2	2						
Pediatrics	55	51	42	3	6	1	2		1
Pulmonary Disease	8	7	5		2			1	
Surgical Specialties	91	91	85	1	5				
Colon and Rectal Surgery	1	1	1						
General Surgery	17	17	16	1					
Neurological Surgery	1	1	1						
Obstetrics & Gynecology	51	51	47		4				
Ophthalmology	8	8	8						
Orthopedic Surgery	3	3	3						
Otolaryngology	3	3	3						
Plastic Surgery	2	2	2						
Urology	5	5	4		1				
Other Specialties	122	119	90	2	27		1	2	
Aerospace Medicine	1	1			1				
Anatomic/Clinical Pathology	6	5	4		1			1	
Anesthesiology	16	16	14		2				
Child & Adolescent Psychiatry	4	4	3		1				
Diagnostic Radiology	28	28	23		5				
Emergency Medicine	21	21	16	1	4				
General Preventive Medicine	1	1			1				
Neurology	7	6	6					1	
Occupational Medicine	2	2	2						
Other Specialty	1	1	1						
Physical Medicine and Rehabilitation	7	7	6		1				
Psychiatry	19	18	9		9		1		
Public Health and General Preventive Medicine	1	1	1						
Radiation Oncology	3	3	3						
Radiology	3	3	2		1				
Unspecified	2	2		1	1				
Inactive	46								
Not Classified	28								

Note: Excludes Address Unknown.

Subspecialties in this table are condensed into major specialties. See Appendix A.

Table 3.8

Female Physicians by State, Self-Designated Specialty, and Activity, 2010, continued
Illinois

		Patient Care				Other Professional Activity			
				Hospital Based					
Specialty	Total Physicians	Total Patient Care	Office Based	Resid./ Fellows	Phys. Staff	Admin.	Med. Teach.	Research	Other
Total Physicians	14,218	11,363	7,598	2,729	1,036	116	121	113	68
FM/GP	1,621	1,577	1,167	300	110	11	25	3	5
Family Medicine	1,526	1,489	1,096	300	93	7	25	2	3
General Practice	95	88	71		17	4		1	2
Medical Specialties	5,324	5,120	3,476	1,226	418	64	47	76	17
Allergy and Immunology	97	91	74	11	6	1	1	4	
Cardiovascular Disease	116	107	72	25	10	2	3	4	
Dermatology	229	225	167	48	10	2		2	
Gastroenterology	78	75	47	22	6		2	1	
Internal Medicine	2,815	2,703	1,804	670	229	42	24	38	8
Pediatric Cardiology	35	31	19	9	3	1		2	1
Pediatrics	1,873	1,813	1,246	420	147	13	17	23	7
Pulmonary Disease	81	75	47	21	7	3		2	1
Surgical Specialties	1,714	1,685	1,143	430	112	5	12	9	3
Colon and Rectal Surgery	7	7	5	1	1				
General Surgery	275	271	124	123	24		1	2	1
Neurological Surgery	16	16	8	5	3				
Obstetrics & Gynecology	1,000	984	729	191	64	5	6	5	
Ophthalmology	200	193	157	28	8		3	2	2
Orthopedic Surgery	51	51	30	18	3				
Otolaryngology	73	73	39	29	5				
Plastic Surgery	48	47	27	19	1		1		
Thoracic Surgery	6	6	6						
Urology	38	37	18	16	3		1		
Other Specialties	3,122	2,981	1,812	773	396	36	37	25	43
Aerospace Medicine	1					1			
Anatomic/Clinical Pathology	354	321	188	75	58	5	6	4	18
Anesthesiology	555	543	333	142	68	1	7	2	2
Child & Adolescent Psychiatry	124	117	90	18	9	2	3		2
Diagnostic Radiology	260	254	155	68	31	1	2		3
Emergency Medicine	445	438	250	118	70	1	4	1	1
Forensic Pathology	13	9	8		1		2		2
General Preventive Medicine	21	18	13	5		1		1	1
Medical Genetics	12	11	6	3	2			1	
Neurology	202	194	124	52	18		1	6	1
Nuclear Medicine	12	12	7	2	3				
Occupational Medicine	30	22	20		2	4		1	3
Other Specialty	55	43	23	14	6	5	1	3	3
Physical Medicine and Rehabilitation	198	193	107	49	37	2	1	1	1
Psychiatry	548	525	373	77	75	8	9	2	4
Public Health and General Preventive Medicine	10	3	2		1	5		2	
Radiation Oncology	48	48	33	11	4				
Radiology	51	50	38	6	6		1		
Transplant Surgery	1							1	
Unspecified	181	179	42	133	4				2
Vascular Medicine	1	1			1				
Inactive	872								
Not Classified	1,565								

Note: Excludes Address Unknown.

Subspecialties in this table are condensed into major specialties. See Appendix A.

Table 3.8

Female Physicians by State, Self-Designated Specialty, and Activity, 2010, continued
Indiana

		Patient Care				Other Professional Activity			
				Hospital Based					
Specialty	Total Physicians	Total Patient Care	Office Based	Resid./ Fellows	Phys. Staff	Admin.	Med. Teach.	Research	Other
Total Physicians	4,308	3,659	2,683	598	378	34	26	36	24
FM/GP	769	755	580	115	60	4	6	1	3
Family Medicine	750	737	564	115	58	4	6	1	2
General Practice	19	18	16		2				1
Medical Specialties	1,508	1,456	1,032	240	184	14	8	23	7
Allergy and Immunology	12	11	11					1	
Cardiovascular Disease	33	30	24	4	2		1	2	
Dermatology	65	65	51	11	3				
Gastroenterology	21	20	10	8	2			1	
Internal Medicine	664	636	465	91	80	8	4	10	6
Pediatric Cardiology	10	10	7	2	1				
Pediatrics	680	662	454	119	89	6	3	8	1
Pulmonary Disease	23	22	10	5	7			1	
Surgical Specialties	558	548	411	105	32	2	8		
Colon and Rectal Surgery	3	3	3						
General Surgery	86	83	49	30	4		3		
Neurological Surgery	7	7	4	2	1				
Obstetrics & Gynecology	350	343	269	52	22	2	5		
Ophthalmology	46	46	38	7	1				
Orthopedic Surgery	15	15	9	5	1				
Otolaryngology	25	25	17	7	1				
Plastic Surgery	15	15	14		1				
Thoracic Surgery	3	3	2		1				
Urology	8	8	6	2					
Other Specialties	944	900	660	138	102	14	4	12	14
Anatomic/Clinical Pathology	99	87	60	16	11	3	2	3	4
Anesthesiology	202	201	154	27	20				1
Child & Adolescent Psychiatry	44	43	34	4	5		1		
Diagnostic Radiology	84	83	68	12	3	1			
Emergency Medicine	131	131	95	18	18				
Forensic Pathology	2	1	1						1
General Preventive Medicine	5	4	3		1			1	
Medical Genetics	5	5	3	2					
Neurology	68	62	47	11	4		1	3	2
Nuclear Medicine	3	2	1	1					1
Occupational Medicine	10	8	8			2			
Other Specialty	30	27	13	13	1	1		1	1
Physical Medicine and Rehabilitation	39	37	27	6	4	1			1
Psychiatry	145	134	99	7	28	4		4	3
Public Health and General Preventive Medicine	1					1			
Radiation Oncology	26	26	19	3	4				
Radiology	30	30	26	1	3				
Unspecified	20	19	2	17		1			
Inactive	270								
Not Classified	259								

Note: Excludes Address Unknown.

Subspecialties in this table are condensed into major specialties. See Appendix A.

Table 3.8

Female Physicians by State, Self-Designated Specialty, and Activity, 2010, continued
Iowa

		Patient Care				Other Professional Activity			
				Hospital Based					
Specialty	Total Physicians	Total Patient Care	Office Based	Resid./ Fellows	Phys. Staff	Admin.	Med. Teach.	Research	Other
Total Physicians	1,715	1,416	956	300	160	17	18	19	2
FM/GP	387	379	284	65	30	3	3	1	1
Family Medicine	378	371	277	65	29	2	3	1	1
General Practice	9	8	7		1	1			
Medical Specialties	506	483	325	99	59	7	8	8	
Allergy and Immunology	10	8	6	2		1		1	
Cardiovascular Disease	17	17	12	3	2				
Dermatology	27	27	19	6	2				
Gastroenterology	8	8	5	2	1				
Internal Medicine	216	207	140	44	23	3	2	4	
Pediatric Cardiology	6	5	2	2	1		1		
Pediatrics	208	199	137	37	25	3	5	1	
Pulmonary Disease	14	12	4	3	5			2	
Surgical Specialties	215	210	141	45	24	1	2	2	
Colon and Rectal Surgery	1	1	1						
General Surgery	37	37	21	10	6				
Neurological Surgery	2	2	1	1					
Obstetrics & Gynecology	110	105	78	15	12	1	2	2	
Ophthalmology	37	37	27	9	1				
Orthopedic Surgery	9	9	7	1	1				
Otolaryngology	13	13	3	7	3				
Plastic Surgery	3	3	2		1				
Urology	3	3	1	2					
Other Specialties	364	344	206	91	47	6	5	8	1
Anatomic/Clinical Pathology	52	49	33	12	4	1	1	1	
Anesthesiology	64	63	39	19	5		1		
Child & Adolescent Psychiatry	18	18	15	3					
Diagnostic Radiology	20	19	16	2	1	1			
Emergency Medicine	26	26	14	7	5				
Forensic Pathology	1	1			1				
General Preventive Medicine	7	7	5	2					
Medical Genetics	2	2	1		1				
Neurology	35	34	18	11	5			1	
Nuclear Medicine	1					1			
Occupational Medicine	6	5	4		1			1	
Other Specialty	14	13	4	7	2	1			
Physical Medicine and Rehabilitation	12	11	10		1	1			
Psychiatry	61	55	32	6	17	1	3	2	
Public Health and General Preventive Medicine	3							2	1
Radiation Oncology	15	15	10	4	1				
Radiology	5	5	2	1	2				
Unspecified	22	21	3	17	1			1	
Inactive	94								
Not Classified	149								

Note: Excludes Address Unknown.

Subspecialties in this table are condensed into major specialties. See Appendix A.

Table 3.8

Female Physicians by State, Self-Designated Specialty, and Activity, 2010, continued
Kansas

		Patient Care				Other Professional Activity			
				Hospital Based					
Specialty	Total Physicians	Total Patient Care	Office Based	Resid./ Fellows	Phys. Staff	Admin.	Med. Teach.	Research	Other
Total Physicians	2,075	1,731	1,234	307	190	16	22	8	8
FM/GP	386	373	291	51	31	4	7	1	1
Family Medicine	370	359	283	51	25	2	7	1	1
General Practice	16	14	8		6	2			
Medical Specialties	649	630	452	101	77	4	10	2	3
Allergy and Immunology	11	11	7	2	2				
Cardiovascular Disease	17	17	15	1	1				
Dermatology	28	28	19	9					
Gastroenterology	7	7	5	2					
Internal Medicine	296	285	199	50	36	2	6	2	1
Pediatric Cardiology	3	3	3						
Pediatrics	275	267	196	34	37	2	4		2
Pulmonary Disease	12	12	8	3	1				
Surgical Specialties	279	276	200	62	14	1	2		
Colon and Rectal Surgery	1	1	1						
General Surgery	57	55	30	19	6	1	1		
Neurological Surgery	2	2	1	1					
Obstetrics & Gynecology	158	157	124	28	5		1		
Ophthalmology	26	26	24		2				
Orthopedic Surgery	12	12	6	6					
Otolaryngology	9	9	3	6					
Plastic Surgery	7	7	7						
Thoracic Surgery	1	1	1						
Urology	6	6	3	2	1				
Other Specialties	471	452	291	93	68	7	3	5	4
Anatomic/Clinical Pathology	57	53	33	7	13	1		1	2
Anesthesiology	77	77	57	14	6				
Child & Adolescent Psychiatry	29	28	18	4	6	1			
Diagnostic Radiology	46	46	32	11	3				
Emergency Medicine	44	44	29	3	12				
Forensic Pathology	1	1	1						
General Preventive Medicine	1	1	1						
Medical Genetics	1								1
Neurology	33	33	21	7	5				
Nuclear Medicine	1	1			1				
Occupational Medicine	3	2	1		1				1
Other Specialty	6	4	3	1			1	1	
Physical Medicine and Rehabilitation	20	20	16	1	3				
Psychiatry	100	92	60	17	15	3	2	3	
Public Health and General Preventive Medicine	2					2			
Radiation Oncology	10	10	8	1	1				
Radiology	7	7	6		1				
Unspecified	33	33	5	27	1				
Inactive	125								
Not Classified	165								

Note: Excludes Address Unknown.

Subspecialties in this table are condensed into major specialties. See Appendix A.

Table 3.8

Female Physicians by State, Self-Designated Specialty, and Activity, 2010, continued
Kentucky

		Patient Care				Other Professional Activity			
				Hospital Based					
Specialty	Total Physicians	Total Patient Care	Office Based	Resid./ Fellows	Phys. Staff	Admin.	Med. Teach.	Research	Other
Total Physicians	3,025	2,517	1,837	449	231	18	32	15	7
FM/GP	398	389	315	45	29	4	4	1	
Family Medicine	380	371	298	45	28	4	4	1	
General Practice	18	18	17		1				
Medical Specialties	1,079	1,048	780	178	90	4	16	8	3
Allergy and Immunology	18	18	17		1				
Cardiovascular Disease	26	26	17	5	4				
Dermatology	56	56	49	6	1				
Gastroenterology	15	14	12	2				1	
Internal Medicine	473	456	324	81	51	2	8	6	1
Pediatric Cardiology	2	2	2						
Pediatrics	473	460	349	79	32	2	8	1	2
Pulmonary Disease	16	16	10	5	1				
Surgical Specialties	385	380	275	83	22	2	2	1	
Colon and Rectal Surgery	4	4	3		1				
General Surgery	67	65	32	27	6		1	1	
Neurological Surgery	4	4	3	1					
Obstetrics & Gynecology	230	227	178	38	11	2	1		
Ophthalmology	30	30	24	5	1				
Orthopedic Surgery	17	17	9	5	3				
Otolaryngology	9	9	5	4					
Plastic Surgery	15	15	13	2					
Thoracic Surgery	1	1	1						
Urology	8	8	7	1					
Other Specialties	727	700	467	143	90	8	10	5	4
Anatomic/Clinical Pathology	79	77	48	13	16	1			1
Anesthesiology	127	121	88	14	19	1	5		
Child & Adolescent Psychiatry	38	36	29	6	1		1	1	
Diagnostic Radiology	62	62	45	10	7				
Emergency Medicine	90	88	59	13	16	1	1		
Forensic Pathology	8	5	2	1	2				3
General Preventive Medicine	2	2		2					
Medical Genetics	3	3	3						
Neurology	40	38	22	14	2	1		1	
Nuclear Medicine	1	1	1						
Occupational Medicine	5	4	4					1	
Other Specialty	13	11	5	6		1		1	
Physical Medicine and Rehabilitation	33	33	24	6	3				
Psychiatry	150	146	98	30	18	2	1	1	
Public Health and General Preventive Medicine	2	1			1	1			
Radiation Oncology	13	13	11		2				
Radiology	18	17	16		1		1		
Transplant Surgery	1	1	1						
Unspecified	42	41	11	28	2		1		
Inactive	193								
Not Classified	243								

Note: Excludes Address Unknown.

Subspecialties in this table are condensed into major specialties. See Appendix A.

Table 3.8

Female Physicians by State, Self-Designated Specialty, and Activity, 2010, continued
Lousiana

		Patient Care				Other Professional Activity			
				Hospital Based					
Specialty	Total Physicians	Total Patient Care	Office Based	Resid./ Fellows	Phys. Staff	Admin.	Med. Teach.	Research	Other
Total Physicians	3,649	3,032	1,953	771	308	21	50	14	6
FM/GP	392	385	276	68	41	1	5	1	
Family Medicine	369	362	257	68	37	1	5	1	
General Practice	23	23	19		4				
Medical Specialties	1,394	1,342	880	321	141	13	28	10	1
Allergy and Immunology	18	17	13	4			1		
Cardiovascular Disease	33	32	20	11	1		1		
Dermatology	83	83	61	20	2				
Gastroenterology	17	16	10	5	1			1	
Internal Medicine	597	570	333	163	74	8	14	4	1
Pediatric Cardiology	3	3	3						
Pediatrics	615	595	424	111	60	5	10	5	
Pulmonary Disease	28	26	16	7	3		2		
Surgical Specialties	571	563	356	183	24		6	1	1
Colon and Rectal Surgery	5	5	3	2					
General Surgery	83	80	26	51	3		1	1	1
Neurological Surgery	6	6	2	3	1				
Obstetrics & Gynecology	317	314	222	80	12		3		
Ophthalmology	61	60	43	14	3		1		
Orthopedic Surgery	21	20	8	11	1		1		
Otolaryngology	47	47	30	15	2				
Plastic Surgery	15	15	12	3					
Thoracic Surgery	3	3	2		1				
Urology	13	13	8	4	1				
Other Specialties	766	742	441	199	102	7	11	2	4
Anatomic/Clinical Pathology	93	86	56	13	17		3	1	3
Anesthesiology	127	125	68	34	23		2		
Child & Adolescent Psychiatry	36	35	26	9			1		
Diagnostic Radiology	70	69	37	22	10		1		
Emergency Medicine	125	125	69	41	15				
Forensic Pathology	1	1			1				
General Preventive Medicine	5	5	4	1					
Medical Genetics	2	1	1				1		
Neurology	66	63	41	15	7		3		
Nuclear Medicine	2	2	1		1				
Occupational Medicine	2	2	1		1				
Other Specialty	18	17	6	11					1
Physical Medicine and Rehabilitation	27	27	22	3	2				
Psychiatry	151	146	87	38	21	5			
Public Health and General Preventive Medicine	3					2		1	
Radiation Oncology	8	8	8						
Radiology	11	11	8		3				
Unspecified	19	19	6	12	1				
Inactive	193								
Not Classified	333								

Note: Excludes Address Unknown.

Subspecialties in this table are condensed into major specialties. See Appendix A.

Table 3.8

Female Physicians by State, Self-Designated Specialty, and Activity, 2010, continued
Maine

		Patient Care				Other Professional Activity			
				Hospital Based					
Specialty	Total Physicians	Total Patient Care	Office Based	Resid./ Fellows	Phys. Staff	Admin.	Med. Teach.	Research	Other
Total Physicians	1,247	1,033	759	130	144	13	12	10	6
FM/GP	248	240	176	39	25	2	4	1	1
Family Medicine	246	239	175	39	25	1	4	1	1
General Practice	2	1	1			1			
Medical Specialties	388	374	296	36	42	4	4	4	2
Allergy and Immunology	2	2	2						
Cardiovascular Disease	9	9	8	1					
Dermatology	7	7	7						
Gastroenterology	2	1	1					1	
Internal Medicine	216	205	161	18	26	3	3	3	2
Pediatric Cardiology	2	2	2						
Pediatrics	137	135	104	17	14	1	1		
Pulmonary Disease	13	13	11		2				
Surgical Specialties	169	162	115	26	21	1	4	2	
Colon and Rectal Surgery	1	1	1						
General Surgery	43	43	20	13	10				
Neurological Surgery	1	1	1						
Obstetrics & Gynecology	92	88	70	13	5	1	3		
Ophthalmology	13	12	9		3		1		
Orthopedic Surgery	12	11	9		2			1	
Otolaryngology	2	2	1		1				
Plastic Surgery	3	3	3						
Thoracic Surgery	1							1	
Urology	1	1	1						
Other Specialties	269	257	172	29	56	6		3	3
Anatomic/Clinical Pathology	13	12	10		2				1
Anesthesiology	39	39	29	5	5				
Child & Adolescent Psychiatry	24	20	17	2	1	1		3	
Diagnostic Radiology	24	24	14	5	5				
Emergency Medicine	53	52	25	7	20	1			
Forensic Pathology	1								1
Medical Genetics	1	1			1				
Neurology	14	14	13		1				
Occupational Medicine	3	3	2		1				
Other Specialty	3	1	1			2			
Physical Medicine and Rehabilitation	9	9	4	1	4				
Psychiatry	74	72	48	9	15	2			
Public Health and General Preventive Medicine	1								1
Radiation Oncology	2	2	2						
Radiology	2	2	2						
Unspecified	6	6	5		1				
Inactive	105								
Not Classified	68								

Note: Excludes Address Unknown.

Subspecialties in this table are condensed into major specialties. See Appendix A.

Table 3.8

Female Physicians by State, Self-Designated Specialty, and Activity, 2010, continued
Maryland

		Patient Care				Other Professional Activity			
				Hospital Based					
Specialty	Total Physicians	Total Patient Care	Office Based	Resid./ Fellows	Phys. Staff	Admin.	Med. Teach.	Research	Other
Total Physicians	9,493	7,144	4,824	1,382	938	179	93	273	82
FM/GP	614	586	494	38	54	11	8	5	4
Family Medicine	577	550	466	38	46	11	8	5	3
General Practice	37	36	28		8				1
Medical Specialties	3,725	3,402	2,308	664	430	80	51	158	34
Allergy and Immunology	62	52	36	10	6		2	8	
Cardiovascular Disease	92	84	59	17	8	1	1	6	
Dermatology	133	128	103	17	8		1	1	3
Gastroenterology	64	59	38	18	3	1	1	3	
Internal Medicine	1,917	1,745	1,143	391	211	45	27	88	12
Pediatric Cardiology	17	16	5	7	4		1		
Pediatrics	1,373	1,255	886	190	179	33	18	48	19
Pulmonary Disease	67	63	38	14	11			4	
Surgical Specialties	1,114	1,077	693	262	122	5	4	17	11
Colon and Rectal Surgery	7	5	5					1	1
General Surgery	167	163	65	81	17		1	2	1
Neurological Surgery	14	12	6	4	2	1		1	
Obstetrics & Gynecology	621	599	433	101	65	3	3	8	8
Ophthalmology	147	142	96	27	19			4	1
Orthopedic Surgery	48	48	21	21	6				
Otolaryngology	44	44	24	14	6				
Plastic Surgery	33	31	27	4		1		1	
Thoracic Surgery	6	6	3	1	2				
Urology	27	27	13	9	5				
Other Specialties	2,318	2,079	1,329	418	332	83	30	93	33
Anatomic/Clinical Pathology	239	199	109	49	41	6	4	18	12
Anesthesiology	324	314	210	46	58	1	6	3	
Child & Adolescent Psychiatry	141	135	110	8	17	3	1	2	
Diagnostic Radiology	183	180	119	24	37	1	1	1	
Emergency Medicine	218	213	148	24	41	2	1		2
Forensic Pathology	11	8	4	1	3			1	2
General Preventive Medicine	93	68	42	21	5	8	3	11	3
Medical Genetics	15	11	4	5	2			4	
Neurology	151	129	79	29	21	2	2	17	1
Nuclear Medicine	13	11	5	6		2			
Occupational Medicine	22	13	10		3	7		1	1
Other Specialty	53	33	14	14	5	6		11	3
Physical Medicine and Rehabilitation	95	85	50	24	11	4	2	3	1
Psychiatry	513	478	343	72	63	16	6	10	3
Public Health and General Preventive Medicine	41	4	4			23	1	9	4
Radiation Oncology	42	39	27	5	7	1		1	1
Radiology	50	47	33	6	8		3		
Unspecified	114	112	18	84	10	1		1	
Inactive	579								
Not Classified	1,143								

Note: Excludes Address Unknown.

Subspecialties in this table are condensed into major specialties. See Appendix A.

Table 3.8

Female Physicians by State, Self-Designated Specialty, and Activity, 2010, continued
Massachusetts

		Patient Care				Other Professional Activity			
				Hospital Based					
Specialty	Total Physicians	Total Patient Care	Office Based	Resid./ Fellows	Phys. Staff	Admin.	Med. Teach.	Research	Other
Total Physicians	12,920	10,073	6,206	2,557	1,310	115	87	283	67
FM/GP	700	676	537	87	52	11	7	1	5
Family Medicine	675	656	524	87	45	9	7		3
General Practice	25	20	13		7	2		1	2
Medical Specialties	5,298	4,983	3,175	1,188	620	50	43	194	28
Allergy and Immunology	41	30	17	10	3	1		10	
Cardiovascular Disease	152	134	73	37	24		2	12	4
Dermatology	197	191	133	42	16	2	1	3	
Gastroenterology	93	88	57	20	11			5	
Internal Medicine	2,925	2,736	1,757	632	347	31	28	116	14
Pediatric Cardiology	43	43	22	16	5				
Pediatrics	1,749	1,671	1,067	398	206	15	12	42	9
Pulmonary Disease	98	90	49	33	8	1		6	1
Surgical Specialties	1,395	1,366	820	409	137	10	7	10	2
Colon and Rectal Surgery	6	6	4	1	1				
General Surgery	304	297	108	161	28	2	2	2	1
Neurological Surgery	15	15	6	9					
Obstetrics & Gynecology	686	668	469	125	74	8	4	5	1
Ophthalmology	173	171	115	44	12			2	
Orthopedic Surgery	70	69	33	30	6			1	
Otolaryngology	50	50	35	8	7				
Plastic Surgery	41	40	28	8	4		1		
Thoracic Surgery	12	12	8	2	2				
Urology	38	38	14	21	3				
Other Specialties	3,232	3,048	1,674	873	501	44	30	78	32
Anatomic/Clinical Pathology	346	316	162	103	51	7	2	9	12
Anesthesiology	474	461	245	161	55	1	9	2	1
Child & Adolescent Psychiatry	183	175	128	26	21	1	1	5	1
Diagnostic Radiology	306	297	156	95	46	1	4	3	1
Emergency Medicine	333	328	164	100	64	3	2		
Forensic Pathology	4	3	3						1
General Preventive Medicine	25	20	11	7	2	1		4	
Medical Genetics	18	15	6	5	4			3	
Neurology	266	249	119	81	49	2	1	13	1
Nuclear Medicine	9	5	2		3		2	1	1
Occupational Medicine	14	7	6		1	3		2	2
Other Specialty	50	34	18	8	8	4	1	7	4
Physical Medicine and Rehabilitation	99	97	51	27	19	2			
Psychiatry	796	750	460	152	138	13	8	22	3
Public Health and General Preventive Medicine	11	3	1		2	5		1	2
Radiation Oncology	67	67	40	15	12				
Radiology	114	108	62	25	21	1		3	2
Transplant Surgery	2	2	2						
Unspecified	115	111	38	68	5			3	1
Inactive	636								
Not Classified	1,659								

Note: Excludes Address Unknown.

Subspecialties in this table are condensed into major specialties. See Appendix A.

Table 3.8

Female Physicians by State, Self-Designated Specialty, and Activity, 2010, continued
Michigan

		Patient Care				Other Professional Activity			
				Hospital Based					
Specialty	Total Physicians	Total Patient Care	Office Based	Resid./ Fellows	Phys. Staff	Admin.	Med. Teach.	Research	Other
Total Physicians	8,932	7,353	4,844	1,806	703	80	100	66	33
FM/GP	1,153	1,118	843	194	81	12	19	3	1
Family Medicine	1,112	1,080	808	194	78	9	19	3	1
General Practice	41	38	35		3	3			
Medical Specialties	3,275	3,155	2,156	712	287	26	47	43	4
Allergy and Immunology	49	49	35	10	4				
Cardiovascular Disease	63	63	38	21	4				
Dermatology	126	126	89	31	6				
Gastroenterology	59	57	37	16	4		1	1	
Internal Medicine	1,687	1,614	1,103	374	137	22	24	25	2
Pediatric Cardiology	24	24	10	10	4				
Pediatrics	1,227	1,185	820	241	124	4	21	15	2
Pulmonary Disease	40	37	24	9	4		1	2	
Surgical Specialties	1,206	1,191	730	375	86	3	7	4	1
Colon and Rectal Surgery	7	7	7						
General Surgery	225	221	93	112	16		3	1	
Neurological Surgery	15	15	5	7	3				
Obstetrics & Gynecology	694	686	467	168	51	3	3	2	
Ophthalmology	128	126	85	36	5		1		1
Orthopedic Surgery	47	47	22	21	4				
Otolaryngology	35	35	16	14	5				
Plastic Surgery	34	33	24	8	1			1	
Thoracic Surgery	4	4	2	2					
Urology	17	17	9	7	1				
Other Specialties	1,998	1,889	1,115	525	249	39	27	16	27
Aerospace Medicine	1							1	
Anatomic/Clinical Pathology	216	192	110	52	30	7	4	4	9
Anesthesiology	233	226	139	52	35	1	3	3	
Child & Adolescent Psychiatry	104	96	71	7	18	3	4	1	
Diagnostic Radiology	200	195	99	71	25		2		3
Emergency Medicine	338	333	184	113	36	2	2		1
Forensic Pathology	3	3	2		1				
General Preventive Medicine	10	8	6	2		1			1
Medical Genetics	6	6	5		1				
Neurology	122	112	76	26	10		4	3	3
Nuclear Medicine	12	11	5		6		1		
Occupational Medicine	21	19	15		4	2			
Other Specialty	31	28	13	11	4	3			
Physical Medicine and Rehabilitation	98	95	64	20	11		1		2
Psychiatry	383	358	243	65	50	13	5	3	4
Public Health and General Preventive Medicine	9	1	1			6		1	1
Radiation Oncology	44	43	26	8	9	1			
Radiology	49	46	34	6	6		1		2
Transplant Surgery	2	2	2						
Unspecified	116	115	20	92	3				1
Inactive	510								
Not Classified	790								

Note: Excludes Address Unknown.

Subspecialties in this table are condensed into major specialties. See Appendix A.

Table 3.8

Female Physicians by State, Self-Designated Specialty, and Activity, 2010, continued
Minnesota

		Patient Care				Other Professional Activity			
				Hospital Based					
Specialty	Total Physicians	Total Patient Care	Office Based	Resid./ Fellows	Phys. Staff	Admin.	Med. Teach.	Research	Other
Total Physicians	5,540	4,772	3,535	931	306	46	39	49	18
FM/GP	1,110	1,089	926	114	49	6	12	2	1
Family Medicine	1,095	1,075	915	114	46	5	12	2	1
General Practice	15	14	11		3	1			
Medical Specialties	1,925	1,850	1,330	390	130	18	17	35	5
Allergy and Immunology	23	22	18	4				1	
Cardiovascular Disease	74	73	52	18	3			1	
Dermatology	107	106	86	17	3		1		
Gastroenterology	43	40	30	9	1		1	2	
Internal Medicine	891	850	591	191	68	12	7	19	3
Pediatric Cardiology	12	12	10	2					
Pediatrics	734	709	516	140	53	5	8	10	2
Pulmonary Disease	41	38	27	9	2	1		2	
Surgical Specialties	706	701	511	167	23		4	1	
Colon and Rectal Surgery	12	12	12						
General Surgery	123	120	55	59	6		2	1	
Neurological Surgery	16	16	9	6	1				
Obstetrics & Gynecology	362	360	313	41	6		2		
Ophthalmology	65	65	47	13	5				
Orthopedic Surgery	52	52	31	20	1				
Otolaryngology	36	36	21	13	2				
Plastic Surgery	13	13	9	3	1				
Thoracic Surgery	5	5	3	1	1				
Urology	22	22	11	11					
Other Specialties	1,183	1,132	768	260	104	22	6	11	12
Anatomic/Clinical Pathology	150	141	94	35	12	4	1	1	3
Anesthesiology	121	120	75	34	11			1	
Child & Adolescent Psychiatry	54	53	44	5	4			1	
Diagnostic Radiology	144	142	107	23	12				2
Emergency Medicine	153	151	95	36	20	1	1		
Forensic Pathology	7	4	3		1				3
General Preventive Medicine	16	15	11	3	1	1			
Medical Genetics	6	6	5		1				
Neurology	95	91	60	25	6	1	1	2	
Nuclear Medicine	2	2	2						
Occupational Medicine	18	10	10			5	1		2
Other Specialty	29	23	8	14	1	3		2	1
Physical Medicine and Rehabilitation	73	68	48	16	4	2		3	
Psychiatry	207	202	140	38	24	3	1	1	
Public Health and General Preventive Medicine	5	3	2		1	2			
Radiation Oncology	22	22	16	4	2				
Radiology	25	23	22		1		1		1
Transplant Surgery	1	1	1						
Unspecified	55	55	25	27	3				
Inactive	273								
Not Classified	343								

Note: Excludes Address Unknown.

Subspecialties in this table are condensed into major specialties. See Appendix A.

Table 3.8

Female Physicians by State, Self-Designated Specialty, and Activity, 2010, continued
Mississippi

		Patient Care				Other Professional Activity			
				Hospital Based					
Specialty	Total Physicians	Total Patient Care	Office Based	Resid./ Fellows	Phys. Staff	Admin.	Med. Teach.	Research	Other
Total Physicians	1,326	1,080	751	190	139	19	12	7	11
FM/GP	196	184	140	24	20	5	4	1	2
Family Medicine	185	175	131	24	20	4	4	1	1
General Practice	11	9	9			1			1
Medical Specialties	460	443	324	67	52	7	4	5	1
Allergy and Immunology	5	4	3	1					1
Cardiovascular Disease	9	8	5	1	2	1			
Dermatology	15	15	13		2				
Gastroenterology	7	7	6	1					
Internal Medicine	209	203	132	37	34	2		4	
Pediatric Cardiology	1	1	1						
Pediatrics	207	198	158	27	13	4	4	1	
Pulmonary Disease	7	7	6		1				
Surgical Specialties	182	178	118	46	14	1	3		
Colon and Rectal Surgery	1	1	1						
General Surgery	29	27	12	10	5	1	1		
Obstetrics & Gynecology	108	107	80	22	5		1		
Ophthalmology	16	15	12	2	1		1		
Orthopedic Surgery	7	7	4	2	1				
Otolaryngology	12	12	4	6	2				
Plastic Surgery	3	3	2	1					
Thoracic Surgery	1	1	1						
Urology	5	5	2	3					
Other Specialties	291	275	169	53	53	6	1	1	8
Anatomic/Clinical Pathology	50	43	23	13	7	1			6
Anesthesiology	52	52	35	9	8				
Child & Adolescent Psychiatry	18	18	12	3	3				
Diagnostic Radiology	25	25	16	6	3				
Emergency Medicine	25	22	14	4	4	1	1		1
Forensic Pathology	1	1			1				
General Preventive Medicine	2	2	2						
Neurology	25	24	17	3	4			1	
Nuclear Medicine	2	1			1	1			
Other Specialty	2	2	2						
Physical Medicine and Rehabilitation	7	7	7						
Psychiatry	62	61	32	9	20	1			
Public Health and General Preventive Medicine	5	3	2		1	2			
Radiology	6	6	5		1				
Unspecified	9	8	2	6					1
Inactive	96								
Not Classified	101								

Note: Excludes Address Unknown.

Subspecialties in this table are condensed into major specialties. See Appendix A.

Table 3.8

Female Physicians by State, Self-Designated Specialty, and Activity, 2010, continued
Missouri

		Patient Care				Other Professional Activity			
				Hospital Based					
Specialty	Total Physicians	Total Patient Care	Office Based	Resid./ Fellows	Phys. Staff	Admin.	Med. Teach.	Research	Other
Total Physicians	4,958	4,056	2,545	1,077	434	33	52	45	13
FM/GP	512	501	409	61	31	5	5		1
Family Medicine	497	486	395	61	30	5	5		1
General Practice	15	15	14		1				
Medical Specialties	1,934	1,867	1,137	509	221	16	22	26	3
Allergy and Immunology	33	32	23	7	2				1
Cardiovascular Disease	41	38	23	12	3	1		2	
Dermatology	95	95	66	25	4				
Gastroenterology	37	36	21	14	1			1	
Internal Medicine	857	825	515	212	98	10	9	13	
Pediatric Cardiology	12	11	5	3	3		1		
Pediatrics	826	797	462	229	106	5	12	10	2
Pulmonary Disease	33	33	22	7	4				
Surgical Specialties	652	647	399	211	37	1	4		
Colon and Rectal Surgery	5	5	5						
General Surgery	111	110	54	50	6		1		
Neurological Surgery	9	9	3	4	2				
Obstetrics & Gynecology	352	348	249	83	16	1	3		
Ophthalmology	61	61	39	19	3				
Orthopedic Surgery	37	37	12	21	4				
Otolaryngology	35	35	14	17	4				
Plastic Surgery	24	24	11	12	1				
Thoracic Surgery	5	5	5						
Urology	13	13	7	5	1				
Other Specialties	1,101	1,041	600	296	145	11	21	19	9
Anatomic/Clinical Pathology	129	116	70	37	9	4	4	1	4
Anesthesiology	184	181	113	42	26		2	1	
Child & Adolescent Psychiatry	60	54	35	7	12	1		5	
Diagnostic Radiology	124	118	62	41	15		4	1	1
Emergency Medicine	131	129	63	38	28		2		
Forensic Pathology	5	4	1	1	2				1
General Preventive Medicine	7	7	5		2				
Medical Genetics	6	2		1	1	1	2	1	
Neurology	89	82	39	37	6	1	1	5	
Nuclear Medicine	7	5	2	2	1		1	1	
Occupational Medicine	6	5	5			1			
Other Specialty	17	15	7	6	2			1	1
Physical Medicine and Rehabilitation	48	46	35	6	5	1	1		
Psychiatry	193	187	121	41	25	2	2	1	1
Public Health and General Preventive Medicine	1	1			1				
Radiation Oncology	22	22	18	2	2				
Radiology	32	28	17	3	8		2	1	1
Unspecified	40	39	7	32				1	
Inactive	244								
Not Classified	515								

Note: Excludes Address Unknown.

Subspecialties in this table are condensed into major specialties. See Appendix A.

Table 3.8

Female Physicians by State, Self-Designated Specialty, and Activity, 2010, continued
Montana

		Patient Care				Other Professional Activity			
				Hospital Based					
Specialty	Total Physicians	Total Patient Care	Office Based	Resid./ Fellows	Phys. Staff	Admin.	Med. Teach.	Research	Other
Total Physicians	629	525	423	21	81	7	7	1	1
FM/GP	159	155	126	14	15	2	2		
Family Medicine	156	153	124	14	15	1	2		
General Practice	3	2	2			1			
Medical Specialties	181	177	145	1	31	1	2		1
Allergy and Immunology	4	4	3		1				
Cardiovascular Disease	5	5	5						
Dermatology	10	10	8		2				
Gastroenterology	2	2	2						
Internal Medicine	89	88	69	1	18		1		
Pediatrics	65	62	52		10	1	1		1
Pulmonary Disease	6	6	6						
Surgical Specialties	84	81	74	2	5	2	1		
General Surgery	17	17	13	1	3				
Obstetrics & Gynecology	46	44	42		2	1	1		
Ophthalmology	4	3	3			1			
Orthopedic Surgery	7	7	7						
Otolaryngology	4	4	3	1					
Plastic Surgery	1	1	1						
Thoracic Surgery	1	1	1						
Urology	4	4	4						
Other Specialties	117	112	78	4	30	2	2	1	
Anatomic/Clinical Pathology	9	9	7		2				
Anesthesiology	19	18	16		2		1		
Child & Adolescent Psychiatry	6	6	5		1				
Diagnostic Radiology	8	8	4		4				
Emergency Medicine	23	22	12		10	1			
General Preventive Medicine	1	1	1						
Medical Genetics	1	1			1				
Neurology	5	5	5						
Occupational Medicine	1	1			1				
Other Specialty	4	3	2		1			1	
Physical Medicine and Rehabilitation	5	5	4		1				
Psychiatry	25	23	18		5	1	1		
Radiation Oncology	4	4	3		1				
Radiology	1	1	1						
Unspecified	5	5		4	1				
Inactive	61								
Not Classified	27								

Note: Excludes Address Unknown.

Subspecialties in this table are condensed into major specialties. See Appendix A.

Table 3.8

Female Physicians by State, Self-Designated Specialty, and Activity, 2010, continued
Nebraska

		Patient Care				Other Professional Activity			
				Hospital Based					
Specialty	Total Physicians	Total Patient Care	Office Based	Resid./ Fellows	Phys. Staff	Admin.	Med. Teach.	Research	Other
Total Physicians	1,373	1,175	791	273	111	13	13	9	4
FM/GP	241	234	184	38	12	4	3		
Family Medicine	237	230	182	38	10	4	3		
General Practice	4	4	2		2				
Medical Specialties	479	463	302	114	47	5	5	4	2
Allergy and Immunology	5	5	3	2					
Cardiovascular Disease	15	15	11	3	1				
Dermatology	9	9	9						
Gastroenterology	7	7	4	3					
Internal Medicine	238	232	138	71	23	1	2	2	1
Pediatric Cardiology	1	1			1				
Pediatrics	196	188	134	32	22	4	1	2	1
Pulmonary Disease	8	6	3	3			2		
Surgical Specialties	190	185	122	52	11	2	1	2	
Colon and Rectal Surgery	3	2	2			1			
General Surgery	32	31	15	15	1			1	
Neurological Surgery	2	2	2						
Obstetrics & Gynecology	103	101	68	26	7		1	1	
Ophthalmology	20	19	15	2	2	1			
Orthopedic Surgery	6	6	5	1					
Otolaryngology	14	14	8	5	1				
Plastic Surgery	7	7	6	1					
Thoracic Surgery	1	1		1					
Urology	2	2	1	1					
Other Specialties	304	293	183	69	41	2	4	3	2
Anatomic/Clinical Pathology	39	35	19	12	4		1	2	1
Anesthesiology	63	61	41	12	8	1	1		
Child & Adolescent Psychiatry	21	21	15	3	3				
Diagnostic Radiology	35	33	19	7	7		1		1
Emergency Medicine	29	29	16	8	5				
General Preventive Medicine	2	1	1					1	
Medical Genetics	2	2		1	1				
Neurology	20	19	14	5			1		
Nuclear Medicine	4	4	1	2	1				
Occupational Medicine	2	1			1	1			
Other Specialty	4	4	3		1				
Physical Medicine and Rehabilitation	10	10	7		3				
Psychiatry	52	52	39	8	5				
Radiation Oncology	4	4	4						
Radiology	8	8	4	2	2				
Unspecified	9	9		9					
Inactive	52								
Not Classified	107								

Note: Excludes Address Unknown.

Subspecialties in this table are condensed into major specialties. See Appendix A.

Table 3.8

Female Physicians by State, Self-Designated Specialty, and Activity, 2010, continued
Nevada

		Patient Care				Other Professional Activity			
				Hospital Based					
Specialty	Total Physicians	Total Patient Care	Office Based	Resid./ Fellows	Phys. Staff	Admin.	Med. Teach.	Research	Other
Total Physicians	1,418	1,119	933	88	98	18	9	4	4
FM/GP	179	175	151	9	15		2		2
Family Medicine	170	166	143	9	14		2		2
General Practice	9	9	8		1				
Medical Specialties	528	511	421	50	40	10	5	2	
Allergy and Immunology	4	3	3					1	
Cardiovascular Disease	15	15	15						
Dermatology	13	13	12		1				
Gastroenterology	5	5	5						
Internal Medicine	287	274	220	28	26	9	4		
Pediatric Cardiology	2	2	2						
Pediatrics	197	194	160	22	12	1	1	1	
Pulmonary Disease	5	5	4		1				
Surgical Specialties	174	172	147	16	9	1	1		
Colon and Rectal Surgery	1	1	1						
General Surgery	31	31	22	6	3				
Neurological Surgery	3	3	3						
Obstetrics & Gynecology	103	101	91	7	3	1	1		
Ophthalmology	13	13	12		1				
Orthopedic Surgery	4	4	2	2					
Otolaryngology	4	4	3		1				
Plastic Surgery	7	7	6	1					
Thoracic Surgery	2	2	2						
Urology	6	6	5		1				
Other Specialties	273	261	214	13	34	7	1	2	2
Anatomic/Clinical Pathology	19	18	16		2	1			
Anesthesiology	41	40	37		3		1		
Child & Adolescent Psychiatry	16	15	11	1	3			1	
Diagnostic Radiology	27	26	25		1				1
Emergency Medicine	47	46	38	3	5	1			
Forensic Pathology	5	4	4			1			
General Preventive Medicine	6	5	4		1	1			
Medical Genetics	1							1	
Neurology	19	19	15	1	3				
Occupational Medicine	2	2	1		1				
Other Specialty	4	4	2		2				
Physical Medicine and Rehabilitation	14	12	10		2	2			
Psychiatry	53	52	34	7	11				1
Public Health and General Preventive Medicine	1					1			
Radiation Oncology	9	9	9						
Radiology	4	4	4						
Unspecified	5	5	4	1					
Inactive	130								
Not Classified	134								

Note: Excludes Address Unknown.

Subspecialties in this table are condensed into major specialties. See Appendix A.

Table 3.8

Female Physicians by State, Self-Designated Specialty, and Activity, 2010, continued
New Hampshire

		Patient Care				Other Professional Activity			
				Hospital Based					
Specialty	Total Physicians	Total Patient Care	Office Based	Resid./ Fellows	Phys. Staff	Admin.	Med. Teach.	Research	Other
Total Physicians	1,330	1,088	769	174	145	9	8	10	4
FM/GP	169	168	140	8	20		1		
Family Medicine	168	167	139	8	20		1		
General Practice	1	1	1						
Medical Specialties	476	461	338	60	63	2	4	6	3
Allergy and Immunology	5	5	5						
Cardiovascular Disease	12	12	9	3					
Dermatology	12	12	7	4	1				
Gastroenterology	4	4	2	1	1				
Internal Medicine	255	248	175	34	39	1	1	4	1
Pediatric Cardiology	2	2	2						
Pediatrics	172	164	130	15	19	1	3	2	2
Pulmonary Disease	14	14	8	3	3				
Surgical Specialties	212	209	148	39	22	1	1	1	
General Surgery	47	46	25	15	6			1	
Neurological Surgery	5	5	4		1				
Obstetrics & Gynecology	118	117	89	14	14		1		
Ophthalmology	13	13	12	1					
Orthopedic Surgery	12	12	6	5	1				
Otolaryngology	4	4	3	1					
Plastic Surgery	6	5	4	1		1			
Thoracic Surgery	1	1	1						
Urology	6	6	4	2					
Other Specialties	262	250	143	67	40	6	2	3	1
Anatomic/Clinical Pathology	32	30	16	10	4			1	1
Anesthesiology	36	36	18	10	8				
Child & Adolescent Psychiatry	16	16	11	4	1				
Diagnostic Radiology	24	24	15	6	3				
Emergency Medicine	32	32	21	1	10				
Forensic Pathology	1	1		1					
General Preventive Medicine	12	11	2	9		1			
Neurology	15	15	8	5	2				
Occupational Medicine	5	2	2			3			
Other Specialty	5	5	3		2				
Physical Medicine and Rehabilitation	7	7	5	2					
Psychiatry	63	59	38	16	5	1	1	2	
Public Health and General Preventive Medicine	1					1			
Radiation Oncology	3	3	1		2				
Radiology	3	2			2		1		
Unspecified	7	7	3	3	1				
Inactive	94								
Not Classified	117								

Note: Excludes Address Unknown.

Subspecialties in this table are condensed into major specialties. See Appendix A.

Table 3.8

Female Physicians by State, Self-Designated Specialty, and Activity, 2010, continued
New Jersey

		Patient Care				Other Professional Activity			
				Hospital Based					
Specialty	Total Physicians	Total Patient Care	Office Based	Resid./ Fellows	Phys. Staff	Admin.	Med. Teach.	Research	Other
Total Physicians	10,238	8,032	5,840	1,196	996	112	99	123	84
FM/GP	650	618	492	83	43	4	20	5	3
Family Medicine	605	577	463	83	31	3	20	3	2
General Practice	45	41	29		12	1		2	1
Medical Specialties	4,341	4,127	3,015	592	520	60	49	68	37
Allergy and Immunology	66	64	55	7	2	1			1
Cardiovascular Disease	95	90	67	14	9	1	1	1	2
Dermatology	138	137	129	4	4			1	
Gastroenterology	60	57	47	3	7	1		1	1
Internal Medicine	2,208	2,065	1,430	397	238	41	27	46	29
Pediatric Cardiology	20	19	11	1	7		1		
Pediatrics	1,685	1,630	1,225	161	244	15	18	18	4
Pulmonary Disease	69	65	51	5	9	1	2	1	
Surgical Specialties	1,133	1,109	841	194	74	7	8	6	3
Colon and Rectal Surgery	5	5	5						
General Surgery	178	176	87	72	17	1		1	
Neurological Surgery	6	6	4	2					
Obstetrics & Gynecology	688	672	542	81	49	6	5	3	2
Ophthalmology	134	130	118	9	3		1	2	1
Orthopedic Surgery	35	35	25	9	1				
Otolaryngology	29	27	19	7	1		2		
Plastic Surgery	34	34	24	8	2				
Thoracic Surgery	4	4	4						
Urology	20	20	13	6	1				
Other Specialties	2,326	2,178	1,492	327	359	41	22	44	41
Aerospace Medicine	1	1			1				
Anatomic/Clinical Pathology	220	189	121	30	38	8	4	6	13
Anesthesiology	435	425	310	43	72		2	4	4
Child & Adolescent Psychiatry	138	131	102	12	17	2	1	3	1
Diagnostic Radiology	220	212	165	36	11		2	3	3
Emergency Medicine	202	200	118	40	42		2		
Forensic Pathology	7	3	2		1	2		1	1
General Preventive Medicine	21	18	14	3	1			2	1
Medical Genetics	7	5	3		2		1		1
Neurology	147	135	101	20	14	2	3	4	3
Nuclear Medicine	10	9	6		3				1
Occupational Medicine	18	12	9		3	5			1
Other Specialty	51	28	18	4	6	7	1	12	3
Physical Medicine and Rehabilitation	144	141	106	13	22	1		1	1
Psychiatry	528	503	329	63	111	12	5	5	3
Public Health and General Preventive Medicine	6	2	2			2			2
Radiation Oncology	39	38	28	4	6			1	
Radiology	57	54	46	1	7			1	2
Transplant Surgery	1							1	
Unspecified	74	72	12	58	2		1		1
Inactive	814								
Not Classified	974								

Note: Excludes Address Unknown.

Subspecialties in this table are condensed into major specialties. See Appendix A.

Table 3.8

Female Physicians by State, Self-Designated Specialty, and Activity, 2010, continued
New Mexico

		Patient Care				Other Professional Activity			
				Hospital Based					
Specialty	Total Physicians	Total Patient Care	Office Based	Resid./ Fellows	Phys. Staff	Admin.	Med. Teach.	Research	Other
Total Physicians	1,920	1,526	1,103	239	184	28	26	18	16
FM/GP	359	350	272	46	32	1	3	3	2
Family Medicine	349	341	264	46	31	1	3	2	2
General Practice	10	9	8		1			1	
Medical Specialties	607	576	409	81	86	11	13	5	2
Allergy and Immunology	2	2	2						
Cardiovascular Disease	18	18	16		2				
Dermatology	19	19	14	5					
Gastroenterology	12	12	6	4	2				
Internal Medicine	306	290	205	38	47	6	8	2	
Pediatric Cardiology	1	1	1						
Pediatrics	239	224	158	32	34	5	5	3	2
Pulmonary Disease	10	10	7	2	1				
Surgical Specialties	208	204	156	36	12	1	2		1
Colon and Rectal Surgery	1	1	1						
General Surgery	48	48	34	11	3				
Neurological Surgery	2	2	1	1					
Obstetrics & Gynecology	120	118	98	16	4		2		
Ophthalmology	9	9	9						
Orthopedic Surgery	14	13	5	4	4				1
Otolaryngology	6	6	3	2	1				
Plastic Surgery	3	3	3						
Urology	5	4	2	2		1			
Other Specialties	440	396	266	76	54	15	8	10	11
Aerospace Medicine	2	1	1			1			
Anatomic/Clinical Pathology	55	46	30	13	3		1	4	4
Anesthesiology	54	54	39	11	4				
Child & Adolescent Psychiatry	24	21	15	3	3	1	1	1	
Diagnostic Radiology	26	23	14	8	1		1		2
Emergency Medicine	75	73	49	12	12	1	1		
Forensic Pathology	1	1	1						
General Preventive Medicine	7	6	2		4			1	
Medical Genetics	2	1	1						1
Neurology	27	26	16	7	3			1	
Nuclear Medicine	1	1			1				
Occupational Medicine	7	6	5		1	1			
Other Specialty	11	6	3	2	1	3		1	1
Physical Medicine and Rehabilitation	14	14	12	1	1				
Psychiatry	106	97	65	15	17	1	4	2	2
Public Health and General Preventive Medicine	7	1	1			6			
Radiation Oncology	5	5	4		1				
Radiology	6	6	4	1	1				
Unspecified	10	8	4	3	1	1			1
Inactive	140								
Not Classified	166								

Note: Excludes Address Unknown.

Subspecialties in this table are condensed into major specialties. See Appendix A.

Table 3.8

Female Physicians by State, Self-Designated Specialty, and Activity, 2010, continued
New York

		Patient Care				Other Professional Activity			
				Hospital Based					
Specialty	Total Physicians	Total Patient Care	Office Based	Resid./ Fellows	Phys. Staff	Admin.	Med. Teach.	Research	Other
Total Physicians	29,467	22,612	13,429	6,375	2,808	352	290	335	136
FM/GP	1,451	1,413	1,079	233	101	18	18	1	1
Family Medicine	1,385	1,350	1,027	233	90	15	18	1	1
General Practice	66	63	52		11	3			
Medical Specialties	11,531	10,936	6,581	3,112	1,243	165	154	214	62
Allergy and Immunology	138	132	95	25	12		1	5	
Cardiovascular Disease	312	302	180	94	28	3	1	6	
Dermatology	471	461	351	96	14	2	5	2	1
Gastroenterology	200	192	109	71	12		3	5	
Internal Medicine	6,028	5,693	3,267	1,800	626	96	80	120	39
Pediatric Cardiology	71	66	31	15	20		2	3	
Pediatrics	4,097	3,887	2,444	942	501	62	60	67	21
Pulmonary Disease	214	203	104	69	30	2	2	6	1
Surgical Specialties	3,389	3,332	2,016	1,031	285	16	22	14	5
Colon and Rectal Surgery	26	26	19	3	4				
General Surgery	606	603	227	310	66	1	1		1
Neurological Surgery	40	40	22	17	1				
Obstetrics & Gynecology	1,818	1,773	1,189	428	156	14	17	10	4
Ophthalmology	411	404	300	81	23		4	3	
Orthopedic Surgery	139	138	46	82	10			1	
Otolaryngology	151	151	78	59	14				
Plastic Surgery	97	97	82	11	4				
Thoracic Surgery	26	25	16	8	1	1			
Urology	75	75	37	32	6				
Other Specialties	7,354	6,931	3,753	1,999	1,179	153	96	106	68
Aerospace Medicine	1	1			1				
Anatomic/Clinical Pathology	660	597	303	166	128	18	10	12	23
Anesthesiology	1,045	1,016	596	275	145	8	11	8	2
Child & Adolescent Psychiatry	429	405	276	59	70	7	7	8	2
Diagnostic Radiology	707	691	385	211	95	3	4		9
Emergency Medicine	786	774	333	299	142	7	4	1	
Forensic Pathology	19	13	11	2		2			4
General Preventive Medicine	88	74	50	21	3	7	3	2	2
Medical Genetics	11	8	2	4	2		1	2	
Neurology	533	505	268	181	56	9	7	12	
Nuclear Medicine	40	36	21	6	9	1	2		1
Occupational Medicine	19	13	11		2	5		1	
Other Specialty	145	108	38	52	18	13	1	17	6
Physical Medicine and Rehabilitation	379	359	229	70	60	7	5	3	5
Psychiatry	1,927	1,814	1,005	427	382	45	33	27	8
Public Health and General Preventive Medicine	43	18	13		5	14	1	8	2
Radiation Oncology	108	104	63	26	15		1	2	1
Radiology	153	142	97	9	36	4	4	2	1
Transplant Surgery	2	2	1		1				
Unspecified	258	250	51	191	8	3	2	1	2
Vascular Medicine	1	1			1				
Inactive	2,079								
Not Classified	3,663								

Note: Excludes Address Unknown.

Subspecialties in this table are condensed into major specialties. See Appendix A.

Table 3.8

Female Physicians by State, Self-Designated Specialty, and Activity, 2010, continued
North Carolina

		Patient Care				Other Professional Activity			
				Hospital Based					
Specialty	Total Physicians	Total Patient Care	Office Based	Resid./ Fellows	Phys. Staff	Admin.	Med. Teach.	Research	Other
Total Physicians	8,132	6,667	4,780	1,296	591	78	97	95	32
FM/GP	1,151	1,117	905	136	76	13	15	2	4
Family Medicine	1,132	1,100	889	136	75	12	15	2	3
General Practice	19	17	16		1	1			1
Medical Specialties	2,995	2,840	2,055	517	268	32	47	70	6
Allergy and Immunology	34	31	24	6	1			3	
Cardiovascular Disease	58	55	34	14	7	1	2		
Dermatology	155	155	127	22	6				
Gastroenterology	49	45	34	5	6	1	1	1	1
Internal Medicine	1,400	1,318	921	243	154	19	17	43	3
Pediatric Cardiology	9	9	7	1	1				
Pediatrics	1,239	1,178	878	210	90	11	27	21	2
Pulmonary Disease	51	49	30	16	3			2	
Surgical Specialties	1,032	1,017	715	248	54	1	10	4	
General Surgery	166	163	78	76	9	1	1	1	
Neurological Surgery	14	14	4	7	3				
Obstetrics & Gynecology	623	612	473	109	30		9	2	
Ophthalmology	99	99	87	11	1				
Orthopedic Surgery	34	34	16	16	2				
Otolaryngology	56	55	33	16	6			1	
Plastic Surgery	20	20	13	5	2				
Thoracic Surgery	5	5	2	3					
Urology	15	15	9	5	1				
Other Specialties	1,791	1,693	1,105	395	193	32	25	19	22
Anatomic/Clinical Pathology	149	134	84	37	13		2	5	8
Anesthesiology	246	239	131	78	30	2	4	1	
Child & Adolescent Psychiatry	108	101	77	17	7	2	2	2	1
Diagnostic Radiology	141	137	98	27	12		3	1	
Emergency Medicine	277	272	167	63	42	1	4		
Forensic Pathology	4	4	3	1					
General Preventive Medicine	40	36	27	6	3	2		2	
Medical Genetics	9	8	3	2	3	1			
Neurology	119	114	82	25	7	2	1	1	1
Nuclear Medicine	5	4	3		1			1	
Occupational Medicine	10	4	3		1	5			1
Other Specialty	41	34	17	14	3	3		2	2
Physical Medicine and Rehabilitation	87	82	52	24	6	2	2	1	
Psychiatry	412	392	280	64	48	7	7	3	3
Public Health and General Preventive Medicine	10	4	4			5			1
Radiation Oncology	42	41	32	4	5				1
Radiology	42	39	29	6	4				3
Unspecified	49	48	13	27	8				1
Inactive	435								
Not Classified	728								

Note: Excludes Address Unknown.

Subspecialties in this table are condensed into major specialties. See Appendix A.

Table 3.8

Female Physicians by State, Self-Designated Specialty, and Activity, 2010, continued
North Dakota

Specialty	Total Physicians	Patient Care				Other Professional Activity			
				Hospital Based					
		Total Patient Care	Office Based	Resid./ Fellows	Phys. Staff	Admin.	Med. Teach.	Research	Other
Total Physicians	441	400	287	56	57	4	4		2
FM/GP	136	133	92	30	11	2	1		
Family Medicine	133	130	89	30	11	2	1		
General Practice	3	3	3						
Medical Specialties	120	117	86	12	19	2	1		
Cardiovascular Disease	1	1	1						
Dermatology	7	7	6		1				
Gastroenterology	1	1	1						
Internal Medicine	67	64	41	12	11	2	1		
Pediatrics	43	43	36		7				
Pulmonary Disease	1	1	1						
Surgical Specialties	62	61	46	7	8		1		
General Surgery	15	14	6	5	3		1		
Obstetrics & Gynecology	33	33	29	1	3				
Ophthalmology	3	3	3						
Orthopedic Surgery	4	4	4						
Otolaryngology	4	4	2	1	1				
Plastic Surgery	3	3	2		1				
Other Specialties	92	89	63	7	19		1		2
Anatomic/Clinical Pathology	14	13	9		4		1		
Anesthesiology	9	9	5	1	3				
Child & Adolescent Psychiatry	11	10	6		4				1
Diagnostic Radiology	4	4	3		1				
Emergency Medicine	8	8	7		1				
Neurology	9	9	7	1	1				
Other Specialty	1	1	1						
Physical Medicine and Rehabilitation	5	5	3		2				
Psychiatry	26	26	20	3	3				
Radiation Oncology	1	1	1						
Radiology	2	1	1						1
Unspecified	2	2		2					
Inactive	16								
Not Classified	15								

Note: Excludes Address Unknown.

Subspecialties in this table are condensed into major specialties. See Appendix A.

Table 3.8

Female Physicians by State, Self-Designated Specialty, and Activity, 2010, continued
Ohio

		Patient Care				Other Professional Activity			
				Hospital Based					
Specialty	Total Physicians	Total Patient Care	Office Based	Resid./ Fellows	Phys. Staff	Admin.	Med. Teach.	Research	Other
Total Physicians	10,859	8,806	5,634	2,247	925	76	105	101	36
FM/GP	1,273	1,241	954	198	89	11	14	5	2
Family Medicine	1,212	1,182	910	198	74	10	14	5	1
General Practice	61	59	44		15	1			1
Medical Specialties	4,111	3,950	2,474	1,027	449	31	57	63	10
Allergy and Immunology	37	35	23	7	5		1	1	
Cardiovascular Disease	83	76	50	15	11	1	3	3	
Dermatology	160	159	109	43	7		1		
Gastroenterology	62	59	38	12	9		3		
Internal Medicine	1,903	1,833	1,187	470	176	19	25	20	6
Pediatric Cardiology	28	25	11	5	9		1	2	
Pediatrics	1,781	1,710	1,024	460	226	11	22	34	4
Pulmonary Disease	57	53	32	15	6		1	3	
Surgical Specialties	1,336	1,317	819	422	76	5	11	2	1
Colon and Rectal Surgery	6	6	4		2				
General Surgery	260	251	116	118	17	4	5		
Neurological Surgery	25	25	9	14	2				
Obstetrics & Gynecology	738	731	518	179	34	1	4	1	1
Ophthalmology	130	128	89	30	9		1	1	
Orthopedic Surgery	53	53	21	27	5				
Otolaryngology	48	48	21	25	2				
Plastic Surgery	34	33	18	13	2		1		
Thoracic Surgery	9	9	6	1	2				
Urology	33	33	17	15	1				
Other Specialties	2,404	2,298	1,387	600	311	29	23	31	23
Anatomic/Clinical Pathology	303	271	164	66	41	6	8	7	11
Anesthesiology	378	374	226	93	55	2		1	1
Child & Adolescent Psychiatry	126	123	93	14	16	1	1		1
Diagnostic Radiology	200	198	129	42	27	1		1	
Emergency Medicine	328	320	191	89	40	2	3	2	1
Forensic Pathology	8	8	6	1	1				
General Preventive Medicine	14	13	10	2	1	1			
Medical Genetics	13	10	6	2	2			3	
Neurology	161	156	78	59	19		1	3	1
Nuclear Medicine	5	5	5						
Occupational Medicine	25	20	15		5	1		2	2
Other Specialty	76	62	22	36	4	2	1	8	3
Physical Medicine and Rehabilitation	89	89	58	21	10				
Psychiatry	454	436	286	91	59	9	5	3	1
Public Health and General Preventive Medicine	7	2	1		1	3	2		
Radiation Oncology	43	42	25	8	9		1		
Radiology	70	66	48	5	13		1	1	2
Transplant Surgery	2	2			2				
Unspecified	100	99	22	71	6	1			
Vascular Medicine	2	2	2						
Inactive	625								
Not Classified	1,110								

Note: Excludes Address Unknown.

Subspecialties in this table are condensed into major specialties. See Appendix A.

Table 3.8

Female Physicians by State, Self-Designated Specialty, and Activity, 2010, continued
Oklahoma

		Patient Care				Other Professional Activity			
				Hospital Based					
Specialty	Total Physicians	Total Patient Care	Office Based	Resid./ Fellows	Phys. Staff	Admin.	Med. Teach.	Research	Other
Total Physicians	1,842	1,546	1,126	281	139	17	28	8	12
FM/GP	306	296	213	60	23	3	4		3
Family Medicine	288	280	199	60	21	3	4		1
General Practice	18	16	14		2				2
Medical Specialties	621	598	453	98	47	2	13	6	2
Allergy and Immunology	7	7	7						
Cardiovascular Disease	12	12	11		1				
Dermatology	29	29	21	7	1				
Gastroenterology	13	13	10	2	1				
Internal Medicine	284	275	208	43	24	1	4	3	1
Pediatric Cardiology	4	4	4						
Pediatrics	262	248	186	43	19	1	9	3	1
Pulmonary Disease	10	10	6	3	1				
Surgical Specialties	251	247	185	50	12		3	1	
Colon and Rectal Surgery	4	4	3		1				
General Surgery	50	50	36	11	3				
Neurological Surgery	3	3	3						
Obstetrics & Gynecology	144	140	105	27	8		3	1	
Ophthalmology	26	26	22	4					
Orthopedic Surgery	9	9	8	1					
Otolaryngology	5	5		5					
Plastic Surgery	4	4	3	1					
Thoracic Surgery	1	1	1						
Urology	5	5	4	1					
Other Specialties	433	405	275	73	57	12	8	1	7
Anatomic/Clinical Pathology	46	41	30	7	4	1	2		2
Anesthesiology	57	53	41	6	6		3		1
Child & Adolescent Psychiatry	27	25	14	2	9	1	1		
Diagnostic Radiology	47	46	36	7	3				1
Emergency Medicine	34	33	20	2	11	1			
Forensic Pathology	1								1
General Preventive Medicine	3	3	2		1				
Medical Genetics	1	1	1						
Neurology	25	25	16	5	4				
Nuclear Medicine	3	2	1	1		1			
Occupational Medicine	7	4	4			3			
Other Specialty	3	2	1	1		1			
Physical Medicine and Rehabilitation	14	14	14						
Psychiatry	116	110	70	22	18	3	2	1	
Public Health and General Preventive Medicine	2	1	1						1
Radiation Oncology	12	11	10	1		1			
Radiology	10	9	9						1
Unspecified	24	24	4	19	1				
Vascular Medicine	1	1	1						
Inactive	118								
Not Classified	113								

Note: Excludes Address Unknown.

Subspecialties in this table are condensed into major specialties. See Appendix A.

Table 3.8

Female Physicians by State, Self-Designated Specialty, and Activity, 2010, continued
Oregon

		Patient Care				Other Professional Activity			
				Hospital Based					
Specialty	Total Physicians	Total Patient Care	Office Based	Resid./ Fellows	Phys. Staff	Admin.	Med. Teach.	Research	Other
Total Physicians	3,975	3,293	2,560	442	291	35	21	32	20
FM/GP	585	567	477	59	31	6	3	4	5
Family Medicine	574	558	468	59	31	5	3	3	5
General Practice	11	9	9			1		1	
Medical Specialties	1,411	1,374	1,059	189	126	11	8	16	2
Allergy and Immunology	6	6	6						
Cardiovascular Disease	39	38	25	7	6	1			
Dermatology	68	68	55	10	3				
Gastroenterology	26	26	23	3					
Internal Medicine	805	781	573	122	86	7	5	10	2
Pediatric Cardiology	7	7	4	2	1				
Pediatrics	440	431	360	42	29	3	3	3	
Pulmonary Disease	20	17	13	3	1			3	
Surgical Specialties	573	569	451	89	29	1	1	2	
Colon and Rectal Surgery	3	3	1	2					
General Surgery	114	113	67	37	9			1	
Neurological Surgery	11	11	9	1	1				
Obstetrics & Gynecology	320	317	279	26	12	1	1	1	
Ophthalmology	47	47	38	5	4				
Orthopedic Surgery	19	19	17	1	1				
Otolaryngology	29	29	17	10	2				
Plastic Surgery	17	17	12	5					
Thoracic Surgery	2	2	2						
Urology	11	11	9	2					
Other Specialties	832	783	573	105	105	17	9	10	13
Anatomic/Clinical Pathology	69	60	46	7	7			3	6
Anesthesiology	144	139	103	17	19	1	4		
Child & Adolescent Psychiatry	38	38	35	1	2				
Diagnostic Radiology	59	58	45	9	4				1
Emergency Medicine	134	132	84	18	30		2		
Forensic Pathology	5	3	3				1		1
General Preventive Medicine	12	8	7	1		2		2	
Medical Genetics	3	2	1	1				1	
Neurology	55	54	41	8	5	1			
Nuclear Medicine	3	3	1	1	1				
Occupational Medicine	8	6	6			2			
Other Specialty	18	12	8	2	2	3		1	2
Physical Medicine and Rehabilitation	32	30	25	2	3	2			
Psychiatry	173	166	122	20	24	3	2	1	1
Public Health and General Preventive Medicine	10	3	2		1	3		2	2
Radiation Oncology	23	23	19	2	2				
Radiology	18	18	15	1	2				
Unspecified	27	27	9	15	3				
Vascular Medicine	1	1	1						
Inactive	266								
Not Classified	308								

Note: Excludes Address Unknown.

Subspecialties in this table are condensed into major specialties. See Appendix A.

Table 3.8

Female Physicians by State, Self-Designated Specialty, and Activity, 2010, continued
Pennsylvania

		Patient Care				Other Professional Activity			
				Hospital Based					
Specialty	Total Physicians	Total Patient Care	Office Based	Resid./ Fellows	Phys. Staff	Admin.	Med. Teach.	Research	Other
Total Physicians	13,822	10,798	6,614	3,007	1,177	156	146	187	79
FM/GP	1,390	1,333	965	280	88	16	29	5	7
Family Medicine	1,336	1,282	921	280	81	15	29	3	7
General Practice	54	51	44		7	1		2	
Medical Specialties	5,068	4,793	2,980	1,294	519	65	60	123	27
Allergy and Immunology	62	57	39	14	4			4	1
Cardiovascular Disease	151	145	92	45	8		1	4	1
Dermatology	223	219	166	45	8		2	2	
Gastroenterology	120	114	78	30	6	1	1	2	2
Internal Medicine	2,612	2,458	1,492	698	268	45	26	69	14
Pediatric Cardiology	41	38	14	17	7	1		2	
Pediatrics	1,756	1,664	1,042	414	208	18	30	35	9
Pulmonary Disease	103	98	57	31	10			5	
Surgical Specialties	1,695	1,651	946	591	114	14	16	8	6
Colon and Rectal Surgery	10	10	6	1	3				
General Surgery	367	360	135	192	33	2	2	2	1
Neurological Surgery	16	16	7	9					
Obstetrics & Gynecology	872	843	533	249	61	9	12	5	3
Ophthalmology	212	207	151	49	7	2	1	1	1
Orthopedic Surgery	64	63	27	33	3	1			
Otolaryngology	73	71	37	31	3		1		1
Plastic Surgery	38	38	24	13	1				
Thoracic Surgery	15	15	9	4	2				
Urology	28	28	17	10	1				
Other Specialties	3,213	3,021	1,723	842	456	61	41	51	39
Anatomic/Clinical Pathology	336	299	143	90	66	10	9	3	15
Anesthesiology	451	433	260	109	64	5	8	4	1
Child & Adolescent Psychiatry	158	148	108	25	15	2	3	4	1
Diagnostic Radiology	366	358	207	105	46		3	2	3
Emergency Medicine	383	374	166	135	73	5	2	2	
Forensic Pathology	9	5	4	1					4
General Preventive Medicine	21	18	15		3	1		2	
Medical Genetics	14	13	5	6	2			1	
Neurology	230	218	119	78	21	3	2	7	
Nuclear Medicine	23	20	12	5	3	1	1	1	
Occupational Medicine	21	13	10		3	6			2
Other Specialty	74	56	24	27	5	3	3	9	3
Physical Medicine and Rehabilitation	178	174	115	29	30	2		1	1
Psychiatry	651	611	406	112	93	14	9	11	6
Public Health and General Preventive Medicine	12	2	1		1	5		2	3
Radiation Oncology	58	57	31	17	9	1			
Radiology	90	89	60	14	15		1		
Transplant Surgery	1	1	1						
Unspecified	136	131	35	89	7	3		2	
Vascular Medicine	1	1	1						
Inactive	988								
Not Classified	1,468								

Note: Excludes Address Unknown.

Subspecialties in this table are condensed into major specialties. See Appendix A.

Table 3.8

Female Physicians by State, Self-Designated Specialty, and Activity, 2010, continued
Puerto Rico

		Patient Care				Other Professional Activity			
				Hospital Based					
Specialty	Total Physicians	Total Patient Care	Office Based	Resid./ Fellows	Phys. Staff	Admin.	Med. Teach.	Research	Other
Total Physicians	4,134	3,049	2,219	499	331	75	48	15	15
FM/GP	672	639	536	12	91	22	7		4
Family Medicine	282	267	230	12	25	10	4		1
General Practice	390	372	306		66	12	3		3
Medical Specialties	1,186	1,119	775	225	119	33	22	6	6
Allergy and Immunology	2	2	1	1					
Cardiovascular Disease	21	21	18	2	1				
Dermatology	41	41	30	8	3				
Gastroenterology	28	25	15	8	2	1	1	1	
Internal Medicine	493	478	299	136	43	4	7	1	3
Pediatric Cardiology	2	2	2						
Pediatrics	579	531	397	65	69	28	13	4	3
Pulmonary Disease	20	19	13	5	1		1		
Surgical Specialties	232	225	157	53	15	3	2	1	1
General Surgery	36	35	23	11	1	1			
Neurological Surgery	2	2		2					
Obstetrics & Gynecology	138	133	91	31	11	1	2	1	1
Ophthalmology	36	36	29	4	3				
Orthopedic Surgery	8	7	4	3		1			
Otolaryngology	5	5	3	2					
Plastic Surgery	3	3	3						
Thoracic Surgery	1	1	1						
Urology	3	3	3						
Other Specialties	1,112	1,066	751	209	106	17	17	8	4
Anatomic/Clinical Pathology	48	42	32	8	2		4	1	1
Anesthesiology	43	41	31	4	6		1		1
Child & Adolescent Psychiatry	37	34	27	4	3	1	2		
Diagnostic Radiology	61	57	41	9	7	2	2		
Emergency Medicine	44	43	23	15	5		1		
Forensic Pathology	3	3	3						
General Preventive Medicine	8	5	5			2		1	
Medical Genetics	3	1	1				1	1	
Neurology	53	50	31	12	7		2	1	
Nuclear Medicine	13	12	9	3		1			
Occupational Medicine	14	12	10		2	2			
Other Specialty	19	15	10	1	4	3	1		
Physical Medicine and Rehabilitation	99	98	73	14	11		1		
Psychiatry	160	151	110	19	22	3	2	3	1
Public Health and General Preventive Medicine	1					1			
Radiation Oncology	6	5	5			1			
Radiology	20	19	18		1			1	
Unspecified	480	478	322	120	36	1			1
Inactive	189								
Not Classified	743								

Note: Excludes Address Unknown.

Subspecialties in this table are condensed into major specialties. See Appendix A.

Table 3.8

Female Physicians by State, Self-Designated Specialty, and Activity, 2010, continued
Rhode Island

		Patient Care				Other Professional Activity			
				Hospital Based					
Specialty	Total Physicians	Total Patient Care	Office Based	Resid./ Fellows	Phys. Staff	Admin.	Med. Teach.	Research	Other
Total Physicians	1,601	1,264	723	404	137	15	15	25	6
FM/GP	119	117	86	26	5	2			
Family Medicine	115	113	82	26	5	2			
General Practice	4	4	4						
Medical Specialties	659	633	362	200	71	3	9	12	2
Allergy and Immunology	1	1	1						
Cardiovascular Disease	17	17	10	5	2				
Dermatology	37	36	18	16	2	1			
Gastroenterology	11	11	6	1	4				
Internal Medicine	327	316	180	103	33	1	2	8	
Pediatric Cardiology	5	5	4	1					
Pediatrics	251	238	134	74	30	1	7	3	2
Pulmonary Disease	10	9	9					1	
Surgical Specialties	208	199	117	69	13	3	2	4	
Colon and Rectal Surgery	2	2	2						
General Surgery	43	40	18	21	1	1		2	
Neurological Surgery	4	4	1	2	1				
Obstetrics & Gynecology	121	115	74	32	9	2	2	2	
Ophthalmology	11	11	7	2	2				
Orthopedic Surgery	12	12	4	8					
Otolaryngology	6	6	6						
Plastic Surgery	4	4	3	1					
Thoracic Surgery	1	1	1						
Urology	4	4	1	3					
Other Specialties	339	315	158	109	48	7	4	9	4
Anatomic/Clinical Pathology	33	26	12	6	8	2	1	2	2
Anesthesiology	33	32	25	2	5	1			
Child & Adolescent Psychiatry	20	19	10	7	2		1		
Diagnostic Radiology	34	32	18	9	5			1	1
Emergency Medicine	54	54	22	26	6				
Forensic Pathology	1								1
General Preventive Medicine	4	4	3	1					
Medical Genetics	1	1			1				
Neurology	25	23	15	8			2		
Occupational Medicine	3	3	2		1				
Other Specialty	20	17	4	13				3	
Physical Medicine and Rehabilitation	3	3			3				
Psychiatry	87	81	37	31	13	3		3	
Public Health and General Preventive Medicine	1					1			
Radiation Oncology	7	7	5	1	1				
Radiology	3	3	2		1				
Unspecified	10	10	3	5	2				
Inactive	82								
Not Classified	194								

Note: Excludes Address Unknown.

Subspecialties in this table are condensed into major specialties. See Appendix A.

Table 3.8

Female Physicians by State, Self-Designated Specialty, and Activity, 2010, continued
South Carolina

		Patient Care				Other Professional Activity			
				Hospital Based					
Specialty	Total Physicians	Total Patient Care	Office Based	Resid./ Fellows	Phys. Staff	Admin.	Med. Teach.	Research	Other
Total Physicians	3,103	2,700	1,906	537	257	23	35	22	12
FM/GP	511	495	363	101	31	6	6	2	2
Family Medicine	492	479	349	101	29	5	6	2	
General Practice	19	16	14		2	1			2
Medical Specialties	1,099	1,062	761	188	113	4	18	12	3
Allergy and Immunology	16	15	14	1			1		
Cardiovascular Disease	22	22	16	4	2				
Dermatology	50	50	44	5	1				
Gastroenterology	9	9	7	2					
Internal Medicine	482	462	325	74	63	3	7	9	1
Pediatric Cardiology	8	8	4	3	1				
Pediatrics	493	477	336	95	46	1	10	3	2
Pulmonary Disease	19	19	15	4					
Surgical Specialties	444	438	311	103	24		5		1
Colon and Rectal Surgery	1	1			1				
General Surgery	59	59	27	31	1				
Neurological Surgery	5	5	3	2					
Obstetrics & Gynecology	288	283	218	47	18		4		1
Ophthalmology	44	44	35	8	1				
Orthopedic Surgery	13	13	6	6	1				
Otolaryngology	14	13	7	5	1		1		
Plastic Surgery	11	11	10		1				
Thoracic Surgery	2	2	2						
Urology	7	7	3	4					
Other Specialties	738	705	471	145	89	13	6	8	6
Anatomic/Clinical Pathology	79	70	49	16	5	3	2	1	3
Anesthesiology	106	102	77	19	6	1	2	1	
Child & Adolescent Psychiatry	70	69	51	10	8			1	
Diagnostic Radiology	54	53	38	11	4				1
Emergency Medicine	96	94	63	13	18	2			
Forensic Pathology	4	4	2	1	1				
General Preventive Medicine	6	6	3	2	1				
Medical Genetics	2	2	1	1					
Neurology	29	27	18	7	2		1	1	
Nuclear Medicine	4	4	3		1				
Occupational Medicine	4	4	2		2				
Other Specialty	14	12	5	6	1			2	
Physical Medicine and Rehabilitation	21	21	17	1	3				
Psychiatry	194	187	107	45	35	2	1	2	2
Public Health and General Preventive Medicine	6	1	1			5			
Radiation Oncology	15	15	15						
Radiology	14	14	12	1	1				
Unspecified	20	20	7	12	1				
Inactive	140								
Not Classified	171								

Note: Excludes Address Unknown.

Subspecialties in this table are condensed into major specialties. See Appendix A.

Table 3.8

Female Physicians by State, Self-Designated Specialty, and Activity, 2010, continued
South Dakota

Specialty	Total Physicians	Patient Care: Total Patient Care	Patient Care: Office Based	Hospital Based: Resid./ Fellows	Hospital Based: Phys. Staff	Other Professional Activity: Admin.	Other Professional Activity: Med. Teach.	Other Professional Activity: Research	Other Professional Activity: Other
Total Physicians	489	432	345	38	49	3	3	1	2
FM/GP	143	139	109	18	12	1	3		
Family Medicine	139	136	106	18	12		3		
General Practice	4	3	3			1			
Medical Specialties	138	135	110	6	19	2		1	
Allergy and Immunology	1	1	1						
Cardiovascular Disease	3	3	3						
Dermatology	13	13	11		2				
Gastroenterology	3	3	3						
Internal Medicine	72	69	51	6	12	2		1	
Pediatric Cardiology	1	1			1				
Pediatrics	44	44	40		4				
Pulmonary Disease	1	1	1						
Surgical Specialties	68	68	58		10				
General Surgery	10	10	8		2				
Obstetrics & Gynecology	43	43	36		7				
Ophthalmology	6	6	6						
Orthopedic Surgery	2	2	2						
Otolaryngology	4	4	3		1				
Plastic Surgery	2	2	2						
Urology	1	1	1						
Other Specialties	92	90	68	14	8				2
Anatomic/Clinical Pathology	12	10	7	3					2
Anesthesiology	7	7	5		2				
Child & Adolescent Psychiatry	8	8	6	2					
Diagnostic Radiology	13	13	11	1	1				
Emergency Medicine	13	13	11		2				
General Preventive Medicine	1	1	1						
Medical Genetics	1	1	1						
Neurology	6	6	6						
Occupational Medicine	1	1	1						
Physical Medicine and Rehabilitation	3	3	3						
Psychiatry	17	17	11	3	3				
Radiation Oncology	3	3	3						
Radiology	1	1	1						
Unspecified	6	6	1	5					
Inactive	27								
Not Classified	21								

Note: Excludes Address Unknown.

Subspecialties in this table are condensed into major specialties. See Appendix A.

Table 3.8

Female Physicians by State, Self-Designated Specialty, and Activity, 2010, continued
Tennessee

		Patient Care				Other Professional Activity			
				Hospital Based					
Specialty	Total Physicians	Total Patient Care	Office Based	Resid./ Fellows	Phys. Staff	Admin.	Med. Teach.	Research	Other
Total Physicians	4,810	4,003	2,808	857	338	38	40	42	22
FM/GP	539	521	425	65	31	6	9	3	
Family Medicine	522	504	411	65	28	6	9	3	
General Practice	17	17	14		3				
Medical Specialties	1,948	1,877	1,314	410	153	16	21	31	3
Allergy and Immunology	21	21	13	8					
Cardiovascular Disease	34	33	27	5	1			1	
Dermatology	77	77	57	16	4				
Gastroenterology	22	22	12	7	3				
Internal Medicine	886	852	593	176	83	7	12	12	3
Pediatric Cardiology	17	16	9	6	1			1	
Pediatrics	848	815	570	186	59	8	9	16	
Pulmonary Disease	43	41	33	6	2	1		1	
Surgical Specialties	679	673	459	185	29	2	2	2	
Colon and Rectal Surgery	4	4	4						
General Surgery	135	135	53	77	5				
Neurological Surgery	5	5	3	2					
Obstetrics & Gynecology	401	396	304	77	15	1	2	2	
Ophthalmology	63	63	51	10	2				
Orthopedic Surgery	18	18	10	6	2				
Otolaryngology	17	17	10	6	1				
Plastic Surgery	16	16	13	2	1				
Thoracic Surgery	7	6	3		3	1			
Urology	13	13	8	5					
Other Specialties	979	932	610	197	125	14	8	6	19
Anatomic/Clinical Pathology	136	118	80	28	10	2	2	2	12
Anesthesiology	149	148	95	32	21	1			
Child & Adolescent Psychiatry	37	34	24	7	3	1	2		
Diagnostic Radiology	104	103	70	21	12				1
Emergency Medicine	112	110	72	17	21		1		1
Forensic Pathology	8	7	6		1				1
General Preventive Medicine	13	11	5	4	2	1	1		
Medical Genetics	5	5	3		2				
Neurology	72	70	51	15	4		1	1	
Nuclear Medicine	7	7	4	3					
Occupational Medicine	8	6	5		1	2			
Other Specialty	21	17	10	5	2	1		2	1
Physical Medicine and Rehabilitation	27	26	20	1	5				1
Psychiatry	185	183	125	28	30	1	1		
Public Health and General Preventive Medicine	9	3	3			5		1	
Radiation Oncology	12	12	7	1	4				
Radiology	33	33	24	3	6				
Unspecified	41	39	6	32	1				2
Inactive	259								
Not Classified	406								

Note: Excludes Address Unknown.

Subspecialties in this table are condensed into major specialties. See Appendix A.

Table 3.8

Female Physicians by State, Self-Designated Specialty, and Activity, 2010, continued
Texas

Specialty	Total Physicians	Patient Care: Total Patient Care	Patient Care: Office Based	Hospital Based: Resid./Fellows	Hospital Based: Phys. Staff	Other Professional Activity: Admin.	Other Professional Activity: Med. Teach.	Other Professional Activity: Research	Other Professional Activity: Other
Total Physicians	17,982	14,749	10,451	3,022	1,276	153	193	118	55
FM/GP	2,141	2,080	1,686	274	120	28	28	2	3
Family Medicine	2,061	2,002	1,620	274	108	26	28	2	3
General Practice	80	78	66		12	2			
Medical Specialties	6,654	6,438	4,607	1,254	577	45	86	72	13
Allergy and Immunology	105	100	83	13	4			5	
Cardiovascular Disease	153	149	100	36	13		2	2	
Dermatology	332	328	230	69	29	1	3		
Gastroenterology	106	102	77	19	6	1	1	2	
Internal Medicine	2,899	2,790	1,991	519	280	22	43	38	6
Pediatric Cardiology	51	51	30	11	10				
Pediatrics	2,917	2,832	2,041	569	222	20	36	23	6
Pulmonary Disease	91	86	55	18	13	1	1	2	1
Surgical Specialties	2,508	2,458	1,699	646	113	16	26	6	2
Colon and Rectal Surgery	14	14	13		1				
General Surgery	415	408	198	186	24		6	1	
Neurological Surgery	20	20	13	6	1				
Obstetrics & Gynecology	1,471	1,442	1,085	306	51	7	17	4	1
Ophthalmology	246	238	184	40	14	3	3	1	1
Orthopedic Surgery	84	83	41	33	9	1			
Otolaryngology	113	110	76	31	3	3			
Plastic Surgery	75	74	47	21	6	1			
Thoracic Surgery	8	8	4	2	2				
Urology	62	61	38	21	2	1			
Other Specialties	3,965	3,773	2,459	848	466	64	53	38	37
Aerospace Medicine	7	4	3		1	2			1
Anatomic/Clinical Pathology	540	492	294	127	71	8	16	7	17
Anesthesiology	782	767	535	159	73	3	11	1	
Child & Adolescent Psychiatry	228	214	156	35	23	8	4		2
Diagnostic Radiology	350	346	230	74	42		2	1	1
Emergency Medicine	373	362	250	63	49	3	5	1	2
Forensic Pathology	17	13	10	2	1	1			3
General Preventive Medicine	27	24	17	4	3	2		1	
Medical Genetics	23	20	13	2	5	1		2	
Neurology	271	260	165	76	19	2	3	6	
Nuclear Medicine	18	16	9	2	5			2	
Occupational Medicine	22	15	14		1	6	1		
Other Specialty	57	48	28	17	3	2	1	3	3
Physical Medicine and Rehabilitation	199	195	148	22	25	3		1	
Psychiatry	700	669	429	140	100	14	3	8	6
Public Health and General Preventive Medicine	14	4	3		1	7	1	2	
Radiation Oncology	84	83	48	19	16		1		
Radiology	97	91	65	7	19		3	2	1
Transplant Surgery	2	1	1				1		
Unspecified	154	149	41	99	9	2	1	1	1
Inactive	851								
Not Classified	1,863								

Note: Excludes Address Unknown.

Subspecialties in this table are condensed into major specialties. See Appendix A.

Table 3.8

Female Physicians by State, Self-Designated Specialty, and Activity, 2010, continued
Utah

		Patient Care				Other Professional Activity			
				Hospital Based					
Specialty	Total Physicians	Total Patient Care	Office Based	Resid./ Fellows	Phys. Staff	Admin.	Med. Teach.	Research	Other
Total Physicians	1,504	1,238	825	303	110	13	15	19	8
FM/GP	162	158	126	22	10	2	2		
Family Medicine	159	156	125	22	9	1	2		
General Practice	3	2	1		1	1			
Medical Specialties	554	529	356	133	40	4	4	15	2
Allergy and Immunology	3	3	3						
Cardiovascular Disease	10	9	6	2	1		1		
Dermatology	25	21	14	6	1		1	3	
Gastroenterology	12	12	8	4					
Internal Medicine	200	192	130	43	19	2	1	5	
Pediatric Cardiology	5	5	3	1	1				
Pediatrics	284	274	183	73	18	2	1	5	2
Pulmonary Disease	15	13	9	4				2	
Surgical Specialties	213	208	136	59	13	3		1	1
Colon and Rectal Surgery	2	2	2						
General Surgery	47	46	22	19	5	1			
Neurological Surgery	6	6	2	4					
Obstetrics & Gynecology	109	107	82	19	6	1			1
Ophthalmology	15	14	10	4				1	
Orthopedic Surgery	12	12	5	6	1				
Otolaryngology	2	2	1	1					
Plastic Surgery	12	11	8	2	1	1			
Thoracic Surgery	1	1	1						
Urology	7	7	3	4					
Other Specialties	364	343	207	89	47	4	9	3	5
Aerospace Medicine	1	1	1						
Anatomic/Clinical Pathology	37	33	17	13	3		2		2
Anesthesiology	45	41	28	12	1		3		1
Child & Adolescent Psychiatry	19	18	16	1	1	1			
Diagnostic Radiology	25	23	13	8	2		1		1
Emergency Medicine	64	63	40	8	15		1		
General Preventive Medicine	12	12	6	5	1				
Medical Genetics	5	5	1	2	2				
Neurology	43	41	28	9	4			2	
Nuclear Medicine	1	1	1						
Occupational Medicine	4	4	4						
Other Specialty	8	8	2	6					
Physical Medicine and Rehabilitation	15	15	9	4	2				
Psychiatry	56	56	31	11	14				
Public Health and General Preventive Medicine	4					3		1	
Radiation Oncology	10	10	6	3	1				
Radiology	6	4	3	1			2		
Unspecified	9	8	1	6	1				1
Inactive	71								
Not Classified	140								

Note: Excludes Address Unknown.

Subspecialties in this table are condensed into major specialties. See Appendix A.

Table 3.8

Female Physicians by State, Self-Designated Specialty, and Activity, 2010, continued
Vermont

		Patient Care				Other Professional Activity			
				Hospital Based					
Specialty	Total Physicians	Total Patient Care	Office Based	Resid./ Fellows	Phys. Staff	Admin.	Med. Teach.	Research	Other
Total Physicians	911	747	493	146	108	9	12	10	5
FM/GP	153	151	118	17	16	1	1		
Family Medicine	151	149	116	17	16	1	1		
General Practice	2	2	2						
Medical Specialties	305	287	193	60	34	3	6	7	2
Allergy and Immunology	3	3	3						
Cardiovascular Disease	5	5	2	2	1				
Dermatology	12	12	8	4					
Gastroenterology	2	2	1		1				
Internal Medicine	164	151	99	33	19	1	5	5	2
Pediatric Cardiology	1	1			1				
Pediatrics	107	104	78	17	9	2	1		
Pulmonary Disease	11	9	2	4	3			2	
Surgical Specialties	117	116	75	27	14		1		
General Surgery	23	23	10	11	2				
Neurological Surgery	2	2	1	1					
Obstetrics & Gynecology	63	62	44	11	7		1		
Ophthalmology	10	10	9		1				
Orthopedic Surgery	9	9	6	1	2				
Otolaryngology	5	5	1	3	1				
Plastic Surgery	3	3	3						
Urology	2	2	1		1				
Other Specialties	208	193	107	42	44	5	4	3	3
Anatomic/Clinical Pathology	34	31	10	16	5	2		1	
Anesthesiology	28	27	14	7	6		1		
Child & Adolescent Psychiatry	13	13	9	2	2				
Diagnostic Radiology	17	15	8	3	4	1	1		
Emergency Medicine	16	16	4		12				
Forensic Pathology	1	1	1						
General Preventive Medicine	3	2	2			1			
Medical Genetics	2	2	1		1				
Neurology	13	12	4	6	2				1
Occupational Medicine	1	1	1						
Other Specialty	5	3	3				1	1	
Physical Medicine and Rehabilitation	7	6	4	1	1	1			
Psychiatry	56	54	39	5	10			1	1
Public Health and General Preventive Medicine	1								1
Radiation Oncology	2	2	2						
Radiology	4	4	4						
Unspecified	5	4	1	2	1		1		
Inactive	60								
Not Classified	68								

Note: Excludes Address Unknown.

Subspecialties in this table are condensed into major specialties. See Appendix A.

Table 3.8

Female Physicians by State, Self-Designated Specialty, and Activity, 2010, continued
Virginia

		Patient Care				Other Professional Activity			
				Hospital Based					
Specialty	Total Physicians	Total Patient Care	Office Based	Resid./ Fellows	Phys. Staff	Admin.	Med. Teach.	Research	Other
Total Physicians	8,076	6,731	4,895	1,113	723	83	74	50	44
FM/GP	1,074	1,042	832	128	82	9	17		6
Family Medicine	1,016	987	794	128	65	9	14		6
General Practice	58	55	38		17		3		
Medical Specialties	2,968	2,858	2,126	429	303	34	29	27	20
Allergy and Immunology	55	50	41	8	1		2	1	2
Cardiovascular Disease	61	58	45	10	3			1	2
Dermatology	140	139	118	14	7				1
Gastroenterology	53	52	37	6	9		1		
Internal Medicine	1,374	1,316	948	209	159	18	14	16	10
Pediatric Cardiology	13	12	11		1			1	
Pediatrics	1,232	1,193	896	177	120	14	12	8	5
Pulmonary Disease	40	38	30	5	3	2			
Surgical Specialties	1,105	1,085	787	207	91	3	10	4	3
Colon and Rectal Surgery	7	7	3	1	3				
General Surgery	173	168	80	60	28	1	3	1	
Neurological Surgery	13	13	8	4	1				
Obstetrics & Gynecology	659	648	517	94	37	2	5	1	3
Ophthalmology	115	113	95	12	6		1	1	
Orthopedic Surgery	41	41	26	12	3				
Otolaryngology	43	43	28	11	4				
Plastic Surgery	30	29	18	6	5		1		
Thoracic Surgery	5	5	3	1	1				
Urology	19	18	9	6	3			1	
Other Specialties	1,835	1,746	1,150	349	247	37	18	19	15
Aerospace Medicine	2	1	1			1			
Anatomic/Clinical Pathology	171	156	98	37	21	3	5	2	5
Anesthesiology	257	254	168	39	47		3		
Child & Adolescent Psychiatry	88	85	66	9	10	2	1		
Diagnostic Radiology	166	163	123	21	19		1	1	1
Emergency Medicine	276	274	177	50	47	2			
Forensic Pathology	7	6	4	1	1	1			
General Preventive Medicine	24	16	15		1	2	2	3	1
Medical Genetics	9	9	4	1	4				
Neurology	112	106	75	26	5	1		4	1
Nuclear Medicine	7	6	6					1	
Occupational Medicine	10	4	2		2	4	1		1
Other Specialty	47	41	27	13	1	1		4	1
Physical Medicine and Rehabilitation	92	88	62	18	8	3		1	
Psychiatry	394	379	255	63	61	7	4	2	2
Public Health and General Preventive Medicine	17	5	3		2	10		1	1
Radiation Oncology	26	26	19	4	3				
Radiology	36	35	24	3	8		1		
Unspecified	94	92	21	64	7				2
Inactive	554								
Not Classified	540								

Note: Excludes Address Unknown.

Subspecialties in this table are condensed into major specialties. See Appendix A.

Table 3.8

Female Physicians by State, Self-Designated Specialty, and Activity, 2010, continued
Virgin Islands

		Patient Care				Other Professional Activity			
				Hospital Based					
Specialty	Total Physicians	Total Patient Care	Office Based	Resid./ Fellows	Phys. Staff	Admin.	Med. Teach.	Research	Other
Total Physicians	70	55	44		11				
FM/GP	8	8	7		1				
Family Medicine	8	8	7		1				
Medical Specialties	24	24	19		5				
Allergy and Immunology	1	1	1						
Dermatology	1	1	1						
Internal Medicine	13	13	12		1				
Pediatrics	9	9	5		4				
Surgical Specialties	14	14	13		1				
General Surgery	2	2	2						
Obstetrics & Gynecology	10	10	9		1				
Ophthalmology	1	1	1						
Orthopedic Surgery	1	1	1						
Other Specialties	9	9	5		4				
Anesthesiology	2	2	1		1				
Diagnostic Radiology	1	1	1						
Emergency Medicine	3	3	1		2				
General Preventive Medicine	1	1	1						
Psychiatry	1	1			1				
Unspecified	1	1	1						
Inactive	7								
Not Classified	8								

Note: Excludes Address Unknown.

Subspecialties in this table are condensed into major specialties. See Appendix A.

Table 3.8

Female Physicians by State, Self-Designated Specialty, and Activity, 2010, continued
Washington

		Patient Care				Other Professional Activity			
				Hospital Based					
Specialty	Total Physicians	Total Patient Care	Office Based	Resid./ Fellows	Phys. Staff	Admin.	Med. Teach.	Research	Other
Total Physicians	6,588	5,411	4,170	786	455	57	56	86	36
FM/GP	1,251	1,214	1,016	134	64	9	18	5	5
Family Medicine	1,216	1,181	988	134	59	7	18	5	5
General Practice	35	33	28		5	2			
Medical Specialties	2,202	2,100	1,611	292	197	19	19	55	9
Allergy and Immunology	19	17	14	1	2	1		1	
Cardiovascular Disease	34	32	25	5	2			2	
Dermatology	108	107	97	6	4	1			
Gastroenterology	46	44	37	6	1			2	
Internal Medicine	1,182	1,125	859	152	114	13	11	28	5
Pediatric Cardiology	7	7	5	1	1				
Pediatrics	766	730	548	112	70	4	8	20	4
Pulmonary Disease	40	38	26	9	3			2	
Surgical Specialties	805	795	605	131	59	1	3	5	1
Colon and Rectal Surgery	3	3	2		1				
General Surgery	177	175	100	63	12		1	1	
Neurological Surgery	12	12	7	4	1				
Obstetrics & Gynecology	396	389	332	28	29	1	2	3	1
Ophthalmology	73	73	64	5	4				
Orthopedic Surgery	42	42	27	11	4				
Otolaryngology	43	43	28	10	5				
Plastic Surgery	29	29	27	2					
Thoracic Surgery	6	5	3	2				1	
Urology	24	24	15	6	3				
Other Specialties	1,388	1,302	938	229	135	28	16	21	21
Aerospace Medicine	1	1	1						
Anatomic/Clinical Pathology	124	114	78	27	9	2	2	2	4
Anesthesiology	266	257	194	45	18	3	5	1	
Child & Adolescent Psychiatry	53	49	34	9	6	1	1	1	1
Diagnostic Radiology	137	133	98	19	16		2		2
Emergency Medicine	160	156	118	12	26	2	1	1	
Forensic Pathology	3	1	1						2
General Preventive Medicine	26	23	22		1	1	1	1	
Medical Genetics	8	5	5					2	1
Neurology	96	92	63	24	5			1	3
Nuclear Medicine	9	8	4	4				1	
Occupational Medicine	16	13	10		3	2			1
Other Specialty	28	17	15	2		6		2	3
Physical Medicine and Rehabilitation	68	65	43	12	10	1	1		1
Psychiatry	272	259	183	48	28	4	2	5	2
Public Health and General Preventive Medicine	12	3	3			5	1	3	
Radiation Oncology	21	21	14	4	3				
Radiology	37	36	29	5	2			1	
Transplant Surgery	1	1	1						
Unspecified	50	48	22	18	8	1			1
Inactive	466								
Not Classified	476								

Note: Excludes Address Unknown.

Subspecialties in this table are condensed into major specialties. See Appendix A.

Table 3.8

Female Physicians by State, Self-Designated Specialty, and Activity, 2010, continued
West Virginia

		Patient Care				Other Professional Activity			
				Hospital Based					
Specialty	Total Physicians	Total Patient Care	Office Based	Resid./ Fellows	Phys. Staff	Admin.	Med. Teach.	Research	Other
Total Physicians	1,189	940	637	201	102	12	19	5	8
FM/GP	212	202	149	38	15	3	6		1
Family Medicine	204	194	143	38	13	3	6		1
General Practice	8	8	6		2				
Medical Specialties	384	367	257	71	39	2	11	3	1
Allergy and Immunology	3	3	3						
Cardiovascular Disease	7	7	5	2					
Dermatology	14	13	10	2	1		1		
Gastroenterology	5	5	4	1					
Internal Medicine	178	169	108	32	29	1	6	1	1
Pediatric Cardiology	1	1	1						
Pediatrics	166	160	119	32	9	1	3	2	
Pulmonary Disease	10	9	7	2			1		
Surgical Specialties	136	135	86	39	10				1
General Surgery	33	33	19	12	2				
Neurological Surgery	1	1		1					
Obstetrics & Gynecology	74	74	49	20	5				
Ophthalmology	14	13	9	2	2				1
Orthopedic Surgery	4	4	2	1	1				
Otolaryngology	3	3	1	2					
Plastic Surgery	3	3	3						
Thoracic Surgery	2	2	2						
Urology	2	2	1	1					
Other Specialties	252	236	145	53	38	7	2	2	5
Aerospace Medicine	1	1			1				
Anatomic/Clinical Pathology	48	42	24	5	13	3			3
Anesthesiology	22	22	16	4	2				
Child & Adolescent Psychiatry	17	16	11	3	2	1			
Diagnostic Radiology	27	27	18	6	3				
Emergency Medicine	31	29	17	5	7		1	1	
General Preventive Medicine	6	6	2	3	1				
Medical Genetics	1	1	1						
Neurology	21	20	13	7			1		
Occupational Medicine	3	2	2					1	
Other Specialty	8	6	3	3		2			
Physical Medicine and Rehabilitation	6	6	6						
Psychiatry	47	47	26	14	7				
Public Health and General Preventive Medicine	2					1			1
Radiology	4	3	2		1				1
Unspecified	8	8	4	3	1				
Inactive	79								
Not Classified	126								

Note: Excludes Address Unknown.

Subspecialties in this table are condensed into major specialties. See Appendix A.

Table 3.8

Female Physicians by State, Self-Designated Specialty, and Activity, 2010, continued
Wisconsin

		Patient Care				Other Professional Activity			
				Hospital Based					
Specialty	Total Physicians	Total Patient Care	Office Based	Resid./ Fellows	Phys. Staff	Admin.	Med. Teach.	Research	Other
Total Physicians	4,942	4,220	3,065	794	361	35	60	42	17
FM/GP	925	901	748	101	52	5	14	2	3
Family Medicine	911	888	739	101	48	5	14	2	2
General Practice	14	13	9		4				1
Medical Specialties	1,709	1,640	1,177	333	130	20	22	24	3
Allergy and Immunology	29	28	21	6	1			1	
Cardiovascular Disease	48	46	38	8				2	
Dermatology	93	93	67	20	6				
Gastroenterology	22	22	15	5	2				
Internal Medicine	802	765	543	150	72	11	9	14	3
Pediatric Cardiology	16	16	7	6	3				
Pediatrics	675	648	473	133	42	9	12	6	
Pulmonary Disease	24	22	13	5	4		1	1	
Surgical Specialties	654	645	465	145	35		5	4	
Colon and Rectal Surgery	3	3	3						
General Surgery	136	134	67	60	7			2	
Neurological Surgery	10	10	7	3					
Obstetrics & Gynecology	353	348	280	49	19		4	1	
Ophthalmology	67	66	54	7	5			1	
Orthopedic Surgery	19	19	13	4	2				
Otolaryngology	27	26	20	5	1		1		
Plastic Surgery	15	15	5	9	1				
Thoracic Surgery	4	4	4						
Urology	20	20	12	8					
Other Specialties	1,086	1,034	675	215	144	10	19	12	11
Anatomic/Clinical Pathology	118	105	71	18	16	4	2	1	6
Anesthesiology	199	189	113	37	39	1	7	2	
Child & Adolescent Psychiatry	50	50	41	6	3				
Diagnostic Radiology	106	106	62	31	13				
Emergency Medicine	106	105	71	15	19	1			
Forensic Pathology	4	3	3			1			
General Preventive Medicine	4	3	3						1
Medical Genetics	5	4	3	1			1		
Neurology	76	75	54	15	6			1	
Nuclear Medicine	10	10	6	4					
Occupational Medicine	11	10	8		2		1		
Other Specialty	25	20	8	9	3		1	4	
Physical Medicine and Rehabilitation	73	71	47	11	13				2
Psychiatry	214	203	148	32	23	2	5	4	
Public Health and General Preventive Medicine	3	1			1	1			1
Radiation Oncology	21	21	15	5	1				
Radiology	25	23	17	4	2		2		
Unspecified	36	35	5	27	3				1
Inactive	283								
Not Classified	285								

Note: Excludes Address Unknown.

Subspecialties in this table are condensed into major specialties. See Appendix A.

Table 3.8

Female Physicians by State, Self-Designated Specialty, and Activity, 2010, continued
Wyoming

		Patient Care				Other Professional Activity			
				Hospital Based					
Specialty	Total Physicians	Total Patient Care	Office Based	Resid./ Fellows	Phys. Staff	Admin.	Med. Teach.	Research	Other
Total Physicians	277	243	201	17	25	2	2	1	1
FM/GP	87	85	65	13	7		2		
Family Medicine	84	83	63	13	7		1		
General Practice	3	2	2				1		
Medical Specialties	73	73	60	3	10				
Allergy and Immunology	1	1	1						
Dermatology	5	5	5						
Gastroenterology	1	1			1				
Internal Medicine	38	38	30	3	5				
Pediatrics	27	27	23		4				
Pulmonary Disease	1	1	1						
Surgical Specialties	39	38	37		1	1			
General Surgery	6	6	6						
Obstetrics & Gynecology	27	26	25		1	1			
Ophthalmology	3	3	3						
Orthopedic Surgery	2	2	2						
Otolaryngology	1	1	1						
Other Specialties	50	47	39	1	7	1		1	1
Anatomic/Clinical Pathology	7	5	4		1			1	1
Anesthesiology	6	6	5		1				
Child & Adolescent Psychiatry	3	3	3						
Diagnostic Radiology	2	2	2						
Emergency Medicine	6	6	5		1				
Neurology	1	1	1						
Other Specialty	2	2	2						
Physical Medicine and Rehabilitation	4	4	4						
Psychiatry	17	16	12		4	1			
Radiology	1	1	1						
Unspecified	1	1		1					
Inactive	20								
Not Classified	8								

Note: Excludes Address Unknown.

Subspecialties in this table are condensed into major specialties. See Appendix A.

Table 3.8

Female Physicians by State, Self-Designated Specialty, and Activity, 2010, continued
Pacific Islands

		Patient Care				Other Professional Activity			
				Hospital Based					
Specialty	Total Physicians	Total Patient Care	Office Based	Resid./ Fellows	Phys. Staff	Admin.	Med. Teach.	Research	Other
Total Physicians	63	51	39	1	11				1
FM/GP	12	12	11		1				
Family Medicine	11	11	10		1				
General Practice	1	1	1						
Medical Specialties	21	21	18		3				
Internal Medicine	8	8	7		1				
Pediatrics	13	13	11		2				
Surgical Specialties	5	5	4		1				
Obstetrics & Gynecology	5	5	4		1				
Other Specialties	14	13	6	1	6				1
Anesthesiology	3	3			3				
Emergency Medicine	3	3	2		1				
General Preventive Medicine	1	1		1					
Psychiatry	5	5	3		2				
Public Health and General Preventive Medicine	1								1
Radiation Oncology	1	1	1						
Inactive	4								
Not Classified	7								

Note: Excludes Address Unknown.

Subspecialties in this table are condensed into major specialties. See Appendix A.

Table 3.9

Physicians by State and County, 2010

		Major Professional Activity									
		Patient Care									
			Office-Based Practice								
State / County	Total Physicians	Total Patient Care	FM/GP Practice	Medical Specialties	Surgical Specialties	Other Specialties	Hospital Based Practice	Other Professional Activity	Inactive	Not Classified
Alabama	11,613	9,377	1,113	2,665	1,884	1,662	2,053	368	1,302	566
Autauga	39	34	13	7	1	6	7	1	3	1
Baldwin	461	352	71	94	65	79	43	10	85	14
Barbour	15	13	6	4	3				2	
Bibb	6	6	4				2			
Blount	21	17	9	5		2	1		4	
Bullock	10	7	1	5	1				2	1
Butler	19	16		6	6		4		3	
Calhoun	224	190	31	65	54	27	13	3	23	8
Chambers	29	24	3	11	6	2	2		2	3
Cherokee	11	9	5	1	1	1	1		2	
Chilton	16	12	5	4	1	1	1		4	
Choctaw	7	5	5						2	
Clarke	16	16	11	2	1		2			
Clay	10	9	5	1	1		2		1	
Cleburne	2	2	1	1						
Coffee	53	46	3	11	17	8	7	1	6	
Colbert	96	79	12	27	19	16	5	2	13	2
Conecuh	8	6	4			1	1		2	
Coosa	1	1	1							
Covington	46	36	12	11	9	4			9	1
Crenshaw	7	5	1	1	1	1	1		2	
Cullman	114	103	22	32	29	16	4		9	2
Dale	41	28	9	7	3	3	6	3	9	1
Dallas	80	58	10	17	13	6	12	1	18	3
De Kalb	57	44	13	10	10	4	7	1	11	1
Elmore	50	38	12	9	4	7	6	2	10	
Escambia	34	26	12	4	3	4	3		8	
Etowah	225	188	33	61	46	38	10	2	30	5
Fayette	12	9	6	1	1		1		3	
Franklin	33	25	10	4	6	3	2	1	7	
Geneva	12	9	6		2		1	2	1	
Greene	6	5	1	1		1	2		1	
Hale	5	4	1			3			1	
Henry	8	6	1	2	1	2			2	
Houston	378	322	25	100	90	83	24	3	46	7
Jackson	54	47	19	7	10	6	5		6	1
Jefferson	4,122	3,200	139	846	540	550	1,125	195	386	341
Lamar	3	3	3							
Lauderdale	181	150	15	57	41	32	5	2	25	4
Lawrence	12	11	3	2	3	1	2		1	
Lee	228	197	27	69	43	29	29	2	22	7
Limestone	63	43	11	12	12	3	5		15	5
Lowndes	3	2		1			1	1		
Macon	21	14	2	1	3	1	7	2	4	1
Madison	986	822	129	232	164	173	124	22	106	36
Marengo	16	14	7		2	3	2		1	1
Marion	27	24	7	7	5	2	3		3	
Marshall	107	91	30	20	18	14	9	4	11	1
Mobile	1,249	1,044	59	320	236	169	260	43	113	49
Monroe	18	11	6	3	1	1		1	6	
Montgomery	719	593	58	193	141	102	99	22	82	22
Morgan	213	179	29	53	50	33	14	2	28	4
Perry	6	4	3	1					1	1
Pickens	9	9	6		2		1			
Pike	31	26	6	10	5	2	3	1	2	2
Randolph	9	8	5			1	2		1	
Russell	31	24	12	5	3	2	2		7	
Saint Clair	36	25	11	10	2	1	1	1	9	1

Table 3.9

Physicians by State and County, 2010, continued

		Major Professional Activity									
		Patient Care									
			Office-Based Practice								
State County	Total Physicians	Total Patient Care	FM/GP Practice	Medical Specialties	Surgical Specialties	Other Specialties	Hospital Based Practice	Other Professional Activity	Inactive	Not Classified
Shelby	542	452	57	139	72	105	79	12	52	26
Sumter	7	6	3	2	1				1	
Talladega	62	49	9	18	15	6	1	1	10	2
Tallapoosa	59	47	9	12	14	5	7	2	9	1
Tuscaloosa	540	443	60	114	85	91	93	21	64	12
Walker	84	72	14	23	21	11	3	1	11	
Washington	6	3	2	1					3	
Wilcox	5	5	3	1			1			
Winston	12	9	5	2	1	1		1	2	
Alaska	1,823	1,502	310	289	275	314	314	66	206	49
Aleutians East	1								1	
Aleutians West	4	4	4							
Anchorage	1,107	895	132	191	184	190	198	51	124	37
Bethel	19	16	8	1			7	1		2
Bristol Bay	1	1				1				
Dillingham	13	13	9	1			3			
Fairbanks North Star	215	181	27	39	37	44	34	7	25	2
Haines	8	5	5						3	
Juneau	93	82	24	12	13	23	10		9	2
Kenai Peninsula	96	78	22	16	14	20	6	3	15	
Ketchikan Gateway	32	25	7	5	3	5	5		7	
Kodiak Island	29	25	14	2	2	3	4		4	
Matanuska Susitna	114	101	26	16	19	22	18	1	7	5
Nome	10	10	6			1	3			
North Slope	2	2					2			
Northwest Arctic	6	5	4				1			1
Prince Wales Ketchikan	7	6	2				4		1	
Sitka	38	31	8	6	2	3	12	3	4	
Skagway Hoonah Angoon	1								1	
Southeast Fairbanks	5	4	2			1	1		1	
Valdez Cordova	7	7	5			1	1			
Wrangell Petersburg	14	10	4		1		5		4	
Yukon Koyukuk	1	1	1							
Arizona	16,944	12,818	1,300	3,780	2,242	3,009	2,487	632	2,653	841
Apache	66	51	8	16	7	9	11	1	7	7
Cochise	136	105	19	34	20	23	9	8	17	6
Coconino	376	304	53	69	63	70	49	11	51	10
Gila	88	59	21	15	9	3	11	3	24	2
Graham	27	19	11	3	2	1	2		4	4
Greenlee	9	6	3	1		1	1		2	1
La Paz	13	10	4	5			1	1	1	1
Maricopa	10,771	8,230	743	2,518	1,473	1,933	1,563	366	1,600	575
Mohave	272	238	27	86	45	60	20	4	23	7
Navajo	119	98	33	17	14	17	17	2	16	3
Pima	4,049	2,984	265	786	471	745	717	211	667	187
Pinal	167	116	26	36	21	22	11	2	39	10
Santa Cruz	52	28	10	7	3	3	5	5	17	2
Yavapai	532	353	55	95	63	86	54	15	158	6
Yuma	267	217	22	92	51	36	16	3	27	20
Arkansas	6,771	5,397	1,025	1,193	935	943	1,301	220	863	291
Arkansas	22	17	11	2	3		1		5	
Ashley	15	15	9	1	4		1			
Baxter	109	95	16	22	28	15	14		11	3
Benton	315	253	62	70	59	36	26	4	46	12
Boone	70	60	22	11	9	10	8		9	1
Bradley	10	9	6		2		1		1	

Table 3.9

Physicians by State and County, 2010, continued

		Major Professional Activity									
		Patient Care									
			Office-Based Practice								
State County	Total Physicians	Total Patient Care	FM/GP Practice	Medical Specialties	Surgical Specialties	Other Specialties	Hospital Based Practice	Other Professional Activity	Inactive	Not Classified
Calhoun	1	1	1							
Carroll	32	23	14	1	6	1	1		8	1
Chicot	18	14	5	3	3	2	1		4	
Clark	24	22	7	6	6	1	2		2	
Clay	7	5	3	1			1		2	
Cleburne	41	26	14	1	5	2	4		14	1
Cleveland	2	1	1						1	
Columbia	26	16	9	3	3		1	1	7	2
Conway	18	15	12	1	1	1			3	
Craighead	323	275	50	75	63	56	31	11	36	1
Crawford	50	43	22	7	3	6	5		7	
Crittenden	51	41	4	21	9	2	5		9	1
Cross	15	10	6	2			2		5	
Dallas	5	5	5							
Desha	9	6	5		1				3	
Drew	11	10	6		1	1	2		1	
Faulkner	169	143	29	35	36	25	18	1	21	4
Franklin	6	5	4		1				1	
Fulton	12	9	6	2			1		3	
Garland	301	217	35	70	40	50	22	7	73	4
Grant	11	5	3			2		1	5	
Greene	45	38	16	6	8	6	2		6	1
Hempstead	18	14	3	4	4		3	1	3	
Hot Spring	12	8	5	3					3	1
Howard	10	9	6	1	1		1		1	
Independence	82	70	21	12	19	10	8		11	1
Izard	8	6	3	1		1	1		2	
Jackson	19	17	6	2	4	1	4		2	
Jefferson	174	137	39	38	27	19	14	6	23	8
Johnson	28	22	14	1	5	1	1		6	
Lafayette	3	2	2					1		
Lawrence	10	8	4	2		1	1		2	
Lee	5	3	3						2	
Little River	8	7	5			1	1		1	
Logan	13	11	5		3	1	2		2	
Lonoke	25	20	11	1	1	4	3		5	
Madison	8	4	3			1			4	
Marion	6	3	2		1				3	
Miller	54	39	9	4	3	4	19		7	8
Mississippi	34	28	10	9	5	1	3		5	1
Monroe	6	5	2	2		1			1	
Montgomery	5	1	1						4	
Nevada	3	3	3							
Newton	5	3	1	1		1			2	
Ouachita	23	19	9	5	4	1			4	
Perry	3	2	1	1					1	
Phillips	23	13	5	4	2	2			8	2
Pike	7	4	3				1		3	
Poinsett	8	5	5						2	1
Polk	26	18	5	4	2	1	6	1	7	
Pope	100	82	18	21	22	13	8	1	17	
Prairie	1								1	
Pulaski	2,879	2,268	166	463	326	455	858	153	251	207
Randolph	14	12	7	2	1		2		2	
Saint Francis	18	18	6	7	3	2				
Saline	127	110	23	25	15	16	31	1	14	2
Scott	3	2		2					1	
Searcy	8	7	3			1	3	1		
Sebastian	428	337	69	98	59	53	58	9	69	13

Table 3.9

Physicians by State and County, 2010, continued

		Major Professional Activity								
		Patient Care								
			Office-Based Practice							
State County	Total Physicians	Total Patient Care	FM/GP Practice	Medical Specialties	Surgical Specialties	Other Specialties	Hospital Based Practice	Other Professional Activity	Inactive	Not Classified
Sevier	13	10	5	3		1	1		3	
Sharp	12	10	7	2		1			2	
Stone	8	8	6		1		1			
Union	103	83	24	16	14	13	16	2	13	5
Van Buren	11	7	3	1	1	1	1	1	3	
Washington	559	464	81	93	102	97	91	17	68	10
White	117	98	25	24	17	21	11	1	17	1
Woodruff	4	3	2	1					1	
Yell	22	18	11		2	2	3		4	
California	118,110	88,369	9,295	26,818	15,007	19,376	17,873	5,121	16,904	7,716
Alameda	5,347	4,061	337	1,446	631	854	793	227	678	381
Alpine	2	1				1		1		
Amador	71	48	11	11	8	12	6	5	17	1
Butte	549	425	71	113	93	94	54	8	105	11
Calaveras	58	39	12	5	8	9	5	3	15	1
Colusa	13	10	4	1	2	1	2		3	
Contra Costa	3,460	2,578	257	939	449	602	331	117	553	212
Del Norte	49	38	8	9	7	10	4		9	2
El Dorado	408	332	65	73	52	101	41	8	52	16
Fresno	2,097	1,661	210	486	300	351	314	68	248	120
Glenn	10	6	2	2	1		1		4	
Humboldt	331	254	57	48	50	70	29	9	64	4
Imperial	161	132	13	50	30	20	19	5	19	5
Inyo	50	34	11	7	6	4	6	1	15	
Kern	1,259	1,038	159	340	173	192	174	30	140	51
Kings	157	128	31	29	19	21	28	3	16	10
Lake	93	76	18	23	13	15	7	1	16	
Lassen	39	28	13	5	6	2	2	2	8	1
Los Angeles	32,420	24,300	2,176	7,520	4,183	5,297	5,124	1,470	4,266	2,384
Madera	190	162	19	64	26	17	36	2	21	5
Marin	1,896	1,256	86	382	206	403	179	119	458	63
Mariposa	12	7	3			2	2		5	
Mendocino	236	168	41	48	32	30	17	9	57	2
Merced	285	239	74	54	39	26	46	6	27	13
Modoc	6	3	2	1					3	
Mono	32	27	2	2	4	10	9		5	
Monterey	1,019	745	134	209	151	154	97	33	222	19
Napa	569	403	45	107	68	120	63	15	144	7
Nevada	288	208	34	50	39	62	23	9	65	6
Orange	10,889	8,327	972	2,661	1,541	1,877	1,276	344	1,654	564
Placer	1,233	959	148	305	170	217	119	24	203	47
Plumas	35	24	12	1	2	3	6		11	
Riverside	3,189	2,307	344	733	469	484	277	83	682	117
Sacramento	4,652	3,597	353	1,005	597	763	879	211	542	302
San Benito	51	41	11	10	9	10	1		8	2
San Bernardino	4,112	3,230	412	859	491	586	882	124	462	296
San Diego	11,602	8,472	848	2,338	1,364	1,936	1,986	656	1,819	655
San Francisco	7,175	5,058	214	1,344	677	1,106	1,717	534	654	929
San Joaquin	1,237	1,014	152	312	195	191	164	25	130	68
San Luis Obispo	930	685	83	156	116	224	106	28	194	23
San Mateo	3,546	2,485	109	824	431	561	560	213	551	297
Santa Barbara	1,431	1,016	119	319	180	261	137	36	346	33
Santa Clara	7,945	5,896	392	1,946	947	1,170	1,441	412	901	736
Santa Cruz	838	633	123	162	100	169	79	28	161	16
Shasta	502	395	79	96	74	105	41	13	85	9
Sierra	1	1	1							
Siskiyou	94	65	19	11	17	11	7	3	25	1
Solano	964	786	103	233	124	156	170	29	99	50
Sonoma	1,573	1,130	239	288	208	266	129	45	355	43

Table 3.9

Physicians by State and County, 2010, continued

		Major Professional Activity								
		Patient Care								
			Office-Based Practice							
State County	Total Physicians	Total Patient Care	FM/GP Practice	Medical Specialties	Surgical Specialties	Other Specialties	Hospital Based Practice	Other Professional Activity	Inactive	Not Classified
Stanislaus	999	807	148	265	149	162	83	20	126	46
Sutter	208	171	34	60	31	32	14	3	28	6
Tehama	62	48	10	12	14	9	3	1	12	1
Trinity	12	6	4		1		1		6	
Tulare	538	441	72	152	85	86	46	6	80	11
Tuolumne	140	109	18	33	16	25	17	2	27	2
Ventura	2,166	1,599	269	489	313	327	201	86	383	98
Yolo	822	613	101	165	83	152	112	44	115	50
Yuba	57	47	11	15	7	7	7		10	
Colorado	15,595	11,932	1,579	3,177	2,125	2,811	2,240	688	2,270	705
Adams	1,026	766	67	224	102	114	259	115	55	90
Alamosa	40	32	8	5	5	8	6	2	6	
Arapahoe	1,940	1,497	143	490	253	364	247	86	280	77
Archuleta	22	12	7	3			2	1	9	
Baca	4	2	1	1					2	
Bent	3								3	
Boulder	1,263	1,007	171	268	204	261	103	44	181	31
Broomfield	104	82	18	26	17	14	7	4	13	5
Chaffee	49	36	16	6	3	6	5		13	
Cheyenne	2	2	1				1			
Clear Creek	3	2		1		1			1	
Conejos	8	6	3			1	2		1	1
Costilla	1								1	
Crowley	2	2	1				1			
Custer	6	2	2						4	
Delta	55	39	15	6	3	6	9		14	2
Denver	3,940	2,984	178	792	448	712	854	219	424	313
Dolores	2	2	1				1			
Douglas	655	504	58	160	121	103	62	26	108	17
Eagle	190	134	18	25	37	31	23	9	43	4
El Paso	1,540	1,222	132	304	252	326	208	47	231	40
Elbert	2	1					1		1	
Fremont	46	34	14	6	5	6	3	1	10	1
Garfield	128	96	22	18	25	21	10	2	27	3
Gilpin	4	3	1		1	1			1	
Grand	23	17	9	2	2	1	3		6	
Gunnison	29	19	7		8	3	1		10	
Hinsdale	5	2		1			1		3	
Huerfano	10	5	3	1		1			5	
Jackson	2	1	1						1	
Jefferson	1,419	1,068	182	339	167	272	108	55	249	47
Kiowa	3	2	1				1		1	
Kit Carson	6	6	6							
La Plata	261	189	31	41	43	56	18	7	59	6
Lake	3	2	2						1	
Larimer	839	657	138	153	131	154	81	22	137	23
Las Animas	21	16	4	1	4	3	4		4	1
Lincoln	3	3	2				1			
Logan	23	20	7	2	6	2	3		2	1
Mesa	461	354	66	70	70	89	59	16	75	16
Mineral	2	1					1	1		
Moffat	13	9	3	1	2	2	1		4	
Montezuma	48	37	14	6	5	6	6	2	8	1
Montrose	103	79	12	18	20	24	5		20	4
Morgan	28	25	11	1	6	1	6		3	
Otero	27	18	8	5	1	1	3	1	8	
Ouray	23	18	5	3	1	9			4	1
Park	8	5	2	2		1			3	

Table 3.9

Physicians by State and County, 2010, continued

			Major Professional Activity							
			Patient Care							
			Office-Based Practice							
State County	Total Physicians	Total Patient Care	FM/GP Practice	Medical Specialties	Surgical Specialties	Other Specialties	Hospital Based Practice	Other Professional Activity	Inactive	Not Classified
Phillips	4	3	3							1
Pitkin	75	53	4	14	13	17	5	2	17	3
Prowers	13	9	3		1		5		3	1
Pueblo	440	355	57	88	64	91	55	9	70	6
Rio Blanco	8	5	2				3	1	2	
Rio Grande	11	8	4	1	1	1	1		3	
Routt	100	70	12	14	23	17	4	1	27	2
Saguache	7	6	2	1	1	1	1		1	
San Juan	1							1		
San Miguel	18	15	5	3		6	1		3	
Sedgwick	4	4	2				2			
Summit	108	67	17	10	15	22	3	2	37	2
Teller	32	24	8	4	3	7	2	3	5	
Weld	370	287	65	61	61	49	51	9	68	6
Yuma	9	6	4		1		1		3	
Connecticut	15,270	11,447	487	3,668	1,911	2,210	3,171	851	1,891	1,081
Fairfield	3,962	3,000	103	1,086	582	626	603	172	563	227
Hartford	4,011	3,077	129	963	533	596	856	231	453	250
Litchfield	458	325	28	116	64	68	49	21	102	10
Middlesex	548	401	44	116	66	83	92	30	90	27
New Haven	5,121	3,769	80	1,072	512	697	1,408	349	468	535
New London	756	548	45	203	101	94	105	38	149	21
Tolland	249	190	35	67	24	30	34	7	42	10
Windham	165	137	23	45	29	16	24	3	24	1
Delaware	2,550	1,988	196	587	336	393	476	96	329	137
Kent	269	217	28	75	41	51	22	8	33	11
New Castle	1,889	1,471	124	410	239	277	421	75	228	115
Sussex	392	300	44	102	56	65	33	13	68	11
District Of Columbia	5,776	4,115	131	898	462	628	1,996	494	501	666
District Of Columbia	5,776	4,115	131	898	462	628	1,996	494	501	666
Florida	58,026	42,785	4,201	13,825	7,933	8,923	7,903	1,829	10,775	2,637
Alachua	2,418	1,820	114	370	197	308	831	162	215	221
Baker	16	15	6	1		3	5		1	
Bay	404	323	31	97	77	80	38	9	55	17
Bradford	19	15	6	4		3	2	1	3	
Brevard	1,418	1,123	133	388	212	265	125	31	232	32
Broward	5,231	3,977	284	1,457	782	901	553	137	864	253
Calhoun	8	8	4	2		1	1			
Charlotte	429	304	26	123	62	68	25	5	110	10
Citrus	329	222	23	86	38	51	24	3	98	6
Clay	383	294	61	85	46	47	55	12	67	10
Collier	1,333	747	54	272	169	181	71	36	531	19
Columbia	125	96	15	30	14	15	22	1	25	3
De Soto	32	21	4	8	3	1	5		9	2
Dixie	4	3	2				1	1		
Duval	3,368	2,702	274	729	449	513	737	111	368	187
Escambia	1,011	797	88	200	154	158	197	39	139	36
Flagler	170	96	20	25	16	18	17	3	68	3
Franklin	10	6	1	2	2	1		1	2	1
Gadsden	41	25	8			6	11	5	11	
Gilchrist	4	4	2	1			1			
Glades	3	1				1			2	
Gulf	18	13	6	1	1	1	4		5	
Hamilton	2	2	1	1						
Hardee	12	10	2	5	2		1		2	
Hendry	21	13	3	4	2	1	3		8	
Hernando	285	232	24	105	47	37	19	5	40	8
Highlands	207	151	16	60	35	26	14	4	41	11

Table 3.9

Physicians by State and County, 2010, continued

		Major Professional Activity								
		Patient Care								
			Office-Based Practice							
State County	Total Physicians	Total Patient Care	FM/GP Practice	Medical Specialties	Surgical Specialties	Other Specialties	Hospital Based Practice	Other Professional Activity	Inactive	Not Classified
Hillsborough	4,604	3,631	241	1,065	613	792	920	180	526	267
Holmes	11	9	4	4	1				2	
Indian River	469	326	28	113	74	83	28	13	124	6
Jackson	53	41	10	12	6	1	12	1	10	1
Jefferson	8	5	2	1	1	1			3	
Lafayette	4	1	1						3	
Lake	666	482	54	185	100	103	40	12	153	19
Lee	1,643	1,086	101	384	262	252	87	40	502	15
Leon	854	626	115	153	118	126	114	55	142	31
Levy	24	15	4	3		6	2	1	8	
Madison	7	4	3			1			3	
Manatee	914	588	62	211	131	131	53	20	293	13
Marion	633	507	58	198	102	113	36	4	107	15
Martin	513	361	33	113	87	88	40	10	138	4
Miami-Dade	10,136	7,235	682	2,272	1,174	1,360	1,747	377	1,690	834
Monroe	247	152	17	37	42	38	18	8	81	6
Nassau	124	64	14	16	11	12	11	6	53	1
Okaloosa	552	452	62	93	97	84	116	10	70	20
Okeechobee	44	42	6	20	9	4	3		2	
Orange	3,422	2,785	277	873	485	595	555	99	378	160
Osceola	328	271	48	105	59	33	26	5	35	17
Palm Beach	4,950	3,390	197	1,299	762	752	380	145	1,281	134
Pasco	738	584	80	230	98	114	62	23	104	27
Pinellas	3,229	2,393	241	824	441	526	361	98	657	81
Polk	1,070	792	89	294	175	154	80	19	219	40
Putnam	84	61	9	18	16	12	6		21	2
Saint Johns	700	510	59	173	82	130	66	29	134	27
Saint Lucie	388	279	39	89	74	61	16	6	90	13
Santa Rosa	337	275	47	73	44	68	43	8	41	13
Sarasota	1,618	1,030	108	372	244	232	74	31	540	17
Seminole	898	735	114	256	125	154	86	24	116	23
Sumter	125	48	5	17	6	14	6	4	71	2
Suwannee	22	16	6	3		2	5	1	5	
Taylor	15	13	1	6	3	1	2		2	
Union	12	10	3		1	3	3		1	1
Volusia	1,150	866	151	245	170	175	125	31	229	24
Wakulla	19	11	6			1	4		7	1
Walton	98	62	10	12	11	15	14	2	32	2
Washington	16	7	6		1			1	6	2
Georgia	24,496	19,195	1,962	5,913	3,725	3,787	3,808	1,091	2,888	1,322
Aiken	1									1
Appling	16	12	1	4	4		3		3	1
Atkinson	1								1	
Bacon	13	11	5	2	3	1			2	
Baldwin	118	89	10	25	16	17	21	2	22	5
Banks	7	7	3	1	2	1				
Barrow	38	32	10	10	5	6	1	2	4	
Bartow	107	91	21	28	21	16	5	1	11	4
Ben Hill	16	13	3	4	2	1	3		3	
Berrien	8	5	2	1	1	1			2	1
Bibb	817	645	59	201	146	107	132	35	101	36
Bleckley	10	7	3		1		3		3	
Brantley	2	2	1				1			
Brooks	4	3		2	1				1	
Bryan	63	51	5	13	10	8	15		3	9
Bulloch	109	94	16	29	24	14	11		12	3
Burke	20	15	7	3	1	3	1	1	4	
Butts	10	8	4	4					2	

Table 3.9

Physicians by State and County, 2010, continued

		Major Professional Activity								
		Patient Care								
			Office-Based Practice							
State County	Total Physicians	Total Patient Care	FM/GP Practice	Medical Specialties	Surgical Specialties	Other Specialties	Hospital Based Practice	Other Professional Activity	Inactive	Not Classified
Calhoun	5	4	3				1		1	
Camden	55	39	7	16	9	2	5	1	12	3
Candler	8	3	2	1					5	
Carroll	207	176	26	58	39	31	22	3	23	5
Catoosa	71	63	15	14	15	13	6	1	6	1
Charlton	2	2	1			1				
Chatham	1,095	861	73	249	180	180	179	34	168	32
Chattooga	11	9	4	1	1	3			2	
Cherokee	200	162	31	52	29	33	17	6	29	3
Clarke	400	332	23	108	90	75	36	14	48	6
Clay	2	1		1					1	
Clayton	268	227	26	87	47	45	22	7	30	4
Clinch	2	2	1	1						
Cobb	1,572	1,261	105	459	276	302	119	43	194	74
Coffee	61	47	7	13	10	8	9	2	8	4
Colquitt	58	49	9	13	12	7	8	1	8	
Columbia	731	566	54	112	48	93	259	31	72	62
Cook	12	11	7		1		3		1	
Coweta	138	116	23	43	27	13	10		20	2
Crawford	11	10	5			1	4		1	
Crisp	38	28	5	13	5	1	4		7	3
Dade	9	6	2	2		2			3	
Dawson	24	19	6	6	1	3	3		5	
Decatur	30	25	3	9	4	4	5		5	
Dekalb	3,699	2,616	137	795	313	545	826	396	314	373
Dodge	27	18	2	6	2	1	7		6	3
Dooly	3	1			1				2	
Dougherty	294	247	30	83	60	43	31	6	32	9
Douglas	138	112	11	51	24	17	9	7	13	6
Early	3	3	2		1					
Effingham	19	19	7	3	6	1	2			
Elbert	16	13	6	3	2		2	1	2	
Emanuel	19	16	5	3	3	1	4		2	1
Evans	11	8	2	2	2	1	1		3	
Fannin	30	23	6	7	5	2	3		6	1
Fayette	344	291	39	103	74	54	21	11	33	9
Floyd	380	311	60	79	73	62	37	6	53	10
Forsyth	171	136	21	53	27	21	14	3	23	9
Franklin	19	15	7	5	2	1			4	
Fulton	5,611	4,388	215	1,296	920	1,025	932	275	590	358
Gilmer	33	24	11	4	5	2	2	1	8	
Glascock	1	1	1							
Glynn	277	203	20	61	51	56	15	4	62	8
Gordon	61	51	12	16	12	7	4	2	7	1
Grady	13	12	6	3	1	1	1		1	
Greene	36	23	6	5	7	3	2	3	10	
Gwinnett	1,262	1,053	124	417	192	200	120	32	110	67
Habersham	44	35	8	14	7	4	2	1	8	
Hall	443	356	27	133	89	77	30	6	75	6
Hancock	5	2	1	1					3	
Haralson	22	17	7	7	2		1		5	
Harris	33	22	9	3	3	4	3	2	8	1
Hart	16	13	5	3	2	1	2		3	
Heard	2	1	1					1		
Henry	274	240	34	90	54	43	19	4	18	12
Houston	219	177	19	62	29	35	32	5	26	11
Irwin	4	3	1	2					1	
Jackson	66	56	9	22	6	9	10		8	2

Table 3.9

Physicians by State and County, 2010, continued

		Major Professional Activity									
		Patient Care									
			Office-Based Practice								
State County	Total Physicians	Total Patient Care	FM/GP Practice	Medical Specialties	Surgical Specialties	Other Specialties	Hospital Based Practice	Other Professional Activity	Inactive	Not Classified
Jasper	10	9	2	1	2	1	3			1
Jeff Davis	6	6	3	2	1					
Jefferson	15	11	3	4	1		3		2	2
Jenkins	5	4	1	1			2		1	
Johnson	5	4	1	2			1	1		
Jones	15	13	3	1		3	6		2	
Lamar	12	10	5	2		2	1		2	
Lanier	3	3	3							
Laurens	149	116	20	34	22	15	25	6	23	4
Lee	36	33	4	11	6	9	3		1	2
Liberty	56	46	4	11	7	6	18	2	5	3
Lincoln	6	3	2				1		3	
Lowndes	219	184	21	59	51	37	16	2	32	1
Lumpkin	25	25	6	5	7	5	2			
Macon	4	3	1		1	1			1	
Madison	8	6	4	1			1		2	
Marion	3	2	1				1		1	
Mcduffie	15	15	6	6	1		2			
Mcintosh	6	3		1		1	1		3	
Meriwether	17	11	4	3	1	1	2		6	
Miller	9	6	3		1		2		3	
Mitchell	15	11	6	2		1	2	1	3	
Monroe	27	20	7	7		3	3		7	
Montgomery	2	1					1		1	
Morgan	18	11	6	3		2			6	1
Murray	11	9	3	4		1	1		2	
Muscogee	721	583	100	128	133	104	118	21	77	40
Newton	72	59	8	28	9	8	6	1	10	2
Oconee	124	103	11	33	13	29	17	2	13	6
Oglethorpe	4	4	3				1			
Paulding	30	26	6	10	3	4	3	1	3	
Peach	12	9	4	2	1		2		2	1
Pickens	49	30	6	9	9	5	1	1	17	1
Pierce	18	13	6	4	1	1	1		5	
Pike	2	2	1	1						
Polk	27	15	7	2	1	3	2	1	10	1
Pulaski	18	13	4	5	2		2		5	
Putnam	16	9	3	2		2	2	1	6	
Rabun	33	17	5	5	4	1	2	2	14	
Randolph	4	2	1			1			2	
Richmond	1,254	962	45	201	180	131	405	79	129	84
Rockdale	138	131	21	55	24	21	10	2	3	2
Screven	6	4	2				2		2	
Seminole	16	16	4	6	5		1			
Spalding	85	61	7	29	15	7	3		22	2
Stephens	46	34	8	12	10	2	2	1	11	
Stewart	5	5	4				1			
Sumter	56	38	6	12	8	6	6		15	3
Tattnall	9	5	2		2		1		4	
Taylor	2	1			1				1	
Telfair	7	6	4	1		1			1	
Terrell	7	2	1		1			1	3	1
Thomas	168	133	10	39	31	38	15	5	28	2
Tift	109	97	10	34	23	23	7	1	11	
Toombs	51	44	5	15	11	6	7		7	
Towns	19	11	6	3		2			7	1
Treutlen	2	1				1			1	
Troup	120	100	3	42	25	23	7	2	17	1
Turner	8	5	2	1	1		1	1	2	

Table 3.9

Physicians by State and County, 2010, continued

		Major Professional Activity								
		Patient Care								
			Office-Based Practice							
State County	Total Physicians	Total Patient Care	FM/GP Practice	Medical Specialties	Surgical Specialties	Other Specialties	Hospital Based Practice	Other Professional Activity	Inactive	Not Classified
Twiggs	1	1	1							
Union	39	30	13	5	5	3	4		9	
Upson	42	34	8	8	12	5	1		8	
Walker	33	24	11	8	2	3			9	
Walton	85	72	19	21	11	14	7	2	5	6
Ware	101	83	8	31	15	14	15	1	13	4
Warren	3	2	1	1					1	
Washington	25	20	6	7	4		3	1	3	1
Wayne	28	24	5	8	6	3	2		4	
White	22	9	6			2	1	2	11	
Whitfield	191	163	16	61	49	27	10	1	23	4
Wilkes	12	8	2	2	1	1	2		4	
Wilkinson	2	2	1	1						
Worth	12	7	2	4			1		5	
Hawaii	4,866	3,668	347	1,087	601	815	818	206	759	233
Hawaii	427	311	63	91	49	85	23	15	93	8
Honolulu	3,857	2,914	208	856	468	627	755	173	558	212
Kauai	188	145	30	37	29	36	13	7	34	2
Maui	394	298	46	103	55	67	27	11	74	11
Idaho	3,215	2,538	498	512	565	588	375	64	526	87
Ada	1,297	1,055	156	253	241	238	167	33	177	32
Adams	3	2		1			1		1	
Bannock	205	158	31	28	31	35	33	5	33	9
Bear Lake	9	6	3	1	2			1	1	1
Benewah	7	6	3		1	1	1		1	
Bingham	32	20	5	2	3	5	5	1	9	2
Blaine	108	67	10	9	15	21	12	2	36	3
Boise	3	2	1	1					1	
Bonner	93	64	14	13	14	18	5	3	23	3
Bonneville	218	181	22	41	50	48	20	2	31	4
Boundary	13	8	5	1			2		3	2
Butte	2	2	1				1			
Canyon	187	141	31	28	38	25	19	4	37	5
Caribou	5	3	1		1	1			2	
Cassia	31	22	7	3	8	2	2		9	
Clearwater	19	14	3		2		9		5	
Custer	1								1	
Elmore	33	27	9	3	10	2	3	2	1	3
Franklin	6	6	3				3			
Fremont	8	3				2	1		5	
Gem	12	8	7				1		4	
Gooding	9	6	4	1		1			3	
Idaho	14	13	5		2		6		1	
Jefferson	5	4	2	1	1				1	
Jerome	12	12	9		1	1	1			
Kootenai	409	335	62	56	58	122	37	4	54	16
Latah	59	48	20	5	7	10	6	2	9	
Lemhi	7	7	2	1	2	1	1			
Lewis	2								2	
Lincoln	1	1	1							
Madison	37	34	11	6	11	3	3		2	1
Minidoka	8	6	3	1	1		1		2	
Nez Perce	108	87	13	20	21	18	15	1	19	1
Oneida	1	1	1							
Owyhee	2	2	2							
Payette	16	13	3	3	4	1	2		3	
Power	1	1	1							
Shoshone	13	7	4	2			1		6	

Table 3.9

Physicians by State and County, 2010, continued

		Major Professional Activity								
		Patient Care								
			Office-Based Practice							
State / County	Total Physicians	Total Patient Care	FM/GP Practice	Medical Specialties	Surgical Specialties	Other Specialties	Hospital Based Practice	Other Professional Activity	Inactive	Not Classified
Teton	14	10	5	1	1	1	2	1	2	1
Twin Falls	166	134	25	30	38	28	13	2	27	3
Valley	33	19	11	1	1	4	2	1	12	1
Washington	6	3	2		1				3	
Illinois	41,724	32,274	3,104	9,482	4,910	6,012	8,766	1,572	4,630	3,248
Adams	190	151	24	45	25	32	25	2	31	6
Alexander	2	2	2							
Bond	18	14	8	2	2	2			3	1
Boone	82	70	15	16	9	19	11	1	8	3
Brown	3	2				2			1	
Bureau	54	40	10	8	10	6	6	1	10	3
Calhoun	5	3	3						2	
Carroll	7	5	5						2	
Cass	2	2	1		1					
Champaign	714	541	60	173	75	101	132	26	107	40
Christian	27	23	11	8	3	1			4	
Clark	9	6	4	1	1				3	
Clay	12	11	4	3	1	2	1		1	
Clinton	26	21	9	4	6	1	1		4	1
Coles	85	69	15	10	14	10	20	4	11	1
Cook	23,404	17,720	1,181	4,974	2,292	3,005	6,268	1,033	2,160	2,491
Crawford	22	17	3	3	3	2	6		4	1
Cumberland	2	1		1					1	
Dekalb	104	79	11	27	25	13	3	2	21	2
Dewitt	17	13	4	4	4		1		4	
Douglas	12	8	6	1			1		4	
Dupage	4,599	3,747	356	1,241	621	905	624	120	517	215
Edgar	12	9	3	3		2	1		3	
Effingham	83	73	13	17	19	13	11		9	1
Fayette	10	7	1	3		1	2		3	
Ford	15	13	6	2	2	1	2		1	1
Franklin	24	20	10	4	2	1	3		4	
Fulton	32	23	9	5	5	1	3		8	1
Gallatin	2	1	1						1	
Greene	10	6	3	2			1		4	
Grundy	52	41	3	13	11	8	6	1	9	1
Hamilton	6	5		1	2	1	1		1	
Hancock	15	12	9		1		2		3	
Hardin	2	2	1				1			
Henderson	4	3	1		1	1			1	
Henry	31	23	12	5	3	1	2	1	7	
Iroquois	30	25	4	10	5	2	4		5	
Jackson	199	152	40	39	22	23	28	6	29	12
Jasper	1	1	1							
Jefferson	105	91	6	32	27	20	6		10	4
Jersey	22	18	4	5	5	2	2		4	
Jo Daviess	18	12	5	2		3	2		6	
Johnson	6	6	2	1	1		2			
Kane	775	614	71	203	138	140	62	21	123	17
Kankakee	179	145	15	49	39	19	23	1	29	4
Kendall	68	51	12	20	7	5	7	1	10	6
Knox	106	84	17	22	21	14	10	1	19	2
La Salle	136	108	21	31	24	11	21	1	25	2
Lake	2,707	2,069	165	698	352	492	362	139	359	140
Lawrence	7	7	4			2	1			
Lee	67	56	9	16	9	4	18	1	8	2
Livingston	29	28	9	8	7	1	3		1	
Logan	20	17	10	2	3	1	1		3	
Macon	289	235	42	59	44	53	37	5	42	7

Table 3.9

Physicians by State and County, 2010, continued

		Major Professional Activity								
		Patient Care								
			Office-Based Practice							
State County	Total Physicians	Total Patient Care	FM/GP Practice	Medical Specialties	Surgical Specialties	Other Specialties	Hospital Based Practice	Other Professional Activity	Inactive	Not Classified
Macoupin	26	21	6	8	4	1	2		2	3
Madison	369	301	37	102	65	52	45	4	57	7
Marion	66	54	7	21	11	14	1	1	8	3
Marshall	8	4	2		1	1			4	
Mason	12	11	2	3	1	3	2		1	
Massac	8	4	3	1				1	2	1
Mcdonough	42	32	10	8	5	3	6		10	
Mchenry	444	351	46	134	76	67	28	6	74	13
Mclean	386	317	46	93	77	76	25	6	56	7
Menard	9	6	2		1	2	1		3	
Mercer	6	6	2	2	1	1				
Monroe	22	18	7	2	4	2	3		4	
Montgomery	28	23	14	1	3	1	4		5	
Morgan	50	37	6	6	15	5	5	1	11	1
Moultrie	7	6	5		1				1	
Ogle	40	35	23	4	3	1	4	1	4	
Peoria	996	803	82	208	144	175	194	46	107	40
Perry	23	17	11	2	2		2		6	
Piatt	11	7	3	1		2	1	1	3	
Pike	14	12	5	2	1	2	2		2	
Pope	2	2				1	1			
Putnam	1	1	1							
Randolph	35	25	9	6	4	1	5	2	6	2
Richland	35	27	3	8	7	6	3	1	7	
Rock Island	305	235	26	76	55	58	20	7	54	9
Saint Clair	540	422	83	112	75	69	83	12	70	36
Saline	39	33	13	7	4	5	4		6	
Sangamon	1,201	980	76	269	162	182	291	45	111	65
Schuyler	3	2	2						1	
Scott	2	2	1	1						
Shelby	9	8	2	3		1	2		1	
Stark	2	1	1						1	
Stephenson	78	63	12	21	13	12	5	3	12	
Tazewell	188	142	28	35	12	26	41	7	32	7
Union	25	21	9	3	4	3	2	1	3	
Vermilion	140	101	19	22	17	18	25	2	31	6
Wabash	13	9	1	4	1	1	2		2	2
Warren	14	13	5	1	1	1	5		1	
Washington	9	5	1	1	2	1			4	
Wayne	10	9	5	2	2				1	
White	8	6	2	2		1	1		2	
Whiteside	85	66	14	17	11	9	15	1	15	3
Will	906	727	93	281	125	133	95	20	118	41
Williamson	164	131	24	34	26	21	26	4	24	5
Winnebago	842	640	102	197	130	129	82	32	142	28
Woodford	43	36	12	9	2	3	10	1	1	5
Indiana	15,898	12,860	1,924	3,297	2,245	2,755	2,639	579	1,884	575
Adams	20	18	10	1	3	2	2		2	
Allen	1,029	854	101	242	175	237	99	28	127	20
Bartholomew	212	176	30	47	41	45	13	4	29	3
Benton	4	3	2	1					1	
Blackford	10	7	5	1			1		3	
Boone	437	349	33	94	40	102	80	25	32	31
Brown	10	2	2					2	6	
Carroll	9	7	6	1					2	
Cass	48	38	9	5	7	9	8	1	7	2
Clark	168	148	24	42	31	43	8		18	2
Clay	17	14	7	5	1		1		3	

Table 3.9

Physicians by State and County, 2010, continued

State County	Total Physicians	Major Professional Activity Patient Care Total Patient Care	Office-Based Practice FM/GP Practice	Medical Specialties	Surgical Specialties	Other Specialties	Hospital Based Practice	Other Professional Activity	Inactive	Not Classified
Clinton	27	22	8	4	3	3	4		4	1
Crawford	1								1	
Daviess	19	14	5	4	1	1	3		5	
De Kalb	43	32	18	2	3	6	3		11	
Dearborn	57	48	10	13	8	7	10		9	
Decatur	23	16	4	6		3	3	1	4	2
Delaware	342	271	32	85	44	38	72	11	43	17
Dubois	84	72	14	18	20	11	9		9	3
Elkhart	303	238	55	40	56	56	31	5	54	6
Fayette	24	22	4	5	4	2	7		2	
Floyd	173	140	26	42	23	41	8	3	24	6
Fountain	6	4	2			1	1		2	
Franklin	8	7	3	1	2		1		1	
Fulton	17	13	5	3	1		4		4	
Gibson	22	20	6	4	4	3	3		2	
Grant	101	79	15	18	18	14	14	1	19	2
Greene	16	13	6		2	3	2	1	1	1
Hamilton	1,637	1,371	125	389	245	367	245	53	159	54
Hancock	145	129	31	31	17	34	16	4	11	1
Harrison	34	26	12	3	2	3	6	1	6	1
Hendricks	263	227	30	55	32	51	59	7	20	9
Henry	57	43	9	9	7	4	14	1	12	1
Howard	160	131	25	38	33	23	12	1	25	3
Huntington	41	35	11	10	6	5	3		4	2
Jackson	58	51	19	6	11	7	8		7	
Jasper	22	17	13	2	1	1			5	
Jay	12	9	6	1	1	1			3	
Jefferson	62	47	13	8	9	3	14	1	13	1
Jennings	13	11	5	4			2		1	1
Johnson	305	252	47	76	40	55	34	9	39	5
Knox	81	68	10	18	12	13	15		13	
Kosciusko	77	52	18	2	14	7	11	1	22	2
La Porte	178	136	22	31	35	32	16	3	38	1
Lagrange	18	15	10	1	3	1			3	
Lake	974	790	108	261	165	167	89	13	148	23
Lawrence	61	44	8	16	13	3	4	2	14	1
Madison	201	166	53	32	24	39	18	6	28	1
Marion	4,320	3,368	260	787	482	621	1,218	293	369	290
Marshall	47	36	23	3	3	3	4	3	7	1
Martin	4	3	1	2				1		
Miami	24	17	4	2	4	4	3		7	
Monroe	388	303	43	74	62	90	34	11	67	7
Montgomery	44	35	11	8	9	4	3	1	8	
Morgan	88	77	14	18	18	11	16	4	7	
Newton	3	2		1		1			1	
Noble	28	25	11	5	3	2	4		3	
Ohio	1								1	
Orange	15	11	7	1			3		3	1
Owen	8	5	1	1		1	2		2	1
Parke	9	7	6				1	2		
Perry	13	11	8	1		1	1	1	1	
Pike	2	2	2							
Porter	324	258	37	82	52	54	33	6	55	5
Posey	11	10	6	1		1	2		1	
Pulaski	6	6	5				1			
Putnam	30	28	12	3	6	3	4		1	1
Randolph	13	12	4	2		1	5		1	
Ripley	42	33	9	8	7	5	4	1	5	3
Rush	12	10	5	1	1	1	2		2	

Table 3.9

Physicians by State and County, 2010, continued

		Major Professional Activity								
		Patient Care								
			Office-Based Practice							
State County	Total Physicians	Total Patient Care	FM/GP Practice	Medical Specialties	Surgical Specialties	Other Specialties	Hospital Based Practice	Other Professional Activity	Inactive	Not Classified
Scott	21	20	10	2	2	2	4		1	
Shelby	32	26	7	8	6	1	4	1	5	
Spencer	7	7	3				4			
St Joseph	753	641	109	165	109	169	89	15	81	16
Starke	10	10	6		2	1	1			
Steuben	28	21	11	1	3	3	3		6	1
Sullivan	9	7	4	2		1			1	1
Switzerland	3	2	1	1					1	
Tippecanoe	452	364	46	112	78	85	43	12	68	8
Tipton	13	13	7	1	3		2			
Union	2	2	1		1					
Vanderburgh	606	492	88	116	108	106	74	19	81	14
Vermillion	11	6	4			2			3	2
Vigo	329	275	48	80	50	55	42	12	31	11
Wabash	27	20	9	2		3	6	2	5	
Warren	3	2					2			1
Warrick	256	228	33	69	42	45	39	3	17	8
Washington	21	19	7	6	1	2	3		2	
Wayne	169	135	17	46	25	27	20	6	26	2
Wells	44	31	11	7	7	4	2		13	
White	18	14	8		1	2	3		4	
Whitley	23	19	8	2	3	1	5	2	2	
Iowa	6,677	5,118	911	1,084	871	937	1,315	286	907	366
Adair	4	3	2				1		1	
Adams	3	3	2	1						
Allamakee	13	10	7	1		1	1		3	
Appanoose	13	12	6	2	2	1	1		1	
Audubon	1	1	1							
Benton	8	5	1	2			2		3	
Black Hawk	327	272	60	65	48	65	34	4	42	9
Boone	22	12	8		1	2	1		9	1
Bremer	28	19	10	1	3		5	1	7	1
Buchanan	14	12	5	2		3	2	1	1	
Buena Vista	19	13	10	1	1	1			6	
Butler	3	3	1			1	1			
Calhoun	9	5	3		2				4	
Carroll	28	23	7	4	4	3	5		5	
Cass	15	11	6		3	1	1		4	
Cedar	10	7	3			1	3		3	
Cerro Gordo	170	135	25	27	23	30	30	2	31	2
Cherokee	13	9	3	1		1	4	2	2	
Chickasaw	6	1	1						3	2
Clarke	3	1	1						2	
Clay	27	27	7	1	13	4	2			
Clayton	12	9	5		2	1	1		3	
Clinton	71	62	12	22	13	10	5	1	7	1
Crawford	9	6	5				1		3	
Dallas	45	33	7	3	9	6	8	2	6	4
Davis	5	2	1		1				3	
Decatur	5	3	2				1		2	
Delaware	13	7	5				2		6	
Des Moines	88	71	14	14	17	15	11		16	1
Dickinson	30	20	6		5	6	3		10	
Dubuque	267	218	19	76	54	50	19	5	39	5
Emmet	9	6	6						3	
Fayette	9	4	2		1	1			5	
Floyd	10	9	4		2	1	2		1	
Franklin	1	1	1							
Fremont	5	2	2						3	

Table 3.9

Physicians by State and County, 2010, continued

		Major Professional Activity								
		Patient Care								
			Office-Based Practice							
State County	Total Physicians	Total Patient Care	FM/GP Practice	Medical Specialties	Surgical Specialties	Other Specialties	Hospital Based Practice	Other Professional Activity	Inactive	Not Classified
Greene	9	4	3	1					5	
Grundy	5	3	1		1		1		2	
Guthrie	4	4	2			1	1			
Hamilton	9	6	3	2			1	1	1	1
Hancock	3	3					3			
Hardin	12	11	7				4		1	
Harrison	7	5	3	1			1		1	1
Henry	25	15	6	3	4	1	1	1	9	
Howard	8	6	4		1		1		2	
Humboldt	5	5	2	1		2				
Ida	4	4	3				1			
Iowa	13	10	5	2		1	2		2	1
Jackson	12	10	4	1	2	1	2		2	
Jasper	19	15	9		4	2		1	2	1
Jefferson	22	17	10	1	1	3	2	3	2	
Johnson	1,966	1,377	68	204	143	221	741	176	146	267
Jones	11	9	7			1	1		1	1
Keokuk	1	1			1					
Kossuth	9	7	3	1			3		2	
Lee	55	44	8	10	9	5	12	2	9	
Linn	478	380	90	80	76	91	43	12	76	10
Louisa	2	1		1					1	
Lucas	2	2	2							
Lyon	3	2	2						1	
Madison	2	2	1			1				
Mahaska	22	18	10	1	2	1	4		4	
Marion	38	28	13	5	4	1	5	2	7	1
Marshall	60	44	14	12	11	5	2		16	
Mills	16	14	6	2		2	4	1	1	
Mitchell	3	1	1						2	
Monona	11	8	4		1		3		3	
Monroe	4	3	3						1	
Montgomery	10	6	2	2	2				4	
Muscatine	38	33	8	8	9	2	6	2	3	
Obrien	11	9	6	1	2				2	
Page	22	15	7	1	1	3	3	1	5	1
Palo Alto	6	2	2						4	
Plymouth	18	12	8		1	1	2		6	
Pocahontas	3	2	1				1		1	
Polk	1,159	927	93	273	198	190	173	45	157	30
Pottawattamie	117	91	17	30	21	13	10	2	23	1
Poweshiek	28	19	11		3	1	4		9	
Ringgold	5	3	1	1			1		2	
Sac	9	5	4				1		3	1
Scott	414	345	62	87	73	80	43	10	51	8
Shelby	9	8	5	1	1		1		1	
Sioux	30	26	16	1	3	1	5		4	
Story	197	163	26	49	29	39	20		30	4
Tama	5	3	1			1	1	1	1	
Union	9	8	5		1		2		1	
Van Buren	1	1	1							
Wapello	66	55	3	22	8	14	8		9	2
Warren	24	18	6	4	1	6	1		6	
Washington	17	14	9	2	2		1		2	1
Wayne	5	4	3			1			1	
Webster	69	53	10	11	19	8	5		14	2
Winnebago	5	4	3			1			1	
Winneshiek	34	29	13	2	5	6	3		5	
Woodbury	198	157	28	38	26	27	38	8	27	6

Table 3.9

Physicians by State and County, 2010, continued

		Major Professional Activity								
		Patient Care								
			Office-Based Practice							
State County	Total Physicians	Total Patient Care	FM/GP Practice	Medical Specialties	Surgical Specialties	Other Specialties	Hospital Based Practice	Other Professional Activity	Inactive	Not Classified
Worth	1	1	1							
Wright	12	9	5		2		2		2	1
Kansas	7,558	5,884	925	1,391	1,046	1,203	1,319	266	1,053	355
Allen	5	3	2		1			1	1	
Anderson	7	3	2			1			4	
Atchison	19	15	6	1	4	2	2		3	1
Barber	4	1					1		3	
Barton	35	27	8	7	7	4	1		8	
Bourbon	19	14	5	2	2	3	2		5	
Brown	14	13	7	1	1	1	3		1	
Butler	86	73	19	14	7	18	15	2	7	4
Cherokee	11	9	2	1	2		4		2	
Cheyenne	4	2	2						2	
Clark	4	3	3						1	
Clay	13	12	10				2	1		
Cloud	12	3	1		1	1			7	2
Coffey	5	3	2				1			2
Comanche	1	1	1							
Cowley	32	24	12	4	4	1	3		7	1
Crawford	54	41	9	13	11	2	6	1	11	1
Decatur	6	6	3		2	1				
Dickinson	13	9	6				3		3	1
Doniphan	4	2					2		2	
Douglas	262	191	36	53	31	41	30	6	55	10
Edwards	2	2	1	1						
Elk	1	1	1							
Ellis	81	61	2	16	14	16	13	1	13	6
Ellsworth	4	3	1	1			1		1	
Finney	45	37	7	8	11	5	6		6	2
Ford	47	39	12	11	9	5	2		6	2
Franklin	20	15	9	3	1	1	1		5	
Geary	33	27	6	6	3	3	9		2	4
Gove	6	5	5						1	
Graham	2	2		1	1					
Grant	4	3	1	1			1		1	
Gray	1	1	1							
Greeley	2	2	1			1				
Greenwood	4	2	2					1	1	
Hamilton	3	1			1				2	
Harper	5	4	1	1		2		1		
Harvey	85	57	17	11	19	5	5	2	24	2
Haskell	2	2	1				1			
Hodgeman	1	1	1							
Jackson	15	12	9			1	2		2	1
Jefferson	16	13	7	2		1	3		3	
Jewell	1	1	1							
Johnson	2,787	2,178	194	574	406	561	443	106	354	149
Kearny	3	3	2				1			
Kingman	1								1	
Kiowa	2	2				1	1			
Labette	43	36	6	3	11	8	8	1	3	3
Lane	1	1					1			
Leavenworth	98	77	17	13	10	8	29	4	16	1
Linn	2	2	2							
Logan	3	2	1	1					1	
Lyon	51	39	11	11	7	7	3	1	11	
Marion	10	4	3	1				1	5	
Marshall	7	5	3	1	1				2	

Table 3.9

Physicians by State and County, 2010, continued

		Major Professional Activity									
		Patient Care									
			Office-Based Practice								
State County	Total Physicians	Total Patient Care	FM/GP Practice	Medical Specialties	Surgical Specialties	Other Specialties	Hospital Based Practice	Other Professional Activity	Inactive	Not Classified
Mcpherson	35	27	18		2	2	5		8	
Meade	3	2	1				1		1	
Miami	29	20	9	2		4	5	2	7	
Mitchell	8	7	3	1	2		1		1	
Montgomery	40	35	9	8	10	5	3		4	1
Morris	9	7	5		1	1			2	
Morton	7	6			2	2	2		1	
Nemaha	7	7	6				1			
Neosho	17	13	6	2	5				4	
Ness	1	1	1							
Norton	4	2	1				1		2	
Osage	6	4	3	1					2	
Osborne	2	2	2							
Ottawa	7	5	4			1			2	
Pawnee	16	11	1	2		3	5	1	3	1
Phillips	2	2	2							
Pottawatomie	20	14	9	1		2	2	1	4	1
Pratt	13	12	4	2	3	1	2		1	
Rawlins	3	2	2						1	
Reno	146	113	21	39	25	20	8	1	28	4
Republic	7	6	5		1				1	
Rice	5	5	4				1			
Riley	165	133	23	31	31	30	18	2	21	9
Rooks	4	3	3						1	
Rush	3	1		1					2	
Russell	7	3	2		1				3	1
Saline	167	133	25	29	35	30	14	5	26	3
Scott	4	3	3						1	
Sedgwick	1,453	1,167	189	269	209	224	276	54	172	60
Seward	37	29	2	9	6	7	5		8	
Shawnee	543	397	39	120	71	94	73	26	116	4
Sheridan	2	1	1						1	
Sherman	4	4	2				2			
Smith	5	4	2		1		1		1	
Stafford	2	1					1		1	
Stanton	2	1	1						1	
Stevens	1	1		1						
Sumner	9	8	4		2	1	1		1	
Thomas	6	3	3						3	
Trego	5	5	1	2			2			
Wabaunsee	2	2	1	1						
Wallace	1								1	
Washington	3	3	2		1					
Wichita	2								1	1
Wilson	10	8	5	1	1	1			2	
Woodson	1	1					1			
Wyandotte	735	575	40	107	70	75	283	45	37	78
Kentucky	11,417	9,182	1,121	2,569	1,655	1,885	1,952	365	1,284	586
Adair	15	12	5	3		1	3		3	
Allen	8	7	3	2		2			1	
Anderson	16	15	5	5	3	2		1		
Ballard	1	1	1							
Barren	93	81	18	16	20	14	13	1	7	4
Bath	5	4	1			2	1		1	
Bell	46	33	5	13	7	4	4	2	10	1
Boone	189	150	37	41	26	26	20	4	25	10
Bourbon	25	23	13	2	1	5	2	1		1
Boyd	240	206	24	58	46	55	23	5	20	9

Table 3.9

Physicians by State and County, 2010, continued

State County	Total Physicians	Major Professional Activity: Patient Care: Total Patient Care	Office-Based Practice: FM/GP Practice	Office-Based Practice: Medical Specialties	Office-Based Practice: Surgical Specialties	Office-Based Practice: Other Specialties	Hospital Based Practice	Other Professional Activity	Inactive	Not Classified
Boyle	110	91	12	26	27	20	6	2	17	
Bracken	3	3	1			1	1			
Breathitt	22	18	3	8	5	2			2	2
Breckinridge	8	6	4	1			1		2	
Bullitt	29	27	10	6	1	3	7	1	1	
Butler	3	3	1	1		1				
Caldwell	14	11	5	2	2		2		3	
Calloway	70	58	9	15	21	11	2		10	2
Campbell	159	121	23	33	25	29	11	5	26	7
Carlisle	1	1	1							
Carroll	6	5	2	1		1	1		1	
Carter	12	8	4	1		1	2		2	2
Casey	4	2	1		1				2	
Christian	133	106	13	28	27	23	15	4	20	3
Clark	56	51	6	16	10	6	13	1	2	2
Clay	15	12	3	2	4		3		2	1
Clinton	7	7	3	2	1		1			
Crittenden	4	4	3			1				
Cumberland	5	4	3				1		1	
Daviess	228	187	14	65	49	41	18	4	35	2
Edmonson	3	3	1	1	1					
Elliott	1									1
Estill	7	6	2	3		1			1	
Fayette	2,277	1,766	104	419	272	354	617	111	213	187
Fleming	14	13	7	4		2			1	
Floyd	60	52	10	23	5	4	10		6	2
Franklin	80	53	8	20	18	4	3	6	17	4
Fulton	15	11	2	4	1		4		4	
Gallatin	2	2	1	1						
Garrard	9	6	4	1		1			3	
Grant	17	13	10	1			2		4	
Graves	40	33	6	11	6	4	6		7	
Grayson	35	30	9	7	4	2	8	1	3	1
Green	7	5	2	1	1		1		2	
Greenup	36	30	5	14	1	6	4		5	1
Hancock	2	1				1			1	
Hardin	224	193	20	62	34	48	29	4	21	6
Harlan	37	30	6	9	6	3	6	1	5	1
Harrison	26	17	8	5	3	1			8	1
Hart	9	7	3	4					2	
Henderson	73	58	10	21	12	10	5	2	11	2
Henry	11	9	4	1		3	1		2	
Hickman	2	1	1						1	
Hopkins	157	128	34	27	21	12	34	4	20	5
Jackson	3	3	1	1		1				
Jefferson	3,907	3,112	200	879	558	704	771	164	399	232
Jessamine	121	94	16	26	9	23	20	4	15	8
Johnson	37	30	8	6	8	5	3		6	1
Kenton	461	399	57	110	78	89	65	12	40	10
Knott	7	5	3	2					2	
Knox	13	11	5	2		2	2		1	1
Larue	4	3	1		1	1				1
Laurel	85	74	13	26	15	13	7		3	8
Lawrence	13	10	4	2		3	1		2	1
Lee	3	3	2	1						
Leslie	7	3	1				2	1	3	
Letcher	26	25	5	10	4	2	4		1	
Lewis	6	4	1	2		1			1	1
Lincoln	19	17	11	1	1	3	1	1	1	

Table 3.9

Physicians by State and County, 2010, continued

State County	Total Physicians	Major Professional Activity Patient Care Total Patient Care	Office-Based Practice FM/GP Practice	Medical Specialties	Surgical Specialties	Other Specialties	Hospital Based Practice	Other Professional Activity	Inactive	Not Classified
Livingston	11	9	4	1	3	1			1	1
Logan	23	18	4	5	4	2	3		5	
Lyon	4	3	2				1		1	
Madison	130	105	21	34	22	15	13	1	18	6
Magoffin	2	1	1					1		
Marion	21	17	3	6	3	1	4		3	1
Marshall	29	21	7	4	2	3	5		8	
Martin	5	3	3						1	1
Mason	48	45	10	15	9	7	4		3	
Mccracken	263	215	21	72	54	54	14	3	39	6
Mccreary	11	10	6	1	1	1	1		1	
Mclean	1	1	1							
Meade	12	8	4	1		1	2		3	1
Menifee	1	1					1			
Mercer	16	9	4	4			1	1	5	1
Metcalfe	3	2	2						1	
Monroe	9	6	3	2		1			2	1
Montgomery	26	23	4	10	4	2	3		3	
Morgan	8	6	4	1			1		1	1
Muhlenberg	28	24	5	6	8	3	2	1	2	1
Nelson	42	31	7	8	7	5	4	1	9	1
Nicholas	6	4	1	2			1		2	
Ohio	14	9	4	1		3	1		3	2
Oldham	119	98	7	35	12	32	12	2	10	9
Owen	5	4	4						1	
Owsley	1	1	1							
Pendleton	5	5	2	1		2				
Perry	100	84	12	29	14	16	13	2	7	7
Pike	148	122	12	41	22	25	22	1	19	6
Powell	5	4	1			2	1		1	
Pulaski	146	120	13	44	26	24	13		19	7
Robertson	1	1			1					
Rockcastle	14	10	6	2			2		2	2
Rowan	69	59	10	11	10	13	15		8	2
Russell	20	15	7	1	1	1	5		4	1
Scott	74	60	10	16	14	13	7	3	8	3
Shelby	58	47	11	7	10	15	4		10	1
Simpson	13	11	8	2		1			2	
Spencer	8	7	4	2			1		1	
Taylor	38	34	6	10	11	4	3	1	2	1
Todd	3	3	3							
Trigg	12	8	3	1		2	2		4	
Trimble	3	2	1				1			1
Union	10	9	4	2	1	2			1	
Warren	303	263	28	99	61	52	23		40	
Washington	10	9	2	3		4			1	
Wayne	10	9	5	2			2		1	
Webster	4	3	1				2		1	
Whitley	84	64	12	25	12	11	4	2	16	2
Wolfe	3	2		1		1		1		
Woodford	55	40	9	8	8	12	3	3	11	1
Louisiana	13,587	10,946	1,074	2,846	2,118	1,899	3,009	427	1,396	818
Acadia	52	40	14	9	9	4	4	1	8	3
Allen	19	15	6	4	2	1	2		3	1
Ascension	112	100	24	28	8	14	26		8	4
Assumption	9	8	4	1			3		1	
Avoyelles	35	31	13	6	6	2	4		3	1
Beauregard	41	35	9	10	10	2	4		2	4
Bienville	5	3	2				1		2	

Table 3.9

Physicians by State and County, 2010, continued

		Major Professional Activity								
		Patient Care								
			Office-Based Practice							
State County	Total Physicians	Total Patient Care	FM/GP Practice	Medical Specialties	Surgical Specialties	Other Specialties	Hospital Based Practice	Other Professional Activity	Inactive	Not Classified
Bossier	163	142	23	37	19	20	43	2	15	4
Caddo	1,784	1,432	88	300	249	206	589	70	131	151
Calcasieu	435	353	65	101	73	67	47	7	64	11
Caldwell	7	7	2	2	1	1	1			
Cameron	1							1		
Catahoula	3	2	2						1	
Claiborne	11	8	4	3		1			3	
Concordia	16	12	3	2	4	1	2		3	1
De Soto	14	10	4	2	1	1	2		3	1
East Baton Rouge	1,746	1,424	117	415	326	301	265	53	206	63
East Carroll	6	3		1			2		2	1
East Feliciana	18	14	3	2		5	4	1	3	
Evangeline	46	38	12	12	7	3	4		8	
Franklin	10	9	3	1	2	1	2		1	
Grant	9	7	3		1	1	2		2	
Iberia	122	95	19	33	22	13	8	1	22	4
Iberville	34	26	7	10	3	3	3	1	7	
Jackson	5	4	1	1	1		1			1
Jefferson	2,064	1,681	95	481	307	281	517	63	179	141
Jefferson Davis	33	26	9	7	3	1	6		6	1
La Salle	11	11	6	2	1	1	1			
Lafayette	851	719	73	216	162	154	114	15	82	35
Lafourche	158	141	23	38	45	19	16		14	3
Lincoln	93	82	14	29	19	16	4		7	4
Livingston	53	44	13	11	4	9	7		5	4
Madison	8	8	4	3			1			
Morehouse	25	18	10		4	1	3	1	6	
Natchitoches	46	38	13	12	6	4	3	1	7	
Orleans	2,699	2,026	70	410	297	338	911	148	231	294
Ouachita	447	373	55	103	69	70	76	10	47	17
Plaquemines	16	10	2	1		3	4	1	3	2
Pointe Coupee	17	13	7	1	4		1		4	
Rapides	462	359	45	89	85	62	78	13	75	15
Red River	3	3	2			1				
Richland	23	20	8	5	4	1	2		3	
Sabine	12	8	4	3		1			3	1
Saint Bernard	16	12	3	3	1	1	4		2	2
Saint Charles	43	33	2	10	5	4	12	1	6	3
Saint Helena	4	4	4							
Saint James	24	21	6	5	4	1	5		2	1
Saint Landry	148	130	29	35	39	19	8		17	1
Saint Martin	25	23	4	3	4	8	4		1	1
Saint Mary	67	53	14	15	14	3	7	1	12	1
Saint Tammany	871	730	36	232	167	187	108	20	98	23
St John The Baptist	55	49	7	15	13	7	7		4	2
Tangipahoa	149	123	16	41	33	11	22	4	17	5
Tensas	1								1	
Terrebonne	215	179	23	47	47	27	35	6	26	4
Union	7	5	1	3		1			2	
Vermilion	49	38	8	12	11	2	5	2	8	1
Vernon	50	42	7	13	8	6	8		5	3
Washington	47	36	9	7	5	5	10	2	8	1
Webster	48	37	17	7	8	3	2	1	9	1
West Baton Rouge	10	9	1	2	1	2	3		1	
West Carroll	7	3	1	1			1		2	2
West Feliciana	14	13	3	2	2	3	3	1		
Winn	13	8	2	2	2		2		5	

Table 3.9

Physicians by State and County, 2010, continued

State County	Total Physicians	Major Professional Activity Patient Care Total Patient Care	Office-Based Practice FM/GP Practice	Medical Specialties	Surgical Specialties	Other Specialties	Hospital Based Practice	Other Professional Activity	Inactive	Not Classified
Maine	4,426	3,337	488	872	550	649	778	195	741	153
Androscoggin	294	229	35	65	36	45	48	17	33	15
Aroostook	165	132	27	26	33	15	31	4	21	8
Cumberland	1,707	1,325	116	376	204	299	330	89	219	74
Franklin	72	53	15	9	10	6	13	1	17	1
Hancock	180	122	35	23	22	17	25	8	47	3
Kennebec	402	298	66	54	49	48	81	26	68	10
Knox	171	105	10	29	18	26	22	9	52	5
Lincoln	124	71	23	16	14	9	9	1	52	
Oxford	66	48	9	13	8	5	13	1	14	3
Penobscot	574	457	48	140	63	103	103	25	70	22
Piscataquis	32	28	9	2	9	1	7		4	
Sagadahoc	72	41	7	17	4	6	7	1	29	1
Somerset	72	57	18	12	11	4	12	2	10	3
Waldo	93	71	14	10	13	19	15	2	18	2
Washington	55	38	8	6	8	5	11	1	15	1
York	347	262	48	74	48	41	51	8	72	5
Maryland	27,334	19,430	1,062	5,903	2,955	3,797	5,713	2,389	3,170	2,345
Allegany	206	159	11	54	33	43	18	5	37	5
Anne Arundel	1,527	1,166	101	373	229	240	223	63	224	74
Baltimore	3,921	2,861	104	951	583	615	608	218	612	230
Baltimore City	5,916	4,164	91	913	418	647	2,095	550	337	865
Calvert	162	131	12	49	30	23	17	4	19	8
Caroline	15	10	4	2		2	2		4	1
Carroll	270	204	27	79	36	30	32	8	51	7
Cecil	133	93	26	16	14	20	17	6	29	5
Charles	170	138	15	72	20	17	14	2	19	11
Dorchester	61	47	5	15	6	9	12	2	9	3
Frederick	552	399	63	123	68	80	65	44	77	32
Garrett	35	25	11	1	6	5	2	1	9	
Harford	469	355	34	126	66	68	61	23	72	19
Howard	2,082	1,576	96	543	181	373	383	128	174	204
Kent	74	41	10	14	9	6	2	3	30	
Montgomery	8,840	5,840	244	1,781	825	1,244	1,746	1,232	1,062	706
Prince Georges	1,697	1,333	118	481	239	188	307	64	160	140
Queen Annes	51	33	9	9	2	5	8	2	16	
Saint Marys	136	102	16	40	19	15	12	6	21	7
Somerset	23	17	1	9	2	3	2	1	5	
Talbot	229	139	7	44	30	30	28	12	72	6
Washington	349	270	34	94	58	55	29	11	59	9
Wicomico	319	259	10	96	72	61	20	3	51	6
Worcester	97	68	13	18	9	18	10	1	21	7
Massachusetts	35,334	25,842	1,123	7,726	3,169	4,927	8,897	2,236	3,459	3,797
Barnstable	860	541	40	197	104	116	84	35	268	16
Berkshire	633	445	24	135	69	106	111	28	106	54
Bristol	1,005	791	68	302	147	161	113	20	160	34
Dukes	76	40	6	6	4	9	15	6	30	
Essex	2,091	1,600	148	576	290	335	251	81	327	83
Franklin	136	98	24	31	15	19	9		36	2
Hampden	1,513	1,231	32	403	201	211	384	54	157	71
Hampshire	728	575	68	191	50	136	130	19	117	17
Middlesex	9,388	6,943	238	2,263	846	1,555	2,041	632	963	850
Nantucket	22	9	3	1	2	1	2	1	12	
Norfolk	4,412	3,241	95	1,053	439	696	958	276	430	465
Plymouth	1,028	809	68	301	130	161	149	28	154	37
Suffolk	10,357	7,126	102	1,517	586	1,066	3,855	903	408	1,920
Worcester	3,085	2,393	207	750	286	355	795	153	291	248

Table 3.9

Physicians by State and County, 2010, continued

		Major Professional Activity								
		Patient Care								
			Office-Based Practice							
State County	Total Physicians	Total Patient Care	FM/GP Practice	Medical Specialties	Surgical Specialties	Other Specialties	Hospital Based Practice	Other Professional Activity	Inactive	Not Classified
Michigan	29,331	22,764	2,226	6,192	3,532	4,162	6,652	1,157	3,494	1,916
Alcona	8	4	4						3	1
Alger	9	8	4	1	2		1		1	
Allegan	77	54	13	14	4	14	9	4	18	1
Alpena	78	60	10	13	12	17	8	1	15	2
Antrim	22	11	4	2		4	1		11	
Arenac	7	6	1	3			2		1	
Baraga	8	6	3	2			1		2	
Barry	53	40	11	8	12	7	2		12	1
Bay	158	126	12	38	35	33	8		30	2
Benzie	28	11	3	2	2	1	3	2	15	
Berrien	354	278	51	86	47	60	34	5	65	6
Branch	54	36	2	11	6	10	7		17	1
Calhoun	235	182	36	53	40	32	21	7	44	2
Cass	20	13	3	2	4	2	2		6	1
Charlevoix	65	40	14	5	8	9	4		23	2
Cheboygan	25	18	5	3	1	7	2		7	
Chippewa	43	33	11	4	5	6	7		7	3
Clare	17	15	5	3	2	1	4		2	
Clinton	46	34	8	8	5	5	8	1	8	3
Crawford	18	13	2	4	4	1	2		4	1
Delta	53	40	15	9	7	3	6	2	9	2
Dickinson	72	60	11	12	15	8	14	2	10	
Eaton	90	66	17	19	4	7	19	2	17	5
Emmet	200	139	14	47	34	34	10	6	53	2
Genesee	1,043	823	118	262	108	115	220	29	122	69
Gladwin	11	7	5	1			1		4	
Gogebic	26	24	9	5	6	2	2			2
Grand Traverse	405	317	27	104	73	82	31	12	71	5
Gratiot	58	50	8	14	11	10	7		5	3
Hillsdale	27	21	5	9	2	1	4		5	1
Houghton	59	48	15	8	6	12	7		9	2
Huron	44	34	4	10	9	5	6	1	8	1
Ingham	1,001	720	69	197	125	152	177	91	133	57
Ionia	25	14	9	2	1	2		1	9	1
Iosco	21	16	4	4	5	1	2	1	4	
Iron	14	11	3	3	1	2	2	1	2	
Isabella	77	67	4	24	14	16	9	1	7	2
Jackson	220	173	28	58	38	27	22	3	39	5
Kalamazoo	1,066	812	68	229	131	171	213	58	149	47
Kalkaska	5	4	3			1			1	
Kent	2,013	1,678	159	459	321	359	380	55	213	67
Keweenaw	3								3	
Lake	3	2		1		1		1		
Lapeer	62	43	8	15	7	6	7	3	15	1
Leelanau	46	19	2	3	2	8	4		26	1
Lenawee	107	73	13	24	13	15	8	1	31	2
Livingston	218	168	25	45	25	27	46	8	29	13
Luce	10	7		3			4	1	2	
Mackinac	13	11	6	3		1	1		2	
Macomb	1,170	971	143	358	184	121	165	21	123	55
Manistee	40	28	2	7	7	7	5	1	11	
Marquette	279	221	40	53	39	42	47	7	44	7
Mason	37	31	7	6	9	8	1		6	
Mecosta	43	35	8	9	8	3	7	2	5	1
Menominee	15	13	4	2	2	3	2		1	1
Midland	236	187	41	38	35	39	34	10	35	4
Missaukee	6	4	1	3					2	
Monroe	168	134	26	37	27	24	20	7	20	7

Table 3.9

Physicians by State and County, 2010, continued

		Major Professional Activity								
		Patient Care								
			Office-Based Practice							
State County	Total Physicians	Total Patient Care	FM/GP Practice	Medical Specialties	Surgical Specialties	Other Specialties	Hospital Based Practice	Other Professional Activity	Inactive	Not Classified
Montcalm	29	16	8	2	1	4	1		13	
Montmorency	7	6	4	1	1			1		
Muskegon	286	215	43	57	42	46	27	7	61	3
Newaygo	42	31	15	6	5	3	2		11	
Oakland	7,150	5,717	362	1,675	923	1,102	1,655	218	768	447
Oceana	16	10	6		1	1	2		5	1
Ogemaw	28	25	6	7	5	5	2		3	
Ontonagon	7	4	2		1		1		3	
Osceola	8	7	1	2			4		1	
Oscoda	2								2	
Otsego	40	29	6	7	5	3	8	1	8	2
Ottawa	414	299	56	77	65	75	26	10	99	6
Presque Isle	4	2	1			1			2	
Roscommon	23	16	8	4	2	1	1		5	2
Saginaw	607	505	83	119	86	80	137	23	61	18
Saint Clair	223	187	38	52	42	36	19	3	29	4
Saint Joseph	64	51	17	7	11	7	9		13	
Sanilac	31	21	4	4	6	3	4		9	1
Schoolcraft	9	5	2			1	2		4	
Shiawassee	58	41	8	11	11	6	5		16	1
Tuscola	36	28	4	11	1	6	6	1	6	1
Van Buren	95	77	21	21	10	13	12	1	17	
Washtenaw	4,241	3,149	107	707	337	577	1,421	310	310	472
Wayne	5,529	4,210	285	1,063	509	660	1,693	234	519	566
Wexford	71	54	16	14	10	8	6	1	13	3
Minnesota	18,143	14,377	2,426	3,636	2,082	2,757	3,476	717	2,193	856
Aitkin	20	16	9		2	1	4		3	1
Anoka	473	384	101	107	66	55	55	11	60	18
Becker	55	42	19	4	9	5	5	2	11	
Beltrami	92	74	18	16	16	13	11	3	13	2
Benton	46	36	8	13	3	8	4		9	1
Big Stone	8	7	6				1		1	
Blue Earth	191	150	25	36	39	32	18	5	32	4
Brown	47	44	19	5	10	5	5		3	
Carlton	46	37	23	3	4	3	4	1	7	1
Carver	185	164	51	40	27	23	23	3	18	
Cass	23	15	10		1	2	2		8	
Chippewa	12	9	5		1		3		3	
Chisago	51	44	20	7	7	6	4	1	6	
Clay	35	23	7	4	1	2	9	1	11	
Clearwater	7	5	2	1		1	1		2	
Cook	10	4	4					1	4	1
Cottonwood	13	10	7	1			2		2	1
Crow Wing	179	140	33	26	30	28	23	2	32	5
Dakota	726	586	150	164	75	94	103	21	96	23
Dodge	14	12	7			2	3		2	
Douglas	92	70	24	17	16	4	9	1	20	1
Faribault	8	3	2		1				4	1
Fillmore	11	7	5	1		1			4	
Freeborn	54	41	8	5	7	7	14		13	
Goodhue	98	73	20	12	14	11	16	4	19	2
Grant	1									1
Hennepin	6,217	4,854	533	1,327	797	1,053	1,144	335	737	291
Houston	21	16	7	2	1	4	2	1	3	1
Hubbard	41	27	13	6	2	3	3	1	13	
Isanti	50	37	19	4	4	2	8	3	10	
Itasca	81	66	31	8	13	7	7	2	12	1
Jackson	5	3		1	1		1		2	

Table 3.9

Physicians by State and County, 2010, continued

State County	Total Physicians	Major Professional Activity: Patient Care: Total Patient Care	Office-Based Practice: FM/GP Practice	Office-Based Practice: Medical Specialties	Office-Based Practice: Surgical Specialties	Office-Based Practice: Other Specialties	Hospital Based Practice	Other Professional Activity	Inactive	Not Classified
Kanabec	20	17	13		1		3		3	
Kandiyohi	126	93	31	24	17	12	9	6	25	2
Kittson	3								3	
Koochiching	18	8	4			2	2	1	9	
Lac Qui Parle	9	6	4	1			1		2	1
Lake	24	13	9	1	1	1	1	1	10	
Lake Of The Woods	2	1	1						1	
Le Sueur	8	7	4	1	1		1		1	
Lincoln	5	4	3	1					1	
Lyon	25	22	9	1	8	1	3		3	
Mahnomen	2	2	2							
Marshall	2	1	1						1	
Martin	42	37	14	6	12	3	2		5	
Mcleod	51	44	24	5	4	3	8	2	5	
Meeker	18	16	10	2	2	1	1		2	
Mille Lacs	37	33	20	3	1	3	6	2	2	
Morrison	33	30	13	5	6	3	3	1	2	
Mower	51	39	11	8	5	5	10	1	11	
Murray	6	3	2	1					3	
Nicollet	61	44	20	10	1	6	7	3	14	
Nobles	29	23	7	5	4	2	5		6	
Norman	3	1	1						2	
Olmsted	3,530	2,783	78	678	248	562	1,217	136	280	331
Otter Tail	88	63	21	12	10	12	8	2	22	1
Pennington	24	20	6	6	6		2		4	
Pine	12	10	8	1	1				2	
Pipestone	8	5	4		1				3	
Polk	32	23	9	7	2	1	4		7	2
Pope	15	10	9		1				4	1
Ramsey	2,208	1,764	251	530	232	371	380	99	255	90
Red Lake	1								1	
Redwood	10	9	9						1	
Renville	10	9	7				2		1	
Rice	120	103	43	16	21	11	12	1	15	1
Rock	13	11	10				1		2	
Roseau	15	11	8				3		3	1
Saint Louis	851	669	134	168	113	137	117	15	137	30
Scott	149	122	53	22	13	21	13	5	17	5
Sherburne	42	38	15	9	7	2	5	2	2	
Sibley	5	5	2	2			1			
Stearns	477	412	78	116	82	89	47	12	48	5
Steele	67	53	24	12	11	1	5	1	10	3
Stevens	15	11	4	1	2	1	3		3	1
Swift	5	5	4				1			
Todd	24	20	16	2	1	1			4	
Traverse	1	1	1							
Wabasha	33	26	14	1	4	2	5		7	
Wadena	16	11	9		1		1		5	
Waseca	11	9	7				2		2	
Washington	676	572	151	139	101	107	74	25	57	22
Watonwan	6	5	4			1			1	
Wilkin	4	2					2	1	1	
Winona	69	52	13	11	5	12	11		14	3
Wright	109	90	39	18	9	11	13	3	14	2
Yellow Medicine	10	10	6	1	1	1	1			
Mississippi	6,149	4,900	651	1,256	970	876	1,147	181	828	240
Adams	71	54	10	19	10	11	4	2	12	3
Alcorn	66	59	10	16	16	10	7	1	4	2
Amite	6	4	2		1		1		1	1

Table 3.9

Physicians by State and County, 2010, continued

		Major Professional Activity								
		Patient Care								
			Office-Based Practice							
State County	Total Physicians	Total Patient Care	FM/GP Practice	Medical Specialties	Surgical Specialties	Other Specialties	Hospital Based Practice	Other Professional Activity	Inactive	Not Classified
Attala	16	13	10	2		1			2	1
Benton	3	3				1	2			
Bolivar	44	38	9	10	10	4	5		5	1
Calhoun	3	3	3							
Carroll	5	4		2			2		1	
Chickasaw	10	10	1	3		1	5			
Choctaw	2	1	1						1	
Claiborne	4	3	2		1				1	
Clarke	6	5	3			1	1		1	
Clay	23	17	2	6	7		2		6	
Coahoma	46	38	5	13	11	2	7	2	4	2
Copiah	16	15	10	2	1	2			1	
Covington	7	4	3			1			3	
Desoto	127	105	12	41	35	11	6	4	12	6
Forrest	453	379	44	119	93	85	38	12	53	9
Franklin	5	5	5							
George	15	11	4	1	2	1	3	1	2	1
Greene	3	1				1			2	
Grenada	31	27	3	9	11	1	3		4	
Hancock	58	40	9	5	7	7	12	1	16	1
Harrison	477	394	25	101	88	78	102	9	64	10
Hinds	1,370	1,053	67	248	182	186	370	81	163	73
Holmes	15	12	7	2			3		1	2
Humphreys	6	5	2	3						1
Itawamba	10	6	5			1			3	1
Jackson	320	260	25	73	47	55	60	7	41	12
Jasper	4	3	2	1					1	
Jefferson	6	6	3	1			2			
Jefferson Davis	4	3	2	1					1	
Jones	106	82	12	25	26	10	9	4	18	2
Kemper	1	1		1						
Lafayette	128	90	11	29	24	14	12	2	34	2
Lamar	17	14	5	1	2	3	3		3	
Lauderdale	257	219	26	65	54	47	27		32	6
Lawrence	9	7	5				2		2	
Leake	10	9	3	2		1	3		1	
Lee	343	285	23	99	62	63	38	7	44	7
Leflore	62	50	4	13	11	8	14	2	9	1
Lincoln	46	39	3	14	15	6	1		7	
Lowndes	122	102	12	31	26	21	12	1	18	1
Madison	566	441	47	93	49	94	158	25	49	51
Marion	25	19	8	5	3	2	1		5	1
Marshall	10	7	2	2	1	1	1	1	2	
Monroe	44	34	8	7	6	3	10	1	9	
Montgomery	13	11	8	1			2		2	
Neshoba	25	20	9	4	1	2	4		3	2
Newton	4	3		2			1		1	
Noxubee	8	5	1	2			2		2	1
Oktibbeha	62	52	13	10	13	10	6		8	2
Panola	20	16	6	3	3	3	1		4	
Pearl River	44	28	10	6	5	3	4	1	13	2
Perry	4	2	2						1	1
Pike	80	66	5	13	24	14	10		13	1
Pontotoc	12	7	5			1	1		5	
Prentiss	20	19	6	5	5	2	1		1	
Quitman	6	4	2	1	1				2	
Rankin	478	399	36	66	69	81	147	10	45	24
Scott	10	5	3	1	1				5	
Sharkey	2	1	1						1	

Table 3.9

Physicians by State and County, 2010, continued

		Major Professional Activity								
		Patient Care								
			Office-Based Practice							
State County	Total Physicians	Total Patient Care	FM/GP Practice	Medical Specialties	Surgical Specialties	Other Specialties	Hospital Based Practice	Other Professional Activity	Inactive	Not Classified
Simpson	16	13	10	2	1				2	1
Smith	5	4	2		1	1			1	
Stone	14	9	3	3	1	1	1		4	1
Sunflower	18	12	8	1	1	1	1	1	4	1
Tallahatchie	6	4	2			2			2	
Tate	16	11	3	5	1		2		3	2
Tippah	11	8	6			1	1		3	
Tishomingo	8	6	5		1				2	
Tunica	4	2	1	1					1	1
Union	29	20	6	6	7	1		1	8	
Walthall	10	9	3	5		1			1	
Warren	89	64	14	19	12	4	15	3	21	1
Washington	97	77	11	27	18	12	9	1	17	2
Wayne	11	10	2	2	3		3		1	
Webster	7	3	1	1			1		4	
Wilkinson	7	5	2	2	1			1	1	
Winston	10	7	4				3		3	
Yalobusha	10	7	2	3		1	1		3	
Yazoo	15	11	4			2	5		3	1
Missouri	16,802	13,190	1,128	3,510	2,125	2,337	4,090	682	1,731	1,199
Adair	14	13	3	3	3	1	3	1		
Andrew	3	1			1				2	
Atchison	2	1	1						1	
Audrain	37	32	5	6	8	3	10		4	1
Barry	32	25	14	3	2	1	5	1	4	2
Barton	5	4	1		1	1	1		1	
Bates	3	2	1				1		1	
Benton	6	6	2	1		2	1			
Bollinger	2	1					1		1	
Boone	1,420	1,074	70	200	135	188	481	72	130	144
Buchanan	200	170	17	47	38	40	28	6	18	6
Butler	125	103	17	30	23	12	21	2	18	2
Caldwell	1								1	
Callaway	37	29	11	4	2	3	9		6	2
Camden	70	56	12	9	16	9	10	1	13	
Cape Girardeau	298	260	30	64	62	63	41	4	30	4
Carroll	5	2	1	1					2	1
Carter	2	1			1				1	
Cass	52	35	14	7	5	6	3		16	1
Cedar	7	3			2		1		4	
Chariton	1									1
Christian	89	75	9	13	11	26	16	2	9	3
Clay	392	329	42	98	77	50	62	11	33	19
Clinton	12	11	6	2	2		1	1		
Cole	179	144	13	42	39	32	18	7	24	4
Cooper	9	8	5	1		1	1		1	
Crawford	8	7	3		1	3			1	
Dade	4	3	3						1	
Dallas	1	1				1				
Daviess	1									1
Dekalb	1	1	1							
Dent	5	4	2	1			1		1	
Douglas	4	3	2	1					1	
Dunklin	39	32	11	8	6	2	5	1	2	4
Franklin	130	116	31	36	25	15	9	3	11	
Gasconade	12	7	3	1			3	2	3	
Gentry	5	5	1	1	1		2			
Greene	913	763	82	223	166	173	119	16	124	10

Table 3.9

Physicians by State and County, 2010, continued

State County	Total Physicians	Major Professional Activity Patient Care Total Patient Care	Office-Based Practice FM/GP Practice	Medical Specialties	Surgical Specialties	Other Specialties	Hospital Based Practice	Other Professional Activity	Inactive	Not Classified
Grundy	10	7	5	1			1		3	
Harrison	6	6	5			1				
Henry	19	16	9	1	2	3	1		2	1
Hickory	3	2		2					1	
Holt	2	2	2							
Howard	6	5	2			1	2		1	
Howell	68	58	18	11	10	8	11		7	3
Iron	8	5	1	1	1	2			3	
Jackson	2,045	1,620	131	433	216	264	576	89	199	137
Jasper	305	255	19	80	51	45	60	3	40	7
Jefferson	121	98	10	33	15	15	25	2	17	4
Johnson	46	44	14	8	7	6	9	2		
Knox	1								1	
Laclede	27	27	10	7	3	2	5			
Lafayette	11	8	4			2	2		2	1
Lawrence	37	32	13	1		5	13	1	3	1
Lewis	1	1	1							
Lincoln	7	7	4	1	2					
Linn	6	6	2	3			1			
Livingston	12	7	2	2	1	1	1		5	
Macon	7	5	5						2	
Madison	6	5	1	2	2				1	
Maries	4	3	1			1	1		1	
Marion	73	60	4	24	14	7	11		10	3
Mcdonald	3	1	1						2	
Mercer	1	1	1							
Miller	9	7	5	1		1			2	
Mississippi	3	3	3							
Moniteau	4	2	2						2	
Monroe	1								1	
Montgomery	5	3		1			2	1	1	
Morgan	6	3	1	2					3	
New Madrid	3	3	2	1						
Newton	22	13	4	2	3	1	3		9	
Nodaway	29	28	8	5	7	5	3		1	
Oregon	3	3	1			2				
Ozark	1	1	1							
Pemiscot	11	11		3	2		6			
Perry	15	11	5	1	2	2	1		3	1
Pettis	48	37	6	10	11	6	4	2	9	
Phelps	76	65	11	24	12	9	9	1	6	4
Pike	11	6	2	1		1	2		5	
Platte	182	150	21	33	27	34	35	6	15	11
Polk	32	26	12	4	6	1	3	1	4	1
Pulaski	28	23	9	2	1	4	7	1	2	2
Ralls	2	2		1		1				
Randolph	16	9		4	3	2			7	
Ray	9	6	2	2	1		1		3	
Reynolds	2	2		2						
Ripley	4	3	1	1		1				1
Saint Charles	416	345	48	128	70	40	59	6	50	15
Saint Clair	6	5	4	1						1
Saint Francois	76	56	13	22	5	6	10	2	13	5
Saint Louis	5,609	4,356	178	1,463	792	895	1,028	196	679	378
Saint Louis City	2,905	2,163	38	334	201	297	1,293	233	98	411
Sainte Genevieve	12	9	2	3	2		2		3	
Saline	19	15	9	1	3		2		3	1
Scotland	3	3	1				2			

Table 3.9

Physicians by State and County, 2010, continued

		Major Professional Activity									
		Patient Care									
			Office-Based Practice								
State County	Total Physicians	Total Patient Care	FM/GP Practice	Medical Specialties	Surgical Specialties	Other Specialties	Hospital Based Practice	Other Professional Activity	Inactive	Not Classified
Scott	55	43	8	10	7	5	13	1	10	1
Shannon	3	3		1		1	1			
Shelby	2	1				1			1	
Stoddard	16	15	6	5	2	1	1		1	
Stone	20	13	3	4	2	1	3		7	
Taney	87	72	21	14	10	9	18	4	8	3
Texas	14	11	5	1	1	1	3		2	1
Vernon	23	15	3	3	2	6	1		8	
Warren	7	6	2	1		2	1		1	
Washington	5	4				1	3		1	
Wayne	5	4	3	1					1	
Webster	29	21	6	5	2	6	2		8	
Wright	7	5	4	1				1		1
Montana	2,658	1,990	377	452	418	446	297	66	550	52
Beaverhead	15	13	3	3	2	2	3		1	1
Big Horn	22	19	8		1	2	8	1	2	
Blaine	5	4	1	2			1			1
Broadwater	8	4	2		1	1			4	
Carbon	16	8	5			2	1	1	7	
Cascade	239	181	24	51	38	51	17	6	51	1
Custer	25	18	3	9	3		3	1	6	
Dawson	12	10	4	2	3	1			2	
Deer Lodge	15	11	3	1	1	2	4		4	
Fallon	1	1	1							
Fergus	20	17	8	3	1		5	1	2	
Flathead	307	220	39	49	56	62	14	6	73	8
Gallatin	291	193	44	46	41	47	15	7	84	7
Glacier	18	13	8	1	1	1	2	1	4	
Golden Valley	1	1		1						
Granite	1	1					1			
Hill	29	21	5	3	8	1	4		7	1
Jefferson	26	19	4	4	2	7	2	2	5	
Lake	47	26	15	1	6	1	3		19	2
Lewis And Clark	200	157	18	33	28	36	42	6	36	1
Liberty	4	3	3					1		
Lincoln	30	20	11	1	3	1	4	1	9	
Madison	13	6	3	1			2		7	
Meagher	1	1					1			
Mineral	4	3	1	1		1			1	
Missoula	429	326	37	88	70	85	46	9	86	8
Musselshell	4	2					2		2	
Park	31	21	10	2	6	2	1	1	9	
Phillips	1	1	1							
Pondera	5	4	3				1		1	
Powell	11	10	6			1	3		1	
Prairie	1	1	1							
Ravalli	79	57	17	11	9	12	8	6	15	1
Richland	17	14	2	3	3	3	3		3	
Roosevelt	5	3	3						1	1
Rosebud	6	5	5						1	
Sanders	10	9	3		2	1	3		1	
Sheridan	1	1	1							
Silver Bow	81	62	8	19	17	10	8	2	17	
Stillwater	6	4	2		1		1		2	
Sweet Grass	3	1	1						2	
Teton	4	2	2					1	1	
Toole	6	5	4				1		1	

Table 3.9

Physicians by State and County, 2010, continued

		Major Professional Activity								
		Patient Care								
			Office-Based Practice							
State County	Total Physicians	Total Patient Care	FM/GP Practice	Medical Specialties	Surgical Specialties	Other Specialties	Hospital Based Practice	Other Professional Activity	Inactive	Not Classified
Treasure	1								1	
Valley	10	9	2	1	5		1	1		
Yellowstone	597	483	56	116	110	114	87	12	82	20
Nebraska	5,150	4,061	695	910	713	711	1,032	199	628	262
Adams	84	63	14	17	20	11	1	3	16	2
Antelope	5	4	3	1					1	
Boone	8	8	6	1			1			
Box Butte	7	7	4			1	2			
Boyd	5	4	4						1	
Brown	2	1		1					1	
Buffalo	136	121	19	36	37	21	8		14	1
Burt	4	2	2						2	
Butler	9	6	6						3	
Cass	23	20	5	2	2	6	5		3	
Cedar	4	4	2			1	1			
Chase	1	1	1							
Cherry	6	5	3	1			1		1	
Cheyenne	10	7	5				2		3	
Clay	2	1	1						1	
Colfax	4	1					1	1	2	
Cuming	5	3	3						2	
Custer	12	9	8				1		2	1
Dakota	5	3	2		1				2	
Dawes	11	7	6				1		4	
Dawson	20	19	13		3	1	2		1	
Deuel	2	2		1	1					
Dixon	2	1	1							1
Dodge	58	47	13	11	14	7	2	1	10	
Douglas	2,928	2,279	200	533	387	404	755	142	305	202
Dundy	2	1					1		1	
Fillmore	5	5	5							
Franklin	3	2	1				1		1	
Frontier	1	1					1			
Furnas	3	2	2						1	
Gage	29	21	12	5	1		3	1	4	3
Garden	2								2	
Garfield	2	1	1						1	
Gosper	1	1		1						
Hall	122	101	18	28	27	19	9	2	16	3
Hamilton	15	11	8	1		2			4	
Harlan	2	1	1						1	
Holt	14	12	9	1			2	1	1	
Hooker	2	2	2							
Howard	5	4	2				2		1	
Jefferson	5	5	5							
Johnson	4	4	3				1			
Kearney	6	5	1				4		1	
Keith	8	8	4	1	1		2			
Knox	7	5	5						2	
Lancaster	778	609	104	179	121	140	65	26	125	18
Lincoln	89	68	14	15	13	18	8	1	12	8
Madison	83	71	16	12	14	15	14	1	8	3
Merrick	3	3	3							
Morrill	4	1	1						2	1
Nance	1								1	
Nemaha	8	7	5				2		1	
Nuckolls	6	5	5						1	
Otoe	12	8	6				2		4	

Table 3.9

Physicians by State and County, 2010, continued

		Major Professional Activity									
		Patient Care									
			Office-Based Practice								
State County	Total Physicians	Total Patient Care	FM/GP Practice	Medical Specialties	Surgical Specialties	Other Specialties	Hospital Based Practice	Other Professional Activity	Inactive	Not Classified
Pawnee	2	2	2							
Perkins	4	4	4							
Phelps	12	10	7	2	1			1	1	
Pierce	9	8	6	1		1			1	
Platte	36	31	10	4	11	3	3		5	
Polk	2	2	1				1			
Red Willow	12	10	7		2		1		2	
Richardson	3	2	2						1	
Rock	2	1	1						1	
Saline	10	7	4				3	1	2	
Sarpy	275	234	37	42	31	34	90	13	12	16
Saunders	14	10	6			2	2	1	3	
Scotts Bluff	100	80	16	11	19	19	15	1	19	
Seward	15	12	7		1	1	3		3	
Sheridan	7	5	3		1		1		2	
Sherman	2	1	1						1	
Sioux	1								1	
Stanton	1	1				1				
Thayer	6	5	2				3		1	
Thurston	9	8	4	1	1		2		1	
Valley	5	3	1			2			1	1
Washington	22	17	4	2	2	2	7	2	2	1
Wayne	6	4	4						1	1
Webster	3	3	3							
York	17	12	9		2		1	1	4	
Nevada	5,899	4,558	497	1,431	861	1,163	606	148	896	297
Carson City	152	128	16	35	31	35	11	4	19	1
Churchill	26	21	6	3	4	1	7		3	2
Clark	4,088	3,149	299	1,075	576	798	401	99	634	206
Douglas	106	73	14	15	14	19	11	3	27	3
Elko	58	47	9	13	15	6	4	1	9	1
Humboldt	10	10	4	1		1	4			
Lander	3	2	1	1					1	
Lincoln	2	2	2							
Lyon	18	13	7	2		1	3		4	1
Mineral	7	6	2	2			2		1	
Nye	31	19	8	4		4	3	1	10	1
Pershing	2								2	
Storey	1	1		1						
Washoe	1,382	1,075	125	277	218	297	158	40	185	82
White Pine	13	12	4	2	3	1	2		1	
New Hampshire	4,563	3,492	407	928	588	635	934	164	686	221
Belknap	170	122	8	37	31	31	15	5	39	4
Carroll	134	82	12	14	16	13	27	4	45	3
Cheshire	197	131	29	32	25	23	22	5	60	1
Coos	87	67	17	12	7	14	17	1	17	2
Grafton	1,263	945	46	157	100	120	522	72	125	121
Hillsborough	1,078	868	98	311	166	189	104	34	146	30
Merrimack	558	419	71	106	85	80	77	22	90	27
Rockingham	685	552	83	174	109	106	80	12	98	23
Strafford	273	218	29	66	40	44	39	6	43	6
Sullivan	118	88	14	19	9	15	31	3	23	4
New Jersey	30,976	23,757	1,205	8,445	4,145	4,710	5,252	1,420	3,825	1,974
Atlantic	693	541	27	179	128	109	98	19	103	30
Bergen	5,270	4,023	107	1,449	744	916	807	225	716	306
Burlington	1,288	1,011	97	344	163	244	163	52	171	54
Camden	1,949	1,511	103	463	249	281	415	80	226	132
Cape May	148	93	9	22	21	30	11	2	51	2

Table 3.9

Physicians by State and County, 2010, continued

		Major Professional Activity									
		Patient Care									
			Office-Based Practice								
State County	Total Physicians	Total Patient Care	FM/GP Practice	Medical Specialties	Surgical Specialties	Other Specialties	Hospital Based Practice	Other Professional Activity	Inactive	Not Classified
Cumberland	211	168	14	71	40	25	18	6	33	4
Essex	3,689	2,780	85	892	510	514	779	212	420	277
Gloucester	370	296	43	93	40	56	64	14	35	25
Hudson	1,345	1,034	64	354	135	144	337	29	130	152
Hunterdon	469	355	80	90	58	72	55	36	63	15
Mercer	1,622	1,176	59	444	216	253	204	132	207	107
Middlesex	3,177	2,491	116	887	329	418	741	146	256	284
Monmouth	2,762	2,204	87	826	404	488	399	83	327	148
Morris	2,178	1,630	62	598	293	351	326	129	282	137
Ocean	966	726	31	350	159	119	67	24	192	24
Passaic	1,155	914	42	375	167	135	195	36	137	68
Salem	65	42	7	12	11	7	5	2	18	3
Somerset	1,613	1,249	92	416	195	268	278	100	172	92
Sussex	229	164	11	61	35	39	18	4	51	10
Union	1,583	1,213	51	478	218	220	246	84	199	87
Warren	194	136	18	41	30	21	26	5	36	17
New Mexico	5,759	4,311	634	1,091	631	885	1,070	271	841	336
Bernalillo	3,139	2,364	217	581	332	480	754	184	357	234
Catron	4	3	2			1			1	
Chaves	134	111	27	31	22	18	13	1	16	6
Cibola	26	21	10	5	4		2		3	2
Colfax	24	14	5	3	3	2	1	1	8	1
Curry	63	53	6	25	11	7	4		7	3
De Baca	1	1	1							
Dona Ana	374	291	65	78	51	56	41	10	53	20
Eddy	70	53	7	12	16	7	11	1	13	3
Grant	79	61	10	19	11	16	5	2	16	
Guadalupe	2	2	1	1						
Hidalgo	2	1			1				1	
Lea	58	47	6	17	7	8	9		8	3
Lincoln	36	24	6	5	3	5	5		12	
Los Alamos	66	48	13	22	6	7		2	14	2
Luna	27	23	4	6	5	2	6	1	3	
Mckinley	169	134	31	26	15	12	50	5	24	6
Mora	1								1	
Otero	86	65	18	15	11	10	11	3	14	4
Quay	6	6	4	2						
Rio Arriba	45	36	12	3	6	9	6		8	1
Roosevelt	13	12	3	4	2	2	1		1	
San Juan	206	163	26	41	32	31	33	4	27	12
San Miguel	47	41	8	15	4	8	6	1	5	
Sandoval	233	173	42	49	12	46	24	13	40	7
Santa Fe	660	433	72	99	62	135	65	35	168	24
Sierra	18	9	1	5	1	2			8	1
Socorro	19	15	5	2	1	2	5		3	1
Taos	103	72	18	15	12	14	13	5	23	3
Torrance	1	1	1							
Union	6	5	2	1		1	1	1		
Valencia	41	29	11	9	1	4	4	2	7	3
New York	86,293	64,089	2,876	18,505	9,320	11,709	21,679	4,154	10,115	7,935
Albany	1,872	1,445	65	396	252	271	461	97	200	130
Allegany	42	29	6	7	8	4	4	1	10	2
Bronx	3,749	2,734	101	700	215	312	1,406	215	274	526
Broome	637	465	39	133	101	91	101	26	126	20
Cattaraugus	134	101	18	39	18	16	10	2	29	2
Cayuga	94	64	2	25	17	12	8	2	27	1
Chautauqua	199	148	22	47	31	38	10	1	44	6
Chemung	270	207	15	65	37	53	37	10	49	4

Table 3.9

Physicians by State and County, 2010, continued

		Major Professional Activity								
		Patient Care								
			Office-Based Practice							
State County	Total Physicians	Total Patient Care	FM/GP Practice	Medical Specialties	Surgical Specialties	Other Specialties	Hospital Based Practice	Other Professional Activity	Inactive	Not Classified
Chenango	69	46	14	5	10	7	10	5	14	4
Clinton	222	178	14	58	35	46	25	3	32	9
Columbia	120	83	13	19	12	21	18	6	26	5
Cortland	71	56	13	18	10	8	7		14	1
Delaware	48	34	12	10	3	3	6	1	9	4
Dutchess	908	697	49	235	149	161	103	32	154	25
Erie	3,841	2,868	170	760	466	517	955	208	479	286
Essex	44	23	10	4	2	5	2	1	19	1
Franklin	103	71	11	21	10	14	15	3	25	4
Fulton	70	52	11	16	11	7	7	1	16	1
Genesee	80	60	6	16	12	15	11		18	2
Greene	42	29	6	12	2	6	3	1	11	1
Hamilton	3	1	1					1	1	
Herkimer	48	35	9	14	4	3	5		12	1
Jefferson	233	168	15	37	35	40	41	5	52	8
Kings	7,871	5,851	202	1,697	570	720	2,662	302	575	1,143
Lewis	28	24	9	5	4	2	4		4	
Livingston	71	55	15	16	13	5	6	4	12	
Madison	110	95	23	20	20	19	13	2	11	2
Monroe	3,932	2,932	147	837	401	460	1,087	236	452	312
Montgomery	87	64	11	23	11	9	10	3	20	
Nassau	9,436	7,378	202	2,440	1,231	1,354	2,151	333	1,128	597
New York	21,452	15,251	226	3,493	2,116	3,081	6,335	1,450	1,978	2,773
Niagara	293	221	41	67	46	31	36	3	60	9
Oneida	616	477	68	139	93	94	83	9	104	26
Onondaga	2,435	1,884	162	420	310	355	637	118	284	149
Ontario	321	243	22	80	45	50	46	7	62	9
Orange	930	745	41	337	129	162	76	24	123	38
Orleans	32	26	3	8	6	4	5		6	
Oswego	112	92	19	31	19	11	12	2	17	1
Otsego	347	282	9	83	70	54	66	10	42	13
Putnam	222	169	5	64	34	42	24	10	39	4
Queens	6,416	4,706	195	1,559	480	671	1,801	190	801	719
Rensselaer	300	228	29	68	33	38	60	20	40	12
Richmond	1,965	1,507	34	513	210	236	514	60	211	187
Rockland	1,332	1,013	37	392	165	223	196	56	196	67
Saint Lawrence	183	146	16	42	30	28	30	4	26	7
Saratoga	502	408	70	107	72	82	77	14	58	22
Schenectady	526	393	49	106	76	89	73	19	94	20
Schoharie	22	16	5	6	1	2	2	1	5	
Schuyler	27	19	4	4	2	3	6	1	6	1
Seneca	22	15	4	4	2	4	1		6	1
Steuben	165	129	21	40	23	19	26	3	30	3
Suffolk	5,118	3,823	216	1,164	638	844	961	202	801	292
Sullivan	121	90	11	31	17	13	18	2	25	4
Tioga	42	33	12	4	3	6	8		8	1
Tompkins	307	235	38	66	36	61	34	10	57	5
Ulster	386	304	82	68	45	64	45	9	55	18
Warren	268	209	30	69	49	39	22	9	47	3
Washington	41	26	10	7	1	3	5	1	14	
Wayne	83	56	8	22	11	7	8	1	23	3
Westchester	7,190	5,286	157	1,817	859	1,166	1,287	416	1,040	448
Wyoming	51	40	11	14	8	4	3		8	3
Yates	32	24	10	5	1	4	4	2	6	
North Carolina	27,850	21,593	2,481	6,118	3,752	4,225	5,017	1,213	3,425	1,619
Alamance	274	215	24	82	44	37	28	7	45	7
Alexander	15	11	6	1	1	2	1	1	3	
Alleghany	21	14	8	3	1	1	1	1	5	1

Table 3.9

Physicians by State and County, 2010, continued

		Major Professional Activity								
		Patient Care								
			Office-Based Practice							
State County	Total Physicians	Total Patient Care	FM/GP Practice	Medical Specialties	Surgical Specialties	Other Specialties	Hospital Based Practice	Other Professional Activity	Inactive	Not Classified
Anson	15	14	8	4		1	1		1	
Ashe	36	23	14		3	5	1	1	11	1
Avery	18	10	4	1	3		2		8	
Beaufort	85	54	11	11	10	9	13		29	2
Bertie	6	5	3	1			1		1	
Bladen	25	19	8	4	3	1	3	2	3	1
Brunswick	139	96	18	31	15	13	19	3	39	1
Buncombe	1,275	966	139	281	171	194	181	35	247	27
Burke	195	153	28	33	32	34	26	3	34	5
Cabarrus	440	379	61	127	67	70	54	6	38	17
Caldwell	97	78	21	12	15	17	13	2	16	1
Camden	9	6		1	2	2	1		3	
Carteret	152	115	16	23	28	23	25	1	33	3
Caswell	9	5		2		2	1		4	
Catawba	437	360	55	94	91	94	26	8	62	7
Chatham	101	54	14	17	3	9	11	5	36	6
Cherokee	37	31	5	10	6	6	4		6	
Chowan	32	27	6	5	10	4	2		5	
Clay	13	12	3	1	1	3	4		1	
Cleveland	168	132	19	50	27	25	11	1	34	1
Columbus	57	49	10	16	15	4	4	1	7	
Craven	271	221	17	89	48	50	17	5	38	7
Cumberland	820	679	91	191	122	104	171	23	78	40
Currituck	12	8	2	1		3	2	1	3	
Dare	62	45	12	10	9	8	6	1	13	3
Davidson	115	91	22	29	23	10	7		22	2
Davie	72	47	9	13	4	14	7	3	19	3
Duplin	31	28	10	9	4	3	2	1	2	
Durham	3,349	2,381	79	454	241	358	1,249	250	220	498
Edgecombe	43	31	8	11	6	4	2	2	9	1
Forsyth	2,324	1,808	120	407	241	328	712	118	210	188
Franklin	28	21	4	10	3	1	3	1	6	
Gaston	374	322	45	111	66	72	28	1	44	7
Gates	2	1		1						1
Graham	5	2	2						2	1
Granville	67	48	20	9	7	4	8	5	10	4
Greene	2	2	1	1						
Guilford	1,470	1,198	143	401	269	242	143	42	189	41
Halifax	79	64	10	27	13	10	4	1	12	2
Harnett	70	61	11	21	9	14	6	1	5	3
Haywood	142	104	21	28	18	22	15	1	36	1
Henderson	305	217	34	63	46	44	30	8	72	8
Hertford	43	35	9	6	10	5	5	1	5	2
Hoke	13	10	3		1	1	5	1	1	1
Hyde	2	1				1			1	
Iredell	340	297	42	95	79	57	24	4	37	2
Jackson	116	79	22	20	14	12	11	2	33	2
Johnston	107	90	33	20	21	6	10	2	14	1
Jones	12	12	1	9	1	1				
Lee	89	66	12	19	11	16	8	5	16	2
Lenoir	108	79	12	32	15	16	4	3	25	1
Lincoln	77	66	20	18	12	8	8	1	8	2
Macon	101	72	12	18	11	24	7	1	28	
Madison	17	12	7	2		1	2		5	
Martin	19	16	6	5	3	1	1	1	2	
Mcdowell	38	30	9	7	8	2	4		8	
Mecklenburg	3,159	2,660	236	873	505	574	472	100	308	91
Mitchell	31	24	10	3	6	1	4		5	2
Montgomery	12	10	4	3		1	2	1	1	

Table 3.9

Physicians by State and County, 2010, continued

		Major Professional Activity								
		Patient Care								
			Office-Based Practice							
State County	Total Physicians	Total Patient Care	FM/GP Practice	Medical Specialties	Surgical Specialties	Other Specialties	Hospital Based Practice	Other Professional Activity	Inactive	Not Classified
Moore	407	318	15	93	71	84	55	12	69	8
Nash	169	146	19	46	41	27	13	3	20	
New Hanover	856	676	55	222	146	156	97	20	134	26
Northampton	7	4	2	1		1			3	
Onslow	269	206	32	38	40	28	68	3	33	27
Orange	2,306	1,565	85	368	170	367	575	274	214	253
Pamlico	11	8	3	3	1	1			3	
Pasquotank	95	76	10	25	23	16	2	1	15	3
Pender	31	20	8	5		6	1		9	2
Perquimans	6	5	2	1		2			1	
Person	45	32	4	11	4	6	7	3	9	1
Pitt	1,103	852	58	216	114	162	302	78	67	106
Polk	54	29	7	6	4	9	3	1	24	
Randolph	143	114	32	41	16	17	8	4	20	5
Richmond	44	32	7	13	7	2	3	1	9	2
Robeson	149	124	22	33	27	19	23	2	17	6
Rockingham	87	75	19	22	15	8	11	1	10	1
Rowan	243	184	22	47	39	32	44	6	46	7
Rutherford	98	80	17	24	14	16	9	2	15	1
Sampson	54	47	15	14	10	6	2	1	6	
Scotland	65	59	14	22	11	7	5		5	1
Stanly	78	62	11	21	15	9	6		15	1
Stokes	22	18	7	1	2	5	3		2	2
Surry	101	85	24	26	21	4	10	2	11	3
Swain	19	18	9	5	1		3		1	
Transylvania	88	49	11	17	8	5	8	5	34	
Union	276	237	44	76	46	51	20	6	26	7
Vance	60	49	13	14	10	8	4		10	1
Wake	2,753	2,172	243	722	420	505	282	111	319	151
Warren	7	5	3		1		1		2	
Washington	8	6	4	1	1				2	
Watauga	174	124	19	40	31	29	5	4	44	2
Wayne	208	169	29	52	31	35	22	4	30	5
Wilkes	68	54	13	19	14	6	2	2	11	1
Wilson	115	94	7	39	22	17	9	1	19	1
Yadkin	23	18	9	1	2	4	2	1	4	
Yancey	25	15	7	7		1		2	8	
North Dakota	1,832	1,514	273	338	265	269	369	61	216	41
Adams	15	14	7	3	1	2	1		1	
Barnes	13	9	5	2	2				4	
Benson	1	1					1			
Bottineau	5	4	2	1			1		1	
Bowman	3	2	2						1	
Burleigh	362	296	39	65	59	66	67	12	39	15
Cass	685	571	60	161	94	110	146	25	75	14
Cavalier	3	1	1						2	
Dickey	4	4		2	1		1			
Divide	2	2	1	1						
Emmons	2	2	1				1			
Foster	5	3	1				2		2	
Grand Forks	278	235	47	38	42	44	64	17	20	6
Griggs	1								1	
Kidder	1									1
Lamoure	1	1		1						
Mchenry	2	1				1			1	
Mcintosh	2	2			1		1			
Mckenzie	2	2	1				1			

Table 3.9

Physicians by State and County, 2010, continued

		Major Professional Activity								
		Patient Care								
			Office-Based Practice							
State County	Total Physicians	Total Patient Care	FM/GP Practice	Medical Specialties	Surgical Specialties	Other Specialties	Hospital Based Practice	Other Professional Activity	Inactive	Not Classified
Mclean	4	2					2		1	1
Mercer	6	6	5		1					
Morton	21	18	9		4	3	2		3	
Mountrail	5	5	4	1						
Nelson	2	1	1						1	
Pembina	6	5	1	1	1		2		1	
Pierce	4	4	3		1					
Ramsey	24	21	8	8	3	2			3	
Ransom	9	6	4				2		3	
Renville	2								2	
Richland	26	17	6	1	5	1	4	1	8	
Rolette	15	11	4	2		1	4	1	3	
Sioux	1	1					1			
Stark	34	27	6	6	5	2	8		7	
Stutsman	29	27	13	3	5	3	3		2	
Towner	3							1	2	
Traill	4	3	2	1					1	
Walsh	13	9	6		1	1	1		4	
Ward	186	161	21	38	28	27	47	4	17	4
Wells	3	2	1				1		1	
Williams	48	38	12	3	11	6	6		10	
Ohio	35,925	27,702	2,763	7,341	4,361	5,076	8,161	1,340	4,190	2,693
Adams	16	11	2	5		1	3		5	
Allen	256	206	28	53	52	53	20	4	41	5
Ashland	63	48	11	13	10	7	7		14	1
Ashtabula	89	59	12	22	12	7	6	1	27	2
Athens	60	45	9	11	11	8	6	2	11	2
Auglaize	82	65	16	21	7	14	7	1	11	5
Belmont	86	66	11	19	15	9	12	2	17	1
Brown	29	21	11	4	4		2		6	2
Butler	534	428	76	141	72	79	60	11	74	21
Carroll	15	12	4	2	1	2	3		3	
Champaign	17	13	6	5		2			3	1
Clark	221	175	28	57	39	37	14	9	35	2
Clermont	299	233	34	73	33	50	43	7	48	11
Clinton	83	67	17	15	8	11	16	3	6	7
Columbiana	102	79	16	26	19	10	8		20	3
Coshocton	27	23	2	7	9	1	4		4	
Crawford	36	22	2	6	7	1	6	2	12	
Cuyahoga	8,989	6,624	253	1,608	874	1,088	2,801	370	868	1,127
Darke	37	30	19	4	2	1	4	1	5	1
Defiance	50	39	13	8	11	5	2	1	9	1
Delaware	618	516	80	155	79	133	69	19	53	30
Erie	141	110	11	36	24	33	6	3	24	4
Fairfield	235	195	45	52	27	46	25	7	23	10
Fayette	19	14	7	3	2		2		5	
Franklin	5,088	3,975	358	956	620	690	1,351	224	454	435
Fulton	49	33	15	8	3	6	1	1	11	4
Gallia	99	83	6	37	17	20	3	4	11	1
Geauga	238	185	16	50	32	46	41	5	38	10
Greene	497	397	59	76	32	65	165	18	38	44
Guernsey	64	48	6	16	14	6	6		14	2
Hamilton	5,081	3,862	230	1,011	619	748	1,254	277	544	398
Hancock	151	121	13	37	32	26	13	1	25	4
Hardin	18	13	4	3		3	3		5	
Harrison	11	10	3	2	1		4		1	
Henry	17	14	9	1	1	2	1		3	
Highland	34	28	11	6	3	3	5		5	1

Table 3.9

Physicians by State and County, 2010, continued

		Major Professional Activity								
		Patient Care								
			Office-Based Practice							
State County	Total Physicians	Total Patient Care	FM/GP Practice	Medical Specialties	Surgical Specialties	Other Specialties	Hospital Based Practice	Other Professional Activity	Inactive	Not Classified
Hocking	19	13	5	3	2	2	1		6	
Holmes	29	24	13	2	2	6	1	1	4	
Huron	79	63	26	8	15	10	4	2	14	
Jackson	18	13	4	2	3	1	3	1	4	
Jefferson	96	73	9	26	18	12	8		18	5
Knox	70	50	9	15	9	6	11	3	17	
Lake	370	298	23	103	60	61	51	5	51	16
Lawrence	71	55	11	14	8	8	14	3	6	7
Licking	183	146	32	36	25	39	14	5	30	2
Logan	53	40	12	5	6	2	15	4	6	3
Lorain	549	413	49	146	65	81	72	5	101	30
Lucas	1,902	1,481	160	383	255	300	383	72	224	125
Madison	43	35	11	9	4	4	7		6	2
Mahoning	758	588	43	182	99	92	172	24	99	47
Marion	123	100	9	31	27	19	14	3	17	3
Medina	291	234	44	68	46	39	37	7	36	14
Meigs	6	4	3			1			2	
Mercer	37	28	8	6	5	3	6	1	7	1
Miami	130	102	22	24	14	21	21	3	22	3
Monroe	2	1	1						1	
Montgomery	2,037	1,609	194	454	251	303	407	87	252	89
Morgan	1	1	1							
Morrow	10	7	5		1		1		3	
Muskingum	162	130	19	42	34	25	10		29	3
Noble	3	1	1						2	
Ottawa	56	38	16	4	3	9	6	2	16	
Paulding	8	6	3	1			2		2	
Perry	7	5	3	1			1	1	1	
Pickaway	51	39	11	8	7	6	7	3	9	
Pike	25	16	4	5		1	6		8	1
Portage	195	156	16	37	21	33	49	5	32	2
Preble	11	9	5	4					2	
Putnam	19	17	10	3	1	1	2		2	
Richland	228	173	14	63	39	38	19	2	51	2
Ross	135	116	27	24	21	18	26	1	16	2
Sandusky	53	41	19	8	6	5	3	1	10	1
Scioto	125	99	11	29	14	24	21	2	21	3
Seneca	56	46	8	12	11	13	2		7	3
Shelby	47	39	13	8	8	4	6	1	7	
Stark	950	755	81	263	136	133	142	25	132	38
Summit	1,872	1,498	150	405	238	266	439	66	206	102
Trumbull	293	215	19	71	44	51	30	8	69	1
Tuscarawas	112	81	18	20	19	11	13	2	27	2
Union	39	33	6	9	11	5	2		5	1
Van Wert	27	23	10	4	5	3	1		3	1
Vinton	2	2	1			1				
Warren	526	442	58	140	51	111	82	14	41	29
Washington	99	79	14	22	15	18	10		18	2
Wayne	160	129	26	36	38	16	13	2	24	5
Williams	42	37	14	9	8	1	5		5	
Wood	279	220	44	47	22	59	48	6	40	13
Wyandot	15	9	5		2	1	1		6	
Oklahoma	7,619	6,030	863	1,514	1,122	1,198	1,333	269	1,044	276
Adair	16	14	6	3		2	3		2	
Atoka	1									1
Beaver	3	3	2				1			
Beckham	32	28	7	6	6	4	5	1	3	
Blaine	9	6	5		1				3	
Bryan	34	27	3	11	9	2	2		7	

Table 3.9

Physicians by State and County, 2010, continued

			Major Professional Activity							
		Patient Care								
			Office-Based Practice							
State County	Total Physicians	Total Patient Care	FM/GP Practice	Medical Specialties	Surgical Specialties	Other Specialties	Hospital Based Practice	Other Professional Activity	Inactive	Not Classified
Caddo	7	4	2	1			1	1	2	
Canadian	98	75	26	14	9	8	18	4	15	4
Carter	81	66	3	19	19	11	14	2	12	1
Cherokee	64	52	8	7	10	8	19	3	7	2
Choctaw	8	6	3		2		1		2	
Cimarron	3	2	2						1	
Cleveland	462	371	51	87	46	88	99	10	60	21
Comanche	263	206	39	40	44	40	43	7	32	18
Cotton	3	3	2		1					
Craig	17	11	7			1	3		4	2
Creek	34	26	11	6	1	3	5		6	2
Custer	32	25	11	3	5		6		7	
Delaware	36	28	14	2	7	1	4	1	7	
Dewey	2	2	2							
Ellis	6	4	4						2	
Garfield	115	90	17	21	22	22	8		22	3
Garvin	8	5	3	1			1		3	
Grady	42	32	5	10	6	7	4	1	8	1
Grant	1								1	
Greer	9	5	2			1	2		4	
Harmon	1	1	1							
Harper	1	1	1							
Haskell	4	4	2	1	1					
Hughes	2								2	
Jackson	33	25	4	6	6	3	6		6	2
Jefferson	2	1	1						1	
Johnston	6	2	1	1					4	
Kay	60	44	14	9	11	9	1	3	13	
Kingfisher	11	7	3	1			3		3	1
Kiowa	9	8	4	1	1	2			1	
Latimer	18	17	3	4	4	1	5		1	
Le Flore	16	11	2		4	1	4		5	
Lincoln	13	9	7	1		1			4	
Logan	20	17	2	5		4	6		2	1
Love	4	2	2					1	1	
Major	5	5	4				1			
Marshall	3	2	1	1					1	
Mayes	20	19	7	4	3	1	4		1	
Mcclain	22	22	9	3		2	8			
Mccurtain	17	15	6	4	4	1			2	
Mcintosh	8	6	3	2			1		2	
Murray	7	5	3				2		2	
Muskogee	124	94	9	38	20	10	17	1	29	
Noble	8	3	3						4	1
Nowata	3	3	1	1		1				
Okfuskee	5	3	3						2	
Oklahoma	3,163	2,525	246	602	462	562	653	162	332	144
Okmulgee	21	15	4	6	2	1	2	1	5	
Osage	8	5	1			2	2		3	
Ottawa	26	21	2	2	6	2	9		5	
Pawnee	4	2	1				1		1	1
Payne	115	85	17	30	20	12	6		27	3
Pittsburg	67	48	7	13	13	8	7		15	4
Pontotoc	82	65	8	15	12	11	19	1	15	1
Pottawatomie	79	59	13	15	12	7	12	1	17	2
Pushmataha	2	2	1		1					
Roger Mills	3	1	1						2	
Rogers	66	52	12	8	15	3	14		14	
Seminole	8	5	2	3					3	

Table 3.9

Physicians by State and County, 2010, continued

		Major Professional Activity								
		Patient Care								
			Office-Based Practice							
State County	Total Physicians	Total Patient Care	FM/GP Practice	Medical Specialties	Surgical Specialties	Other Specialties	Hospital Based Practice	Other Professional Activity	Inactive	Not Classified
Sequoyah	13	8	4	1	1	1	1	1	4	
Stephens	44	38	17	4	10	2	5		6	
Texas	13	13	2	6	4		1			
Tillman	6	5	2		1		2		1	
Tulsa	1,939	1,548	163	468	297	332	288	65	268	58
Wagoner	29	22	7	6	1	3	5	2	5	
Washington	89	69	11	18	19	15	6	1	17	2
Washita	1	1	1							
Woods	8	7	2	1		1	3			1
Woodward	25	17	8	3	4	2			8	
Oregon	13,007	9,737	1,252	2,709	1,771	2,150	1,855	506	2,082	682
Baker	23	19	9	1	4	3	2		4	
Benton	337	248	33	88	42	66	19	10	70	9
Clackamas	1,166	877	86	260	167	227	137	40	222	27
Clatsop	71	52	11	9	12	7	13	1	18	
Columbia	20	14	5	7	1	1			4	2
Coos	172	120	18	39	29	15	19	3	44	5
Crook	14	9	6		1	1	1	1	4	
Curry	31	17	8	1	1	2	5	4	10	
Deschutes	597	430	51	116	102	121	40	16	133	18
Douglas	216	155	21	53	30	31	20	4	54	3
Grant	11	10	8		1		1		1	
Harney	9	6	4				2		3	
Hood River	104	83	26	11	14	18	14	5	11	5
Jackson	692	502	79	168	104	109	42	18	155	17
Jefferson	30	22	8	3	3	1	7		6	2
Josephine	146	108	26	28	26	17	11	1	32	5
Klamath	167	122	38	19	21	22	22	5	30	10
Lake	6	4	3				1		2	
Lane	1,092	851	155	249	175	232	40	24	206	11
Lincoln	89	54	11	13	11	8	11	1	33	1
Linn	171	127	52	27	20	13	15	3	40	1
Malheur	41	35	5	7	9	9	5		6	
Marion	716	553	117	137	115	123	61	29	125	9
Morrow	4	4	1	1		1	1			
Multnomah	4,760	3,557	236	934	543	766	1,078	269	482	452
Polk	107	75	18	16	11	23	7	5	23	4
Tillamook	55	42	13	4	6	9	10	2	11	
Umatilla	97	70	19	14	20	12	5	1	24	2
Union	54	45	7	9	9	10	10	1	7	1
Wallowa	17	13	7	2		3	1		4	
Wasco	61	45	6	9	15	7	8	2	8	6
Washington	1,734	1,329	134	442	252	272	229	59	259	87
Yamhill	197	139	31	42	27	21	18	2	51	5
Pennsylvania	44,988	33,568	2,845	9,002	5,068	6,252	10,401	2,271	5,856	3,293
Adams	129	100	28	27	14	24	7	3	24	2
Allegheny	8,167	6,101	340	1,569	851	1,086	2,255	409	853	804
Armstrong	68	51	7	24	9	7	4		14	3
Beaver	260	198	30	55	37	45	31	10	43	9
Bedford	32	21	7	4	3	3	4	1	7	3
Berks	883	666	91	178	131	119	147	28	158	31
Blair	343	274	38	85	58	50	43	6	57	6
Bradford	276	218	24	49	41	28	76	6	39	13
Bucks	1,741	1,298	104	459	243	268	224	102	275	66
Butler	301	225	18	78	35	47	47	11	53	12
Cambria	417	316	43	72	52	47	102	13	62	26
Cameron	5	2		1			1		2	1
Carbon	58	43	9	13	9	10	2	1	13	1

Table 3.9

Physicians by State and County, 2010, continued

		Major Professional Activity								
		Patient Care								
			Office-Based Practice							
State County	Total Physicians	Total Patient Care	FM/GP Practice	Medical Specialties	Surgical Specialties	Other Specialties	Hospital Based Practice	Other Professional Activity	Inactive	Not Classified
Centre	358	276	34	84	49	72	37	14	53	15
Chester	1,547	1,103	125	385	191	242	160	89	296	59
Clarion	27	17	4	7	2	2	2	3	4	3
Clearfield	137	114	8	33	23	21	29	1	21	1
Clinton	41	30	7	10	5	3	5		7	4
Columbia	120	93	19	27	16	15	16	3	18	6
Crawford	133	108	20	29	26	18	15	4	19	2
Cumberland	720	557	71	186	106	117	77	18	130	15
Dauphin	1,625	1,261	72	216	151	193	629	102	109	153
Delaware	2,953	2,147	121	744	314	457	511	197	426	183
Elk	48	34	7	2	8	8	9		13	1
Erie	595	448	78	107	100	73	90	17	115	15
Fayette	184	145	29	46	29	24	17	2	32	5
Franklin	247	189	43	53	38	35	20	4	50	4
Fulton	6	6	4		2					
Greene	26	21	6	9	6				4	1
Huntingdon	45	34	8	6	4	10	6		11	
Indiana	120	94	15	31	21	11	16	3	21	2
Jefferson	50	33	9	4	10	2	8	1	15	1
Juniata	9	8	6				2		1	
Lackawanna	609	465	22	164	93	100	86	17	107	20
Lancaster	1,085	824	188	208	139	161	128	37	189	35
Lawrence	111	85	17	25	18	15	10	3	22	1
Lebanon	333	246	38	38	34	49	87	9	56	22
Lehigh	1,224	969	97	251	195	192	234	33	157	65
Luzerne	770	584	73	181	116	102	112	26	126	34
Lycoming	270	204	47	52	32	36	37	8	51	7
Mckean	62	45	8	12	9	7	9		14	3
Mercer	217	153	19	42	35	35	22	1	57	6
Mifflin	54	45	9	13	12	7	4	2	7	
Monroe	248	189	22	58	39	49	21	9	42	8
Montgomery	5,349	3,755	233	1,154	573	909	886	383	870	341
Montour	599	481	9	105	63	59	245	18	38	62
Northampton	906	733	59	218	143	133	180	33	104	36
Northumberland	78	54	13	16	4	11	10	2	19	3
Perry	21	15	8	3		1	3		6	
Philadelphia	8,383	6,175	157	1,207	592	879	3,340	558	528	1,122
Pike	61	43	9	15	7	7	5		18	
Potter	23	19	2	3	6	2	6		3	1
Schuylkill	181	141	15	52	25	32	17	3	33	4
Snyder	38	30	11	6	2	4	7		8	
Somerset	102	72	17	13	14	10	18	3	25	2
Sullivan	6								6	
Susquehanna	39	22	3	5	3	7	4	2	14	1
Tioga	48	38	14	6	5	4	9		10	
Union	148	119	10	25	32	30	22	6	17	6
Venango	96	76	10	27	20	15	4	4	15	1
Warren	84	60	9	10	10	14	17	1	21	2
Washington	424	326	58	99	50	73	46	12	72	14
Wayne	65	48	7	20	8	8	5	1	13	3
Westmoreland	743	581	109	176	90	124	82	18	132	12
Wyoming	19	14	6	5	2	1			5	
York	921	726	121	200	113	139	153	34	126	35
Puerto Rico	12,154	9,133	1,684	2,283	1,127	2,072	1,967	429	997	1,595
Adjuntas	24	20	6	3		5	6		1	3
Aguada	84	61	16	20		12	13	1	5	17
Aguadilla	188	153	37	33	18	37	28	4	11	20
Aguas Buenas	25	20	6	3		5	6	2	1	2

Table 3.9

Physicians by State and County, 2010, continued

		Major Professional Activity								
		Patient Care								
			Office-Based Practice							
State County	Total Physicians	Total Patient Care	FM/GP Practice	Medical Specialties	Surgical Specialties	Other Specialties	Hospital Based Practice	Other Professional Activity	Inactive	Not Classified
Aibonito	74	61	14	19	12	5	11	3	2	8
Anasco	55	41	10	8	3	12	8	1	4	9
Arecibo	376	280	70	59	23	72	56	6	33	57
Arroyo	31	28	8	3		8	9			3
Barceloneta	31	20	6	3	2	5	4	1	1	9
Barranquitas	33	23	5	6	2	4	6	1	2	7
Bayamon	915	706	129	178	85	161	153	30	51	128
Cabo Rojo	127	100	35	17	10	21	17	1	12	14
Caguas	603	500	102	149	61	99	89	10	39	54
Camuy	41	26	10	4		6	6		3	12
Canovanas	49	39	19	7	1	5	7	1	2	7
Carolina	316	236	65	49	19	55	48	4	18	58
Catano	29	22	8	1		8	5	1	5	1
Cayey	103	88	17	25	11	18	17	1	8	6
Ceiba	20	16	7	5	1	2	1		1	3
Ciales	20	15	10	1	1	1	2		3	2
Cidra	50	36	7	10	3	14	2	2	3	9
Coamo	39	29	8	8	1	6	6	1	3	6
Comerio	18	14	8			3	3		1	3
Corozal	46	31	11	7	3	8	2	1	3	11
Culebra	2	2	1			1				
Dorado	116	94	11	23	13	28	19	2	8	12
Fajardo	117	88	19	18	14	23	14	4	12	13
Florida	6	2	2							4
Guanica	27	19	5	5	1	3	5		2	6
Guayama	127	98	23	23	12	24	16	3	9	17
Guayanilla	37	22	11	4		3	4		1	14
Guaynabo	833	612	67	155	88	162	140	44	86	91
Gurabo	99	78	19	24	4	15	16	2	6	13
Hatillo	50	37	14	5	3	7	8	1	4	8
Hormigueros	43	31	4	6	6	7	8	2		10
Humacao	204	162	26	47	20	45	24	4	16	22
Isabela	74	53	22	8	1	13	9		7	14
Jayuya	19	15	7	5		1	2	1		3
Juana Diaz	43	31	7	8	3	6	7		1	11
Juncos	60	46	11	11	2	9	13	1	1	12
Lajas	38	21	6	7	1	2	5	1	8	8
Lares	65	38	22	6		6	4	1	4	22
Las Marias	4	3	2				1			1
Las Piedras	50	41	12	9	3	8	9	2		7
Loiza	7	5	1	1		3			1	1
Luquillo	37	26	4	6	1	8	7	1	2	8
Manati	147	123	22	28	25	27	21	5	6	13
Maricao	4	2	1				1		1	1
Maunabo	13	9	3	3		1	2		1	3
Mayaguez	558	430	69	115	77	90	79	6	54	68
Moca	60	41	13	9	3	7	9	2	3	14
Morovis	30	22	5	8	1	4	4		1	7
Naguabo	16	12	4	2		2	4			4
Naranjito	19	15	6	3		5	1			4
Orocovis	20	16	6	2	1	4	3	1	1	2
Patillas	27	22	6	7	1	3	5	1	3	1
Penuelas	27	21	4	9		4	4			6
Ponce	909	676	86	207	97	148	138	32	77	124
Quebradillas	34	18	4	6	1	2	5	1	5	10
Rincon	18	17	5	3		9			1	
Rio Grande	1									1
Sabana Grande	51	39	11	12	3	6	7	1	5	6

Table 3.9

Physicians by State and County, 2010, continued

State / County	Total Physicians	Major Professional Activity: Patient Care: Total Patient Care	Office-Based Practice: FM/GP Practice	Office-Based Practice: Medical Specialties	Office-Based Practice: Surgical Specialties	Office-Based Practice: Other Specialties	Hospital Based Practice	Other Professional Activity	Inactive	Not Classified
Salinas	20	15	6	3		3	3	1	1	3
San German	117	89	15	34	11	13	16	1	9	18
San Juan	3,868	2,841	325	711	442	642	721	215	399	413
San Lorenzo	36	27	11	7	1	6	2	3	3	3
San Sebastian	73	46	8	11	1	14	12		10	17
Santa Isabel	23	14	5	3	1	3	2		1	8
Toa Alta	82	65	16	17	1	20	11	1	2	14
Toa Baja	157	123	35	23	9	30	26	4	7	23
Trujillo Alto	160	117	25	25	12	26	29	8	8	27
Utuado	34	28	11	5		7	5	1	2	3
Vega Alta	38	30	8	10	2	5	5		1	7
Vega Baja	108	76	33	8	6	20	9	2	8	22
Vieques	6	3			1	2		2		1
Villalba	15	12	2	2	2	1	5	1		2
Yabucoa	19	14	3	3		6	2		2	3
Yauco	109	81	26	18	1	16	20	1	6	21
Rhode Island	4,622	3,515	163	1,063	521	571	1,197	204	524	379
Bristol	300	232	7	93	26	54	52	7	52	9
Kent	532	414	27	128	85	95	79	15	80	23
Newport	263	183	18	53	28	33	51	8	64	8
Providence	3,149	2,400	91	677	328	327	977	159	259	331
Washington	378	286	20	112	54	62	38	15	69	8
South Carolina	12,240	9,851	1,315	2,558	1,819	1,989	2,170	400	1,579	410
Abbeville	23	18	10	2	2	1	3		5	
Aiken	252	192	26	41	40	49	36	3	45	12
Allendale	9	9	7		1	1				
Anderson	372	306	53	66	53	74	60	7	48	11
Bamberg	11	10	7		1		2		1	
Barnwell	12	8	2	4	1	1		1	1	2
Beaufort	613	343	33	98	92	73	47	12	252	6
Berkeley	172	159	27	38	18	45	31	1	9	3
Calhoun	4	3		2			1		1	
Charleston	3,068	2,467	133	582	381	563	808	155	284	162
Cherokee	46	37	16	5	9	4	3		9	
Chester	23	18	4	4	5	2	3	1	4	
Chesterfield	30	24	13	4	2	1	4		5	1
Clarendon	33	31	10	7	7	3	4		2	
Colleton	51	39	8	10	8	6	7		11	1
Darlington	76	61	23	17	12	5	4	3	11	1
Dillon	22	19	6	5	1		7	1	2	
Dorchester	118	91	32	19	18	11	11	4	20	3
Edgefield	18	13	6	1	2	1	3		5	
Fairfield	19	15	6	2	2	1	4	1	2	1
Florence	446	390	65	113	82	81	49	10	31	15
Georgetown	145	103	21	27	21	24	10	3	35	4
Greenville	1,626	1,363	156	383	260	244	320	38	170	55
Greenwood	259	213	52	44	42	34	41	13	27	6
Hampton	16	11	3	2	3		3		4	1
Horry	532	449	57	146	97	110	39	7	64	12
Jasper	22	15	4	5	3	2	1		6	1
Kershaw	113	96	13	24	23	18	18	2	11	4
Lancaster	91	72	15	23	19	11	4	3	13	3
Laurens	55	49	21	9	11	5	3	1	5	
Lee	4	3	3						1	
Lexington	508	423	69	107	80	89	78	6	61	18

Table 3.9

Physicians by State and County, 2010, continued

State County	Total Physicians	Major Professional Activity: Patient Care: Total Patient Care	Office-Based Practice: FM/GP Practice	Office-Based Practice: Medical Specialties	Office-Based Practice: Surgical Specialties	Office-Based Practice: Other Specialties	Hospital Based Practice	Other Professional Activity	Inactive	Not Classified
Marion	37	30	7	8	7	2	6		7	
Marlboro	17	15	6	3	1	2	3		2	
Mccormick	5	4	3			1			1	
Newberry	42	38	16	7	3	7	5	1	3	
Oconee	161	120	26	22	26	32	14	2	34	5
Orangeburg	130	106	22	36	20	11	17	3	17	4
Pickens	182	149	46	35	27	23	18	1	29	3
Richland	1,615	1,288	110	362	210	245	361	91	184	52
Saluda	2	2	2							
Spartanburg	680	566	96	137	127	103	103	24	77	13
Sumter	180	145	23	43	33	32	14	3	25	7
Union	32	25	8	7	4	2	4		6	1
Williamsburg	8	6	5				1		1	1
York	360	307	44	108	65	70	20	3	48	2
South Dakota	2,098	1,691	331	390	344	326	300	65	299	43
Beadle	22	19	6	4	6	2	1		3	
Bennett	1	1					1			
Bon Homme	4	4	3		1					
Brookings	35	27	8	5	7		7		8	
Brown	90	72	19	11	17	17	8	3	14	1
Brule	13	10	6		2		2		3	
Buffalo	2	1	1					1		
Butte	6	5	2			1	2		1	
Charles Mix	9	7	3	1			3		1	1
Clark	1								1	
Clay	18	16	7	3		4	2		1	1
Codington	68	55	13	12	13	10	7	1	10	2
Custer	12	10	8			1	1		2	
Davison	41	36	7	11	8	7	3		5	
Day	3	3	2				1			
Deuel	3	3	1	1			1			
Dewey	4	4	2			1	1			
Douglas	3	1	1						1	1
Edmunds	5	4			3	1			1	
Fall River	18	11	3	1	2		5	1	6	
Faulk	1	1					1			
Grant	9	8	6		2				1	
Gregory	5	5	4		1					
Haakon	2	2	1				1			
Hamlin	2	1	1						1	
Hand	3	3	3							
Hanson	3	1			1				2	
Hughes	27	22	7	6	6	2	1		4	1
Hutchinson	12	9	7	1		1			3	
Jerauld	3	3	2			1				
Kingsbury	3	2	1	1					1	
Lake	17	13	8	2		3			4	
Lawrence	54	36	14	6	9	3	4	1	17	
Lincoln	258	224	28	57	52	46	41	4	21	9
Lyman	1	1	1							
Marshall	2	2	1	1						
Mccook	3	1	1						2	
Mcpherson	3	2	2						1	
Meade	37	27	8	2		3	14	3	6	1
Minnehaha	666	546	73	144	92	113	124	33	71	16
Moody	2	2				1	1			
Pennington	380	285	38	79	60	65	43	15	71	9
Perkins	1								1	

Table 3.9

Physicians by State and County, 2010, continued

		Major Professional Activity									
		Patient Care									
			Office-Based Practice								
State County	Total Physicians	Total Patient Care	FM/GP Practice	Medical Specialties	Surgical Specialties	Other Specialties	Hospital Based Practice	Other Professional Activity	Inactive	Not Classified
Potter	1	1					1			
Roberts	12	11	5	3	1	2			1	
Sanborn	1								1	
Shannon	8	8		3	1	1	3			
Spink	8	5	2	2			1		3	
Stanley	4	3		1			2		1	
Todd	7	6	1	1		1	3	1		
Tripp	9	9	6		3					
Turner	7	7	1		1	2	3			
Union	83	74	6	13	33	22		1	7	1
Walworth	7	4	2	1			1		3	
Yankton	99	78	10	18	23	16	11	1	20	
Tennessee	19,035	15,143	1,646	4,464	2,816	2,849	3,368	712	2,177	1,003
Anderson	205	164	30	45	39	38	12	6	34	1
Bedford	35	29	11	7	5	2	4		6	
Benton	6	5	3		1		1		1	
Bledsoe	6	3	2	1				1	1	1
Blount	242	187	28	69	32	38	20	3	48	4
Bradley	154	128	17	41	31	25	14	2	24	
Campbell	43	35	8	16	3	4	4		6	2
Cannon	9	5	3		1	1			4	
Carroll	29	28	13	2	7	3	3		1	
Carter	51	39	12	8	11	4	4	1	10	1
Cheatham	27	23	9	4		5	5		3	1
Chester	4	4	2	1	1					
Claiborne	23	20	7	6	5		2	1	2	
Clay	3	1		1					2	
Cocke	24	23	12	7	2		2			1
Coffee	117	97	14	27	24	17	15	2	16	2
Crockett	6	4	1	2		1			2	
Cumberland	110	81	11	33	21	10	6	1	25	3
Davidson	4,185	3,184	105	823	562	593	1,101	240	386	375
Decatur	9	8	3	1	1	1	2			1
Dekalb	17	12	10			1	1		5	
Dickson	55	47	14	12	10	7	4		5	3
Dyer	66	49	8	18	12	5	6		15	2
Fayette	15	13	7	1	1		4		2	
Fentress	15	11	3	4	1		3		2	2
Franklin	53	42	13	10	10	4	5	1	6	4
Gibson	44	38	18	9	5	1	5		6	
Giles	33	21	8	6	4	2	1		11	1
Grainger	7	3		2		1			4	
Greene	109	88	23	24	18	11	12	4	16	1
Grundy	7	7	1	3	1	1	1			
Hamblen	132	109	18	39	22	21	9	1	20	2
Hamilton	1,454	1,153	91	363	245	229	225	50	201	50
Hancock	4	2	1			1			1	1
Hardeman	16	10	5	3		2			6	
Hardin	18	17	7	5	2	2	1	1		
Hawkins	32	22	10	10	1	1		1	7	2
Haywood	12	8	4	3	1				4	
Henderson	15	11	6	3	1	1			3	1
Henry	58	43	7	13	10	10	3		14	1
Hickman	6	5	3	1		1			1	
Houston	4	4	3			1				
Humphreys	11	9	4	3	2				2	
Jackson	4	3		1	1	1			1	
Jefferson	58	42	12	16	5	7	2	1	12	3

Table 3.9

Physicians by State and County, 2010, continued

		Major Professional Activity								
		Patient Care								
			Office-Based Practice							
State County	Total Physicians	Total Patient Care	FM/GP Practice	Medical Specialties	Surgical Specialties	Other Specialties	Hospital Based Practice	Other Professional Activity	Inactive	Not Classified
Johnson	17	10	5	1		2	2		7	
Knox	2,044	1,687	177	552	342	343	273	51	244	62
Lake	4	4			1	1	2			
Lauderdale	8	5	2	1	1		1		2	1
Lawrence	33	25	9	8	5	3			5	3
Lewis	6	5	2	2	1				1	
Lincoln	32	26	18	4	3	1			6	
Loudon	66	47	11	12	4	13	7	1	18	
Macon	8	6	2	4					2	
Madison	467	392	41	137	100	67	47	9	53	13
Marion	24	21	6	7	4	2	2	1	2	
Marshall	16	15	6	3	2	3	1		1	
Maury	213	177	23	55	42	37	20	3	25	8
Mcminn	57	47	13	10	14	8	2	1	9	
Mcnairy	20	18	8	4	5		1		1	1
Meigs	5	4	2	1			1		1	
Monroe	31	27	10	4	6	4	3		4	
Montgomery	236	195	21	58	43	40	33	3	29	9
Moore	1	1				1				
Morgan	1	1	1							
Obion	45	36	9	8	9	7	3	1	8	
Overton	30	24	7	6	5	4	2		4	2
Perry	3	2	1	1					1	
Pickett	2	2	1	1						
Polk	15	14	4	5		2	3		1	
Putnam	195	158	19	53	35	35	16	2	31	4
Rhea	18	15	5	5	2	2	1	1	2	
Roane	39	30	14	8	4	3	1	2	7	
Robertson	63	54	13	16	14	5	6		8	1
Rutherford	425	358	33	117	79	66	63	12	45	10
Scott	14	11	3	4	2	1	1	1	1	1
Sequatchie	8	6	4			2			2	
Sevier	79	63	26	13	12	7	5		15	1
Shelby	3,776	3,022	212	905	513	546	846	149	359	246
Smith	13	10	8		2				3	
Stewart	3	2	2						1	
Sullivan	704	566	101	169	121	101	74	30	93	15
Sumner	257	206	37	70	42	38	19	3	37	11
Tipton	48	40	10	14	7	3	6	3	4	1
Trousdale	4	3	2		1				1	
Unicoi	13	10	6	2	1	1			3	
Union	7	7	1	5			1			
Van Buren	3	1	1						2	
Warren	40	33	10	9	8	4	2		7	
Washington	991	787	74	192	115	122	284	40	98	66
Wayne	8	8	5	2			1			
Weakley	37	32	8	13	6	2	3		5	
White	20	14	5	5	2		2	1	5	
Williamson	1,199	950	81	292	135	298	144	76	96	77
Wilson	154	129	20	43	30	23	13	6	13	6
Texas	60,991	48,536	5,512	13,413	8,701	9,741	11,169	2,196	6,104	4,155
Anderson	60	47	6	16	13	10	2		13	
Andrews	11	9	3	1	3		2	1	1	
Angelina	155	135	18	52	30	24	11	1	17	2
Aransas	28	13	5	3	1	4			15	
Archer	4	4	1	1	1	1				
Atascosa	25	22	5	6	3	5	3	1	2	
Austin	17	10	2	3		4	1		7	
Bailey	7	6	5		1				1	

Table 3.9

Physicians by State and County, 2010, continued

State / County	Total Physicians	Major Professional Activity: Patient Care: Total Patient Care	Office-Based Practice: FM/GP Practice	Office-Based Practice: Medical Specialties	Office-Based Practice: Surgical Specialties	Office-Based Practice: Other Specialties	Hospital Based Practice	Other Professional Activity	Inactive	Not Classified
Bandera	21	10	1	4		2	3	1	10	
Bastrop	50	39	15	8	3	9	4	1	10	
Baylor	4	3	1	1			1			1
Bee	22	20	8	4	4	3	1		2	
Bell	1,309	1,075	75	215	123	143	519	50	120	64
Bexar	6,480	5,083	457	1,262	780	961	1,623	309	608	480
Blanco	11	7	3			2	2	1	3	
Bosque	18	9	4	3	1	1		1	8	
Bowie	286	239	36	73	62	53	15	2	40	5
Brazoria	800	634	76	176	55	100	227	21	47	98
Brazos	482	397	80	104	89	81	43	24	45	16
Brewster	18	11	3		2	2	4	1	5	1
Briscoe	2	2	1		1					
Brooks	1								1	
Brown	61	53	9	16	16	9	3	1	6	1
Burleson	7	6	2	1		2	1		1	
Burnet	59	46	13	10	5	9	9		12	1
Caldwell	27	22	9	5	2	5	1	1	3	1
Calhoun	19	15	5	5	1	1	3		4	
Callahan	4	1	1						3	
Cameron	580	478	60	185	103	68	62	15	61	26
Camp	8	6	5	1					2	
Cass	12	11	10		1					1
Castro	4	4	4							
Chambers	9	7	4	1		2			1	1
Cherokee	53	45	6	7	7	17	8	2	6	
Childress	11	10	9		1				1	
Clay	9	4	3			1			4	1
Cochran	2	1	1					1		
Coke	3	3				2	1			
Coleman	8	4	4						4	
Collin	2,009	1,719	190	589	321	422	197	23	138	129
Colorado	28	21	12	2	7			1	6	
Comal	236	183	43	38	33	46	23	11	34	8
Comanche	10	7	4	1	1		1		3	
Concho	1	1				1				
Cooke	25	20	6	4	4	3	3		4	1
Coryell	25	20	6	5	1	4	4	1	3	1
Crane	5	4		1	1		2		1	
Crosby	2	2	1	1						
Culberson	1	1					1			
Dallam	5	5	3	1			1			
Dallas	8,308	6,505	390	1,780	1,116	1,422	1,797	346	752	705
Dawson	7	4	1	1	1		1		2	1
De Witt	7	4	3	1					3	
Deaf Smith	6	5	3		2				1	
Delta	1	1				1				
Denton	1,133	958	137	304	204	198	115	21	100	54
Dimmit	6	6	3	2		1				
Donley	1	1	1							
Eastland	8	4	2			1	1		4	
Ector	302	246	28	76	51	27	64	12	21	23
Edwards	2	1	1						1	
El Paso	1,614	1,278	108	355	241	213	361	59	152	125
Ellis	123	106	23	33	32	11	7	1	15	1
Erath	47	40	10	13	11	6			7	
Falls	10	8	1		1	2	4		2	
Fannin	20	15	4	1	2		8	1	3	1

Table 3.9

Physicians by State and County, 2010, continued

		Major Professional Activity									
		Patient Care									
			Office-Based Practice								
State County	Total Physicians	Total Patient Care	FM/GP Practice	Medical Specialties	Surgical Specialties	Other Specialties	Hospital Based Practice	Other Professional Activity	Inactive	Not Classified
Fayette	22	17	3	2	9		3		4	1
Fisher	2	2	2							
Floyd	4	4	3	1						
Fort Bend	1,362	1,117	166	342	146	223	240	38	96	111
Franklin	5	4	2	1		1			1	
Freestone	5	4	4						1	
Frio	9	7	4			1	2		2	
Gaines	5	5	2	1	2					
Galveston	1,357	976	79	178	101	152	466	116	99	166
Garza	2	2	1		1					
Gillespie	104	75	16	19	19	12	9	1	28	
Goliad	3	2		1	1				1	
Gonzales	14	9	4	3		2			5	
Gray	23	18	3	9	5		1		5	
Grayson	244	204	26	63	46	51	18	2	35	3
Gregg	339	297	36	100	74	60	27	2	34	6
Grimes	14	8	4	3			1		6	
Guadalupe	135	103	19	18	17	10	39	9	17	6
Hale	23	18	6	7	3	2			5	
Hall	2	2	1	1						
Hamilton	12	10	6	1		1	2		2	
Hansford	3	2	1				1			1
Hardeman	4	3		2		1			1	
Hardin	22	20	10	4	3	3			2	
Harris	13,347	10,410	805	2,777	1,718	2,079	3,031	592	1,099	1,246
Harrison	53	44	7	12	11	8	6		8	1
Haskell	2	1	1						1	
Hays	211	161	32	45	33	34	17	4	41	5
Hemphill	4	3	3						1	
Henderson	74	60	22	8	16	11	3		12	2
Hidalgo	913	799	147	304	151	118	79	6	64	44
Hill	23	15	10	2	2		1		6	2
Hockley	13	12	4	4	2		2		1	
Hood	66	44	5	14	10	8	7	4	16	2
Hopkins	36	31	9	6	9	2	5		5	
Houston	12	12	6		1	3	2			
Howard	50	38	4	7	9	5	13	2	9	1
Hudspeth	1								1	
Hunt	62	49	14	13	10	9	3	1	11	1
Hutchinson	15	13	5	3	5				2	
Irion	1	1	1							
Jack	3	2	1				1		1	
Jackson	6	5	1		2		2		1	
Jasper	26	22	11	7	2	1	1		4	
Jeff Davis	3	1	1						2	
Jefferson	601	502	59	168	111	135	29	8	71	20
Jim Hogg	1	1	1							
Jim Wells	30	28	9	11	5	1	2		1	1
Johnson	155	122	29	35	24	17	17	1	25	7
Jones	9	8	5	1	1		1		1	
Karnes	7	7	5	1		1				
Kaufman	71	57	16	13	6	9	13	2	12	
Kendall	226	163	15	35	21	54	38	11	40	12
Kent	1							1		
Kerr	189	117	12	39	22	24	20	6	63	3
Kimble	4	3	2			1			1	
Kinney	1								1	
Kleberg	27	20	7	8	2	2	1		6	1
Knox	2	2	1				1			

Table 3.9

Physicians by State and County, 2010, continued

		Major Professional Activity								
		Patient Care								
			Office-Based Practice							
State County	Total Physicians	Total Patient Care	FM/GP Practice	Medical Specialties	Surgical Specialties	Other Specialties	Hospital Based Practice	Other Professional Activity	Inactive	Not Classified
Lamar	114	90	6	31	25	25	3	3	19	2
Lamb	7	5	4				1		2	
Lampasas	18	17	11			4	2		1	
Lavaca	20	17	10	2	1	3	1		2	1
Lee	4	3	2	1					1	
Leon	9	3	2		1			2	4	
Liberty	44	33	11	11	7	2	2	1	10	
Limestone	10	9	6	2			1		1	
Llano	33	22	10	3	5	2	2	2	9	
Lubbock	1,142	895	90	220	162	171	252	47	121	79
Lynn	5	4	3		1				1	
Madison	3	3	2				1			
Marion	5	1					1		3	1
Martin	3	3	2			1				
Mason	1								1	
Matagorda	35	25	6	9	8	2		4	5	1
Maverick	32	26	4	12	7	2	1		3	3
Mcculloch	6	3	1				2		2	1
Mclennan	549	446	92	82	94	100	78	25	65	13
Mcmullen	1	1				1				
Medina	23	17	12	1		3	1		6	
Menard	1	1	1							
Midland	260	228	17	77	49	53	32	6	19	7
Milam	16	12	6	2	1	1	2	2	2	
Mills	5	2	1		1				3	
Mitchell	3	2					2		1	
Montague	12	10	5	1	2	1	1		2	
Montgomery	920	762	126	251	153	162	70	20	97	41
Moore	11	9	5	1	1	1	1			2
Morris	3	2	1	1					1	
Motley	1								1	
Nacogdoches	146	129	24	33	40	22	10		16	1
Navarro	56	40	9	14	13	3	1	1	13	2
Newton	7	4	2		1	1			3	
Nolan	10	8	2	2	2	2			1	1
Nueces	960	784	89	234	165	170	126	16	124	36
Ochiltree	6	5	3		1		1		1	
Oldham	1									1
Orange	43	34	12	8	5	8	1	2	6	1
Palo Pinto	22	18	5	5	6	1	1		4	
Panola	13	10	5	2	1		2		3	
Parker	108	78	16	18	13	20	11	3	19	8
Parmer	5	4	4						1	
Pecos	7	6	4	1			1		1	
Polk	64	40	9	12	8	4	7	7	17	
Potter	471	386	32	123	90	71	70	18	44	23
Presidio	3	2	1			1				1
Rains	4	3	1	2					1	
Randall	255	209	37	50	36	48	38	9	25	12
Reagan	2	1	1						1	
Real	1								1	
Red River	9	4		2	1		1	1	3	1
Reeves	3	2		1			1		1	
Refugio	1	1	1							
Robertson	4	3		1		1	1		1	
Rockwall	155	127	21	20	31	30	25	4	17	7
Runnels	7	6	5				1		1	
Rusk	37	29	11	3	5	7	3	1	7	
Sabine	5	4	1	1		1	1		1	

Table 3.9

Physicians by State and County, 2010, continued

State / County	Total Physicians	Major Professional Activity: Patient Care: Total Patient Care	Office-Based Practice: FM/GP Practice	Office-Based Practice: Medical Specialties	Office-Based Practice: Surgical Specialties	Office-Based Practice: Other Specialties	Hospital Based Practice	Other Professional Activity	Inactive	Not Classified
San Augustine	5	4	2	2					1	
San Jacinto	5	3	1	1	1			1		1
San Patricio	32	28	10	7	1	7	3		4	
San Saba	4	2	2						1	1
Schleicher	3	2	1				1		1	
Scurry	12	10	6	2			2		2	
Shackelford	1	1	1							
Shelby	13	11	6	2	2		1		2	
Smith	875	726	85	205	156	163	117	29	104	16
Somervell	10	8	5		2	1			1	1
Starr	23	19	9	5	1	2	2	1	1	2
Stephens	7	5	5					1	1	
Stonewall	1	1	1							
Sutton	4	4	3			1				
Swisher	4	2	1				1		2	
Tarrant	3,531	2,897	342	883	655	637	380	95	364	175
Taylor	319	256	38	76	65	51	26	5	47	11
Terry	11	7	4	1	1		1	1	3	
Throckmorton	1	1	1							
Titus	46	41	5	12	16	8			5	
Tom Green	263	218	25	62	48	52	31	1	36	8
Travis	3,445	2,753	299	822	551	704	377	132	374	186
Trinity	3	3	1	2						
Tyler	13	7	4			1	2		5	1
Upshur	20	15	9	2		4		1	3	1
Upton	2	1	1						1	
Uvalde	25	22	10	5	4	1	2		3	
Val Verde	46	40	8	11	12	1	8	1	2	3
Van Zandt	16	11	4	2	1	4			5	
Victoria	221	178	22	58	41	43	14	3	32	8
Walker	68	51	11	14	11	8	7	3	11	3
Waller	12	11	3	4		2	2		1	
Ward	5	4	2	2						1
Washington	54	40	10	11	12	4	3	1	12	1
Webb	261	202	38	69	45	27	23	6	36	17
Wharton	54	43	9	14	14	4	2		11	
Wheeler	5	5	3	1		1				
Wichita	348	277	48	69	51	55	54	8	46	17
Wilbarger	20	16	4	3	1	2	6	1	2	1
Willacy	7	7	5	2						
Williamson	770	586	107	167	114	108	90	16	107	61
Wilson	25	18	10		2	1	5		6	1
Winkler	3	3	3							
Wise	49	42	13	8	13	3	5		5	2
Wood	31	24	12	7	4	1			7	
Yoakum	4	4	2	1	1					
Young	16	14	9	1	3		1		1	1
Zapata	4	3				1	2			1
Zavala	4	4	3	1						
Utah	6,865	5,334	648	1,242	1,019	1,153	1,272	289	835	407
Beaver	9	7	6			1			1	1
Box Elder	40	31	11	7	8	2	3	2	7	
Cache	192	152	23	38	40	32	19	1	36	3
Carbon	25	22	5	4	8	2	3	1	1	1
Davis	514	419	69	92	80	106	72	6	65	24
Duchesne	20	18	1	6	7	2	2		1	1
Emery	1	1	1							
Garfield	1	1	1							

Table 3.9

Physicians by State and County, 2010, continued

		Major Professional Activity								
		Patient Care								
			Office-Based Practice							
State County	Total Physicians	Total Patient Care	FM/GP Practice	Medical Specialties	Surgical Specialties	Other Specialties	Hospital Based Practice	Other Professional Activity	Inactive	Not Classified
Grand	23	18	7	3	1	2	5		5	
Iron	47	36	6	11	8	6	5		7	4
Juab	9	8	3		3		2		1	
Kane	6	2	1				1		4	
Millard	8	6	5				1		2	
Morgan	14	13	2	2	1	6	2		1	
Piute	1								1	
Rich	1								1	
Salt Lake	4,147	3,188	254	766	548	680	940	236	415	308
San Juan	7	7	4			2	1			
Sanpete	25	19	11		1	3	4	1	5	
Sevier	11	10	6	1			3		1	
Summit	206	143	14	30	27	47	25	9	37	17
Tooele	36	30	9	4	6	6	5	1	5	
Uintah	25	24	7	3	7	3	4			1
Utah	743	610	116	141	132	128	93	16	92	25
Wasatch	31	22	8	2	4	5	3		6	3
Washington	299	219	31	57	54	54	23	4	69	7
Wayne	2	1			1				1	
Weber	422	327	47	75	83	66	56	12	71	12
Vermont	2,752	2,016	272	477	289	343	635	143	441	152
Addison	110	76	21	18	17	4	16	2	30	2
Bennington	150	115	16	31	27	21	20	11	22	2
Caledonia	65	49	13	8	10	5	13	4	12	
Chittenden	1,346	1,016	92	217	118	174	415	76	140	114
Essex	4	4	1	1		1	1			
Franklin	70	53	7	19	14	9	4	3	14	
Grand Isle	21	11		2		7	2	5	4	1
Lamoille	67	45	15	8	5	11	6	2	18	2
Orange	73	46	5	15	7	5	14	6	21	
Orleans	64	45	7	11	8	6	13	1	18	
Rutland	191	130	25	33	22	24	26	5	50	6
Washington	188	140	29	38	24	26	23	7	33	8
Windham	142	113	22	26	15	25	25	1	28	
Windsor	261	173	19	50	22	25	57	20	51	17
Virgin Islands	209	171	21	42	47	25	36	2	25	11
Saint Croix	90	70	8	17	20	9	16	2	13	5
Saint John	5	5	2	1	1		1			
SaintThomas	114	96	11	24	26	16	19		12	6
Virginia	25,571	19,819	2,258	5,498	3,311	3,894	4,858	1,015	3,460	1,277
Accomack	33	21	6	6	2	4	3	1	11	
Albemarle	797	596	49	149	64	107	227	36	111	54
Alexandria City	526	396	28	121	79	83	85	21	68	41
Alleghany	34	26	2	10	6	3	5	1	7	
Amelia	3	1					1		2	
Amherst	14	6	6						7	1
Appomattox	3	2	1	1					1	
Arlington	875	646	36	175	102	141	192	56	89	84
Augusta	119	97	18	22	27	21	9		20	2
Bath	4	2	2						2	
Bedford	103	71	26	9	12	14	10	2	29	1
Bland	2	2				2				
Botetourt	50	36	10	7	3	7	9	3	10	1
Bristol	13	8	4			1	3		5	
Brunswick	8	6	3	2		1			2	
Buchanan	19	12	2	8		1	1		5	2

Table 3.9

Physicians by State and County, 2010, continued

		Major Professional Activity								
		Patient Care								
			Office-Based Practice							
State County	Total Physicians	Total Patient Care	FM/GP Practice	Medical Specialties	Surgical Specialties	Other Specialties	Hospital Based Practice	Other Professional Activity	Inactive	Not Classified
Buckingham	6	5	2	2			1		1	
Buena Vista City	2	2	1	1						
Campbell	17	13	11			2			4	
Caroline	12	8	2	2	1		3	1	3	
Carroll	13	10	7	1	1	1			3	
Charles City	4	3	1	2					1	
Charlotte	6	5	3			1	1		1	
Charlottesville City	1,400	1,020	24	147	82	173	594	112	88	180
Chesapeake City	663	561	75	149	102	85	150	17	53	32
Chesterfield	1,048	842	121	229	132	183	177	31	119	56
Clarke	25	16	3	7		1	5	3	6	
Colonial Heights City	73	63	10	29	14	7	3	1	9	
Covington City	10	5	1		2	1	1		5	
Craig	1	1	1							
Culpeper	60	47	7	16	13	7	4		13	
Cumberland	3	2	1		1				1	
Danville City	147	118	13	42	31	20	12	3	24	2
Dickenson	10	8	3	3	2				2	
Dinwiddie	5	2	2						3	
Essex	20	18	2	6	4	4	2		2	
Fairfax	4,451	3,467	279	1,165	620	738	665	214	546	224
Fairfax City	155	122	12	54	20	23	13	4	20	9
Falls Church City	117	97	11	39	17	18	12	2	13	5
Fauquier	115	92	13	26	21	24	8	4	18	1
Floyd	10	6	2		1	2	1		4	
Fluvanna	41	28	4	9	1	2	12	4	4	5
Franklin	65	49	17	11	5	5	11	2	14	
Franklin City	35	29	9	7	4	5	4	1	5	
Frederick	129	112	12	25	19	39	17	1	14	2
Fredericksburg City	193	172	9	65	45	36	17	1	19	1
Galax City	47	42	8	12	7	5	10	1	4	
Giles	19	13	7	2	2		2		5	1
Gloucester	69	50	6	17	14	6	7	2	16	1
Goochland	72	51	11	8	10	15	7	3	17	1
Grayson	8	8	4	2		1	1			
Greene	14	9	3	2		2	2	2	3	
Greensville	20	17	8	4	1	1	3		2	1
Halifax	72	59	9	23	13	9	5	1	12	
Hampton City	236	185	32	42	28	42	41	9	38	4
Hanover	200	170	26	61	30	32	21	4	18	8
Harrisonburg City	242	192	35	52	43	46	16	4	42	4
Henrico	1,848	1,357	121	410	274	273	279	61	348	82
Henry	11	8	4		2		2		3	
Highland	4	2	1	1					2	
Hopewell City	34	30	6	14	2	5	3		4	
Isle Of Wight	65	51	11	10	5	17	8	2	9	3
James City	427	296	36	69	48	78	65	20	102	9
King And Queen	6	4	1	1		1	1		2	
King George	11	7	3		2	2		2	1	1
King William	11	7	7						4	
Lancaster	63	41	9	10	11	6	5		21	1
Lee	18	15	6	5	3	1			2	1
Lexington City	53	37	11	9	6	4	7		15	1
Loudoun	716	548	74	186	91	109	88	43	90	35
Louisa	17	6	5	1				1	10	
Lunenburg	5	3	2	1					2	
Lynchburg City	433	338	40	102	71	76	49	11	81	3
Madison	15	10	5	2	1	1	1		4	1
Manassas City	134	115	25	30	28	22	10	3	15	1

Table 3.9

Physicians by State and County, 2010, continued

		Major Professional Activity								
		Patient Care								
			Office-Based Practice							
State County	Total Physicians	Total Patient Care	FM/GP Practice	Medical Specialties	Surgical Specialties	Other Specialties	Hospital Based Practice	Other Professional Activity	Inactive	Not Classified
Martinsville City	103	80	10	28	15	18	9	1	21	1
Mathews	14	3		1	1		1	2	8	1
Mecklenburg	57	44	14	9	7	6	8	1	11	1
Middlesex	16	11	8	1		1	1		5	
Montgomery	189	152	26	34	34	33	25	5	28	4
Nelson	32	15	6	2		3	4	3	13	1
New Kent	18	9	3	2		2	2		5	4
Newport News City	468	383	55	96	85	48	99	7	70	8
Norfolk City	1,253	998	37	288	166	169	338	48	133	74
Northampton	47	35	3	14	8	7	3	1	11	
Northumberland	22	7	3	2		2			13	2
Norton City	40	37	6	13	13	3	2		2	1
Nottoway	17	11	9	1			1	2	3	1
Orange	49	35	13	10	2	2	8	3	7	4
Page	21	14	6	1	2	1	4	2	5	
Patrick	13	7	5		1		1		6	
Petersburg City	71	50	10	13	9	9	9		18	3
Pittsylvania	7	5	4	1					2	
Poquoson City	38	30	5	3	4	12	6	5	3	
Portsmouth City	362	268	28	33	23	37	147	16	46	32
Powhatan	27	24	14	5		3	2		2	1
Prince Edward	41	35	7	8	9	4	7		6	
Prince George	13	9	3	3	3				2	2
Prince William	492	387	58	150	61	58	60	9	77	19
Pulaski	47	39	9	12	4	8	6		8	
Radford	52	40	5	12	7	10	6	2	10	
Rappahannock	9	6	3	1		1	1		2	1
Richmond	2	1				1			1	
Richmond City	1,243	940	52	189	98	141	460	99	77	127
Roanoke	497	393	42	74	52	95	130	11	66	27
Roanoke City	520	405	20	112	79	72	122	28	67	20
Rockbridge	8	4	1	1	1		1	1	3	
Rockingham	64	41	11	7	5	14	4	1	22	
Russell	19	17	5	6		2	4		2	
Salem	198	161	14	42	29	24	52	5	27	5
Scott	11	9	6			3		1	1	
Shenandoah	48	39	10	7	8	8	6		9	
Smyth	63	47	9	7	13	6	12	4	12	
Southampton	7	4	1	2			1		3	
Spotsylvania	222	187	27	54	31	59	16	5	22	8
Stafford	128	97	17	31	16	16	17	3	22	6
Staunton City	85	58	5	12	13	16	12	3	22	2
Suffolk City	313	274	26	78	43	57	70	4	21	14
Surry	2	1	1							1
Sussex	4	4	3		1					
Tazewell	114	98	17	32	13	19	17		13	3
Virginia Beach City	1,338	1,065	152	282	194	257	180	42	201	30
Warren	40	34	11	7	5	3	8		5	1
Washington	136	117	18	30	25	28	16	1	17	1
Waynesboro City	75	51	12	16	7	12	4		22	2
Westmoreland	8	4	3			1			4	
Williamsburg City	8	5				3	2		3	
Winchester City	268	227	20	83	68	40	16	4	35	2
Wise	44	38	10	10	6	7	5	1	4	1
Wythe	54	47	10	8	7	12	10		6	1
York	225	195	38	42	18	45	52	5	20	5

Table 3.9

Physicians by State and County, 2010, continued

		Major Professional Activity								
		Patient Care								
			Office-Based Practice							
State County	Total Physicians	Total Patient Care	FM/GP Practice	Medical Specialties	Surgical Specialties	Other Specialties	Hospital Based Practice	Other Professional Activity	Inactive	Not Classified
Washington	21,795	16,274	2,555	4,170	2,587	3,622	3,340	1,064	3,363	1,094
Adams	14	12	6	2	2	1	1		2	
Asotin	50	39	11	9	9	8	2		11	
Benton	403	320	47	107	59	70	37	10	54	19
Chelan	281	225	42	60	42	57	24	8	45	3
Clallam	214	132	38	31	22	25	16	12	67	3
Clark	828	660	121	196	134	130	79	23	115	30
Columbia	4	2	2						2	
Cowlitz	217	159	28	46	29	41	15	1	54	3
Douglas	36	26	10	6	2	5	3		10	
Ferry	6	4	2				2		2	
Franklin	70	66	11	18	18	10	9		4	
Garfield	2	1	1						1	
Grant	82	68	26	18	11	6	7	2	12	
Grays Harbor	80	59	15	14	12	15	3	2	16	3
Island	176	109	14	13	19	25	38	7	57	3
Jefferson	89	50	19	7	7	8	9	9	30	
King	10,518	7,716	914	1,993	1,113	1,732	1,964	701	1,317	784
Kitsap	712	524	89	115	76	124	120	32	142	14
Kittitas	46	33	14	5	6	2	6	1	12	
Klickitat	32	21	12	1	2	5	1	1	9	1
Lewis	105	72	20	18	17	12	5	4	26	3
Lincoln	8	5	2			1	2	2	1	
Mason	50	30	7	4	11	3	5	1	17	2
Okanogan	65	53	30	7	4	7	5	1	11	
Pacific	25	15	5	2	2	2	4	1	9	
Pend Oreille	12	8	2	1	1		4		4	
Pierce	2,206	1,755	230	421	278	358	468	68	298	85
San Juan	61	28	12	4	4	7	1	5	28	
Skagit	357	266	68	67	50	59	22	5	79	7
Skamania	6	4	1		2	1			2	
Snohomish	1,212	925	183	256	166	214	106	33	226	28
Spokane	1,586	1,203	181	315	225	306	176	66	267	50
Stevens	43	32	18	7	5	1	1		11	
Thurston	793	604	129	151	84	146	94	31	129	29
Wahkiakum	3								3	
Walla Walla	250	177	32	43	31	39	32	3	68	2
Whatcom	618	452	112	118	65	126	31	18	137	11
Whitman	65	45	15	14	8	4	4	1	16	3
Yakima	470	374	86	101	71	72	44	16	69	11
West Virginia	4,922	3,819	509	935	668	684	1,023	183	609	311
Barbour	9	7	1	3			3		2	
Berkeley	162	125	18	33	22	21	31	5	30	2
Boone	8	8	4	1	1	1	1			
Braxton	6	6	2	2	1		1			
Brooke	10	7	4	2	1				2	1
Cabell	684	539	56	131	91	91	170	34	43	68
Calhoun	3	3		1			2			
Clay	4	2	2						1	1
Doddridge	2	1		1					1	
Fayette	40	29	11	7	4	2	5		10	1
Gilmer	2	2	2							
Grant	10	9	3	2	1	2	1	1		
Greenbrier	78	51	3	21	11	10	6	2	22	3
Hampshire	13	10	3	3	1		3	1	2	
Hancock	61	48	7	16	9	7	9	1	12	
Hardy	10	6	1		2	3		1	3	
Harrison	186	141	27	39	20	17	38	7	27	11

Table 3.9

Physicians by State and County, 2010, continued

State / County	Total Physicians	Major Professional Activity: Patient Care: Total Patient Care	Office-Based Practice: FM/GP Practice	Office-Based Practice: Medical Specialties	Office-Based Practice: Surgical Specialties	Office-Based Practice: Other Specialties	Hospital Based Practice	Other Professional Activity	Inactive	Not Classified
Jackson	17	10	3		2	2	3		7	
Jefferson	91	60	14	9	8	11	18	7	15	9
Kanawha	940	755	68	219	160	147	161	36	100	49
Lewis	22	18	3	5	5	2	3		4	
Lincoln	6	4	4						1	1
Logan	46	35	6	12	8	1	8	1	6	4
Marion	96	79	12	27	12	12	16		15	2
Marshall	34	27	5	7	8	6	1	1	5	1
Mason	29	26	4	7	8	2	5		3	
Mcdowell	14	11	6	1		2	2		3	
Mercer	136	103	10	28	22	29	14	2	29	2
Mineral	29	20	3	6	2	6	3		7	2
Mingo	30	21	4	8	2	2	5	1	7	1
Monongalia	1,004	772	45	132	105	132	358	58	59	115
Monroe	6	1				1		1	4	
Morgan	10	6	4	2				1	3	
Nicholas	33	29	15	3	5	3	3	1	2	1
Ohio	270	213	26	42	41	55	49	5	47	5
Pendleton	6	5	4	1						1
Pleasants	2	2	1	1						
Pocahontas	8	2	1			1			6	
Preston	30	18	6	3	3	4	2	3	8	1
Putnam	98	84	22	25	8	16	13	1	7	6
Raleigh	223	180	13	62	40	32	33	4	31	8
Randolph	65	51	12	11	13	7	8		11	3
Ritchie	5	2	2						2	1
Roane	14	9	4		1	2	2		5	
Summers	12	9	3	5	1				3	
Taylor	13	10	5				5	2	1	
Tucker	10	6	3	1		1	1		3	1
Tyler	5	4	2	1			1		1	
Upshur	31	21	6	4	5	2	4		9	1
Wayne	55	41	8	9	4	4	16	4	6	4
Webster	4	3	1	1			1		1	
Wetzel	13	10	4	2	2		2		2	1
Wirt	1	1					1			
Wood	221	173	33	39	38	48	15	3	40	5
Wyoming	5	4	3		1				1	
Wisconsin	17,220	13,668	2,048	3,516	2,244	2,796	3,064	650	2,234	668
Adams	6	5	2	2		1			1	
Ashland	59	52	20	8	13	8	3		7	
Barron	99	86	39	10	16	16	5	1	11	1
Bayfield	20	9	4		2	3			11	
Brown	659	565	67	179	146	141	32	8	78	8
Buffalo	8	3	3						5	
Burnett	12	6	4		1		1		6	
Calumet	16	13	8		1	3	1		3	
Chippewa	101	80	28	17	14	16	5	1	18	2
Clark	22	14	7	3	1	1	2		7	1
Columbia	65	52	21	8	8	3	12		13	
Crawford	23	13	8	1	2	1	1	2	8	
Dane	3,154	2,427	259	551	284	484	849	222	355	150
Dodge	102	83	32	12	21	11	7		18	1
Door	82	45	10	16	6	8	5	2	35	
Douglas	33	23	9	6	1	2	5	1	9	
Dunn	45	35	11	7	7	1	9		9	1
Eau Claire	457	386	50	116	86	80	54	9	53	9

Table 3.9

Physicians by State and County, 2010, continued

		Major Professional Activity								
		Patient Care								
			Office-Based Practice							
State County	Total Physicians	Total Patient Care	FM/GP Practice	Medical Specialties	Surgical Specialties	Other Specialties	Hospital Based Practice	Other Professional Activity	Inactive	Not Classified
Florence	6	4		1	1	2			2	
Fond Du Lac	194	158	27	46	28	31	26	2	31	3
Forest	3	3	2	1						
Grant	43	31	19	2	4	2	4	2	8	2
Green	86	61	8	21	11	14	7	2	23	
Green Lake	31	26	8	5	6	4	3	1	4	
Iowa	30	22	12	2	6	1	1	1	7	
Iron	5	3	1	1	1				2	
Jackson	29	25	18	1	1	2	3		2	2
Jefferson	78	64	20	16	15	5	8	1	10	3
Juneau	33	27	15	2	4	3	3	1	5	
Kenosha	251	199	36	57	32	44	30	6	32	14
Kewaunee	14	8	3	2	1	2		1	5	
La Crosse	658	531	58	142	77	110	144	16	90	21
Lafayette	8	7	5			1	1		1	
Langlade	34	26	6	8	5	4	3		8	
Lincoln	38	28	11	4	3	5	5		7	3
Manitowoc	166	130	23	39	33	13	22	2	29	5
Marathon	402	331	58	88	70	83	32	13	50	8
Marinette	83	68	10	23	16	12	7	2	11	2
Marquette	5	2	1			1			2	1
Menominee	4	4	3				1			
Milwaukee	3,794	2,989	235	731	469	553	1,001	185	376	244
Monroe	62	51	21	4	7	3	16	3	7	1
Oconto	28	22	4	4	5	4	5		6	
Oneida	169	137	14	43	38	28	14	2	26	4
Outagamie	438	361	83	99	76	60	43	11	57	9
Ozaukee	468	382	40	121	62	124	35	17	59	10
Pepin	9	5	2	1	1		1		4	
Pierce	43	29	16	1	4	2	6	1	13	
Polk	77	65	32	7	8	8	10	3	9	
Portage	136	109	20	24	23	27	15	4	20	3
Price	15	12	6	3		2	1		3	
Racine	332	279	51	78	55	64	31	4	40	9
Richland	24	19	9	2	2	1	5		4	1
Rock	339	271	46	82	41	43	59	13	48	7
Rusk	16	12	3	6	1		2		3	1
Saint Croix	95	74	31	8	10	14	11	4	12	5
Sauk	99	86	38	13	17	4	14	4	9	
Sawyer	29	22	16		1	3	2		5	2
Shawano	38	31	22	1	4		4		6	1
Sheboygan	224	176	36	47	45	38	10	1	41	6
Taylor	13	11	7	1			3		2	
Trempealeau	33	26	10	3	2	4	7	1	5	1
Vernon	46	38	15	5	5	9	4		7	1
Vilas	28	15	9		2	1	3		11	2
Walworth	122	83	24	16	20	16	7	6	30	3
Washburn	27	18	13	1	3	1			7	2
Washington	191	150	35	46	25	27	17	5	29	7
Waukesha	2,044	1,647	167	497	235	418	330	54	251	92
Waupaca	66	47	31	1	2	6	7		19	
Waushara	16	12	6		2	2	2		4	
Winnebago	483	385	52	101	78	112	42	12	78	8
Wood	552	449	28	173	78	104	66	24	67	12

Table 3.9

Physicians by State and County, 2010, continued

		Major Professional Activity								
		Patient Care								
			Office-Based Practice							
State County	Total Physicians	Total Patient Care	FM/GP Practice	Medical Specialties	Surgical Specialties	Other Specialties	Hospital Based Practice	Other Professional Activity	Inactive	Not Classified
Wyoming	1,242	964	198	186	229	194	157	32	223	23
Albany	87	73	9	8	19	14	23	1	12	1
Big Horn	9	6	4			1	1		3	
Campbell	67	63	12	11	15	15	10		3	1
Carbon	14	13	6		1	2	4		1	
Converse	17	13	3	2	4	1	3	1	3	
Crook	4	2	2						2	
Fremont	107	77	18	11	16	17	15	2	26	2
Goshen	14	12	7		3	1	1		2	
Hot Springs	8	6	3		2		1		2	
Johnson	17	12	6	1	2	2	1		5	
Laramie	268	205	34	58	46	37	30	12	45	6
Lincoln	14	11	6	1	2		2		3	
Natrona	214	172	31	44	36	35	26	4	30	8
Niobrara	1								1	
Park	85	66	20	9	16	13	8	1	16	2
Platte	10	9	4	1	1	2	1		1	
Sheridan	83	65	4	13	20	15	13	2	14	2
Sublette	10	7	5			1	1	1	2	
Sweetwater	37	31	7	4	9	7	4	1	5	
Teton	127	84	6	17	28	24	9	5	38	
Uinta	33	26	3	6	6	7	4	2	4	1
Washakie	7	6	4		2				1	
Weston	9	5	4		1				4	
Pacific Islands	233	187	44	52	27	19	45	7	22	17
American Samoa	9	6	2	2			2	1	2	
Federated States Of Micro	4	3		1		1	1	1		
Guam	186	149	32	45	25	15	32	5	19	13
Marshall Islands	2	2	1	1						
Northern Mariana Islands	28	24	7	3	1	3	10		1	3
Palau	4	3	2		1					1
APOs and FPOs	1,040	814	119	89	89	144	373	39	45	142
APOs and FPOs	1,040	814	119	89	89	144	373	39	45	142

Note: Does not include Address Unknown.

Table 3.10

Physicians by Metropolitan Statistical Area, 2010

		Major Professional Activity								
		Patient Care								
			Office-Based Practice							
Metropolitan Areas	Total Physicians	Total Patient Care	FM/GP Practice	Medical Specialties	Surgical Specialties	Other Specialties	Hospital Based Practice	Other Professional Activity	Inactive	Not Classified
Total Metropolitan Physicians	909,946	695,279	63,240	199,367	114,159	140,273	178,240	40,673	111,866	62,128
Abilene, TX	332	265	44	77	66	51	27	5	51	11
Aguadilla-Isabela-San Sebastián, PR	617	450	133	98	26	110	83	9	45	113
Akron, OH	2,065	1,652	166	441	259	299	487	71	238	104
Albany-Schenectady-Troy, NY	3,222	2,490	218	683	434	482	673	151	397	184
Albany, GA	349	289	37	98	67	52	35	7	41	12
Albuquerque, NM	3,414	2,567	271	639	345	530	782	199	404	244
Alexandria, LA	471	366	48	89	86	63	80	13	77	15
Allentown-Bethlehem-Easton, PA-NJ	2,379	1,879	183	523	377	356	440	72	310	118
Altoona, PA	341	273	37	85	58	50	43	6	56	6
Amarillo, TX	726	595	69	173	126	119	108	27	69	35
Ames, IA	197	163	26	49	29	39	20		30	4
Anchorage, AK	1,221	996	158	207	203	212	216	52	131	42
Anderson, IN	201	166	53	32	24	39	18	6	28	1
Anderson, SC	372	306	53	66	53	74	60	7	48	11
Ann Arbor, MI	4,264	3,168	111	711	339	580	1,427	310	312	474
Anniston-Oxford, AL	224	190	31	65	54	27	13	3	23	8
Appleton, WI	454	374	91	99	77	63	44	11	60	9
Asheville, NC	1,739	1,299	201	374	235	261	228	44	360	36
Athens-Clarke County, GA	505	416	41	127	95	101	52	16	61	12
Atlanta-Sandy Springs-Marietta, GA	14,587	11,357	920	3,718	2,125	2,417	2,177	798	1,492	940
Atlantic City-Hammonton, NJ	693	541	27	179	128	109	98	19	103	30
Auburn-Opelika, AL	228	197	27	69	43	29	29	2	22	7
Augusta-Richmond County, GA-SC	2,291	1,763	144	364	272	277	706	114	255	159
Austin-Round Rock-San Marcos, TX	4,504	3,562	463	1,047	703	860	489	154	535	253
Bakersfield-Delano, CA	1,259	1,038	159	340	173	192	174	30	140	51
Baltimore-Towson, MD	14,238	10,360	462	2,994	1,515	1,979	3,410	992	1,487	1,399
Bangor, ME	556	443	46	135	61	101	100	25	66	22
Barnstable Town, MA	860	541	40	197	104	116	84	35	268	16
Baton Rouge, LA	2,008	1,647	179	471	348	337	312	56	234	71
Battle Creek, MI	235	182	36	53	40	32	21	7	44	2
Bay City, MI	158	126	12	38	35	33	8		30	2
Beaumont-Port Arthur, TX	666	556	81	180	119	146	30	10	79	21
Bellingham, WA	618	452	112	118	65	126	31	18	137	11
Bend, OR	597	430	51	116	102	121	40	16	133	18
Billings, MT	613	491	61	116	110	116	88	13	89	20
Binghamton, NY	679	498	51	137	104	97	109	26	134	21
Birmingham-Hoover, AL	4,815	3,775	239	1,026	634	669	1,207	209	464	367
Bismarck, ND	383	314	48	65	63	69	69	12	42	15
Blacksburg-Christiansburg-Radford, VA	306	243	46	60	47	51	39	7	51	5
Bloomington-Normal, IL	386	317	46	93	77	76	25	6	56	7
Bloomington, IN	412	321	50	75	64	94	38	12	70	9
Boise City-Nampa, ID	1,501	1,208	197	282	279	263	187	37	219	37
Boston-Cambridge-Quincy, MA-NH	28,231	20,488	763	5,949	2,440	3,963	7,373	1,938	2,422	3,383
Boulder, CO	1,253	998	169	263	201	259	106	41	184	30
Bowling Green, KY	306	266	29	100	62	52	23		40	
Bremerton-Silverdale, WA	712	524	89	115	76	124	120	32	142	14
Bridgeport-Stamford-Norwalk, CT	3,962	3,000	103	1,086	582	626	603	172	563	227

Table 3.10

Physicians by Metropolitan Statistical Area, 2010, continued

		Major Professional Activity								
		Patient Care								
			Office-Based Practice							
Metropolitan Areas	Total Physicians	Total Patient Care	FM/GP Practice	Medical Specialties	Surgical Specialties	Other Specialties	Hospital Based Practice	Other Professional Activity	Inactive	Not Classified
Brownsville-Harlingen, TX	580	478	60	185	103	68	62	15	61	26
Brunswick, GA	285	208	21	62	51	57	17	4	65	8
Buffalo-Niagara Falls, NY	4,136	3,091	211	827	512	550	991	211	539	295
Burlington-South Burlington, VT	1,436	1,080	99	238	132	190	421	84	158	114
Burlington, NC	274	215	24	82	44	37	28	7	45	7
Canton-Massillon, OH	965	767	85	265	137	135	145	25	135	38
Cape Coral-Fort Myers, FL	1,643	1,086	101	384	262	252	87	40	502	15
Cape Girardeau-Jackson, MO-IL	302	263	32	64	62	63	42	4	31	4
Carson City, NV	152	128	16	35	31	35	11	4	19	1
Casper, WY	214	172	31	44	36	35	26	4	30	8
Cedar Rapids, IA	497	394	98	82	76	92	46	12	80	11
Champaign-Urbana, IL	740	561	69	176	77	104	135	27	111	41
Charleston-North Charleston-Summerville, SC	3,358	2,717	192	639	417	619	850	160	313	168
Charleston, WV	1,055	852	100	245	169	164	174	37	109	57
Charlotte-Gastonia-Rock Hill, NC-SC	4,624	3,919	438	1,299	749	838	595	116	465	124
Charlottesville, VA	2,275	1,662	86	305	147	287	837	156	217	240
Chattanooga, TN-GA	1,604	1,278	129	397	267	251	234	52	223	51
Cheyenne, WY	268	205	34	58	46	37	30	12	45	6
Chicago-Joliet-Naperville, IL-IN-WI	34,633	26,665	2,132	7,994	3,897	5,035	7,607	1,368	3,632	2,968
Chico, CA	549	425	71	113	93	94	54	8	105	11
Cincinnati-Middletown, OH-KY-IN	7,408	5,763	559	1,578	925	1,147	1,554	331	823	491
Clarksville, TN-KY	384	311	39	87	70	65	50	7	54	12
Cleveland-Elyria-Mentor, OH	10,437	7,754	385	1,975	1,077	1,315	3,002	392	1,094	1,197
Cleveland, TN	169	142	21	46	31	27	17	2	25	
Coeur d'Alene, ID	409	335	62	56	58	122	37	4	54	16
College Station-Bryan, TX	493	406	82	106	89	84	45	24	47	16
Colorado Springs, CO	1,572	1,246	140	308	255	333	210	50	236	40
Columbia, MO	1,426	1,079	72	200	135	189	483	72	131	144
Columbia, SC	2,261	1,827	200	497	315	353	462	100	259	75
Columbus, GA-AL	787	630	122	135	139	110	124	23	93	41
Columbus, IN	212	176	30	47	41	45	13	4	29	3
Columbus, OH	6,267	4,946	548	1,225	774	923	1,476	258	583	480
Corpus Christi, TX	1,020	825	104	244	167	181	129	16	143	36
Corvallis, OR	337	248	33	88	42	66	19	10	70	9
Crestview-Fort Walton Beach-Destin, FL	552	452	62	93	97	84	116	10	70	20
Cumberland, MD-WV	235	179	14	60	35	49	21	5	44	7
Dallas-Fort Worth-Arlington, TX	15,705	12,661	1,191	3,696	2,425	2,779	2,570	497	1,458	1,089
Dalton, GA	202	172	19	65	49	28	11	1	25	4
Danville, IL	140	101	19	22	17	18	25	2	31	6
Danville, VA	154	123	17	43	31	20	12	3	26	2
Davenport-Moline-Rock Island, IA-IL	756	609	102	170	132	140	65	18	112	17
Dayton, OH	2,673	2,116	279	558	297	389	593	108	314	135
Decatur, AL	225	190	32	55	53	34	16	2	29	4
Decatur, IL	289	235	42	59	44	53	37	5	42	7
Deltona-Daytona Beach-Ormond Beach, FL	1,150	866	151	245	170	175	125	31	229	24
Denver-Aurora-Broomfield, CO	9,101	6,912	649	2,034	1,109	1,582	1,538	505	1,135	549

Table 3.10

Physicians by Metropolitan Statistical Area, 2010, continued

Metropolitan Areas	Total Physicians	Total Patient Care	FM/GP Practice	Medical Specialties	Surgical Specialties	Other Specialties	Hospital Based Practice	Other Professional Activity	Inactive	Not Classified
		Major Professional Activity								
		Patient Care								
			Office-Based Practice							
Des Moines-West Des Moines, IA	1,235	984	109	280	208	204	183	47	170	34
Detroit-Warren-Livonia, MI	14,352	11,296	861	3,208	1,690	1,952	3,585	487	1,483	1,086
Dothan, AL	404	341	34	104	93	85	25	6	50	7
Dover, DE	269	217	28	75	41	51	22	8	33	11
Dubuque, IA	267	218	19	76	54	50	19	5	39	5
Duluth, MN-WI	929	729	166	177	118	142	126	17	152	31
Durham-Chapel Hill, NC	5,801	4,032	182	850	418	740	1,842	532	479	758
Eau Claire, WI	571	478	81	134	101	98	64	11	71	11
El Centro, CA	161	132	13	50	30	20	19	5	19	5
El Paso, TX	1,614	1,278	108	355	241	213	361	59	152	125
Elizabethtown, KY	228	196	21	62	35	49	29	4	21	7
Elkhart-Goshen, IN	303	238	55	40	56	56	31	5	54	6
Elmira, NY	270	207	15	65	37	53	37	10	49	4
Erie, PA	590	444	77	105	99	73	90	17	114	15
Eugene-Springfield, OR	1,092	851	155	249	175	232	40	24	206	11
Evansville, IN-KY	972	811	144	211	166	165	125	24	113	24
Fairbanks, AK	215	181	27	39	37	44	34	7	25	2
Fajardo, PR	174	130	30	29	16	33	22	5	15	24
Fargo, ND-MN	720	594	67	165	95	112	155	26	86	14
Farmington, NM	206	163	26	41	32	31	33	4	27	12
Fayetteville-Springdale-Rogers, AR-MO	885	722	147	163	161	134	117	21	120	22
Fayetteville, NC	819	676	92	190	118	103	173	24	79	40
Flagstaff, AZ	376	304	53	69	63	70	49	11	51	10
Flint, MI	1,043	823	118	262	108	115	220	29	122	69
Florence-Muscle Shoals, AL	277	229	27	84	60	48	10	4	38	6
Florence, SC	522	451	88	130	94	86	53	13	42	16
Fond du Lac, WI	194	158	27	46	28	31	26	2	31	3
Fort Collins-Loveland, CO	854	667	140	155	131	160	81	23	141	23
Fort Smith, AR-OK	514	405	101	107	68	61	68	10	86	13
Fort Wayne, IN	1,096	904	120	251	185	242	106	30	142	20
Fresno, CA	2,097	1,661	210	486	300	351	314	68	248	120
Gadsden, AL	225	188	33	61	46	38	10	2	30	5
Gainesville, FL	2,422	1,824	116	371	197	308	832	162	215	221
Gainesville, GA	441	355	27	133	89	76	30	6	74	6
Glens Falls, NY	309	235	40	76	50	42	27	10	61	3
Goldsboro, NC	208	169	29	52	31	35	22	4	30	5
Grand Forks, ND-MN	310	258	56	45	44	45	68	17	27	8
Grand Junction, CO	461	354	66	70	70	89	59	16	75	16
Grand Rapids-Wyoming, MI	2,136	1,765	194	475	339	371	386	56	246	69
Great Falls, MT	239	181	24	51	38	51	17	6	51	1
Greeley, CO	365	286	65	64	64	45	48	11	61	7
Green Bay, WI	694	588	72	185	152	143	36	9	89	8
Greensboro-High Point, NC	1,700	1,387	194	464	300	267	162	47	219	47
Greenville-Mauldin-Easley, SC	1,866	1,564	226	427	298	272	341	40	204	58
Greenville, NC	1,106	855	61	216	114	162	302	78	67	106
Guayama, PR	99	81	19	19	4	21	18	2	5	11
Gulfport-Biloxi, MS	549	443	37	109	96	86	115	10	84	12
Hagerstown-Martinsburg, MD-WV	521	401	56	129	80	76	60	17	92	11
Hanford-Corcoran, CA	157	128	31	29	19	21	28	3	16	10
Harrisburg-Carlisle, PA	2,366	1,833	151	405	257	311	709	120	245	168
Harrisonburg, VA	306	233	46	59	48	60	20	5	64	4

Table 3.10

Physicians by Metropolitan Statistical Area, 2010, continued

Metropolitan Areas	Total Physicians	Total Patient Care	FM/GP Practice	Medical Specialties	Surgical Specialties	Other Specialties	Hospital Based Practice	Other Professional Activity	Inactive	Not Classified
		Major Professional Activity: Patient Care	Office-Based Practice							
Hartford-West Hartford-East Hartford, CT	4,808	3,668	208	1,146	623	709	982	268	585	287
Hattiesburg, MS	470	393	49	120	95	88	41	12	56	9
Hickory-Lenoir-Morganton, NC	744	602	110	140	139	147	66	14	115	13
Hinesville-Fort Stewart, GA	56	46	4	11	7	6	18	2	5	3
Holland-Grand Haven, MI	414	299	56	77	65	75	26	10	99	6
Honolulu, HI	3,857	2,914	208	856	468	627	755	173	558	212
Hot Springs, AR	299	216	35	70	40	50	21	7	72	4
Houma-Bayou Cane-Thibodaux, LA	373	320	46	85	92	46	51	6	40	7
Houston-Sugar Land-Baytown, TX	17,871	13,962	1,273	3,744	2,181	2,725	4,039	789	1,456	1,664
Huntington-Ashland, WV-KY-OH	1,087	872	105	226	150	164	227	46	80	89
Huntsville, AL	1,049	865	140	244	176	176	129	22	121	41
Idaho Falls, ID	223	185	24	42	51	48	20	2	32	4
Indianapolis-Carmel, IN	7,267	5,829	561	1,461	886	1,245	1,676	398	649	391
Iowa City, IA	1,983	1,391	77	206	145	221	742	176	148	268
Ithaca, NY	307	235	38	66	36	61	34	10	57	5
Jackson, MI	220	173	28	58	38	27	22	3	39	5
Jackson, MS	2,446	1,921	170	411	302	363	675	116	260	149
Jackson, TN	471	396	43	138	101	67	47	9	53	13
Jacksonville, FL	4,591	3,585	414	1,004	588	705	874	158	623	225
Jacksonville, NC	239	184	26	36	39	24	59	3	28	24
Janesville, WI	339	271	46	82	41	43	59	13	48	7
Jefferson City, MO	220	175	26	46	41	35	27	7	32	6
Johnson City, TN	1,047	830	90	202	126	126	286	41	109	67
Johnstown, PA	416	316	43	72	52	47	102	13	61	26
Jonesboro, AR	331	280	55	75	63	56	31	11	38	2
Joplin, MO	327	268	23	82	54	46	63	3	49	7
Kalamazoo-Portage, MI	1,161	889	89	250	141	184	225	59	166	47
Kankakee-Bradley, IL	181	147	15	50	39	20	23	1	29	4
Kansas City, MO-KS	6,377	5,027	491	1,274	815	1,005	1,442	264	689	397
Kennewick-Pasco-Richland, WA	473	386	58	125	77	80	46	10	58	19
Killeen-Temple-Fort Hood, TX	1,352	1,112	92	220	124	151	525	51	124	65
Kingsport-Bristol-Bristol, TN-VA	895	721	139	208	147	134	93	33	123	18
Kingston, NY	387	305	83	68	45	64	45	9	55	18
Knoxville, TN	2,568	2,095	248	684	417	433	313	61	345	67
Kokomo, IN	173	144	32	39	36	23	14	1	25	3
La Crosse, WI-MN	679	547	65	144	78	114	146	17	93	22
Lafayette, IN	465	374	54	114	78	85	43	12	71	8
Lafayette, LA	876	742	77	219	166	162	118	15	83	36
Lake Charles, LA	436	353	65	101	73	67	47	8	64	11
Lake Havasu City-Kingman, AZ	272	238	27	86	45	60	20	4	23	7
Lakeland-Winter Haven, FL	1,070	792	89	294	175	154	80	19	219	40
Lancaster, PA	1,085	824	188	208	139	161	128	37	189	35
Lansing-East Lansing, MI	1,137	820	94	224	134	164	204	94	158	65
Laredo, TX	261	202	38	69	45	27	23	6	36	17
Las Cruces, NM	374	291	65	78	51	56	41	10	53	20
Las Vegas-Paradise, NV	4,088	3,149	299	1,075	576	798	401	99	634	206
Lawrence, KS	262	191	36	53	31	41	30	6	55	10
Lawton, OK	263	206	39	40	44	40	43	7	32	18

Table 3.10

Physicians by Metropolitan Statistical Area, 2010, continued

		Major Professional Activity								
		Patient Care								
			Office-Based Practice							
Metropolitan Areas	Total Physicians	Total Patient Care	FM/GP Practice	Medical Specialties	Surgical Specialties	Other Specialties	Hospital Based Practice	Other Professional Activity	Inactive	Not Classified
Lebanon, PA	333	246	38	38	34	49	87	9	56	22
Lewiston-Auburn, ME	294	229	35	65	36	45	48	17	33	15
Lewiston, ID-WA	159	126	24	29	30	26	17	1	31	1
Lexington-Fayette, KY	2,605	2,031	158	487	313	412	661	123	249	202
Lima, OH	291	235	30	68	56	61	20	4	45	7
Lincoln, NE	793	621	111	179	122	141	68	26	128	18
Little Rock-North Little Rock-Conway, AR	3,220	2,552	235	525	378	502	912	156	299	213
Logan, UT-ID	198	158	26	38	40	32	22	1	36	3
Longview, TX	396	341	56	105	79	71	30	4	44	7
Longview, WA	217	159	28	46	29	41	15	1	54	3
Los Angeles-Long Beach-Santa Ana, CA	43,309	32,627	3,148	10,181	5,724	7,174	6,400	1,814	5,920	2,948
Louisville/Jefferson County, KY-IN	4,585	3,674	317	1,032	645	852	828	172	485	254
Lubbock, TX	1,144	897	91	221	162	171	252	47	121	79
Lynchburg, VA	570	430	84	112	83	92	59	13	122	5
Macon, GA	871	689	75	209	146	114	145	35	111	36
Madera-Chowchilla, CA	190	162	19	64	26	17	36	2	21	5
Madison, WI	3,249	2,501	292	561	298	488	862	223	375	150
Manchester-Nashua, NH	1,078	868	98	311	166	189	104	34	146	30
Manhattan, KS	218	174	38	38	34	35	29	3	27	14
Mankato-North Mankato, MN	252	194	45	46	40	38	25	8	46	4
Mansfield, OH	231	174	14	63	39	39	19	2	53	2
Mayagüez, PR	601	461	73	121	83	97	87	8	54	78
McAllen-Edinburg-Mission, TX	913	799	147	304	151	118	79	6	64	44
Medford, OR	692	502	79	168	104	109	42	18	155	17
Memphis, TN-MS-AR	4,046	3,240	251	990	567	563	869	157	392	257
Merced, CA	285	239	74	54	39	26	46	6	27	13
Miami-Fort Lauderdale-Pompano Beach, FL	20,317	14,602	1,163	5,028	2,718	3,013	2,680	659	3,835	1,221
Michigan City-La Porte, IN	181	137	22	31	35	32	17	3	39	2
Midland, TX	307	269	20	99	53	58	39	7	21	10
Milwaukee-Waukesha-West Allis, WI	6,497	5,168	477	1,395	791	1,122	1,383	261	715	353
Minneapolis-St. Paul-Bloomington, MN-WI	11,041	8,772	1,434	2,383	1,352	1,763	1,840	513	1,299	457
Missoula, MT	431	328	37	89	70	86	46	9	86	8
Mobile, AL	1,249	1,044	59	320	236	169	260	43	113	49
Modesto, CA	999	807	148	265	149	162	83	20	126	46
Monroe, LA	454	378	56	106	69	71	76	10	49	17
Monroe, MI	145	115	22	33	25	21	14	7	18	5
Montgomery, AL	811	667	83	210	146	115	113	26	95	23
Morgantown, WV	1,037	793	54	135	108	136	360	61	67	116
Morristown, TN	193	151	29	56	27	28	11	2	35	5
Mount Vernon-Anacortes, WA	357	266	68	67	50	59	22	5	79	7
Muncie, IN	342	271	32	85	44	38	72	11	43	17
Muskegon-Norton Shores, MI	286	215	43	57	42	46	27	7	61	3
Myrtle Beach-North Myrtle Beach-Conway, SC	532	449	57	146	97	110	39	7	64	12
Napa, CA	569	403	45	107	68	120	63	15	144	7
Naples-Marco Island, FL	1,333	747	54	272	169	181	71	36	531	19
Nashville-Davidson--Murfreesboro--Franklin, TN	6,404	4,980	330	1,382	876	1,037	1,355	336	604	484
New Haven-Milford, CT	5,121	3,769	80	1,072	512	697	1,408	349	468	535

Table 3.10

Physicians by Metropolitan Statistical Area, 2010, continued

		Major Professional Activity									
		Patient Care									
			Office-Based Practice								
Metropolitan Areas	Total Physicians	Total Patient Care	FM/GP Practice	Medical Specialties	Surgical Specialties	Other Specialties	Hospital Based Practice	Other Professional Activity	Inactive	Not Classified
New Orleans-Metairie-Kenner, LA	5,764	4,541	215	1,152	790	821	1,563	233	523	467
NewYork-Northern New Jersey-Long Island, NY-NJ-PA	89,234	66,538	2,211	20,629	9,770	12,339	21,589	4,342	9,998	8,356
Niles-Benton Harbor, MI	354	278	51	86	47	60	34	5	65	6
North Port-Bradenton-Sarasota, FL	2,532	1,618	170	583	375	363	127	51	833	30
Norwich-New London, CT	756	548	45	203	101	94	105	38	149	21
Ocala, FL	633	507	58	198	102	113	36	4	107	15
Ocean City, NJ	148	93	9	22	21	30	11	2	51	2
Odessa, TX	255	205	25	54	47	22	57	11	19	20
Ogden-Clearfield, UT	950	759	118	169	164	178	130	18	137	36
Oklahoma City, OK	3,820	3,051	346	722	523	672	788	177	421	171
Olympia, WA	793	604	129	151	84	146	94	31	129	29
Omaha-Council Bluffs, NE-IA	3,402	2,670	278	612	443	463	874	161	350	221
Orlando-Kissimmee-Sanford, FL	5,313	4,273	493	1,419	769	885	707	140	681	219
Oshkosh-Neenah, WI	483	385	52	101	78	112	42	12	78	8
Owensboro, KY	231	189	15	65	49	42	18	4	36	2
Oxnard-Thousand Oaks-Ventura, CA	2,166	1,599	269	489	313	327	201	86	383	98
Palm Bay-Melbourne-Titusville, FL	1,418	1,123	133	388	212	265	125	31	232	32
Palm Coast, FL	170	96	20	25	16	18	17	3	68	3
Panama City-Lynn Haven-Panama City Beach, FL	403	322	31	97	76	80	38	9	55	17
Parkersburg-Marietta-Vienna, WV-OH	322	254	47	62	53	66	26	3	58	7
Pascagoula, MS	335	271	29	74	49	56	63	8	43	13
Pensacola-Ferry Pass-Brent, FL	1,348	1,072	135	273	198	226	240	47	180	49
Peoria, IL	1,237	986	125	252	159	205	245	54	145	52
Philadelphia-Camden-Wilmington, PA-NJ-DE-MD	25,667	18,902	1,140	5,287	2,629	3,640	6,206	1,558	3,102	2,105
Phoenix-Mesa-Glendale, AZ	10,938	8,346	769	2,554	1,494	1,955	1,574	368	1,639	585
Pine Bluff, AR	176	138	40	38	27	19	14	6	24	8
Pittsburgh, PA	10,137	7,622	590	2,046	1,102	1,404	2,480	461	1,195	859
Pittsfield, MA	631	444	24	135	68	106	111	28	105	54
Pocatello, ID	206	159	32	28	31	35	33	5	33	9
Ponce, PR	967	719	95	217	102	155	150	33	78	137
Port St. Lucie, FL	901	640	72	202	161	149	56	16	228	17
Portland-South Portland-Biddeford, ME	2,126	1,628	171	467	256	346	388	98	320	80
Portland-Vancouver-Hillsboro, OR-WA	8,712	6,580	614	1,881	1,126	1,418	1,541	393	1,135	604
Poughkeepsie-Newburgh-Middletown, NY	1,837	1,441	89	572	278	323	179	56	277	63
Prescott, AZ	532	353	55	95	63	86	54	15	158	6
Providence-New Bedford-Fall River, RI-MA	5,627	4,306	231	1,365	668	732	1,310	224	684	413
Provo-Orem, UT	752	618	119	141	135	128	95	16	93	25
Pueblo, CO	440	355	57	88	64	91	55	9	70	6
Punta Gorda, FL	429	304	26	123	62	68	25	5	110	10
Racine, WI	332	279	51	78	55	64	31	4	40	9
Raleigh-Cary, NC	2,888	2,283	280	752	444	512	295	114	339	152
Rapid City, SD	422	316	48	81	60	69	58	18	78	10
Reading, PA	886	668	91	178	131	119	149	28	158	32

Table 3.10

Physicians by Metropolitan Statistical Area, 2010, continued

		Major Professional Activity									
		Patient Care									
			Office-Based Practice								
Metropolitan Areas	Total Physicians	Total Patient Care	FM/GP Practice	Medical Specialties	Surgical Specialties	Other Specialties	Hospital Based Practice	Other Professional Activity	Inactive	Not Classified
Redding, CA	494	388	77	94	73	105	39	13	84	9
Reno-Sparks, NV	1,383	1,076	125	278	218	297	158	40	185	82
Richmond, VA	4,712	3,582	399	969	575	671	968	201	645	284
Riverside-San Bernardino-Ontario, CA	7,301	5,537	756	1,592	960	1,070	1,159	207	1,144	413
Roanoke, VA	1,331	1,045	104	246	168	203	324	49	184	53
Rochester, MN	3,577	2,821	99	679	252	566	1,225	136	289	331
Rochester, NY	4,439	3,312	195	963	476	526	1,152	248	555	324
Rockford, IL	924	710	117	213	139	148	93	33	150	31
Rocky Mount, NC	209	176	26	57	47	31	15	4	28	1
Rome, GA	380	311	60	79	73	62	37	6	53	10
Sacramento--Arden-Arcade--Roseville, CA	7,116	5,502	667	1,548	902	1,234	1,151	287	912	415
Saginaw-Saginaw Township North, MI	607	505	83	119	86	80	137	23	61	18
Salem, OR	823	628	135	153	126	146	68	34	148	13
Salinas, CA	1,019	745	134	209	151	154	97	33	222	19
Salisbury, MD	341	275	11	105	74	63	22	4	56	6
Salt Lake City, UT	4,389	3,361	277	800	581	733	970	246	457	325
San Angelo, TX	264	219	26	62	48	52	31	1	36	8
San Antonio-New Braunfels, TX	7,171	5,599	562	1,364	856	1,082	1,735	342	723	507
San Diego-Carlsbad-San Marcos, CA	11,602	8,472	848	2,338	1,364	1,936	1,986	656	1,819	655
San Francisco-Oakland-Fremont, CA	21,424	15,438	1,003	4,935	2,394	3,526	3,580	1,210	2,894	1,882
San Germán-Cabo Rojo, PR	333	249	67	70	25	42	45	4	34	46
San Jose-Sunnyvale-Santa Clara, CA	7,996	5,937	403	1,956	956	1,180	1,442	412	909	738
San Juan-Caguas-Guaynabo, PR	8,903	6,702	1,156	1,651	857	1,546	1,492	359	741	1,101
San Luis Obispo-Paso Robles, CA	930	685	83	156	116	224	106	28	194	23
Sandusky, OH	141	110	11	36	24	33	6	3	24	4
Santa Barbara-Santa Maria-Goleta, CA	1,431	1,016	119	319	180	261	137	36	346	33
Santa Cruz-Watsonville, CA	838	633	123	162	100	169	79	28	161	16
Santa Fe, NM	660	433	72	99	62	135	65	35	168	24
Santa Rosa-Petaluma, CA	1,573	1,130	239	288	208	266	129	45	355	43
Savannah, GA	1,177	931	85	265	196	189	196	34	171	41
Scranton--Wilkes-Barre, PA	1,397	1,062	101	350	211	202	198	43	238	54
Seattle-Tacoma-Bellevue, WA	13,935	10,396	1,327	2,670	1,557	2,304	2,538	802	1,840	897
Sebastian-Vero Beach, FL	469	326	28	113	74	83	28	13	124	6
Sheboygan, WI	224	176	36	47	45	38	10	1	41	6
Sherman-Denison, TX	244	204	26	63	46	51	18	2	35	3
Shreveport-Bossier City, LA	1,961	1,584	115	339	269	227	634	72	149	156
Sioux City, IA-NE-SD	288	235	37	51	60	49	38	9	36	8
Sioux Falls, SD	934	778	103	201	145	161	168	37	94	25
South Bend-Mishawaka, IN-MI	770	653	112	167	113	171	90	15	86	16
Spartanburg, SC	680	566	96	137	127	103	103	24	77	13
Spokane, WA	1,585	1,202	181	314	225	306	176	66	267	50
Springfield, IL	1,210	986	78	269	163	184	292	45	114	65
Springfield, MA	2,383	1,908	126	625	267	366	524	73	311	91
Springfield, MO	1,064	886	109	245	185	207	140	19	145	14
Springfield, OH	221	175	28	57	39	37	14	9	35	2

Table 3.10

Physicians by Metropolitan Statistical Area, 2010, continued

Metropolitan Areas	Total Physicians	Major Professional Activity: Patient Care: Total Patient Care	Office-Based Practice: FM/GP Practice	Office-Based Practice: Medical Specialties	Office-Based Practice: Surgical Specialties	Office-Based Practice: Other Specialties	Hospital Based Practice	Other Professional Activity	Inactive	Not Classified
St. Cloud, MN	506	434	82	122	85	95	50	12	55	5
St. George, UT	299	219	31	57	54	54	23	4	69	7
St. Joseph, MO-KS	209	175	19	47	39	40	30	6	22	6
St. Louis, MO-IL	10,228	7,913	468	2,231	1,266	1,394	2,554	456	1,003	856
State College, PA	358	276	34	84	49	72	37	14	53	15
Steubenville-Weirton, OH-WV	167	128	20	44	28	19	17	1	32	6
Stockton, CA	1,237	1,014	152	312	195	191	164	25	130	68
Sumter, SC	178	143	22	42	33	32	14	3	25	7
Syracuse, NY	2,657	2,071	204	471	349	385	662	122	312	152
Tallahassee, FL	922	667	131	154	119	134	129	60	163	32
Tampa-St. Petersburg-Clearwater, FL	8,856	6,840	586	2,224	1,199	1,469	1,362	306	1,327	383
Terre Haute, IN	367	303	64	87	51	58	43	12	38	14
Texarkana, TX-Texarkana, AR	340	278	45	77	65	57	34	2	47	13
Toledo, OH	2,286	1,772	235	442	283	374	438	81	291	142
Topeka, KS	582	428	59	124	71	96	78	26	123	5
Trenton-Ewing, NJ	1,622	1,176	59	444	216	253	204	132	207	107
Tucson, AZ	4,049	2,984	265	786	471	745	717	211	667	187
Tulsa, OK	2,101	1,670	199	494	316	344	317	68	302	61
Tuscaloosa, AL	562	461	62	116	87	96	100	21	67	13
Tyler, TX	861	719	83	204	154	162	116	28	99	15
Utica-Rome, NY	664	512	77	153	97	97	88	9	116	27
Valdosta, GA	226	190	24	61	52	37	16	2	33	1
Vallejo-Fairfield, CA	964	786	103	233	124	156	170	29	99	50
Victoria, TX	243	195	27	64	43	44	17	3	37	8
Vineland-Millville-Bridgeton, NJ	211	168	14	71	40	25	18	6	33	4
Virginia Beach-Norfolk-Newport News, VA-NC	5,493	4,373	504	1,111	731	859	1,168	180	726	214
Visalia-Porterville, CA	538	441	72	152	85	86	46	6	80	11
Waco, TX	549	446	92	82	94	100	78	25	65	13
Warner Robins, GA	219	177	19	62	29	35	32	5	26	11
Washington-Arlington-Alexandria, DC-VA-MD-WV	25,484	18,398	1,200	5,528	2,789	3,522	5,359	2,215	2,864	2,007
Waterloo-Cedar Falls, IA	360	294	71	66	52	65	40	5	51	10
Wausau, WI	402	331	58	88	70	83	32	13	50	8
Wenatchee-East Wenatchee, WA	317	251	52	66	44	62	27	8	55	3
Wheeling, WV-OH	390	306	42	68	64	70	62	8	69	7
Wichita Falls, TX	361	285	52	70	52	57	54	8	50	18
Wichita, KS	1,633	1,305	229	294	237	248	297	58	204	66
Williamsport, PA	272	206	48	52	32	37	37	8	51	7
Wilmington, NC	1,026	792	81	258	161	175	117	23	182	29
Winchester, VA-WV	410	349	35	111	88	79	36	6	51	4
Winston-Salem, NC	2,441	1,891	145	422	249	351	724	122	235	193
Worcester, MA	3,083	2,390	205	750	286	355	794	153	292	248
Yakima, WA	470	374	86	101	71	72	44	16	69	11
Yauco, PR	286	210	64	50	11	40	45	3	16	57
York-Hanover, PA	921	726	121	200	113	139	153	34	126	35
Youngstown-Warren-Boardman, OH-PA	1,268	958	81	296	178	178	225	33	223	54
Yuba City, CA	265	218	45	75	38	39	21	3	38	6
Yuma, AZ	267	217	22	92	51	36	16	3	27	20

Note: Does not include Address Unknown.

Table 3.11

Physicians by Micropolitan Statistical Area, 2010

		Major Professional Activity								
		Patient Care								
			Office-Based Practice							
Micropolitan Areas	Total Physicians	Total Patient Care	FM/GP Practice	Medical Specialties	Surgical Specialties	Other Specialties	Hospital Based Practice	Other Professional Activity	Inactive	Not Classified
Total Micropolitan Physicians	54,313	41,871	8,153	11,104	8,667	7,319	6,628	1,204	9,768	1,470
Abbeville, LA	49	38	8	12	11	2	5	2	8	1
Aberdeen, SD	95	76	19	11	20	18	8	3	15	1
Aberdeen, WA	80	59	15	14	12	15	3	2	16	3
Ada, OK	82	65	8	15	12	11	19	1	15	1
Adjuntas, PR	24	20	6	3		5	6		1	3
Adrian, MI	107	73	13	24	13	15	8	1	31	2
Alamogordo, NM	86	65	18	15	11	10	11	3	14	4
Albany-Lebanon, OR	171	127	52	27	20	13	15	3	40	1
Albemarle, NC	76	60	10	20	15	9	6		15	1
Albert Lea, MN	54	41	8	5	7	7	14		13	
Albertville, AL	107	91	30	20	18	14	9	4	11	1
Alexander City, AL	60	48	10	12	14	5	7	2	9	1
Alexandria, MN	90	69	24	16	16	4	9	1	19	1
Alice, TX	30	28	9	11	5	1	2		1	1
Allegan, MI	74	52	13	14	4	14	7	4	17	1
Alma, MI	58	50	8	14	11	10	7		5	3
Alpena, MI	78	60	10	13	12	17	8	1	15	2
Altus, OK	33	25	4	6	6	3	6		6	2
Americus, GA	55	38	6	12	8	6	6		14	3
Amsterdam, NY	86	63	11	23	11	8	10	3	20	
Andrews, TX	11	9	3	1	3		2	1	1	
Angola, IN	28	21	11	1	3	3	3		6	1
Arcadia, FL	32	21	4	8	3	1	5		9	2
Ardmore, OK	85	68	5	19	19	11	14	3	13	1
Arkadelphia, AR	24	22	7	6	6	1	2		2	
Ashland, OH	63	48	11	13	10	7	7		14	1
Ashtabula, OH	89	59	12	22	12	7	6	1	27	2
Astoria, OR	71	52	11	9	12	7	13	1	18	
Atchison, KS	19	15	6	1	4	2	2		3	1
Athens, OH	60	45	9	11	11	8	6	2	11	2
Athens, TN	57	47	13	10	14	8	2	1	9	
Athens, TX	74	60	22	8	16	11	3		12	2
Auburn, IN	43	32	18	2	3	6	3		11	
Auburn, NY	94	64	2	25	17	12	8	2	27	1
Augusta-Waterville, ME	415	309	75	54	49	48	83	26	70	10
Austin, MN	51	39	11	8	5	5	10	1	11	
Bainbridge, GA	30	25	3	9	4	4	5		5	
Baraboo, WI	99	86	38	13	17	4	14	4	9	
Barre, VT	188	140	29	38	24	26	23	7	33	8
Bartlesville, OK	89	69	11	18	19	15	6	1	17	2
Bastrop, LA	25	18	10		4	1	3	1	6	
Batavia, NY	80	60	6	16	12	15	11		18	2
Batesville, AR	82	70	21	12	19	10	8		11	1
Bay City, TX	35	25	6	9	8	2		4	5	1
Beatrice, NE	29	21	12	5	1		3	1	4	3
Beaver Dam, WI	102	83	32	12	21	11	7		18	1
Beckley, WV	223	180	13	62	40	32	33	4	31	8
Bedford, IN	61	44	8	16	13	3	4	2	14	1
Beeville, TX	22	20	8	4	4	3	1		2	
Bellefontaine, OH	53	40	12	5	6	2	15	4	6	3
Bemidji, MN	93	75	19	16	16	13	11	3	13	2
Bennettsville, SC	17	15	6	3	1	2	3		2	
Bennington, VT	150	115	16	31	27	21	20	11	22	2
Berlin, NH-VT	91	71	18	13	7	15	18	1	17	2
Big Rapids, MI	43	35	8	9	8	3	7	2	5	1
Big Spring, TX	50	38	4	7	9	5	13	2	9	1

Table 3.11

Physicians by Micropolitan Statistical Area, 2010, continued

		Major Professional Activity								
		Patient Care								
			Office-Based Practice							
Micropolitan Areas	Total Physicians	Total Patient Care	FM/GP Practice	Medical Specialties	Surgical Specialties	Other Specialties	Hospital Based Practice	Other Professional Activity	Inactive	Not Classified
Bishop, CA	50	34	11	7	6	4	6	1	15	
Blackfoot, ID	32	20	5	2	3	5	5	1	9	2
Bloomsburg-Berwick, PA	719	574	28	132	79	74	261	21	56	68
Bluefield, WV-VA	250	201	27	60	35	48	31	2	42	5
Blytheville, AR	34	28	10	9	5	1	3		5	1
Bogalusa, LA	47	36	9	7	5	5	10	2	8	1
Bonham, TX	20	15	4	1	2		8	1	3	1
Boone, IA	22	12	8		1	2	1		9	1
Boone, NC	174	124	19	40	31	29	5	4	44	2
Borger, TX	15	13	5	3	5				2	
Bozeman, MT	291	193	44	46	41	47	15	7	84	7
Bradford, PA	62	45	8	12	9	7	9		14	3
Brainerd, MN	202	155	43	26	31	30	25	2	40	5
Branson, MO	107	85	24	18	12	10	21	4	15	3
Brenham, TX	54	40	10	11	12	4	3	1	12	1
Brevard, NC	84	48	10	17	8	5	8	5	31	
Brigham City, UT	40	31	11	7	8	2	3	2	7	
Brookhaven, MS	46	39	3	14	15	6	1		7	
Brookings, OR	31	17	8	1	1	2	5	4	10	
Brookings, SD	35	27	8	5	7		7		8	
Brownsville, TN	12	8	4	3	1				4	
Brownwood, TX	61	53	9	16	16	9	3	1	6	1
Bucyrus, OH	36	22	2	6	7	1	6	2	12	
Burley, ID	39	28	10	4	9	2	3		11	
Burlington, IA-IL	92	74	15	14	18	16	11		17	1
Butte-Silver Bow, MT	81	62	8	19	17	10	8	2	17	
Cadillac, MI	77	58	17	17	10	8	6	1	15	3
Calhoun, GA	61	51	12	16	12	7	4	2	7	1
Cambridge, MD	61	47	5	15	6	9	12	2	9	3
Cambridge, OH	64	48	6	16	14	6	6		14	2
Camden, AR	24	20	10	5	4	1			4	
Campbellsville, KY	38	34	6	10	11	4	3	1	2	1
Cañon City, CO	46	34	14	6	5	6	3	1	10	1
Canton, IL	32	23	9	5	5	1	3		8	1
Carbondale, IL	199	152	40	39	22	23	28	6	29	12
Carlsbad-Artesia, NM	70	53	7	12	16	7	11	1	13	3
Cedar City, UT	47	36	6	11	8	6	5		7	4
Cedartown, GA	27	15	7	2	1	3	2	1	10	1
Celina, OH	37	28	8	6	5	3	6	1	7	1
Central City, KY	28	24	5	6	8	3	2	1	2	1
Centralia, IL	66	54	7	21	11	14	1	1	8	3
Centralia, WA	105	72	20	18	17	12	5	4	26	3
Chambersburg, PA	247	189	43	53	38	35	20	4	50	4
Charleston-Mattoon, IL	87	70	15	11	14	10	20	4	12	1
Chester, SC	23	18	4	4	5	2	3	1	4	
Chillicothe, OH	135	116	27	24	21	18	26	1	16	2
Claremont, NH	118	88	14	19	9	15	31	3	23	4
Clarksburg, WV	199	150	30	40	20	17	43	9	29	11
Clarksdale, MS	46	38	5	13	11	2	7	2	4	2
Clearlake, CA	93	76	18	23	13	15	7	1	16	
Cleveland, MS	44	38	9	10	10	4	5		5	1
Clewiston, FL	21	13	3	4	2	1	3		8	
Clinton, IA	71	62	12	22	13	10	5	1	7	1
Clovis, NM	63	53	6	25	11	7	4		7	3
Coamo, PR	59	44	14	11	1	9	9	2	4	9
Coffeyville, KS	40	35	9	8	10	5	3		4	1
Coldwater, MI	54	36	2	11	6	10	7		17	1
Columbia, TN	213	177	23	55	42	37	20	3	25	8

Table 3.11

Physicians by Micropolitan Statistical Area, 2010, continued

		Major Professional Activity								
		Patient Care								
			Office-Based Practice							
Micropolitan Areas	Total Physicians	Total Patient Care	FM/GP Practice	Medical Specialties	Surgical Specialties	Other Specialties	Hospital Based Practice	Other Professional Activity	Inactive	Not Classified
Columbus, MS	123	103	12	32	26	21	12	1	18	1
Columbus, NE	36	31	10	4	11	3	3		5	
Concord, NH	558	419	71	106	85	80	77	22	90	27
Connersville, IN	24	22	4	5	4	2	7		2	
Cookeville, TN	229	185	26	60	41	40	18	2	36	6
Coos Bay, OR	172	120	18	39	29	15	19	3	44	5
Corbin, KY	84	64	12	25	12	11	4	2	16	2
Cordele, GA	38	28	5	13	5	1	4		7	3
Corinth, MS	66	59	10	16	16	10	7	1	4	2
Cornelia, GA	44	35	8	14	7	4	2	1	8	
Corning, NY	165	129	21	40	23	19	26	3	30	3
Corsicana, TX	56	40	9	14	13	3	1	1	13	2
Cortland, NY	71	56	13	18	10	8	7		14	1
Coshocton, OH	27	23	2	7	9	1	4		4	
Crawfordsville, IN	44	35	11	8	9	4	3	1	8	
Crescent City, CA	49	38	8	9	7	10	4		9	2
Crossville, TN	110	81	11	33	21	10	6	1	25	3
Crowley, LA	53	41	15	9	9	4	4	1	8	3
Cullman, AL	114	103	22	32	29	16	4		9	2
Culpeper, VA	61	47	7	16	13	7	4		14	
Danville, KY	129	108	23	27	28	23	7	3	18	
Daphne-Fairhope-Foley, AL	461	352	71	94	65	79	43	10	85	14
Decatur, IN	20	18	10	1	3	2	2		2	
Defiance, OH	50	39	13	8	11	5	2	1	9	1
Del Rio, TX	46	40	8	11	12	1	8	1	2	3
Deming, NM	27	23	4	6	5	2	6	1	3	
DeRidder, LA	41	35	9	10	10	2	4		2	4
Dickinson, ND	34	27	6	6	5	2	8		7	
Dillon, SC	22	19	6	5	1		7	1	2	
Dixon, IL	68	57	10	16	9	4	18	1	8	2
Dodge City, KS	47	39	12	11	9	5	2		6	2
Douglas, GA	62	47	7	13	10	8	9	2	9	4
Dublin, GA	154	120	21	36	22	15	26	7	23	4
DuBois, PA	137	114	8	33	23	21	29	1	21	1
Dumas, TX	11	9	5	1	1	1	1			2
Duncan, OK	44	38	17	4	10	2	5		6	
Dunn, NC	85	74	13	22	14	16	9	2	5	4
Durango, CO	261	189	31	41	43	56	18	7	59	6
Durant, OK	33	27	3	11	9	2	2		6	
Dyersburg, TN	66	49	8	18	12	5	6		15	2
Eagle Pass, TX	32	26	4	12	7	2	1		3	3
East Liverpool-Salem, OH	102	79	16	26	19	10	8		20	3
East Stroudsburg, PA	248	189	22	58	39	49	21	9	42	8
Easton, MD	229	139	7	44	30	30	28	12	72	6
Edwards, CO	193	136	20	25	37	31	23	9	44	4
Effingham, IL	83	73	13	17	19	13	11		9	1
El Campo, TX	54	43	9	14	14	4	2		11	
El Dorado, AR	103	83	24	16	14	13	16	2	13	5
Elizabeth City, NC	110	87	12	27	25	20	3	1	19	3
Elk City, OK	32	28	7	6	6	4	5	1	3	
Elko, NV	58	47	9	13	15	6	4	1	9	1
Ellensburg, WA	46	33	14	5	6	2	6	1	12	
Emporia, KS	51	39	11	11	7	7	3	1	11	
Enid, OK	115	90	17	21	22	22	8		22	3
Enterprise-Ozark, AL	88	70	10	16	20	11	13	3	14	1
Escanaba, MI	53	40	15	9	7	3	6	2	9	2
Espanola, NM	45	36	12	3	6	9	6		8	1
Eufaula, AL-GA	15	13	6	4	3				2	

Table 3.11

Physicians by Micropolitan Statistical Area, 2010, continued

		Major Professional Activity								
		Patient Care								
			Office-Based Practice							
Micropolitan Areas	Total Physicians	Total Patient Care	FM/GP Practice	Medical Specialties	Surgical Specialties	Other Specialties	Hospital Based Practice	Other Professional Activity	Inactive	Not Classified
Eureka-Arcata-Fortuna, CA	331	254	57	48	50	70	29	9	64	4
Evanston, WY	33	26	3	6	6	7	4	2	4	1
Fairmont, MN	42	37	14	6	12	3	2		5	
Fairmont, WV	96	79	12	27	12	12	16		15	2
Fallon, NV	26	21	6	3	4	1	7		3	2
Faribault-Northfield, MN	120	103	43	16	21	11	12	1	15	1
Farmington, MO	76	56	13	22	5	6	10	2	13	5
Fergus Falls, MN	88	63	21	12	10	12	8	2	22	1
Fernley, NV	17	12	6	2		1	3		4	1
Findlay, OH	151	121	13	37	32	26	13	1	25	4
Fitzgerald, GA	20	16	4	6	2	1	3		4	
Forest City, NC	101	81	18	24	14	16	9	3	16	1
Forrest City, AR	18	18	6	7	3	2				
Fort Dodge, IA	69	53	10	11	19	8	5		14	2
Fort Leonard Wood, MO	28	23	9	2	1	4	7	1	2	2
Fort Madison-Keokuk, IA-MO	55	44	8	10	9	5	12	2	9	
Fort Morgan, CO	28	25	11	1	6	1	6		3	
Fort Payne, AL	57	44	13	10	10	4	7	1	11	1
Fort Polk South, LA	50	42	7	13	8	6	8		5	3
Fort Valley, GA	12	9	4	2	1		2		2	1
Frankfort, IN	27	22	8	4	3	3	4		4	1
Frankfort, KY	96	68	13	25	21	6	3	7	17	4
Fredericksburg, TX	104	75	16	19	19	12	9	1	28	
Freeport, IL	78	63	12	21	13	12	5	3	12	
Fremont, NE	58	47	13	11	14	7	2	1	10	
Fremont, OH	72	59	28	10	8	8	5	1	11	1
Gaffney, SC	46	37	16	5	9	4	3		9	
Gainesville, TX	25	20	6	4	4	3	3		4	1
Galesburg, IL	120	97	22	23	22	15	15	1	20	2
Gallup, NM	167	132	31	25	15	12	49	5	24	6
Garden City, KS	45	37	7	8	11	5	6		6	2
Gardnerville Ranchos, NV	107	74	15	15	14	19	11	3	27	3
Georgetown, SC	146	104	22	27	21	24	10	3	35	4
Gettysburg, PA	129	100	28	27	14	24	7	3	24	2
Gillette, WY	67	63	12	11	15	15	10		3	1
Glasgow, KY	96	83	20	16	20	14	13	1	8	4
Gloversville, NY	70	52	11	16	11	7	7	1	16	1
Granbury, TX	76	52	10	14	12	9	7	4	17	3
Grand Island, NE	130	108	23	28	27	19	11	2	17	3
Grants Pass, OR	146	108	26	28	26	17	11	1	32	5
Grants, NM	28	23	10	6	4		3		3	2
Great Bend, KS	35	27	8	7	7	4	1		8	
Greeneville, TN	118	95	25	25	19	12	14	4	18	1
Greensburg, IN	23	16	4	6		3	3	1	4	2
Greenville, MS	97	77	11	27	18	12	9	1	17	2
Greenville, OH	39	31	20	4	2	1	4	1	5	2
Greenwood, MS	67	54	4	15	11	8	16	2	10	1
Greenwood, SC	256	210	49	44	42	34	41	13	27	6
Grenada, MS	31	27	3	9	11	1	3		4	
Guymon, OK	13	13	2	6	4		1			
Hammond, LA	149	123	16	41	33	11	22	4	17	5
Hannibal, MO	75	62	4	25	14	8	11		10	3
Harriman, TN	39	30	14	8	4	3	1	2	7	
Harrisburg, IL	39	33	13	7	4	5	4		6	
Harrison, AR	74	62	22	12	9	11	8		11	1
Hastings, NE	86	64	15	17	20	11	1	3	17	2
Havre, MT	29	21	5	3	8	1	4		7	1
Hays, KS	81	61	2	16	14	16	13	1	13	6

Table 3.11

Physicians by Micropolitan Statistical Area, 2010, continued

		Major Professional Activity								
		Patient Care								
			Office-Based Practice							
Micropolitan Areas	Total Physicians	Total Patient Care	FM/GP Practice	Medical Specialties	Surgical Specialties	Other Specialties	Hospital Based Practice	Other Professional Activity	Inactive	Not Classified
Heber, UT	31	22	8	2	4	5	3		6	3
Helena-West Helena, AR	23	13	5	4	2	2			8	2
Helena, MT	226	176	22	37	30	43	44	8	41	1
Henderson, NC	60	49	13	14	10	8	4		10	1
Hereford, TX	7	5	3		2				1	1
Hilo, HI	427	311	63	91	49	85	23	15	93	8
Hilton Head Island-Beaufort, SC	635	358	37	103	95	75	48	12	258	7
Hobbs, NM	58	47	6	17	7	8	9		8	3
Homosassa Springs, FL	329	222	23	86	38	51	24	3	98	6
Hood River, OR	104	83	26	11	14	18	14	5	11	5
Hope, AR	22	18	6	4	4		4	1	3	
Houghton, MI	62	48	15	8	6	12	7		12	2
Hudson, NY	120	83	13	19	12	21	18	6	26	5
Humboldt, TN	44	38	18	9	5	1	5		6	
Huntingdon, PA	45	34	8	6	4	10	6		11	
Huntington, IN	41	35	11	10	6	5	3		4	2
Huntsville, TX	68	51	11	14	11	8	7	3	11	3
Huron, SD	22	19	6	4	6	2	1		3	
Hutchinson, KS	146	113	21	39	25	20	8	1	28	4
Hutchinson, MN	51	44	24	5	4	3	8	2	5	
Indiana, PA	128	97	15	32	21	12	17	4	25	2
Indianola, MS	18	12	8	1	1	1	1	1	4	1
Iron Mountain, MI-WI	78	64	11	13	16	10	14	2	12	
Jackson, WY-ID	141	94	11	18	29	25	11	6	40	1
Jacksonville, IL	52	39	7	7	15	5	5	1	11	1
Jacksonville, TX	67	52	8	8	9	18	9	3	11	1
Jamestown-Dunkirk-Fredonia, NY	197	146	22	47	31	36	10	1	44	6
Jamestown, ND	29	27	13	3	5	3	3		2	
Jasper, IN	86	74	16	18	20	11	9		9	3
Jayuya, PR	19	15	7	5		1	2	1		3
Jennings, LA	33	26	9	7	3	1	6		6	1
Jesup, GA	28	24	5	8	6	3	2		4	
Juneau, AK	93	82	24	12	13	23	10		9	2
Kahului-Wailuku, HI	394	298	46	103	55	67	27	11	74	11
Kalispell, MT	309	220	39	49	56	62	14	6	75	8
Kapaa, HI	188	145	30	37	29	36	13	7	34	2
Kearney, NE	142	126	20	36	37	21	12		15	1
Keene, NH	197	131	29	32	25	23	22	5	60	1
Kendallville, IN	28	25	11	5	3	2	4		3	
Kennett, MO	39	32	11	8	6	2	5	1	2	4
Kerrville, TX	189	117	12	39	22	24	20	6	63	3
Ketchikan, AK	32	25	7	5	3	5	5		7	
Key West, FL	247	152	17	37	42	38	18	8	81	6
Kill Devil Hills, NC	62	45	12	10	9	8	6	1	13	3
Kingsville, TX	27	20	7	8	2	2	1		6	1
Kinston, NC	107	78	11	32	15	16	4	3	25	1
Kirksville, MO	14	13	3	3	3	1	3	1		
Klamath Falls, OR	167	122	38	19	21	22	22	5	30	10
Kodiak, AK	29	25	14	2	2	3	4		4	
La Follette, TN	40	32	7	16	3	3	3		6	2
La Grande, OR	54	45	7	9	9	10	10	1	7	1
Laconia, NH	170	122	8	37	31	31	15	5	39	4
LaGrange, GA	120	100	3	42	25	23	7	2	17	1
Lake City, FL	125	96	15	30	14	15	22	1	25	3
Lamesa, TX	7	4	1	1	1		1		2	1
Lancaster, SC	91	72	15	23	19	11	4	3	13	3

Table 3.11

Physicians by Micropolitan Statistical Area, 2010, continued

		Major Professional Activity									
		Patient Care									
			Office-Based Practice								
Micropolitan Areas	Total Physicians	Total Patient Care	FM/GP Practice	Medical Specialties	Surgical Specialties	Other Specialties	Hospital Based Practice	Other Professional Activity	Inactive	Not Classified
Laramie, WY	87	73	9	8	19	14	23	1	12	1
Las Vegas, NM	46	40	8	15	4	7	6	1	5	
Laurel, MS	110	85	14	26	26	10	9	4	19	2
Laurinburg, NC	65	59	14	22	11	7	5		5	1
Lawrenceburg, TN	33	25	9	8	5	3			5	3
Lebanon, MO	27	27	10	7	3	2	5			
Lebanon, NH-VT	1,597	1,164	70	222	129	150	593	98	197	138
Levelland, TX	13	12	4	4	2		2		1	
Lewisburg, PA	146	117	9	25	32	29	22	6	17	6
Lewisburg, TN	16	15	6	3	2	3	1		1	
Lewistown, PA	54	45	9	13	12	7	4	2	7	
Lexington Park, MD	129	96	16	35	18	15	12	6	20	7
Lexington, NE	21	20	13	1	3	1	2		1	
Liberal, KS	37	29	2	9	6	7	5		8	
Lincoln, IL	20	17	10	2	3	1	1		3	
Lincolnton, NC	77	66	20	18	12	8	8	1	8	2
Lock Haven, PA	41	30	7	10	5	3	5		7	4
Logansport, IN	48	38	9	5	7	9	8	1	7	2
London, KY	85	74	13	26	15	13	7		3	8
Los Alamos, NM	66	48	13	22	6	7		2	14	2
Lufkin, TX	155	135	18	52	30	24	11	1	17	2
Lumberton, NC	149	124	22	33	27	19	23	2	17	6
Macomb, IL	42	32	10	8	5	3	6		10	
Madison, IN	65	50	14	8	9	4	15	1	13	1
Madisonville, KY	157	128	34	27	21	12	34	4	20	5
Magnolia, AR	26	16	9	3	3		1	1	7	2
Malone, NY	103	71	11	21	10	14	15	3	25	4
Manitowoc, WI	166	130	23	39	33	13	22	2	29	5
Marble Falls, TX	59	46	13	10	5	9	9		12	1
Marinette, WI-MI	98	81	14	25	18	15	9	2	12	3
Marion-Herrin, IL	164	131	24	34	26	21	26	4	24	5
Marion, IN	101	79	15	18	18	14	14	1	19	2
Marion, OH	123	100	9	31	27	19	14	3	17	3
Marquette, MI	279	221	40	53	39	42	47	7	44	7
Marshall, MN	25	22	9	1	8	1	3		3	
Marshall, MO	19	15	9	1	3		2		3	1
Marshall, TX	53	44	7	12	11	8	6		8	1
Marshalltown, IA	60	44	14	12	11	5	2		16	
Marshfield-Wisconsin Rapids, WI	552	449	28	173	78	104	66	24	67	12
Martin, TN	37	32	8	13	6	2	3		5	
Martinsville, VA	114	88	14	28	17	18	11	1	24	1
Maryville, MO	29	28	8	5	7	5	3		1	
Mason City, IA	171	136	26	27	23	30	30	2	31	2
Mayfield, KY	40	33	6	11	6	4	6		7	
Maysville, KY	54	49	11	17	9	8	4		4	1
McAlester, OK	67	48	7	13	13	8	7		15	4
McComb, MS	86	70	7	13	25	14	11		14	2
McMinnville, TN	40	33	10	9	8	4	2		7	
McPherson, KS	35	27	18		2	2	5		8	
Meadville, PA	140	112	21	31	27	18	15	4	22	2
Menomonie, WI	45	35	11	7	7	1	9		9	1
Meridian, MS	264	225	29	66	54	48	28		33	6
Merrill, WI	38	28	11	4	3	5	5		7	3
Mexico, MO	37	32	5	6	8	3	10		4	1
Miami, OK	26	21	2	2	6	2	9		5	
Middlesborough, KY	46	33	5	13	7	4	4	2	10	1

Table 3.11

Physicians by Micropolitan Statistical Area, 2010, continued

		Major Professional Activity								
		Patient Care								
			Office-Based Practice							
Micropolitan Areas	Total Physicians	Total Patient Care	FM/GP Practice	Medical Specialties	Surgical Specialties	Other Specialties	Hospital Based Practice	Other Professional Activity	Inactive	Not Classified
Midland, MI	236	187	41	38	35	39	34	10	35	4
Milledgeville, GA	123	91	11	26	16	17	21	2	25	5
Minden, LA	48	37	17	7	8	3	2	1	9	1
Mineral Wells, TX	21	17	5	5	6		1		4	
Minot, ND	190	162	21	38	28	28	47	4	20	4
Mitchell, SD	41	36	7	11	8	7	3		5	
Moberly, MO	16	9		4	3	2			7	
Monroe, WI	86	61	8	21	11	14	7	2	23	
Montrose, CO	102	79	12	18	20	24	5		19	4
Morehead City, NC	183	138	22	25	30	27	34	1	38	6
Morgan City, LA	67	53	14	15	14	3	7	1	12	1
Moscow, ID	58	48	20	5	7	10	6	2	8	
Moses Lake, WA	82	68	26	18	11	6	7	2	12	
Moultrie, GA	58	49	9	13	12	7	8	1	8	
Mount Airy, NC	98	83	23	25	21	4	10	2	10	3
Mount Pleasant, MI	77	67	4	24	14	16	9	1	7	2
Mount Pleasant, TX	46	41	5	12	16	8			5	
Mount Sterling, KY	32	28	5	10	4	4	5		4	
Mount Vernon, IL	111	96	6	33	29	21	7		11	4
Mount Vernon, OH	70	50	9	15	9	6	11	3	17	
Mountain Home, AR	114	99	18	23	28	15	15		12	3
Mountain Home, ID	33	27	9	3	10	2	3	2	1	3
Murray, KY	70	58	9	15	21	11	2		10	2
Muscatine, IA	40	34	8	9	9	2	6	2	4	
Muskogee, OK	124	94	9	38	20	10	17	1	29	
Nacogdoches, TX	146	129	24	33	40	22	10		16	1
Natchez, MS-LA	87	66	13	21	14	12	6	2	15	4
Natchitoches, LA	46	38	13	12	6	4	3	1	7	
New Bern, NC	293	240	21	101	49	52	17	5	41	7
New Castle, IN	56	42	9	9	7	4	13	1	12	1
New Castle, PA	113	86	17	25	18	16	10	3	23	1
New Iberia, LA	122	95	19	33	22	13	8	1	22	4
New Philadelphia-Dover, OH	111	81	18	20	19	11	13	2	26	2
New Ulm, MN	47	44	19	5	10	5	5		3	
Newberry, SC	42	38	16	7	3	7	5	1	3	
Newport, TN	24	23	12	7	2		2			1
Newton, IA	19	15	9		4	2		1	2	1
Nogales, AZ	52	28	10	7	3	3	5	5	17	2
Norfolk, NE	93	80	22	13	14	17	14	1	9	3
North Platte, NE	89	68	14	15	13	18	8	1	12	8
North Vernon, IN	13	11	5	4			2		1	1
North Wilkesboro, NC	71	56	14	20	14	6	2	2	12	1
Norwalk, OH	57	44	17	6	13	6	2	2	11	
Oak Harbor, WA	176	109	14	13	19	25	38	7	57	3
Oak Hill, WV	40	29	11	7	4	2	5		10	1
Ocean Pines, MD	97	68	13	18	9	18	10	1	21	7
Ogdensburg-Massena, NY	183	146	16	42	30	28	30	4	26	7
Oil City, PA	95	75	10	26	20	15	4	4	15	1
Okeechobee, FL	44	42	6	20	9	4	3		2	
Olean, NY	134	101	18	39	18	16	10	2	29	2
Oneonta, NY	348	283	9	83	70	55	66	10	42	13
Ontario, OR-ID	57	48	8	10	13	10	7		9	
Opelousas-Eunice, LA	148	130	29	35	39	19	8		17	1
Orangeburg, SC	130	106	22	36	20	11	17	3	17	4
Oskaloosa, IA	22	18	10	1	2	1	4		4	
Ottawa-Streator, IL	190	148	31	39	34	17	27	2	35	5
Ottumwa, IA	66	55	3	22	8	14	8		9	2

Table 3.11

Physicians by Micropolitan Statistical Area, 2010, continued

		Major Professional Activity								
		Patient Care								
			Office-Based Practice							
Micropolitan Areas	Total Physicians	Total Patient Care	FM/GP Practice	Medical Specialties	Surgical Specialties	Other Specialties	Hospital Based Practice	Other Professional Activity	Inactive	Not Classified
Owatonna, MN	67	53	24	12	11	1	5	1	10	3
Owosso, MI	58	41	8	11	11	6	5		16	1
Oxford, MS	128	90	11	29	24	14	12	2	34	2
Paducah, KY-IL	283	229	29	74	57	55	14	4	42	8
Pahrump, NV	31	19	8	4		4	3	1	10	1
Palatka, FL	84	61	9	18	16	12	6		21	2
Palestine, TX	60	47	6	16	13	10	2		13	
Pampa, TX	23	18	3	9	5		1		5	
Paragould, AR	45	38	16	6	8	6	2		6	1
Paris, TN	58	43	7	13	10	10	3		14	1
Paris, TX	114	90	6	31	25	25	3	3	19	2
Parsons, KS	43	36	6	3	11	8	8	1	3	3
Payson, AZ	88	59	21	15	9	3	11	3	24	2
Pecos, TX	3	2		1			1		1	
Pella, IA	37	28	13	5	4	1	5	2	6	1
Pendleton-Hermiston, OR	101	74	20	15	20	13	6	1	24	2
Peru, IN	24	17	4	2	4	4	3		7	
Phoenix Lake-Cedar Ridge, CA	140	109	18	33	16	25	17	2	27	2
Picayune, MS	44	28	10	6	5	3	4	1	13	2
Pierre Part, LA	9	8	4	1			3		1	
Pierre, SD	31	25	7	7	6	2	3		5	1
Pittsburg, KS	54	41	9	13	11	2	6	1	11	1
Plainview, TX	23	18	6	7	3	2			5	
Platteville, WI	42	31	19	2	4	2	4	2	7	2
Plattsburgh, NY	222	178	14	58	35	46	25	3	32	9
Plymouth, IN	47	36	23	3	3	3	4	3	7	1
Point Pleasant, WV-OH	129	110	10	44	25	22	9	4	14	1
Ponca City, OK	60	44	14	9	11	9	1	3	13	
Pontiac, IL	29	28	9	8	7	1	3		1	
Poplar Bluff, MO	127	104	17	31	23	12	21	2	19	2
Port Angeles, WA	214	132	38	31	22	25	16	12	67	3
Portales, NM	13	12	3	4	2	2	1		1	
Portsmouth, OH	125	99	11	29	14	24	21	2	21	3
Pottsville, PA	181	141	15	52	25	32	17	3	33	4
Price, UT	25	22	5	4	8	2	3	1	1	1
Prineville, OR	14	9	6		1	1	1	1	4	
Pullman, WA	65	45	15	14	8	4	4	1	16	3
Quincy, IL-MO	191	152	25	45	25	32	25	2	31	6
Raymondville, TX	7	7	5	2						
Red Bluff, CA	70	55	12	14	15	9	5	1	13	1
Red Wing, MN	98	73	20	12	14	11	16	4	19	2
Rexburg, ID	45	37	11	6	11	5	4		7	1
Richmond-Berea, KY	144	115	27	36	22	15	15	1	20	8
Richmond, IN	169	135	17	46	25	27	20	6	26	2
Rio Grande City-Roma, TX	23	19	9	5	1	2	2	1	1	2
Riverton, WY	107	77	18	11	16	17	15	2	26	2
Roanoke Rapids, NC	86	68	12	28	13	11	4	1	15	2
Rochelle, IL	40	35	23	4	3	1	4	1	4	
Rock Springs, WY	37	31	7	4	9	7	4	1	5	
Rockingham, NC	44	32	7	13	7	2	3	1	9	2
Rockland, ME	171	105	10	29	18	26	22	9	52	5
Rolla, MO	76	65	11	24	12	9	9	1	6	4
Roseburg, OR	216	155	21	53	30	31	20	4	54	3
Roswell, NM	134	111	27	31	22	18	13	1	16	6
Ruidoso, NM	36	24	6	5	3	5	5		12	
Russellville, AR	118	97	27	21	24	15	10	1	20	
Ruston, LA	98	86	15	30	20	16	5		7	5

Table 3.11

Physicians by Micropolitan Statistical Area, 2010, continued

Micropolitan Areas	Total Physicians	Major Professional Activity: Patient Care: Total Patient Care	Office-Based Practice: FM/GP Practice	Office-Based Practice: Medical Specialties	Office-Based Practice: Surgical Specialties	Office-Based Practice: Other Specialties	Hospital Based Practice	Other Professional Activity	Inactive	Not Classified
Rutland, VT	191	130	25	33	22	24	26	5	50	6
Safford, AZ	36	25	14	4	2	2	3		6	5
Salina, KS	174	138	29	29	35	31	14	5	28	3
Salisbury, NC	245	186	23	48	39	32	44	6	46	7
Sanford, NC	88	66	12	19	11	16	8	4	16	2
Santa Isabel, PR	23	14	5	3	1	3	2		1	8
Sault Ste. Marie, MI	43	33	11	4	5	6	7		7	3
Sayre, PA	276	218	24	49	41	28	76	6	39	13
Scottsbluff, NE	100	80	16	11	19	19	15	1	19	
Scottsboro, AL	54	47	19	7	10	6	5		6	1
Scottsburg, IN	18	17	9	2	2	1	3		1	
Seaford, DE	392	300	44	102	56	65	33	13	68	11
Searcy, AR	117	98	25	24	17	21	11	1	17	1
Sebring, FL	207	151	16	60	35	26	14	4	41	11
Sedalia, MO	48	37	6	10	11	6	4	2	9	
Selinsgrove, PA	39	31	12	6	2	4	7		8	
Selma, AL	80	58	10	17	13	6	12	1	18	3
Seneca Falls, NY	22	15	4	4	2	4	1		6	1
Seneca, SC	161	120	26	22	26	32	14	2	34	5
Sevierville, TN	79	63	26	13	12	7	5		15	1
Seymour, IN	58	51	19	6	11	7	8		7	
Shawnee, OK	79	59	13	15	12	7	12	1	17	2
Shelby, NC	165	131	18	50	27	25	11		33	1
Shelbyville, TN	33	27	10	7	4	2	4		6	
Shelton, WA	50	30	7	4	11	3	5	1	17	2
Sheridan, WY	83	65	4	13	20	15	13	2	14	2
Show Low, AZ	119	98	33	17	14	17	17	2	16	3
Sidney, OH	47	39	13	8	8	4	6	1	7	
Sierra Vista-Douglas, AZ	136	105	19	34	20	23	9	8	17	6
Sikeston, MO	55	43	8	10	7	5	13	1	10	1
Silver City, NM	79	61	10	19	11	16	5	2	16	
Silverthorne, CO	108	67	17	10	15	22	3	2	37	2
Snyder, TX	12	10	6	2			2		2	
Somerset, KY	146	120	13	44	26	24	13		19	7
Somerset, PA	102	72	17	13	14	10	18	3	25	2
Southern Pines-Pinehurst, NC	407	318	15	93	71	84	55	12	69	8
Spearfish, SD	54	36	14	6	9	3	4	1	17	
Spencer, IA	27	27	7	1	13	4	2			
Spirit Lake, IA	30	20	6		5	6	3		10	
St. Marys, GA	55	39	7	16	9	2	5	1	12	3
St. Marys, PA	48	34	7	2	8	8	9		13	1
Starkville, MS	62	52	13	10	13	10	6		8	2
Statesboro, GA	109	94	16	29	24	14	11		12	3
Statesville-Mooresville, NC	340	297	42	95	79	57	24	4	37	2
Staunton-Waynesboro, VA	279	206	35	50	47	49	25	3	64	6
Stephenville, TX	47	40	10	13	11	6			7	
Sterling, CO	23	20	7	2	6	2	3		2	1
Sterling, IL	85	66	14	17	11	9	15	1	15	3
Stevens Point, WI	136	109	20	24	23	27	15	4	20	3
Stillwater, OK	115	85	17	30	20	12	6		27	3
Storm Lake, IA	19	13	10	1	1	1			6	
Sturgis, MI	64	51	17	7	11	7	9		13	
Sulphur Springs, TX	36	31	9	6	9	2	5		5	
Summerville, GA	11	9	4	1	1	3			2	
Sunbury, PA	78	54	13	16	4	11	10	2	19	3
Susanville, CA	39	28	13	5	6	2	2	2	8	1
Sweetwater, TX	10	8	2	2	2	2			1	1

Table 3.11

Physicians by Micropolitan Statistical Area, 2010, continued

		Major Professional Activity								
		Patient Care								
			Office-Based Practice							
Micropolitan Areas	Total Physicians	Total Patient Care	FM/GP Practice	Medical Specialties	Surgical Specialties	Other Specialties	Hospital Based Practice	Other Professional Activity	Inactive	Not Classified
Tahlequah, OK	64	52	8	7	10	8	19	3	7	2
Talladega-Sylacauga, AL	62	49	9	18	15	6	1	1	10	2
Tallulah, LA	8	8	4	3			1			
Taos, NM	103	72	18	15	12	14	13	5	23	3
Taylorville, IL	24	20	8	8	3	1			4	
The Dalles, OR	61	45	6	9	15	7	8	2	8	6
The Villages, FL	125	48	5	17	6	14	6	4	71	2
Thomaston, GA	42	34	8	8	12	5	1		8	
Thomasville-Lexington, NC	115	91	22	29	23	10	7		22	2
Thomasville, GA	167	132	10	38	31	38	15	5	28	2
Tiffin, OH	56	46	8	12	11	13	2		7	3
Tifton, GA	109	97	10	34	23	23	7	1	11	
Toccoa, GA	46	34	8	12	10	2	2	1	11	
Torrington, CT	458	325	28	116	64	68	49	21	102	10
Traverse City, MI	484	351	35	109	77	92	38	14	113	6
Troy, AL	31	26	6	10	5	2	3	1	2	2
Truckee-Grass Valley, CA	288	208	34	50	39	62	23	9	65	6
Tullahoma, TN	173	142	28	37	35	22	20	3	22	6
Tupelo, MS	361	295	30	98	62	65	40	7	51	8
Tuskegee, AL	22	15	3	1	3	1	7	2	4	1
Twin Falls, ID	178	146	34	30	39	29	14	2	27	3
Ukiah, CA	236	168	41	48	32	30	17	9	57	2
Union City, TN-KY	60	47	11	12	10	7	7	1	12	
Union, SC	32	25	8	7	4	2	4		6	1
Urbana, OH	17	13	6	5		2			3	1
Utuado, PR	34	28	11	5		7	5	1	2	3
Uvalde, TX	25	22	10	5	4	1	2		3	
Valley, AL	29	24	3	11	6	2	2		2	3
Van Wert, OH	27	23	10	4	5	3	1		3	1
Vermillion, SD	17	16	7	3		4	2			1
Vernal, UT	25	24	7	3	7	3	4			1
Vernon, TX	20	16	4	3	1	2	6	1	2	1
Vicksburg, MS	89	64	14	19	12	4	15	3	21	1
Vidalia, GA	53	45	5	15	11	6	8		8	
Vincennes, IN	81	68	10	18	12	13	15		13	
Wabash, IN	27	20	9	2		3	6	2	5	
Wahpeton, ND-MN	30	19	6	1	5	1	6	2	9	
Walla Walla, WA	250	177	32	43	31	39	32	3	68	2
Walterboro, SC	53	39	8	10	8	6	7		13	1
Wapakoneta, OH	47	36	14	6	3	6	7	1	7	3
Warren, PA	84	60	9	10	10	14	17	1	21	2
Warrensburg, MO	46	44	14	8	7	6	9	2		
Warsaw, IN	77	52	18	2	14	7	11	1	22	2
Washington Court House, OH	19	14	7	3	2		2		5	
Washington, IN	19	14	5	4	1	1	3		5	
Washington, NC	85	54	11	11	10	9	13		29	2
Watertown-Fort Atkinson, WI	78	64	20	16	15	5	8	1	10	3
Watertown-Fort Drum, NY	233	168	15	37	35	40	41	5	52	8
Watertown, SD	70	56	14	12	13	10	7	1	11	2
Wauchula, FL	12	10	2	5	2		1		2	
Waycross, GA	119	96	14	35	16	15	16	1	18	4
Weatherford, OK	32	25	11	3	5		6		7	
West Plains, MO	68	58	18	11	10	8	11		7	3
West Point, MS	23	17	2	6	7		2		6	
Whitewater, WI	122	83	24	16	20	16	7	6	30	3
Willimantic, CT	165	137	23	45	29	16	24	3	24	1
Williston, ND	48	38	12	3	11	6	6		10	
Willmar, MN	126	93	31	24	17	12	9	6	25	2

Table 3.11

Physicians by Micropolitan Statistical Area, 2010, continued

		Major Professional Activity								
		Patient Care								
			Office-Based Practice							
Micropolitan Areas	Total Physicians	Total Patient Care	FM/GP Practice	Medical Specialties	Surgical Specialties	Other Specialties	Hospital Based Practice	Other Professional Activity	Inactive	Not Classified
Wilmington, OH	83	67	17	15	8	11	16	3	6	7
Wilson, NC	119	96	8	40	22	17	9	2	20	1
Winfield, KS	32	24	12	4	4	1	3		7	1
Winona, MN	69	52	13	11	5	12	11		14	3
Woodward, OK	25	17	8	3	4	2			8	
Wooster, OH	160	129	26	36	38	16	13	2	24	5
Worthington, MN	29	23	7	5	4	2	5		6	
Yankton, SD	100	78	10	18	23	16	11	1	21	
Yazoo City, MS	16	12	5			2	5		3	1
Zanesville, OH	162	130	19	42	34	25	10		29	3

Note: Does not include Address Unknown.

Table 3.12

Non-Metropolitan Physicians by State, 2010

		Major Professional Activity								
		Patient Care								
			Office-Based Practice							
State	Total Physicians	Total Patient Care	FM/GP Practice	Medical Specialties	Surgical Specialties	Other Specialties	Hospital Based Practice	Other Professional Activity	Inactive	Not Classified
Total Non-Metropolitan Physicians	20,684	15,422	5,705	2,867	2,256	1,914	2,680	413	4,294	555
Alabama	333	266	122	54	42	22	26	3	60	4
Alaska	233	193	80	24	17	27	45	7	30	3
Arizona	79	61	12	21	7	9	12	2	8	8
Arkansas	449	342	200	39	45	19	39	4	100	3
California	345	236	72	34	43	48	39	12	94	3
Colorado	788	564	181	92	99	110	82	14	194	16
Florida	328	227	68	50	27	36	46	9	85	7
Georgia	765	569	193	147	95	53	81	13	169	14
Idaho	346	229	70	30	41	47	41	7	100	10
Illinois	455	356	145	73	47	37	54	4	90	5
Indiana	184	149	85	14	10	9	31	4	29	2
Iowa	590	430	237	32	48	38	75	10	143	7
Kansas	349	256	140	24	30	19	43	6	79	8
Kentucky	989	800	233	222	104	113	128	9	143	37
Louisiana	235	189	72	47	29	14	27		39	7
Maine	864	623	151	122	130	83	137	20	200	21
Maryland	123	76	25	17	15	13	6	4	42	1
Massachusetts	99	50	9	8	6	10	17	7	42	
Michigan	865	621	153	160	113	109	86	15	212	17
Minnesota	664	503	303	51	55	32	62	11	140	10
Mississippi	401	309	138	64	34	25	48	3	80	9
Missouri	463	358	146	60	41	47	64	7	86	12
Montana	439	318	137	42	48	30	61	15	100	6
Nebraska	304	231	171	11	9	6	34	5	64	4
Nevada	37	32	13	6	3	2	8		5	
New Hampshire	134	82	12	14	16	13	27	4	45	3
New Mexico	84	57	21	14	6	9	7	2	22	3
New York	507	359	94	97	57	51	60	15	113	20
North Carolina	891	661	210	157	122	96	76	21	194	15
North Dakota	159	123	60	23	12	6	22	2	32	2
Ohio	294	226	98	43	23	24	38	3	63	2
Oklahoma	288	216	110	31	26	12	37	2	64	6
Oregon	240	170	63	23	25	24	35	3	64	3
Pennsylvania	354	244	64	61	46	30	43	8	88	14
South Carolina	187	155	70	28	24	10	23	1	26	5
South Dakota	194	154	82	18	14	12	28	3	35	2
Tennessee	413	324	147	72	47	28	30	7	72	10
Texas	836	610	323	92	72	51	72	22	187	17
Utah	115	90	43	10	10	10	17	1	22	2
Vermont	449	328	78	71	55	51	73	10	106	5
Virginia	1,122	848	238	220	143	119	128	23	231	20
Washington	365	232	111	32	27	32	30	19	114	
West Virginia	462	333	92	84	60	41	56	8	104	17
Wisconsin	1,147	872	371	135	135	123	108	15	239	21
Wyoming	219	168	74	14	34	23	23	3	46	2
Possessions	457	368	69	95	75	47	82	11	48	30
APOs and FPOs	1,040	814	119	89	89	144	373	39	45	142

Note: Does not include Address Unknown.

Chapter 4

Primary Care Specialties

Chapter 4 provides data for two groups of physicians: (1) physicians in general primary care specialties and (2) physicians in primary care subspecialties. Information is provided on major professional activity, age, sex, board certification, school and year of graduation, and state of location. Data are also presented for International Medical Graduates (IMGs) in primary care and the number of primary care physicians located in metropolitan areas.

General primary care specialties are defined as Family Medicine, General Practice, Internal Medicine, Obstetrics/Gynecology, and Pediatrics, excluding the subspecialties within these general specialties. The primary care subspecialties, which include only the subspecialties of the mentioned groups, are listed in the "Definitions" section of the Introduction and in the footnotes to Tables 4.5, 4.7-4.9, and 4.11-4.16.

The statistics in this chapter focus on the general primary care specialties and primary care subspecialties, but also provide information on the total active physician population, the number of physicians in all other specialties, physicians Not Classified by major professional activity, and Inactive physicians.

Trends in Primary Care

Table 4.1

From 1975 to 2010, the total number of physicians more than doubled, whereas the percentage of primary care physicians increased by 110.3%. During this same period, the proportion in the primary care subspecialties increased by 796.8%. The largest percentage increase in the primary care specialties was in Family Medicine (607.2%), followed by Pediatrics (165.9%). At the same time, physicians in General Practice decreased 79.7%. Among the primary care subspecialties, the highest increase (1899.0%) was in the Pediatric subspecialties. Figure 4.1 displays the trends of the total physician population in comparison with the general primary care specialties and the primary care subspecialties.

Primary care physicians and their subspecialties comprised 41.9% of all active physicians in 1975 and 44.3% in 2010. The largest component, Internal Medicine and subspecialties, represented 14.8% of all active physicians in 1975 and 19.1% in 2010. Figure 4.2 illustrates the percentage of physicians practicing in the general primary care specialties and subspecialties.

Activity and Sex

Table 4.2

Office-Based practice represented a higher percentage of primary care physicians (74.6%) than physicians in the primary care subspecialties (65.5%), with All Other Specialties in between (69.5%). By contrast, Research activities included a higher percentage of the subspecialties (5.3%) compared with the primary care specialties (0.9%). Among the primary care specialties, 76.8% of male physicians were in Office-Based practice; for the subspecialties, 6.0% of male physicians were in Research.

However, a larger percentage of female physicians compared with male physicians were in primary care (42.7% and 25.8%, respectively). In each of the primary care specialties except General Practice, the

Figure 4.1

Trends in Self-Designated Primary Care With and Without Subspecialties, 1975-2010

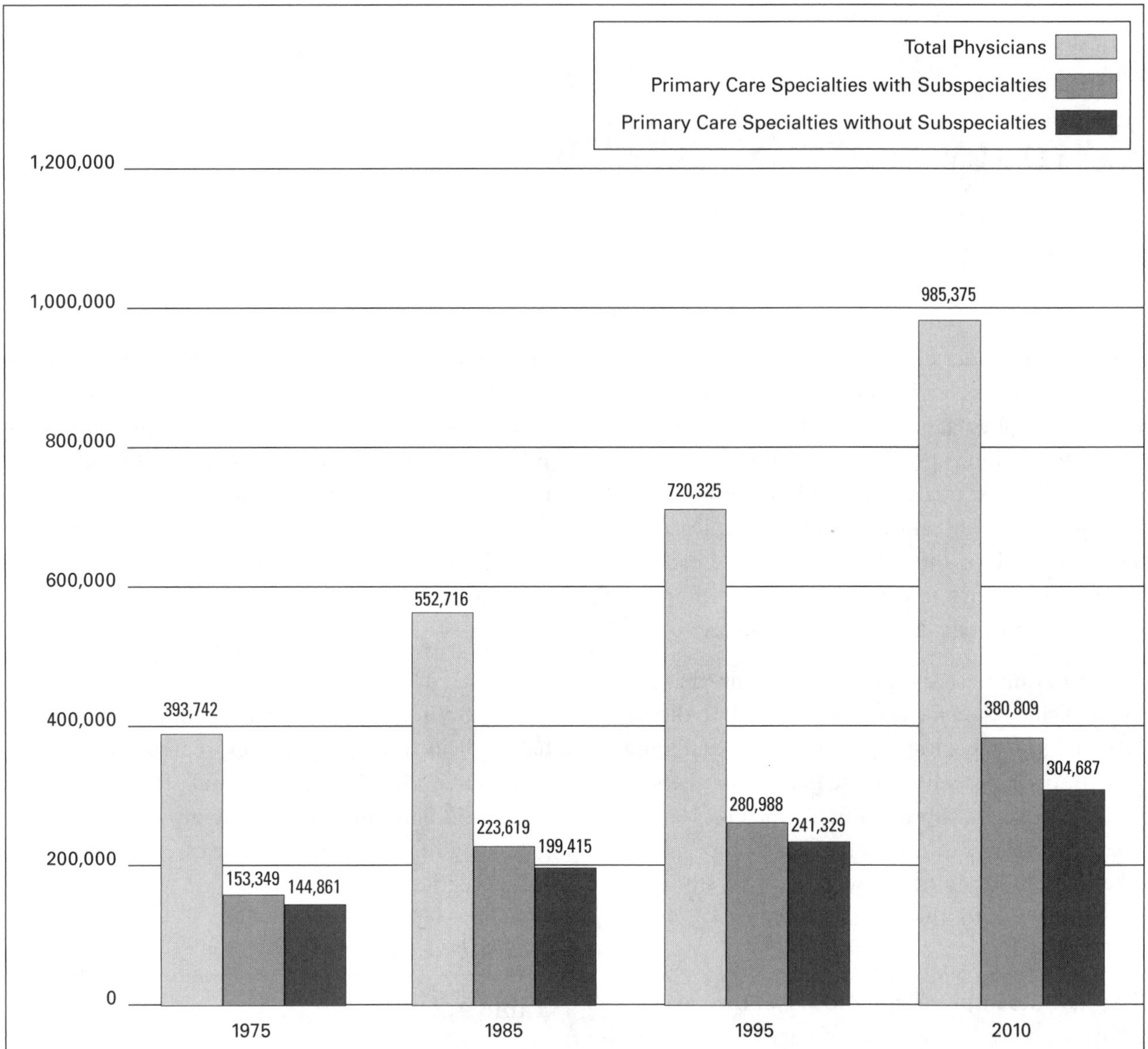

Source: Table 4.1

percentages of female physicians surpassed those of male physicians. This difference was especially apparent for Pediatrics, which represented 11.5% of all female physicians but only 3.5% of male physicians.

Age and Sex

Table 4.3

The largest percentage of active physicians was in the age group 45 to 54 years (25.2%), with the age groups 35 to 44 years and 55 to 64 years having the next largest percentages (24.8% and 20.6%, respectively).

Among primary care physicians, the largest percentage (26.0%) was in the age group 45 to 54 years, whereas the next largest group was 35 to 44 (25.2%). The age group 55 to 64 years included only 21.3% of primary care physicians. Among General Practice physicians, the largest percentage was found in the group 65 years and older (46.7%);

Figure 4.2

Distribution of Self-Designated Primary Care Specialties and Subspecialties, 2010

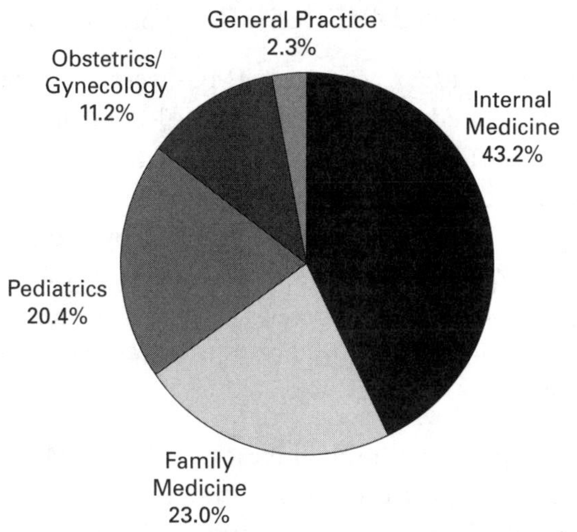

Source: Table 4.2
Note: Includes Primary Care Specialties and Primary Care Subspecialties.

the group 35 to 44 years represented only 3.6% of General Practice physicians.

Primary care accounted for nearly half (41.6%) of female physicians in the age group younger than 35 years. The comparable percentage for male physicians was 26.4%. A similar gender gap existed for the age group 35 to 44 years. In the older age groups, the gender gap is less because of the relatively small female physician population in these groups. For example, in the age group 65 years and older, primary care included 13.5% of male physicians and 20.0% of female physicians.

Board Certification and Sex

Table 4.4

Among all active physicians, 75.7% were board certified. Of the primary care physician population, 75.0% were board certified; in comparison, the proportions were 91.3% for the primary care subspecialties and 76.3% for all other specialties.

Among female physicians in primary care specialties, the highest board certification occurred for Family Medicine, in which 81.0% were certified. The lowest percentage, excluding General Practice, was in Obstetrics/Gynecology (67.8%). A slightly different pattern was observed for male physicians, with Obstetrics/Gynecology showing the highest rate of certification (83.3%), and Internal Medicine (72.5%) showing the lowest.

School and Year of Graduation

Tables 4.5 and 4.6

Table G shows the top 10 schools with the largest numbers of total graduates with the number and percentage of their graduates practicing in the primary care specialties. Two schools had 50% or more of their graduates practicing in primary care: Morehouse University (52.2%), and Mercer University (50.0%).

Three fifths (76.0%) of primary care physicians and 74.7% of all active physicians have graduated since 1980. However, great differences exist with respect to sex. Among primary care physicians, 67.3% of males and 88.3% of females graduated since 1980. This difference reflects the great increase in numbers of female physicians in recent years. Similarly, for all active physicians, 68.5% of male physicians and 87.7% of female physicians graduated since 1980.

Among female physicians, the highest percentage of graduates since 1980 occurred in Family Medicine (92.0%), followed by Obstetrics/Gynecology (91.4%). For male physicians, the highest percentages were in Family Medicine (72.3%), and Internal Medicine (71.4%).

Table G

Top 10 Schools in Number of Graduates and Self-Designated Primary Care Specialists, 2010

School	*Total Graduates*	*Graduates Practicing in Residents*	*Percentage of Graduates in Primary Care*
U of Illinois	14,476	4,334	29.9%
Jefferson Med Coll	14,185	3,805	26.8%
Indiana U	12,938	3,937	30.4%
U of Minnesota	11,900	4,271	35.9%
Wayne State U	10,800	3,278	30.4%
U of Michigan	10,738	2,267	21.1%
SUNY (Brooklyn)	10,727	2,574	24.0%
Ohio State U	10,345	3,042	29.4%
Med Coll of PA	9,851	2,800	28.4%
New York Med Coll	9,611	2,506	26.1%

Source: Table 4.5

Table H

Top 10 States With Largest Number and Percentage of Primary Care Physicians Compared to Total Physicians in State, 2010

State	*Total Physicians in State*	*Number of Primary Care Physicians*	*Percentage of Primary Care Physicians*
CA	118,110	36,759	31.1%
NY	86,293	24,447	28.3%
TX	60,991	19,137	31.4%
FL	58,026	16,351	28.2%
PA	44,988	12,503	27.8%
IL	41,724	13,699	32.8%
OH	35,925	11,030	30.7%
MA	35,334	9,535	27.0%
NJ	30,976	9,592	31.0%
MI	29,331	9,360	31.9%

Source: Table 4.7

State of Location and Sex

Tables 4.7 through 4.9

The 10 states with the largest number of total physicians are shown in Table H, along with the number and percentage of primary care physicians in those states.

Among male physicians in 26 states and the District of Columbia, Internal Medicine was the primary care specialty with the largest number of physicians. In the remaining 24 states, the primary care specialty with the largest number of physicians was Family Medicine. In the Possessions, General Practice represented the largest number of primary care physicians.

Among female physicians in primary care, Family Medicine was the specialty with the largest number of primary care physicians in 25 states. In the remaining 25 states, Internal Medicine had the largest number of physicians in 19 states and the District of Columbia and Pediatrics in 6.

Country of Graduation

Tables 4.10 through 4.13

Table I shows that a higher percentage (35.1%) of IMGs, compared with US Medical Graduates (USMGs) and Canadian Medical Graduates (CMGs), were in the primary care specialties (29.6% and 23.0%, respectively). Among all IMGs, the largest number (43,424) were in Internal Medicine, which represented 48.7% of IMGs in primary care.

Nearly half (42.8%) of female IMGs were in primary care, compared with one third (31.4%) of male IMGs. For female IMGs, Internal Medicine was the specialty representing the largest number of primary care physicians (42.6%), followed by Pediatrics (24.9%). Among male IMGs in primary care, Internal Medicine accounted for the largest number of physicians (52.6%), followed by Family Medicine (21.5%).

The age group with the highest number of IMG primary care physicians was 45 to 54 years, which comprised 24.1% of these physicians. Among IMG male primary care physicians, this age group represented 24.7% of these physicians; for female IMGs, this age group was 23.2% of these physicians.

Graduates of US medical schools (USMGs) have a smaller percentage in primary care compared with IMGs (29.6% and 35.1%, respectively). Moreover, USMGs were found in higher proportions in Family/General Practice (9.6%) compared with IMGs (9.4%); conversely, IMGs were represented in a higher proportion in Internal Medicine (17.1%) compared with USMGs (9.7%). The states with the highest percentages of USMGs in primary care were Alaska (39.4%), North Dakota (37.1%), and South Dakota (36.7%). Lowest percentages were found in Florida (24.6%) and New York (24.8%). Among graduates of Canadian medical schools, only 22.3% were in primary care, and the highest percentage of these was in Family Medicine (11.7%).

Table I

Country of Graduation of Active Physicians, 2010

School	*Total Number*	*Number in Primary Care*	*% Primary Care of Total Physicians*
Total	**985,375**	**304,687**	**30.9**
USMGs	719,122	212,727	29.6
IMGs	254,396	89,236	35.1
CMGs	11,857	2,724	23.0

Source: Table 4.5, 4.11, 4.12, 4.13

Metropolitan Areas

Tables 4.14 through 4.16

Of the 374 Metropolitan Statistical Areas listed in Table 4.14, eight recorded more than 20,000 physicians within their boundaries: New York (89,234), Los Angeles (43,309), Chicago (34,633), Boston (28,231), Philadelphia (25,667), Washington, DC (25,483), San Francisco (21,424) and Miami (20,317). The percentage of primary care physicians in these metropolitan areas ranged from 25.7 (Boston) to 31.9% (Chicago). Although Internal Medicine comprised the primary care specialty with the largest number of physicians in each of these metropolitan areas, the percentage in Internal Medicine of total primary care physicians varied from 53.9% in Boston to 38.5% in Los Angeles.

Table 4.1

Primary Care Physicians by Self-Designated Specialty for Selected Years, 1975-2010

	1975	1980	1985	1990	1995	2000	2010
				Number			
Total Physicians*	393,742	467,679	552,716	615,421	720,325	813,770	985,375
Active Physicians	366,425	435,545	511,090	559,988	646,022	737,504	859,015
Primary Care	144,861	170,705	199,495	213,514	241,329	274,653	304,687
Family Medicine	12,183	27,530	40,021	47,639	59,109	71,102	86,155
General Practice	42,374	32,519	27,030	22,841	16,867	15,210	8,591
Internal Medicine	47,761	58,462	70,691	76,295	88,240	101,353	113,591
Obstetrics/Gynecology	20,797	24,612	28,754	30,220	33,519	35,922	38,520
Pediatrics	21,746	27,582	32,999	36,519	43,594	51,066	57,830
Prim. Care Subspec.	8,488	16,642	24,124	30,911	39,659	52,294	76,122
FM Subspecialties					236	483	1,445
IM Subspecialties	6,570	13,069	18,171	22,054	26,928	34,831	50,730
OBG Subspecialties	934	1,693	2,113	3,477	4,133	4,319	4,277
PD Subspecialties	984	1,880	3,840	5,380	8,362	12,661	19,670
All Other Specialties	186,931	227,569	273,521	302,885	344,455	365,421	414,053
Inactive	21,449	25,744	38,646	52,653	72,326	75,168	125,928
Not Classified	26,145	20,629	13,950	12,678	20,579	45,136	64,153
Address Unknown	5,868	6,390	2,980	2,780	1,977	1,098	432
				Percent Distribution			
Total Physicians*	100.0	100.0	100.0	100.0	100.0	100.0	100.0
Active Physicians	93.1	93.1	92.5	91.0	89.7	90.6	87.2
Primary Care	36.8	36.5	36.1	34.7	33.5	33.8	30.9
Family Medicine	3.1	5.9	7.2	7.7	8.2	8.7	8.7
General Practice	10.8	7.0	4.9	3.7	2.3	1.9	0.9
Internal Medicine	12.1	12.5	12.8	12.4	12.3	12.5	11.5
Obstetrics/Gynecology	5.3	5.3	5.2	4.9	4.7	4.4	3.9
Pediatrics	5.5	5.9	6.0	5.9	6.1	6.3	5.9
Prim. Care Subspec.	2.2	3.6	4.4	5.0	5.5	6.4	7.7
FM Subspecialties	0.0	0.0	0.0	0.0	0.0	0.1	0.1
IM Subspecialties	1.7	2.8	3.3	3.6	3.7	4.3	5.1
OBG Subspecialties	0.2	0.4	0.4	0.6	0.6	0.5	0.4
PD Subspecialties	0.2	0.4	0.7	0.9	1.2	1.6	2.0
All Other Specialties	47.5	48.7	49.5	49.2	47.8	44.9	42.0
Inactive	5.4	5.5	7.0	8.6	10.0	9.2	12.8
Not Classified	6.6	4.4	2.5	2.1	2.9	5.5	6.5
Address Unknown	1.5	1.4	0.5	0.5	0.3	0.1	0.0
				Percent Change			
	1975-2010	1975-1985	1985-1995	1975-1980	1980-1985	1985-1990	1990-2010
Total Physicians*	150.3	40.4	30.3	18.8	18.2	11.3	60.1
Active Physicians	134.4	39.5	26.4	18.9	17.3	9.6	53.4
Primary Care	110.3	37.7	21.0	17.8	16.9	7.0	42.7
Family Medicine	607.2	228.5	47.7	126.0	45.4	19.0	80.8
General Practice	−79.7	−36.2	−37.6	−23.3	−16.9	−15.5	−62.4
Internal Medicine	137.8	48.0	24.8	22.4	20.9	7.9	48.9
Obstetrics/Gynecology	85.2	38.3	16.6	18.3	16.8	5.1	27.5
Pediatrics	165.9	51.7	32.1	26.8	19.6	10.7	58.4
Prim. Care Subspec.	796.8	184.2	64.4	96.1	45.0	28.1	146.3
FM Subspecialties	0.0	0.0	0.0	0.0	0.0	0.0	0.0
IM Subspecialties	672.1	176.6	48.2	98.9	39.0	21.4	130.0
OBG Subspecialties	357.9	126.2	95.6	81.3	24.8	64.6	23.0
PD Subspecialties	1899.0	290.2	117.8	91.1	104.3	40.1	265.6
All Other Specialties	121.5	46.3	25.9	21.7	20.2	10.7	36.7
Inactive	487.1	80.2	87.2	20.0	50.1	36.2	139.2
Not Classified	145.4	−46.6	47.5	−21.1	−32.4	−9.1	406.0
Address Unknown	−92.6	−49.2	−33.7	8.9	−53.4	−6.7	−84.5

Note: Data for 1990 are as of January 1; all others are as of December 31.

**Includes Active, Inactive, and Address Unknown.*

Table 4.2

Physicians by Self-Designated Primary Care Specialty, Activity, and Sex, 2010

		Patient Care				Other Professional Activity			
				Hospital Based					
Specialty	Total Physicians	Total Patient Care	Office Based	Resid./ Fellows	Phys. Staff	Admin.	Med. Teach.	Research	Other
				Both Sexes					
Total Physicians	985,375	752,572	565,024	108,142	79,406	14,009	9,909	13,755	4,617
Active Physicians	859,015	752,572	565,024	108,142	79,406	14,009	9,909	13,755	4,617
Primary Care	304,687	291,916	227,344	38,531	26,041	5,002	3,891	2,736	1,142
Family Medicine	86,155	82,908	68,794	7,930	6,184	1,370	1,428	207	242
General Practice	8,591	8,243	7,202		1,041	192	30	43	83
Internal Medicine	113,591	108,179	77,990	18,950	11,239	2,101	1,230	1,594	487
Obstetrics/Gynecology	38,520	37,540	30,526	4,509	2,505	336	395	176	73
Pediatrics	57,830	55,046	42,832	7,142	5,072	1,003	808	716	257
Prim. Care Subspec.	76,122	69,000	49,883	10,905	8,212	1,431	1,397	4,006	288
FM Subspecialties	1,445	1,395	1,091	210	94	15	25	7	3
IM Subspecialties	50,730	45,470	34,338	6,256	4,876	1,028	900	3,129	203
OBG Subspecialties	4,277	3,951	3,557	7	387	108	123	74	21
PD Subspecialties	19,670	18,184	10,897	4,432	2,855	280	349	796	61
All Other Specialties	414,053	391,656	287,797	58,706	45,153	7,576	4,621	7,013	3,187
Inactive	125,928								
Not Classified	64,153								
Address Unknown	432								
				Male					
Total Physicians	688,468	513,592	399,429	59,089	55,074	11,036	7,134	10,661	3,179
Active Physicians	581,100	513,592	399,429	59,089	55,074	11,036	7,134	10,661	3,179
Primary Care	177,775	168,985	136,602	16,757	15,626	3,686	2,480	1,948	676
Family Medicine	54,212	51,856	44,164	3,527	4,165	1,073	997	135	151
General Practice	6,735	6,487	5,731		756	138	20	33	57
Internal Medicine	73,928	69,963	52,233	10,457	7,273	1,609	818	1,226	312
Obstetrics/Gynecology	19,078	18,408	16,194	852	1,362	260	252	118	40
Pediatrics	23,822	22,271	18,280	1,921	2,070	606	393	436	116
Prim. Care Subspec.	49,545	44,242	33,675	5,372	5,195	1,124	1,010	2,991	178
FM Subspecialties	1,021	984	778	134	72	13	19	4	1
IM Subspecialties	35,163	31,092	24,376	3,448	3,268	823	684	2,430	134
OBG Subspecialties	2,899	2,649	2,398	3	248	82	95	59	14
PD Subspecialties	10,462	9,517	6,123	1,787	1,607	206	212	498	29
All Other Specialties	318,282	300,365	229,152	36,960	34,253	6,226	3,644	5,722	2,325
Inactive	107,072								
Not Classified	35,498								
Address Unknown	296								
				Female					
Total Physicians	296,907	238,980	165,595	49,053	24,332	2,973	2,775	3,094	1,438
Active Physicians	277,915	238,980	165,595	49,053	24,332	2,973	2,775	3,094	1,438
Primary Care	126,912	122,931	90,742	21,774	10,415	1,316	1,411	788	466
Family Medicine	31,943	31,052	24,630	4,403	2,019	297	431	72	91
General Practice	1,856	1,756	1,471		285	54	10	10	26
Internal Medicine	39,663	38,216	25,757	8,493	3,966	492	412	368	175
Obstetrics/Gynecology	19,442	19,132	14,332	3,657	1,143	76	143	58	33
Pediatrics	34,008	32,775	24,552	5,221	3,002	397	415	280	141
Prim. Care Subspec.	26,577	24,758	16,208	5,533	3,017	307	387	1,015	110
FM Subspecialties	424	411	313	76	22	2	6	3	2
IM Subspecialties	15,567	14,378	9,962	2,808	1,608	205	216	699	69
OBG Subspecialties	1,378	1,302	1,159	4	139	26	28	15	7
PD Subspecialties	9,208	8,667	4,774	2,645	1,248	74	137	298	32
All Other Specialties	95,771	91,291	58,645	21,746	10,900	1,350	977	1,291	862
Inactive	18,856								
Not Classified	28,655								
Address Unknown	136								

Table 4.3

Physicians by Self-Designated Primary Care Specialty, Age, and Sex, 2010

Activity	Total Physicians	< 35	35-44	45-54	55-64	≥ 65
			Both Sexes			
Total Physicians	985,375	165,544	214,468	220,858	189,648	194,857
Active Physicians	859,015	165,374	213,002	216,109	176,684	87,846
Primary Care	304,687	55,706	76,899	79,316	64,904	27,862
Family Medicine	86,155	13,201	24,450	23,943	19,009	5,552
General Practice	8,591	61	310	1,290	2,920	4,010
Internal Medicine	113,591	24,214	27,305	29,743	23,263	9,066
Obstetrics/Gynecology	38,520	6,821	10,040	9,807	8,014	3,838
Pediatrics	57,830	11,409	14,794	14,533	11,698	5,396
Prim. Care Subspec.	76,122	13,133	22,043	19,327	15,370	6,249
FM Subspecialties	1,445	436	611	206	145	47
IM Subspecialties	50,730	7,630	15,011	13,246	10,579	4,264
OBG Subspecialties	4,277	27	343	1,180	1,698	1,029
PD Subspecialties	19,670	5,040	6,078	4,695	2,948	909
All Other Specialties	414,053	68,459	87,857	110,928	94,286	52,523
Inactive	125,928	168	1,461	4,749	12,919	106,631
Not Classified	64,153	28,076	26,203	6,538	2,124	1,212
Address Unknown	432	2	5		45	380
			Male			
Total Physicians	688,468	86,505	128,445	152,102	149,078	172,338
Active Physicians	581,100	86,462	127,954	149,698	139,934	77,052
Primary Care	177,775	22,843	36,184	47,327	48,072	23,349
Family Medicine	54,212	5,642	12,824	15,673	15,184	4,889
General Practice	6,735	31	182	893	2,191	3,438
Internal Medicine	73,928	13,213	15,210	19,515	18,065	7,925
Obstetrics/Gynecology	19,078	1,193	3,364	5,237	5,957	3,327
Pediatrics	23,822	2,764	4,604	6,009	6,675	3,770
Prim. Care Subspec.	49,545	6,479	13,116	12,757	11,698	5,495
FM Subspecialties	1,021	291	422	146	121	41
IM Subspecialties	35,163	4,144	9,537	9,213	8,415	3,854
OBG Subspecialties	2,899	10	155	654	1,178	902
PD Subspecialties	10,462	2,034	3,002	2,744	1,984	698
All Other Specialties	318,282	43,320	63,430	85,485	78,715	47,332
Inactive	107,072	42	489	2,404	9,108	95,029
Not Classified	35,498	13,820	15,224	4,129	1,449	876
Address Unknown	296	1	2		36	257
			Female			
Total Physicians	296,907	79,039	86,023	68,756	40,570	22,519
Active Physicians	277,915	78,912	85,048	66,411	36,750	10,794
Primary Care	126,912	32,863	40,715	31,989	16,832	4,513
Family Medicine	31,943	7,559	11,626	8,270	3,825	663
General Practice	1,856	30	128	397	729	572
Internal Medicine	39,663	11,001	12,095	10,228	5,198	1,141
Obstetrics/Gynecology	19,442	5,628	6,676	4,570	2,057	511
Pediatrics	34,008	8,645	10,190	8,524	5,023	1,626
Prim. Care Subspec.	26,577	6,654	8,927	6,570	3,672	754
FM Subspecialties	424	145	189	60	24	6
IM Subspecialties	15,567	3,486	5,474	4,033	2,164	410
OBG Subspecialties	1,378	17	188	526	520	127
PD Subspecialties	9,208	3,006	3,076	1,951	964	211
All Other Specialties	95,771	25,139	24,427	25,443	15,571	5,191
Inactive	18,856	126	972	2,345	3,811	11,602
Not Classified	28,655	14,256	10,979	2,409	675	336
Address Unknown	136	1	3		9	123

Table 4.4

Physicians by Self-Designated Primary Care Specialty and Corresponding Board Certification, 2010

Primary Specialty	Total Physicians	Total Certified	By Corresponding Board Only	By Corresponding Board and Other Boards	By Non-Corresponding Board	Not Board Certified
			Both Sexes			
Total Physicians	985,375	736,142	647,329	38,261	50,552	249,233
Active Physicians	859,015	650,165	572,889	33,085	44,191	208,850
Primary Care	304,687	228,610	219,820	5,143	3,647	76,077
Family Medicine	86,155	71,811	69,967	1,119	725	14,344
General Practice	8,591	1,240			1,240	7,351
Internal Medicine	113,591	80,987	77,244	2,484	1,259	32,604
Obstetrics/Gynecology	38,520	29,064	28,479	425	160	9,456
Pediatrics	57,830	45,508	44,130	1,115	263	12,322
Prim. Care Subspec.	76,122	69,470	52,955	1,201	15,314	6,652
FM Subspecialties	1,445	1,288	1,107	15	166	157
IM Subspecialties	50,730	47,235	34,697	692	11,846	3,495
OBG Subspecialties	4,277	3,960	3,649	89	222	317
PD Subspecialties	19,670	16,987	13,502	405	3,080	2,683
All Other Specialties	414,053	316,019	269,633	25,519	20,867	98,034
Inactive	125,928	85,943	74,412	5,176	6,355	39,985
Not Classified	64,153	36,066	30,481	1,222	4,363	28,087
Address Unknown	432	34	28		6	398
			Male			
Total Physicians	688,468	526,469	458,550	30,649	37,270	161,999
Active Physicians	581,100	451,694	394,012	25,973	31,709	129,406
Primary Care	177,775	135,995	129,607	3,619	2,769	41,780
Family Medicine	54,212	45,951	44,478	894	579	8,261
General Practice	6,735	1,043			1,043	5,692
Internal Medicine	73,928	53,567	50,857	1,796	914	20,361
Obstetrics/Gynecology	19,078	15,885	15,524	283	78	3,193
Pediatrics	23,822	19,549	18,748	646	155	4,273
Prim. Care Subspec.	49,545	45,614	34,636	822	10,156	3,931
FM Subspecialties	1,021	910	787	14	109	111
IM Subspecialties	35,163	32,788	24,013	493	8,282	2,375
OBG Subspecialties	2,899	2,689	2,471	59	159	210
PD Subspecialties	10,462	9,227	7,365	256	1,606	1,235
All Other Specialties	318,282	251,175	214,100	20,803	16,272	67,107
Inactive	107,072	74,755	64,521	4,676	5,558	32,317
Not Classified	35,498	18,910	15,669	729	2,512	16,588
Address Unknown	296	20	17		3	276
			Female			
Total Physicians	296,907	209,673	188,779	7,612	13,282	87,234
Active Physicians	277,915	198,471	178,877	7,112	12,482	79,444
Primary Care	126,912	92,615	90,213	1,524	878	34,297
Family Medicine	31,943	25,860	25,489	225	146	6,083
General Practice	1,856	197			197	1,659
Internal Medicine	39,663	27,420	26,387	688	345	12,243
Obstetrics/Gynecology	19,442	13,179	12,955	142	82	6,263
Pediatrics	34,008	25,959	25,382	469	108	8,049
Prim. Care Subspec.	26,577	23,856	18,319	379	5,158	2,721
FM Subspecialties	424	378	320	1	57	46
IM Subspecialties	15,567	14,447	10,684	199	3,564	1,120
OBG Subspecialties	1,378	1,271	1,178	30	63	107
PD Subspecialties	9,208	7,760	6,137	149	1,474	1,448
All Other Specialties	95,771	64,844	55,533	4,716	4,595	30,927
Inactive	18,856	11,188	9,891	500	797	7,668
Not Classified	28,655	17,156	14,812	493	1,851	11,499
Address Unknown	136	14	11		3	122

Table 4.5

Physicians by Self-Designated Primary Care Specialty and School of Graduation, 2010

School	Total Physicians	Total Primary Care	Family Medicine	General Practice	Internal Medicine	OB/Gyn	Pediatrics	Primary Care Sub-specialties	All Other Specialties	Not Classi-fied	Inactive/ Address Unknown
Total Physicians	985,375	304,687	86,155	8,591	113,591	38,520	57,830	76,122	414,053	64,153	126,360
AL-U Of Alabama	6,847	2,262	664	40	711	385	462	459	3,069	316	741
" -U Of So Alabama	2,071	845	271	16	273	126	159	178	908	93	47
AZ-U Of Arizona	3,424	1,234	451	11	321	176	275	205	1,678	197	110
AR-U Of Arkansas	6,163	2,113	1,094	88	384	249	298	347	2,564	219	920
CA-Loma Linda U	7,206	2,251	987	105	547	324	288	233	3,119	343	1,260
" -Stanford U	4,331	898	182	21	391	81	223	352	1,929	337	815
" -U Of Cal (Davis)	3,367	1,440	582	18	416	174	250	173	1,443	206	105
" -U Of Cal (Irvine)	4,852	1,520	549	112	393	228	238	210	1,803	230	1,089
" -U Of Cal (LA)	7,215	2,270	741	39	722	332	436	480	3,558	386	521
" -U Of Cal (San Diego)	4,033	1,454	419	15	447	200	373	323	1,888	280	88
" -U Of Cal (SF)	7,449	2,210	583	40	843	288	456	404	3,155	500	1,180
" -U Of So Cal (LA)	6,913	2,054	572	56	732	354	340	441	3,187	383	848
CO-U Of Colorado	6,185	1,990	788	51	574	254	323	345	2,570	289	991
CT-U Of Connecticut	2,857	1,009	224	2	363	173	247	261	1,310	203	74
" -Yale U	5,210	973	95	9	473	152	244	512	2,516	338	871
DC-George Wash U	7,349	2,058	441	41	820	319	437	478	3,221	392	1,200
" -Georgetown U	9,020	2,228	459	37	870	410	452	599	4,473	443	1,277
" -Howard U	5,027	1,837	440	65	610	379	343	244	1,886	288	772
FL-Florida St U	336	161	43		46	39	33	9	151	15	
" -U Of Florida	4,694	1,459	450	25	387	268	329	313	2,323	256	343
" -U Of Miami	6,693	1,862	393	41	772	353	303	462	3,444	325	600
" -U Of So Florida	3,138	1,079	315	6	325	192	241	250	1,570	180	59
GA-Emory U	5,468	1,360	214	23	575	213	335	305	2,659	257	887
" -Med Coll Of Georgia	7,910	2,577	744	73	761	464	535	462	3,515	310	1,046
" -Mercer U	1,086	543	193	1	165	87	97	70	398	69	6
" -Morehouse U	867	453	150	2	121	77	103	38	283	87	6
HI-U Of Hawaii	2,082	907	216	24	380	126	161	155	829	132	59
IL-Chgo Med School	7,022	2,026	488	25	788	392	333	425	3,347	453	771
" -Loyola U/Stritch	6,424	1,798	474	39	628	283	374	519	2,796	270	1,041
" -Northwestern U	9,082	1,932	351	26	811	326	418	619	4,224	449	1,858
" -Rush Med Coll	4,227	1,456	486	5	524	189	252	352	2,007	250	162
" -Southern Illinois U	2,300	971	445	6	231	135	154	185	993	117	34
" -U Of Chgo/Pritzker	5,232	1,082	129	13	507	145	288	531	2,487	329	803
" -U Of Illinois	14,476	4,334	1,336	81	1,545	622	750	964	6,092	694	2,392
IN-Indiana U	12,938	3,937	1,688	90	930	518	711	769	5,886	434	1,912
IA-U Of Iowa	8,032	2,515	1,271	54	500	321	369	398	3,377	270	1,472
KS-U Of Kansas	8,321	2,739	1,230	51	721	346	391	587	3,378	293	1,324
KY-U Of Kentucky	3,995	1,430	539	29	381	238	243	266	1,855	186	258
" -U Of Louisville	6,472	2,001	628	66	631	268	408	377	2,768	228	1,098
LA-Lsu (New Orleans)	8,174	2,327	604	85	702	458	478	473	3,874	335	1,165
" -Lsu (Shreveport)	3,237	1,230	412	31	317	251	219	239	1,552	147	69
" -Tulane U	7,906	1,758	369	44	615	337	393	438	3,829	393	1,488
MD-Johns Hopkins	5,995	1,130	96	11	554	108	361	654	2,844	406	961
" -U Of Maryland	7,804	2,153	558	26	895	254	420	519	3,366	365	1,401

Notes:

Total Physicians include Active, Inactive, and Address Unknown.

FM subspecialties include FPG and FSM.

IM subspecialties include AMI, CCM, DIA, END, HEM, HEP, HO, ICE, ID, ILI, IMG, ISM, NEP, NTR, ON, PCC, and RHU.

OBG Subspecialties include: GO, GYN, MFM, OBS, OCC, and REN.

PD subspecialties include ADL, CCP, MPD, NPM, PDA, PDC, PDE, PDI, PDP, PDT, PEM, PG, PHO, PLI, PN, PPR, and PSM.

Table 4.5

Physicians by Self-Designated Primary Care Specialty and School of Graduation, 2010, continued

School	Total Physicians	Total Primary Care	Family Medicine	General Practice	Internal Medicine	OB/Gyn	Pediatrics	Primary Care Sub-specialties	All Other Specialties	Not Classi-fied	Inactive/ Address Unknown
" -Uniformed Services U	4,510	1,197	620	27	153	174	223	231	2,640	398	44
MA-Boston U	6,693	1,812	305	26	798	280	403	464	3,135	433	849
" -Harvard U	9,286	1,782	198	22	981	165	416	945	4,132	690	1,737
" -Tufts U	8,143	2,203	378	31	1,020	289	485	645	3,476	443	1,376
" -U Of Massachusetts	3,245	1,292	378	4	512	118	280	286	1,380	225	62
MI-Michigan State U	3,709	1,657	676	24	415	254	288	270	1,474	177	131
" -U Of Michigan	10,738	2,267	660	45	716	375	471	627	5,235	423	2,186
" -Wayne State U	10,800	3,278	1,029	38	1,138	598	475	735	5,161	492	1,134
MN-Mayo Medical School	1,353	411	184	3	105	46	73	92	742	79	29
" -U Of Minnesota	11,900	4,271	2,223	73	1,087	383	505	762	4,446	370	2,051
MS-U Of Mississippi	4,847	1,726	694	53	456	245	278	346	2,181	143	451
MO-St Louis U	7,461	2,163	521	36	721	347	538	503	3,149	273	1,373
" -U Of Mo (Columbia)	4,629	1,623	652	35	435	225	276	375	1,985	166	480
" -U Of Mo (Kansas City)	2,841	961	325	8	323	146	159	251	1,404	162	63
" -Washington U	6,393	1,307	208	15	554	167	363	578	2,955	325	1,228
NE-Creighton U	5,455	1,719	532	51	498	357	281	311	2,391	180	854
" -U Of Nebraska	6,393	1,980	893	46	452	239	350	345	2,678	213	1,177
NV-U Of Nevada	1,487	577	237	6	155	109	70	73	724	92	21
NH-Dartmouth Med School	2,169	697	194	6	259	90	148	168	1,108	164	32
NJ-N Jersey Med Sch (Newark)	6,510	1,900	359	16	733	361	431	506	3,226	440	438
" -N Jersey Med Sch (Rutgers)	4,524	1,481	399	6	518	234	324	411	2,185	359	88
NM-U Of New Mexico	2,678	1,056	474	16	279	111	176	169	1,191	135	127
NY-Albany Med Coll	5,733	1,604	464	26	545	242	327	464	2,655	291	719
" -Albert Einstein Coll Of Med	7,481	1,958	213	19	939	255	532	748	3,763	517	495
" -Columbia U	8,068	1,349	130	19	675	198	327	682	4,036	540	1,461
" -Cornell U	5,619	996	85	12	519	151	229	529	2,700	350	1,044
" -Mt Sinai School Of Med	4,414	1,185	112	8	522	234	309	423	2,325	379	102
" -New York Med Coll	9,611	2,506	326	35	1,118	488	539	661	4,496	462	1,486
" -New York U	8,899	1,840	123	18	963	259	477	787	4,086	523	1,663
" -Suny (Brooklyn)	10,727	2,574	264	43	1,197	415	655	872	5,040	586	1,655
" -Suny (Buffalo)	6,846	1,880	453	23	653	270	481	531	3,050	347	1,038
" -Suny (Stony Brook)	3,218	1,067	200	4	464	187	212	277	1,520	301	53
" -Suny (Syracuse)	6,918	1,944	607	19	609	235	474	559	3,188	333	894
" -U Of Rochester	5,002	1,293	241	8	569	158	317	409	2,171	279	850
NC-Bowman Gray	4,700	1,408	473	18	401	206	310	300	2,129	212	651
" -Duke University	5,482	1,019	188	14	431	138	248	504	2,610	285	1,064
" -East Carolina U	1,875	841	380	3	154	148	156	154	725	128	27
" -U Of No Carolina	6,437	2,146	689	29	604	345	479	567	2,724	373	627
ND-U Of No Dakota	1,721	790	387	6	145	148	104	81	773	54	23
OH-Case Western Res	6,923	1,785	443	22	679	248	393	539	3,086	409	1,104
" -Northeastern Ohio U	2,780	969	319	1	329	156	164	229	1,340	208	34
" -Ohio State U	10,345	3,042	1,133	46	873	459	531	785	4,478	434	1,606

Notes:

Total Physicians include Active, Inactive, and Address Unknown.

FM subspecialties include FPG and FSM.

IM subspecialties include AMI, CCM, DIA, END, HEM, HEP, HO, ICE, ID, ILI, IMG, ISM, NEP, NTR, ON, PCC, and RHU.

OBG Subspecialties include: GO, GYN, MFM, OBS, OCC, and REN.

PD subspecialties include ADL, CCP, MPD, NPM, PDA, PDC, PDE, PDI, PDP, PDT, PEM, PG, PHO, PLI, PN, PPR, and PSM.

Table 4.5

Physicians by Self-Designated Primary Care Specialty and School of Graduation, 2010, continued

School	Total Physicians	Total Primary Care	Family Medicine	General Practice	Internal Medicine	OB/Gyn	Pediatrics	Primary Care Sub-specialties	All Other Specialties	Not Classi-fied	Inactive/ Address Unknown
" -U Of Cincinnati	7,672	2,297	700	42	726	324	505	536	3,373	295	1,171
" -U of Toledo	4,394	1,662	633	8	493	225	303	303	2,071	276	82
" -Wright State U	2,576	1,216	568	6	304	146	192	168	987	159	46
OK-U Of Oklahoma	6,975	2,082	831	73	568	283	327	411	3,219	233	1,030
OR-U Of Oregon	5,167	1,611	588	50	507	203	263	248	2,059	207	1,042
PA-Jefferson Med Coll	14,185	3,805	1,320	46	1,275	536	628	930	6,354	1,024	2,072
" -Med Coll Of Penn	9,851	2,800	730	60	1,147	401	462	696	4,262	59	2,034
" -Pennsylvania State U	3,751	1,308	448	9	373	187	291	310	1,818	229	86
" -Temple U	9,099	2,431	761	60	848	323	439	632	3,810	510	1,716
" -U Of Pennsylvania	8,441	1,753	269	31	752	234	467	678	3,743	520	1,747
" -U Of Pittsburgh	6,720	1,764	433	20	617	268	426	506	2,935	340	1,175
PR-Ponce Med Sch	1,520	562	112	2	217	129	102	105	662	179	12
" -San Juan Bautista Sch of Med	882	437	131	125	96	13	72	38	319	75	13
" -U Central Del Caribe	2,102	796	151	21	314	146	164	204	839	215	48
" -U Of Puerto Rico	5,121	1,455	248	42	408	294	463	471	2,494	381	320
RI-Brown U	2,674	895	231	1	348	123	192	241	1,238	250	50
SC-Med Coll Of So Carolina	6,466	2,106	792	62	513	325	414	382	2,889	250	839
" -U Of So Carolina	1,812	793	270	1	220	114	188	126	764	106	23
SD-U Of So Dakota	1,617	714	342	10	168	122	72	87	736	48	32
TN-East Tennessee State U	1,532	690	266	5	209	96	114	95	640	79	28
" -Meharry Med Coll	3,898	1,599	461	61	474	375	228	145	1,347	220	587
" -U Of Tennessee	9,095	2,666	760	128	851	442	485	523	3,693	322	1,891
" -Vanderbilt U	4,633	959	113	16	372	169	289	410	2,309	270	685
TX-Baylor Coll Of Med	7,488	1,895	475	49	544	332	495	584	3,664	396	949
" -Texas A&M U	1,549	611	217	5	123	131	135	89	705	128	16
" -Texas Tech U	3,266	1,307	479	15	309	272	232	156	1,504	234	65
" -U Of Tx (Dallas)	8,702	2,440	620	35	833	475	477	612	4,147	506	997
" -U Of Tx (Galveston)	9,282	2,779	950	93	775	454	507	497	4,206	390	1,410
" -U Of Tx (Houston)	5,935	2,108	829	15	525	318	421	471	2,892	369	95
" -U Of Tx (San Antonio)	6,679	2,448	958	40	583	392	475	374	3,256	424	177
UT-U Of Utah	4,567	1,293	529	33	266	200	265	207	2,240	202	625
VT-U Of Vermont	4,201	1,317	384	10	394	195	334	292	1,762	219	611
VA-Eastern Virginia Med Sch	2,995	1,249	425	13	352	187	272	198	1,315	184	49
" -Med Coll Of Va	7,849	2,529	1,003	58	668	361	439	534	3,169	345	1,272
" -U Of Virginia	6,301	1,767	555	25	491	259	437	461	2,813	325	935
WA-U Of Washington	7,248	2,718	1,285	43	746	268	376	423	2,867	338	902
WV-Marshall U	1,284	580	260	4	129	75	112	85	508	92	19
" -West Virginia U	3,627	1,120	423	22	321	150	204	301	1,761	191	254
WI-Med Coll Of Wisconsin	8,345	2,409	842	46	744	310	467	476	3,863	346	1,251
" -U Of Wisconsin	7,027	2,134	831	32	597	233	441	395	3,069	251	1,178
INA-Inactive Schools	601	200	108	17	44	12	19	17	148	14	222
CAN-Canadian Schools	11,857	2,724	1,393	246	524	282	279	777	4,979	1,118	2,259
IMG-Internat'L Schools	254,396	89,236	19,698	4,308	43,424	6,269	15,537	25,111	84,607	25,748	29,694

Notes:

Total Physicians include Active, Inactive, and Address Unknown.

FM subspecialties include FPG and FSM.

IM subspecialties include AMI, CCM, DIA, END, HEM, HEP, HO, ICE, ID, ILI, IMG, ISM, NEP, NTR, ON, PCC, and RHU.

OBG Subspecialties include: GO, GYN, MFM, OBS, OCC, and REN.

PD subspecialties include ADL, CCP, MPD, NPM, PDA, PDC, PDE, PDI, PDP, PDT, PEM, PG, PHO, PLI, PN, PPR, and PSM.

Table 4.6

Physicians by Self-Designated Primary Care Specialty, Year of Graduation, and Sex, 2010

Specialty	Total Physicians	Prior 1950	1950-1959	1960-1969	1970-1979	1980-1989	1990-1999	2000-Present
			Both Sexes					
Total Physicians	985,375	21,910	54,358	100,073	157,998	217,816	211,266	221,954
Active Physicians	859,015	2,482	13,294	57,999	143,228	211,259	209,160	221,593
Primary Care	304,687	818	4,414	17,309	50,540	77,734	81,090	72,782
Family Medicine	86,155	84	832	3,026	13,662	22,552	25,828	20,171
General Practice	8,591	255	900	2,199	2,797	1,843	426	171
Internal Medicine	113,591	271	1,491	5,645	17,879	30,087	29,172	29,046
Obstetrics/Gynecology	38,520	81	471	2,565	6,424	9,153	10,734	9,092
Pediatrics	57,830	127	720	3,874	9,778	14,099	14,930	14,302
Prim. Care Subspec.	76,122	127	831	4,378	13,055	19,263	21,424	17,044
FM Subspecialties	1,445	1	5	28	113	182	479	637
IM Subspecialties	50,730	86	526	3,022	9,033	13,319	14,695	10,049
OBG Subspecialties	4,277	20	183	693	1,453	1,431	427	70
PD Subspecialties	19,670	20	117	635	2,456	4,331	5,823	6,288
All Other Specialties	414,053	1,417	7,877	35,681	78,037	109,318	90,973	90,750
Inactive	125,928	19,293	40,969	41,960	14,689	6,557	2,101	359
Not Classified	64,153	120	172	631	1,596	4,944	15,673	41,017
Address Unknown	432	135	95	114	81		5	2
			Male					
Total Physicians	688,468	19,468	49,158	87,755	129,516	154,028	127,962	120,581
Active Physicians	581,100	2,162	11,939	50,614	118,207	150,544	127,161	120,473
Primary Care	177,775	709	3,909	14,104	39,470	49,139	39,398	31,046
Family Medicine	54,212	79	769	2,625	11,570	15,772	13,880	9,517
General Practice	6,735	223	807	1,831	2,212	1,294	273	95
Internal Medicine	73,928	249	1,352	4,963	14,568	20,431	16,417	15,948
Obstetrics/Gynecology	19,078	73	434	2,137	5,229	5,311	4,080	1,814
Pediatrics	23,822	85	547	2,548	5,891	6,331	4,748	3,672
Prim. Care Subspec.	49,545	108	752	3,854	10,386	12,905	12,718	8,822
FM Subspecialties	1,021		5	24	99	137	310	446
IM Subspecialties	35,163	75	492	2,752	7,482	9,359	9,292	5,711
OBG Subspecialties	2,899	17	161	599	1,098	802	197	25
PD Subspecialties	10,462	16	94	479	1,707	2,607	2,919	2,640
All Other Specialties	318,282	1,245	7,140	32,227	67,251	85,321	65,877	59,221
Inactive	107,072	17,215	37,162	37,061	11,244	3,484	799	107
Not Classified	35,498	100	138	429	1,100	3,179	9,168	21,384
Address Unknown	296	91	57	80	65		2	1
			Female					
Total Physicians	296,907	2,442	5,200	12,318	28,482	63,788	83,304	101,373
Active Physicians	277,915	320	1,355	7,385	25,021	60,715	81,999	101,120
Primary Care	126,912	109	505	3,205	11,070	28,595	41,692	41,736
Family Medicine	31,943	5	63	401	2,092	6,780	11,948	10,654
General Practice	1,856	32	93	368	585	549	153	76
Internal Medicine	39,663	22	139	682	3,311	9,656	12,755	13,098
Obstetrics/Gynecology	19,442	8	37	428	1,195	3,842	6,654	7,278
Pediatrics	34,008	42	173	1,326	3,887	7,768	10,182	10,630
Prim. Care Subspec.	26,577	19	79	524	2,669	6,358	8,706	8,222
FM Subspecialties	424	1		4	14	45	169	191
IM Subspecialties	15,567	11	34	270	1,551	3,960	5,403	4,338
OBG Subspecialties	1,378	3	22	94	355	629	230	45
PD Subspecialties	9,208	4	23	156	749	1,724	2,904	3,648
All Other Specialties	95,771	172	737	3,454	10,786	23,997	25,096	31,529
Inactive	18,856	2,078	3,807	4,899	3,445	3,073	1,302	252
Not Classified	28,655	20	34	202	496	1,765	6,505	19,633
Address Unknown	136	44	38	34	16		3	1

Table 4.7

Physicians by Self-Designated Primary Care Specialty and State of Location, 2010

State	Total Physicians	Total Primary Care	Family Medicine	General Practice	Internal Medicine	OB/Gyn	Pediatrics	Primary Care Sub-specialties	All Other Specialties	Not Classi-fied	Inactive
Total Physicians	985,375	304,687	86,155	8,591	113,591	38,520	57,830	76,122	414,053	64,153	125,928
Alabama	11,613	3,890	1,254	93	1,372	494	677	847	5,008	566	1,302
Alaska	1,823	722	397	24	128	76	97	80	766	49	206
Arizona	16,944	4,993	1,416	127	1,869	649	932	1,212	7,245	841	2,653
Arkansas	6,771	2,380	1,198	93	458	251	380	504	2,733	291	863
California	118,110	36,759	9,556	1,439	13,894	4,610	7,260	7,871	48,860	7,716	16,904
Colorado	15,595	4,890	1,839	70	1,491	649	841	1,136	6,594	705	2,270
Connecticut	15,270	4,473	566	36	2,327	652	892	1,250	6,575	1,081	1,891
Delaware	2,550	749	238	14	236	87	174	236	1,099	137	329
District Of Columbia	5,776	1,507	192	24	710	190	391	611	2,491	666	501
Florida	58,026	16,351	4,204	829	6,213	1,969	3,136	4,283	23,980	2,637	10,775
Georgia	24,496	8,215	2,258	168	2,904	1,215	1,670	1,828	10,243	1,322	2,888
Hawaii	4,866	1,600	356	75	629	222	318	296	1,978	233	759
Idaho	3,215	1,075	567	32	231	134	111	148	1,379	87	526
Illinois	41,724	13,699	3,626	332	5,678	1,680	2,383	3,232	16,915	3,248	4,630
Indiana	15,898	5,325	2,283	130	1,437	647	828	1,321	6,793	575	1,884
Iowa	6,677	2,192	1,119	46	519	202	306	421	2,791	366	907
Kansas	7,558	2,414	1,104	62	620	276	352	526	3,210	355	1,053
Kentucky	11,417	3,594	1,230	105	1,151	453	655	898	5,055	586	1,284
Louisiana	13,587	4,328	1,246	148	1,421	678	835	1,048	5,997	818	1,396
Maine	4,426	1,459	608	20	466	152	213	286	1,787	153	741
Maryland	27,334	7,671	1,194	138	3,570	1,031	1,738	2,530	11,618	2,345	3,170
Massachusetts	35,334	9,535	1,282	105	5,096	984	2,068	3,408	15,135	3,797	3,459
Michigan	29,331	9,360	2,672	170	3,692	1,266	1,560	2,343	12,218	1,916	3,494
Minnesota	18,143	6,047	2,794	59	1,747	582	865	1,539	7,508	856	2,193
Mississippi	6,149	2,016	724	77	585	300	330	415	2,650	240	828
Missouri	16,802	4,981	1,294	87	1,904	657	1,039	1,533	7,358	1,199	1,731
Montana	2,658	839	431	18	206	92	92	132	1,085	52	550
Nebraska	5,150	1,809	845	29	469	194	272	347	2,104	262	628
Nevada	5,899	1,876	531	47	760	247	291	390	2,440	297	896
New Hampshire	4,563	1,455	476	17	523	185	254	317	1,884	221	686
New Jersey	30,976	9,592	1,328	167	4,449	1,288	2,360	2,645	12,940	1,974	3,825
New Mexico	5,759	1,940	770	51	574	209	336	380	2,262	336	841
New York	86,293	24,447	3,407	324	12,039	3,183	5,494	7,004	36,792	7,935	10,115
North Carolina	27,850	8,807	2,862	123	2,998	1,169	1,655	2,290	11,709	1,619	3,425
North Dakota	1,832	699	365	21	184	56	73	126	750	41	216
Ohio	35,925	11,030	3,142	221	4,168	1,362	2,137	3,081	14,931	2,693	4,190
Oklahoma	7,619	2,488	1,004	84	724	300	376	535	3,276	276	1,044
Oregon	13,007	4,186	1,397	81	1,600	484	624	777	5,280	682	2,082
Pennsylvania	44,988	12,503	3,494	221	5,092	1,496	2,200	3,871	19,465	3,293	5,856
Rhode Island	4,622	1,407	221	13	673	184	316	427	1,885	379	524
South Carolina	12,240	4,106	1,564	95	1,135	568	744	868	5,277	410	1,579
South Dakota	2,098	766	392	28	204	74	68	128	862	43	299
Tennessee	19,035	6,122	1,808	145	2,243	813	1,113	1,665	8,068	1,003	2,177
Texas	60,991	19,137	6,075	492	5,853	2,865	3,852	5,088	26,507	4,155	6,104
Utah	6,865	2,060	748	29	538	284	461	452	3,111	407	835
Vermont	2,752	899	318	13	303	96	169	176	1,084	152	441
Virginia	25,571	8,331	2,638	199	2,745	1,129	1,620	1,820	10,683	1,277	3,460
Washington	21,795	6,950	2,923	154	2,079	703	1,091	1,517	8,871	1,094	3,363
West Virginia	4,922	1,575	590	69	508	179	229	348	2,079	311	609
Wisconsin	17,220	5,714	2,370	84	1,779	622	859	1,274	7,330	668	2,234
Wyoming	1,242	462	242	13	97	60	50	45	489	23	223
Possessions	13,636	5,262	997	1,350	1,300	572	1,043	617	4,903	1,765	1,089
Address Unknown	432										

Notes:

Total Physicians include Active, Inactive, and Address Unknown.

FM subspecialties include FPG and FSM.

IM subspecialties include AMI, CCM, DIA, END, HEM, HEP, HO, ICE, ID, ILI, IMG, ISM, NEP, NTR, ON, PCC, and RHU.

OBG subspecialties include GO, GYN, MFM, OBS, OCC, and REN.

PD subspecialties include ADL, CCP, MPD, NPM, PDA, PDC, PDE, PDI, PDP, PDT, PEM, PG, PHO, PLI, PN, PPR, and PSM.

Table 4.8

Male Physicians by Self-Designated Primary Care Specialty and State of Location, 2010

State	Total Physicians	Total Primary Care	Family Medicine	General Practice	Internal Medicine	OB/Gyn	Pediatrics	Primary Care Sub-specialties	All Other Specialties	Not Classi-fied	Inactive
Total Physicians	688,468	177,775	54,212	6,735	73,928	19,078	23,822	49,545	318,282	35,498	107,072
Alabama	8,846	2,600	888	81	1,006	320	305	616	4,140	340	1,150
Alaska	1,237	381	207	20	77	38	39	52	605	30	169
Arizona	12,335	3,000	880	105	1,275	324	416	829	5,697	494	2,315
Arkansas	5,167	1,672	912	83	337	159	181	359	2,190	169	777
California	81,764	20,876	5,767	1,147	8,780	2,244	2,938	5,122	37,212	4,167	14,387
Colorado	10,686	2,633	1,061	60	922	255	335	717	5,044	342	1,950
Connecticut	10,406	2,493	348	26	1,467	288	364	795	4,923	573	1,622
Delaware	1,726	391	113	12	157	34	75	156	835	72	272
District Of Columbia	3,420	716	103	21	406	77	109	340	1,658	331	375
Florida	44,218	10,439	2,791	655	4,421	1,186	1,386	3,073	19,576	1,652	9,478
Georgia	17,342	4,804	1,427	135	1,903	652	687	1,229	8,082	692	2,535
Hawaii	3,479	956	208	64	421	108	155	207	1,578	126	612
Idaho	2,562	717	395	30	142	84	66	109	1,197	59	480
Illinois	27,506	7,495	2,115	237	3,525	729	889	2,070	12,500	1,683	3,758
Indiana	11,590	3,271	1,539	111	978	319	324	895	5,494	316	1,614
Iowa	4,962	1,380	742	37	368	102	131	297	2,255	217	813
Kansas	5,483	1,464	737	46	417	125	139	353	2,548	190	928
Kentucky	8,392	2,283	855	87	789	241	311	629	4,046	343	1,091
Louisiana	9,938	2,739	879	125	998	378	359	699	4,812	485	1,203
Maine	3,179	873	370	18	316	65	104	172	1,413	85	636
Maryland	17,841	4,069	625	101	2,215	466	662	1,548	8,431	1,202	2,591
Massachusetts	22,414	4,841	612	80	2,989	361	799	1,971	10,641	2,138	2,823
Michigan	20,399	5,360	1,576	129	2,411	597	647	1,548	9,381	1,126	2,984
Minnesota	12,603	3,486	1,718	44	1,140	242	342	987	5,697	513	1,920
Mississippi	4,823	1,404	539	66	444	197	158	302	2,246	139	732
Missouri	11,844	2,946	809	72	1,315	325	425	997	5,730	684	1,487
Montana	2,029	529	278	15	146	49	41	81	905	25	489
Nebraska	3,777	1,133	608	25	292	93	115	244	1,669	155	576
Nevada	4,481	1,206	361	38	529	153	125	292	2,054	163	766
New Hampshire	3,233	851	313	16	336	75	111	196	1,490	104	592
New Jersey	20,738	5,305	748	122	2,828	661	946	1,664	9,758	1,000	3,011
New Mexico	3,839	1,060	422	41	358	96	143	231	1,677	170	701
New York	56,826	13,759	2,033	258	7,728	1,520	2,220	4,138	26,621	4,272	8,036
North Carolina	19,718	5,110	1,747	104	1,994	589	676	1,549	9,178	891	2,990
North Dakota	1,391	449	234	18	134	25	38	97	619	26	200
Ohio	25,066	6,353	1,959	160	2,731	660	843	2,033	11,532	1,583	3,565
Oklahoma	5,777	1,648	718	66	535	163	166	372	2,668	163	926
Oregon	9,032	2,295	827	70	960	190	248	500	4,047	374	1,816
Pennsylvania	31,166	7,222	2,188	167	3,277	693	897	2,451	14,800	1,825	4,868
Rhode Island	3,021	747	106	9	429	73	130	269	1,378	185	442
South Carolina	9,137	2,567	1,079	76	783	288	341	621	4,271	239	1,439
South Dakota	1,609	492	253	24	150	32	33	99	724	22	272
Tennessee	14,225	3,922	1,292	128	1,576	437	489	1,160	6,628	597	1,918
Texas	43,009	11,377	4,052	412	3,872	1,463	1,578	3,361	20,726	2,292	5,253
Utah	5,361	1,435	593	26	384	185	247	311	2,584	267	764
Vermont	1,841	481	169	11	193	38	70	101	794	84	381
Virginia	17,495	4,610	1,636	141	1,741	508	584	1,179	8,063	737	2,906
Washington	15,207	3,884	1,716	119	1,221	343	485	983	6,825	618	2,897
West Virginia	3,733	1,037	388	61	379	112	97	251	1,730	185	530
Wisconsin	12,278	3,343	1,470	70	1,168	281	354	873	5,728	383	1,951
Wyoming	965	297	159	10	68	34	26	31	419	15	203
Possessions	9,056	3,374	647	956	897	401	473	386	3,463	955	878
Address Unknown	296										

Notes:

Total Physicians include Active, Inactive, and Address Unknown.

FM subspecialties include FPG and FSM.

IM subspecialties include AMI, CCM, DIA, END, HEM, HEP, HO, ICE, ID, ILI, IMG, ISM, NEP, NTR, ON, PCC, and RHU.

OBG subspecialties include GO, GYN, MFM, OBS, OCC, and REN.

PD subspecialties include ADL, CCP, MPD, NPM, PDA, PDC, PDE, PDI, PDP, PDT, PEM, PG, PHO, PLI, PN, PPR, and PSM.

Table 4.9

Female Physicians by Self-Designated Primary Care Specialty and State of Location, 2010

State	Total Physicians	Total Primary Care	Family Medicine	General Practice	Internal Medicine	OB/Gyn	Pediatrics	Primary Care Sub-specialties	All Other Specialties	Not Classi-fied	Inactive
Total Physicians	296,907	126,912	31,943	1,856	39,663	19,442	34,008	26,577	95,771	28,655	18,856
Alabama	2,767	1,290	366	12	366	174	372	231	868	226	152
Alaska	586	341	190	4	51	38	58	28	161	19	37
Arizona	4,609	1,993	536	22	594	325	516	383	1,548	347	338
Arkansas	1,604	708	286	10	121	92	199	145	543	122	86
California	36,346	15,883	3,789	292	5,114	2,366	4,322	2,749	11,648	3,549	2,517
Colorado	4,909	2,257	778	10	569	394	506	419	1,550	363	320
Connecticut	4,864	1,980	218	10	860	364	528	455	1,652	508	269
Delaware	824	358	125	2	79	53	99	80	264	65	57
District Of Columbia	2,356	791	89	3	304	113	282	271	833	335	126
Florida	13,808	5,912	1,413	174	1,792	783	1,750	1,210	4,404	985	1,297
Georgia	7,154	3,411	831	33	1,001	563	983	599	2,161	630	353
Hawaii	1,387	644	148	11	208	114	163	89	400	107	147
Idaho	653	358	172	2	89	50	45	39	182	28	46
Illinois	14,218	6,204	1,511	95	2,153	951	1,494	1,162	4,415	1,565	872
Indiana	4,308	2,054	744	19	459	328	504	426	1,299	259	270
Iowa	1,715	812	377	9	151	100	175	124	536	149	94
Kansas	2,075	950	367	16	203	151	213	173	662	165	125
Kentucky	3,025	1,311	375	18	362	212	344	269	1,009	243	193
Louisiana	3,649	1,589	367	23	423	300	476	349	1,185	333	193
Maine	1,247	586	238	2	150	87	109	114	374	68	105
Maryland	9,493	3,602	569	37	1,355	565	1,076	982	3,187	1,143	579
Massachusetts	12,920	4,694	670	25	2,107	623	1,269	1,437	4,494	1,659	636
Michigan	8,932	4,000	1,096	41	1,281	669	913	795	2,837	790	510
Minnesota	5,540	2,561	1,076	15	607	340	523	552	1,811	343	273
Mississippi	1,326	612	185	11	141	103	172	113	404	101	96
Missouri	4,958	2,035	485	15	589	332	614	536	1,628	515	244
Montana	629	310	153	3	60	43	51	51	180	27	61
Nebraska	1,373	676	237	4	177	101	157	103	435	107	52
Nevada	1,418	670	170	9	231	94	166	98	386	134	130
New Hampshire	1,330	604	163	1	187	110	143	121	394	117	94
New Jersey	10,238	4,287	580	45	1,621	627	1,414	981	3,182	974	814
New Mexico	1,920	880	348	10	216	113	193	149	585	166	140
New York	29,467	10,688	1,374	66	4,311	1,663	3,274	2,866	10,171	3,663	2,079
North Carolina	8,132	3,697	1,115	19	1,004	580	979	741	2,531	728	435
North Dakota	441	250	131	3	50	31	35	29	131	15	16
Ohio	10,859	4,677	1,183	61	1,437	702	1,294	1,048	3,399	1,110	625
Oklahoma	1,842	840	286	18	189	137	210	163	608	113	118
Oregon	3,975	1,891	570	11	640	294	376	277	1,233	308	266
Pennsylvania	13,822	5,281	1,306	54	1,815	803	1,303	1,420	4,665	1,468	988
Rhode Island	1,601	660	115	4	244	111	186	158	507	194	82
South Carolina	3,103	1,539	485	19	352	280	403	247	1,006	171	140
South Dakota	489	274	139	4	54	42	35	29	138	21	27
Tennessee	4,810	2,200	516	17	667	376	624	505	1,440	406	259
Texas	17,982	7,760	2,023	80	1,981	1,402	2,274	1,727	5,781	1,863	851
Utah	1,504	625	155	3	154	99	214	141	527	140	71
Vermont	911	418	149	2	110	58	99	75	290	68	60
Virginia	8,076	3,721	1,002	58	1,004	621	1,036	641	2,620	540	554
Washington	6,588	3,066	1,207	35	858	360	606	534	2,046	476	466
West Virginia	1,189	538	202	8	129	67	132	97	349	126	79
Wisconsin	4,942	2,371	900	14	611	341	505	401	1,602	285	283
Wyoming	277	165	83	3	29	26	24	14	70	8	20
Possessions	4,580	1,888	350	394	403	171	570	231	1,440	810	211
Address Unknown	136										

Notes:

Total Physicians include Active, Inactive, and Address Unknown.

FM subspecialties include FPG and FSM.

IM subspecialties include AMI, CCM, DIA, END, HEM, HEP, HO, ICE, ID, ILI, IMG, ISM, NEP, NTR, ON, PCC, and RHU.

OBG subspecialties include GO, GYN, MFM, OBS, OCC, and REN.

PD subspecialties include ADL, CCP, MPD, NPM, PDA, PDC, PDE, PDI, PDP, PDT, PEM, PG, PHO, PLI, PN, PPR, and PSM.

Table 4.10

International Medical Graduates by Self-Designated Primary Care Specialty, Age, and Sex, 2010

Specialty	Total Physicians	< 35	35-44	45-54	55-64	≥ 65
			Both Sexes			
Total Physicians	254,396	37,385	57,994	53,973	48,295	56,749
Active Physicians	224,702	37,334	57,708	53,195	45,520	30,945
Primary Care	89,236	16,803	21,187	21,496	18,419	11,331
Family Medicine	19,698	4,102	5,628	4,558	3,550	1,860
General Practice	4,308	36	145	604	1,511	2,012
Internal Medicine	43,424	9,965	11,459	11,048	7,385	3,567
Obstetrics/Gynecology	6,269	841	1,075	934	1,854	1,565
Pediatrics	15,537	1,859	2,880	4,352	4,119	2,327
Prim. Care Subspec.	25,111	4,403	8,560	6,642	3,745	1,761
FM Subspecialties	405	104	193	60	35	13
IM Subspecialties	18,839	3,273	6,927	5,009	2,525	1,105
OBG Subspecialties	712	2	18	82	283	327
PD Subspecialties	5,155	1,024	1,422	1,491	902	316
All Other Specialties	84,607	8,472	16,620	20,727	21,840	16,948
Inactive	29,608	49	282	778	2,774	25,725
Not Classified	25,748	7,656	11,341	4,330	1,516	905
Address Unknown	86	2	4		1	79
			Male			
Total Physicians	173,007	20,739	34,238	36,827	35,861	45,342
Active Physicians	150,005	20,724	34,123	36,349	34,049	24,760
Primary Care	54,403	8,700	10,944	13,417	12,864	8,478
Family Medicine	11,707	1,939	2,841	2,799	2,648	1,480
General Practice	3,195	15	87	420	1,082	1,591
Internal Medicine	28,592	5,813	6,523	7,597	5,730	2,929
Obstetrics/Gynecology	4,042	308	515	628	1,408	1,183
Pediatrics	6,867	625	978	1,973	1,996	1,295
Prim. Care Subspec.	16,729	2,463	5,293	4,719	2,812	1,442
FM Subspecialties	264	74	104	45	31	10
IM Subspecialties	13,033	1,921	4,463	3,692	2,002	955
OBG Subspecialties	524	1	12	63	202	246
PD Subspecialties	2,908	467	714	919	577	231
All Other Specialties	63,774	5,542	11,307	15,406	17,321	14,198
Inactive	22,940	14	113	478	1,811	20,524
Not Classified	15,099	4,019	6,579	2,807	1,052	642
Address Unknown	62	1	2		1	58
			Female			
Total Physicians	81,389	16,646	23,756	17,146	12,434	11,407
Active Physicians	74,697	16,610	23,585	16,846	11,471	6,185
Primary Care	34,833	8,103	10,243	8,079	5,555	2,853
Family Medicine	7,991	2,163	2,787	1,759	902	380
General Practice	1,113	21	58	184	429	421
Internal Medicine	14,832	4,152	4,936	3,451	1,655	638
Obstetrics/Gynecology	2,227	533	560	306	446	382
Pediatrics	8,670	1,234	1,902	2,379	2,123	1,032
Prim. Care Subspec.	8,382	1,940	3,267	1,923	933	319
FM Subspecialties	141	30	89	15	4	3
IM Subspecialties	5,806	1,352	2,464	1,317	523	150
OBG Subspecialties	188	1	6	19	81	81
PD Subspecialties	2,247	557	708	572	325	85
All Other Specialties	20,833	2,930	5,313	5,321	4,519	2,750
Inactive	6,668	35	169	300	963	5,201
Not Classified	10,649	3,637	4,762	1,523	464	263
Address Unknown	24	1	2			21

Table 4.11

International Medical Graduates by Self-Designated Primary Care Specialty and State of Location, 2010

State	Total Physicians	Total Primary Care	Family Medicine	General Practice	Internal Medicine	OB/Gyn	Pediatrics	Primary Care Sub-specialties	All Other Specialties	Not Classi-fied	Inactive
Total Physicians	254,396	89,236	19,698	4,308	43,424	6,269	15,537	25,111	84,607	25,748	29,608
Alabama	1,884	748	241	15	359	18	115	192	634	207	103
Alaska	120	49	25	1	16	2	5	10	39	4	18
Arizona	3,954	1,447	297	34	836	70	210	470	1,257	359	421
Arkansas	1,086	382	203	14	110	6	49	150	371	138	45
California	27,752	10,603	2,638	665	4,433	885	1,982	2,260	9,012	2,422	3,455
Colorado	1,177	338	107	8	152	25	46	132	410	116	181
Connecticut	4,433	1,512	165	20	1,009	141	177	392	1,536	512	481
Delaware	790	249	79	8	107	17	38	86	279	58	118
District Of Columbia	1,175	295	23	9	182	20	61	176	389	205	110
Florida	21,719	7,461	1,686	601	3,273	431	1,470	2,080	6,950	1,420	3,808
Georgia	5,091	2,037	603	54	929	122	329	630	1,480	436	508
Hawaii	746	256	37	13	134	20	52	59	232	45	154
Idaho	146	51	26	3	17	4	1	19	45	8	23
Illinois	14,166	5,415	1,391	246	2,620	341	817	1,217	4,360	1,416	1,758
Indiana	3,384	1,162	417	33	499	65	148	461	1,207	214	340
Iowa	1,367	449	178	9	171	18	73	144	478	172	124
Kansas	1,482	399	95	21	186	17	80	177	630	135	141
Kentucky	2,422	744	207	24	354	41	118	304	957	228	189
Louisiana	2,710	979	286	17	411	70	195	378	888	316	149
Maine	649	220	95	4	89	15	17	65	231	43	90
Maryland	7,439	2,440	296	63	1,419	207	455	706	2,485	794	1,014
Massachusetts	7,850	2,070	230	49	1,373	122	296	783	3,007	1,311	679
Michigan	10,166	3,879	939	104	1,924	306	606	1,068	3,218	1,053	948
Minnesota	2,827	823	327	11	356	38	91	388	1,050	342	224
Mississippi	842	315	86	15	131	16	67	98	314	77	38
Missouri	3,820	1,067	183	30	663	71	120	515	1,401	486	351
Montana	122	43	24	3	8	4	4	10	43	6	20
Nebraska	755	224	109	5	80	6	24	93	299	97	42
Nevada	1,876	763	165	16	410	40	132	180	489	151	293
New Hampshire	734	264	77	6	142	12	27	87	226	56	101
New Jersey	13,762	5,175	593	124	2,715	442	1,301	1,256	4,622	1,081	1,628
New Mexico	1,013	366	140	14	138	17	57	109	359	84	95
New York	34,800	11,766	1,475	185	6,487	1,085	2,534	2,983	11,700	3,985	4,366
North Carolina	3,844	1,414	327	29	817	49	192	418	1,238	403	371
North Dakota	480	205	89	5	97	1	13	62	146	31	36
Ohio	10,362	3,302	650	114	1,890	209	439	1,039	3,519	1,273	1,229
Oklahoma	1,572	595	201	26	253	24	91	187	563	106	121
Oregon	1,214	396	101	9	229	17	40	109	378	166	165
Pennsylvania	11,760	3,767	872	94	2,053	268	480	1,184	4,278	1,320	1,211
Rhode Island	1,213	369	35	9	253	27	45	152	386	129	177
South Carolina	1,689	594	208	12	264	33	77	222	579	121	173
South Dakota	289	106	27	9	60	5	5	44	95	15	29
Tennessee	3,211	1,169	324	22	622	51	150	420	1,065	335	222
Texas	15,166	5,367	1,556	167	2,207	332	1,105	1,908	5,025	1,549	1,317
Utah	597	177	46	4	81	12	34	83	227	67	43
Vermont	260	55	15		30	2	8	34	92	34	45
Virginia	5,616	1,999	498	83	912	150	356	511	1,851	447	808
Washington	2,861	1,002	365	45	430	63	99	299	865	291	404
West Virginia	1,726	573	126	43	265	52	87	156	635	148	214
Wisconsin	3,219	1,109	360	27	551	56	115	393	1,146	245	326
Wyoming	144	73	41	3	16	5	8	12	40	7	12
Possessions	6,828	2,973	414	1,183	661	219	496	200	1,881	1,084	690
Address Unknown	86										

Notes:

Total Physicians include Active, Inactive, and Address Unknown.

FM subspecialties include FPG and FSM.

IM subspecialties include AMI, CCM, DIA, END, HEM, HEP, HO, ICE, ID, ILI, IMG, ISM, NEP, NTR, ON, PCC, and RHU.

OBG subspecialties include GO, GYN, MFM, OBS, OCC, and REN.

PD subspecialties include ADL, CCP, MPD, NPM, PDA, PDC, PDE, PDI, PDP, PDT, PEM, PG, PHO, PLI, PN, PPR, and PSM.

Table 4.12

Graduates of US Medical Schools by Self-Designated Primary Care Specialty and State of Location, 2010

State	Total Physicians	Total Primary Care	Family Medicine	General Practice	Internal Medicine	OB/Gyn	Pediatrics	Primary Care Sub-specialties	All Other Specialties	Not Classi-fied	Inactive
Total Physicians	719,122	212,727	65,064	4,037	69,643	31,969	42,014	50,234	324,467	37,287	94,407
Alabama	9,609	3,088	978	68	1,007	473	562	651	4,334	351	1,185
Alaska	1,691	667	368	21	112	74	92	70	722	45	187
Arizona	12,651	3,468	1,072	84	1,018	574	720	724	5,837	469	2,153
Arkansas	5,640	1,981	983	78	347	243	330	352	2,343	153	811
California	88,449	25,770	6,744	741	9,370	3,685	5,230	5,494	39,044	5,142	12,999
Colorado	14,246	4,513	1,710	58	1,334	621	790	995	6,099	575	2,064
Connecticut	10,658	2,927	386	14	1,314	508	705	848	4,961	558	1,364
Delaware	1,741	498	158	6	128	70	136	148	812	76	207
District Of Columbia	4,540	1,204	167	15	524	169	329	432	2,065	453	386
Florida	35,707	8,778	2,459	213	2,922	1,524	1,660	2,175	16,752	1,193	6,809
Georgia	19,199	6,121	1,628	112	1,966	1,086	1,329	1,184	8,665	877	2,352
Hawaii	4,041	1,323	311	59	490	199	264	233	1,711	187	587
Idaho	3,014	999	527	23	209	130	110	128	1,318	78	491
Illinois	27,230	8,209	2,198	81	3,040	1,335	1,555	1,987	12,421	1,786	2,827
Indiana	12,338	4,103	1,823	85	934	581	680	853	5,528	337	1,517
Iowa	5,228	1,727	928	36	346	184	233	270	2,280	182	769
Kansas	6,018	2,004	1,005	39	433	257	270	347	2,549	219	899
Kentucky	8,865	2,810	1,000	73	795	405	537	588	4,038	349	1,080
Louisiana	10,802	3,332	951	130	1,009	604	638	664	5,069	496	1,241
Maine	3,619	1,193	486	14	370	135	188	213	1,505	107	601
Maryland	19,659	5,189	887	73	2,138	819	1,272	1,807	9,025	1,509	2,129
Massachusetts	26,698	7,302	1,006	53	3,660	840	1,743	2,539	11,831	2,340	2,686
Michigan	18,814	5,424	1,710	62	1,751	954	947	1,254	8,840	840	2,456
Minnesota	14,891	5,132	2,423	45	1,364	535	765	1,129	6,270	454	1,906
Mississippi	5,264	1,684	625	61	453	282	263	316	2,322	161	781
Missouri	12,882	3,898	1,103	55	1,238	585	917	1,006	5,909	700	1,369
Montana	2,518	791	403	15	197	88	88	122	1,035	45	525
Nebraska	4,357	1,578	730	23	389	188	248	249	1,783	162	585
Nevada	3,950	1,095	357	30	348	204	156	207	1,923	143	582
New Hampshire	3,675	1,138	362	9	375	169	223	221	1,600	159	557
New Jersey	17,060	4,385	723	43	1,724	842	1,053	1,374	8,253	880	2,168
New Mexico	4,682	1,561	622	36	435	191	277	267	1,878	247	729
New York	50,456	12,507	1,871	128	5,506	2,067	2,935	3,943	24,639	3,815	5,552
North Carolina	23,750	7,319	2,493	88	2,168	1,113	1,457	1,853	10,378	1,189	3,011
North Dakota	1,263	469	259	13	85	53	59	64	562	8	160
Ohio	25,160	7,654	2,453	96	2,267	1,145	1,693	2,010	11,246	1,343	2,907
Oklahoma	5,995	1,872	789	56	469	274	284	348	2,690	170	915
Oregon	11,546	3,706	1,240	62	1,359	462	583	654	4,818	497	1,871
Pennsylvania	32,856	8,674	2,599	123	3,017	1,222	1,713	2,657	15,014	1,924	4,587
Rhode Island	3,328	1,017	180	4	415	152	266	267	1,467	243	334
South Carolina	10,487	3,499	1,348	83	870	531	667	642	4,669	288	1,389
South Dakota	1,791	658	363	19	144	69	63	84	760	26	263
Tennessee	15,642	4,884	1,449	112	1,613	753	957	1,231	6,932	663	1,932
Texas	45,146	13,573	4,398	299	3,624	2,520	2,732	3,136	21,216	2,556	4,665
Utah	6,189	1,863	690	24	455	271	423	364	2,855	331	776
Vermont	2,389	818	289	13	272	87	157	134	946	113	378
Virginia	19,735	6,262	2,100	110	1,824	971	1,257	1,301	8,745	815	2,612
Washington	18,434	5,836	2,491	101	1,626	631	987	1,186	7,789	759	2,864
West Virginia	3,165	992	462	24	242	123	141	192	1,432	162	387
Wisconsin	13,854	4,559	1,975	52	1,227	563	742	872	6,123	416	1,884
Wyoming	1,091	387	201	8	81	55	42	33	445	16	210
Possessions	6,796	2,286	581	167	639	353	546	416	3,019	680	395
Address Unknown	313										

Notes:

Total Physicians include Active, Inactive, and Address Unknown.

FM subspecialties include FPG and FSM.

IM subspecialties include AMI, CCM, DIA, END, HEM, HEP, HO, ICE, ID, ILI, IMG, ISM, NEP, NTR, ON, PCC, and RHU.

OBG subspecialties include GO, GYN, MFM, OBS, OCC, and REN.

PD subspecialties include ADL, CCP, MPD, NPM, PDA, PDC, PDE, PDI, PDP, PDT, PEM, PG, PHO, PLI, PN, PPR, and PSM.

Table 4.13

Graduates of Canadian Medical Schools by Self-Designated Primary Care Specialty and State of Location, 2010

State	Total Physicians	Total Primary Care	Family Medicine	General Practice	Internal Medicine	OB/Gyn	Pediatrics	Primary Care Sub-specialties	All Other Specialties	Not Classi-fied	Inactive
Total Physicians	11,857	2,724	1,393	246	524	282	279	777	4,979	1,118	2,259
Alabama	120	54	35	10	6	3		4	40	8	14
Alaska	12	6	4	2					5		1
Arizona	339	78	47	9	15	5	2	18	151	13	79
Arkansas	45	17	12	1	1	2	1	2	19		7
California	1,909	386	174	33	91	40	48	117	804	152	450
Colorado	172	39	22	4	5	3	5	9	85	14	25
Connecticut	179	34	15	2	4	3	10	10	78	11	46
Delaware	19	2	1		1			2	8	3	4
District Of Columbia	61	8	2		4	1	1	3	37	8	5
Florida	600	112	59	15	18	14	6	28	278	24	158
Georgia	206	57	27	2	9	7	12	14	98	9	28
Hawaii	79	21	8	3	5	3	2	4	35	1	18
Idaho	55	25	14	6	5			1	16	1	12
Illinois	328	75	37	5	18	4	11	28	134	46	45
Indiana	176	60	43	12	4	1		7	58	24	27
Iowa	82	16	13	1	2			7	33	12	14
Kansas	58	11	4	2	1	2	2	2	31	1	13
Kentucky	130	40	23	8	2	7		6	60	9	15
Louisiana	75	17	9	1	1	4	2	6	40	6	6
Maine	158	46	27	2	7	2	8	8	51	3	50
Maryland	236	42	11	2	13	5	11	17	108	42	27
Massachusetts	786	163	46	3	63	22	29	86	297	146	94
Michigan	351	57	23	4	17	6	7	21	160	23	90
Minnesota	425	92	44	3	27	9	9	22	188	60	63
Mississippi	43	17	13	1	1	2		1	14	2	9
Missouri	100	16	8	2	3	1	2	12	48	13	11
Montana	18	5	4		1				7	1	5
Nebraska	38	7	6	1				5	22	3	1
Nevada	73	18	9	1	2	3	3	3	28	3	21
New Hampshire	154	53	37	2	6	4	4	9	58	6	28
New Jersey	154	32	12		10	4	6	15	65	13	29
New Mexico	64	13	8	1	1	1	2	4	25	5	17
New York	1,037	174	61	11	46	31	25	78	453	135	197
North Carolina	256	74	42	6	13	7	6	19	93	27	43
North Dakota	89	25	17	3	2	2	1		42	2	20
Ohio	403	74	39	11	11	8	5	32	166	77	54
Oklahoma	52	21	14	2	2	2	1		23		8
Oregon	247	84	56	10	12	5	1	14	84	19	46
Pennsylvania	372	62	23	4	22	6	7	30	173	49	58
Rhode Island	81	21	6		5	5	5	8	32	7	13
South Carolina	64	13	8		1	4		4	29	1	17
South Dakota	18	2	2						7	2	7
Tennessee	182	69	35	11	8	9	6	14	71	5	23
Texas	679	197	121	26	22	13	15	44	266	50	122
Utah	79	20	12	1	2	1	4	5	29	9	16
Vermont	103	26	14		1	7	4	8	46	5	18
Virginia	220	70	40	6	9	8	7	8	87	15	40
Washington	500	112	67	8	23	9	5	32	217	44	95
West Virginia	31	10	2	2	1	4	1		12	1	8
Wisconsin	147	46	35	5	1	3	2	9	61	7	24
Wyoming	7	2		2					4		1
Possessions	12	3	2				1	1	3	1	4
Address Unknown	33										

Notes:

Total Physicians include Active, Inactive, and Address Unknown.

FM subspecialties include FPG and FSM.

IM subspecialties include AMI, CCM, DIA, END, HEM, HEP, HO, ICE, ID, ILI, IMG, ISM, NEP, NTR, ON, PCC, and RHU.

OBG subspecialties include GO, GYN, MFM, OBS, OCC, and REN.

PD subspecialties include ADL, CCP, MPD, NPM, PDA, PDC, PDE, PDI, PDP, PDT, PEM, PG, PHO, PLI, PN, PPR, and PSM.

Table 4.14

Physicians by Metropolitan Statistical Area and Self-Designated Primary Care Specialty, 2010

			Primary Care							
Metropolitan Areas	Total Physicians	Total Primary Care	Family Medicine	General Practice	Internal Medicine	OB/Gyn	Pediatrics	Primary Care Sub-specialties	All Other Specialties	Not Classi-fied/ Inactive
Total Metropolitan Physicians	909,945	274,218	71,352	7,298	105,902	35,463	54,203	73,195	388,539	173,993
Abilene, TX	332	111	40	7	31	16	17	20	139	62
Aguadilla-Isabela-San Sebastián, PR	617	267	53	92	61	16	45	15	177	158
Akron, OH	2,065	715	211	10	269	90	135	178	830	342
Albany-Schenectady-Troy, NY	3,222	893	267	24	320	114	168	258	1,490	581
Albany, GA	349	136	47	2	41	20	26	26	134	53
Albuquerque, NM	3,414	1,042	351	18	343	121	209	269	1,455	648
Alexandria, LA	471	169	69	4	51	21	24	24	186	92
Allentown-Bethlehem-Easton, PA-NJ	2,379	778	241	9	304	129	95	178	995	428
Altoona, PA	341	117	50	1	33	17	16	20	142	62
Amarillo, TX	726	279	83	7	91	46	52	51	292	104
Ames, IA	197	66	31	1	18	6	10	13	84	34
Anchorage, AK	1,221	427	211	11	78	61	66	73	548	173
Anderson, IN	201	82	55	3	9	8	7	16	74	29
Anderson, SC	372	150	81	5	31	12	21	20	143	59
Ann Arbor, MI	4,264	967	151	12	475	132	197	477	2,034	786
Anniston-Oxford, AL	224	86	32	2	24	14	14	17	90	31
Appleton, WI	454	182	106	1	42	12	21	18	185	69
Asheville, NC	1,739	543	251	6	146	69	71	129	671	396
Athens-Clarke County, GA	505	152	42	5	51	32	22	38	242	73
Atlanta-Sandy Springs-Marietta, GA	14,587	4,675	1,005	67	1,809	700	1,094	1,224	6,256	2,432
Atlantic City-Hammonton, NJ	693	229	23	4	134	26	42	32	299	133
Auburn-Opelika, AL	228	88	27	4	28	12	17	18	93	29
Augusta-Richmond County, GA-SC	2,291	633	197	14	210	92	120	191	1,053	414
Austin-Round Rock-San Marcos, TX	4,504	1,475	480	33	414	216	332	291	1,950	788
Bakersfield-Delano, CA	1,259	548	166	22	199	77	84	63	457	191
Baltimore-Towson, MD	14,238	4,008	510	57	2,042	531	868	1,266	6,078	2,886
Bangor, ME	556	175	70	2	59	13	31	50	243	88
Barnstable Town, MA	860	226	41	2	121	24	38	32	318	284
Baton Rouge, LA	2,008	682	200	16	222	106	138	152	869	305
Battle Creek, MI	235	86	38		30	11	7	14	89	46
Bay City, MI	158	50	9	3	19	10	9	8	68	32
Beaumont-Port Arthur, TX	666	223	77	11	69	30	36	37	306	100
Bellingham, WA	618	204	116	4	43	16	25	22	244	148
Bend, OR	597	161	55	1	54	23	28	28	257	151
Billings, MT	613	164	82	1	42	18	21	47	293	109
Binghamton, NY	679	220	71	1	97	25	26	35	269	155
Birmingham-Hoover, AL	4,815	1,307	261	16	591	165	274	439	2,238	831
Bismarck, ND	383	112	68	1	16	13	14	28	186	57
Blacksburg-Christiansburg-Radford, VA	306	120	53	2	32	16	17	8	122	56
Bloomington-Normal, IL	386	121	48	1	34	19	19	23	179	63
Bloomington, IN	412	123	52	5	32	19	15	18	192	79
Boise City-Nampa, ID	1,501	522	245	7	132	80	58	97	626	256
Boston-Cambridge-Quincy, MA-NH	28,231	7,250	886	72	3,906	774	1,612	2,841	12,335	5,805
Boulder, CO	1,253	435	186	3	111	70	65	62	542	214

Table 4.14

Physicians by Metropolitan Statistical Area and Self-Designated Primary Care Specialty, 2010, continued

Metropolitan Areas	Total Physicians	Total Primary Care	Primary Care: Family Medicine	Primary Care: General Practice	Primary Care: Internal Medicine	Primary Care: OB/Gyn	Primary Care: Pediatrics	Primary Care Sub-specialties	All Other Specialties	Not Classi-fied/ Inactive
Bowling Green, KY	306	99	29	5	31	15	19	28	139	40
Bremerton-Silverdale, WA	712	229	118	8	55	13	35	37	290	156
Bridgeport-Stamford-Norwalk, CT	3,962	1,218	130	5	664	185	234	254	1,700	790
Brownsville-Harlingen, TX	580	241	66	7	71	31	66	48	204	87
Brunswick, GA	285	68	20	4	18	12	14	18	126	73
Buffalo-Niagara Falls, NY	4,136	1,203	267	19	518	150	249	334	1,765	834
Burlington-South Burlington, VT	1,436	426	127	3	147	50	99	120	618	272
Burlington, NC	274	100	29		41	9	21	20	102	52
Canton-Massillon, OH	965	367	117	4	144	48	54	79	346	173
Cape Coral-Fort Myers, FL	1,643	391	94	15	145	51	86	109	626	517
Cape Girardeau-Jackson, MO-IL	302	70	27	4	23	9	7	33	164	35
Carson City, NV	152	49	18		15	8	8	7	76	20
Casper, WY	214	75	47		12	8	8	10	91	38
Cedar Rapids, IA	497	175	117	5	16	16	21	25	206	91
Champaign-Urbana, IL	740	264	83	4	128	18	31	66	258	152
Charleston-North Charleston-Summerville, SC	3,358	877	246	13	293	134	191	314	1,686	481
Charleston, WV	1,055	339	105	16	116	41	61	96	454	166
Charlotte-Gastonia-Rock Hill, NC-SC	4,624	1,683	506	10	590	238	339	362	1,990	589
Charlottesville, VA	2,275	533	122	10	229	57	115	212	1,073	457
Chattanooga, TN-GA	1,604	519	148	10	189	74	98	131	680	274
Cheyenne, WY	268	83	41	1	20	10	11	18	116	51
Chicago-Joliet-Naperville, IL-IN-WI	34,633	11,058	2,441	274	4,886	1,411	2,046	2,747	14,228	6,600
Chico, CA	549	170	63	13	48	23	23	25	238	116
Cincinnati-Middletown, OH-KY-IN	7,408	2,292	605	39	773	306	569	722	3,080	1,314
Clarksville, TN-KY	384	131	42	3	37	23	26	19	168	66
Cleveland-Elyria-Mentor, OH	10,437	2,675	430	61	1,320	324	540	958	4,513	2,291
Cleveland, TN	169	74	24	2	28	11	9	6	64	25
Coeur d'Alene, ID	409	102	62	2	19	8	11	13	224	70
College Station-Bryan, TX	493	201	106		39	30	26	26	203	63
Colorado Springs, CO	1,572	446	176	9	105	67	89	87	763	276
Columbia, MO	1,426	342	115	3	130	42	52	146	663	275
Columbia, SC	2,261	757	238	22	233	106	158	154	1,016	334
Columbus, GA-AL	787	308	178	10	52	36	32	46	299	134
Columbus, IN	212	79	32	2	19	11	15	8	93	32
Columbus, OH	6,267	1,931	636	29	606	270	390	612	2,661	1,063
Corpus Christi, TX	1,020	367	136	7	74	47	103	64	410	179
Corvallis, OR	337	109	32	6	40	13	18	20	129	79
Crestview-Fort Walton Beach-Destin, FL	552	191	93	6	44	20	28	18	253	90
Cumberland, MD-WV	235	63	15	3	28	6	11	15	106	51
Dallas-Fort Worth-Arlington, TX	15,705	4,834	1,286	92	1,668	817	971	1,364	6,960	2,547
Dalton, GA	202	83	20		27	17	19	10	80	29
Danville, IL	140	53	18	2	20	7	6	5	45	37
Danville, VA	154	49	21		16	7	5	11	66	28
Davenport-Moline-Rock Island, IA-IL	756	250	124	4	63	29	30	42	335	129

Table 4.14

Physicians by Metropolitan Statistical Area and Self-Designated Primary Care Specialty, 2010, continued

		Primary Care								
Metropolitan Areas	Total Physicians	Total Primary Care	Family Medicine	General Practice	Internal Medicine	OB/Gyn	Pediatrics	Primary Care Sub-specialties	All Other Specialties	Not Classified/ Inactive
Dayton, OH	2,673	915	315	12	341	108	139	194	1,115	449
Decatur, AL	225	97	34	1	26	22	14	10	85	33
Decatur, IL	289	107	59		27	11	10	15	118	49
Deltona-Daytona Beach-Ormond Beach, FL	1,150	371	183	9	106	35	38	78	448	253
Denver-Aurora-Broomfield, CO	9,101	2,772	763	37	1,033	389	550	828	3,817	1,684
Des Moines-West Des Moines, IA	1,235	391	144	7	110	45	85	102	538	204
Detroit-Warren-Livonia, MI	14,352	4,549	1,023	89	1,971	681	785	1,179	6,055	2,569
Dothan, AL	404	110	32	2	37	19	20	26	211	57
Dover, DE	269	85	30	2	30	10	13	23	117	44
Dubuque, IA	267	83	23	1	36	11	12	15	125	44
Duluth, MN-WI	929	345	204	4	77	30	30	60	341	183
Durham-Chapel Hill, NC	5,801	1,227	246	3	497	175	306	733	2,604	1,237
Eau Claire, WI	571	200	100	1	53	23	23	37	252	82
El Centro, CA	161	56	12	3	16	10	15	11	70	24
El Paso, TX	1,614	545	140	7	188	87	123	120	672	277
Elizabethtown, KY	228	82	24	5	26	8	19	11	107	28
Elkhart-Goshen, IN	303	103	58	1	19	15	10	13	127	60
Elmira, NY	270	66	18	1	30	8	9	21	130	53
Erie, PA	590	162	94	2	29	16	21	47	252	129
Eugene-Springfield, OR	1,092	368	147	14	109	42	56	62	445	217
Evansville, IN-KY	972	346	180	6	77	41	42	68	421	137
Fairbanks, AK	215	77	31	3	21	9	13	5	106	27
Fajardo, PR	174	75	6	36	17	6	10	5	55	39
Fargo, ND-MN	720	243	79	3	111	17	33	67	310	100
Farmington, NM	206	81	35	1	21	12	12	14	72	39
Fayetteville-Springdale-Rogers, AR-MO	885	347	186	10	66	41	44	50	346	142
Fayetteville, NC	819	327	128	5	101	40	53	54	319	119
Flagstaff, AZ	376	130	58	5	27	21	19	18	167	61
Flint, MI	1,043	475	159	5	206	41	64	75	302	191
Florence-Muscle Shoals, AL	277	88	23	5	34	9	17	17	128	44
Florence, SC	522	213	112	6	47	25	23	36	215	58
Fond du Lac, WI	194	69	29	1	19	8	12	5	86	34
Fort Collins-Loveland, CO	854	289	159	1	55	35	39	51	350	164
Fort Smith, AR-OK	514	222	132	9	41	18	22	32	161	99
Fort Wayne, IN	1,096	323	160	5	77	44	37	87	524	162
Fresno, CA	2,097	748	237	19	257	91	144	121	860	368
Gadsden, AL	225	77	35		20	7	15	11	102	35
Gainesville, FL	2,422	568	146	14	225	48	135	249	1,169	436
Gainesville, GA	441	138	25	7	53	28	25	27	196	80
Glens Falls, NY	309	108	45		26	11	26	13	124	64
Goldsboro, NC	208	76	28	4	23	7	14	19	78	35
Grand Forks, ND-MN	310	134	88	1	24	12	9	21	120	35
Grand Junction, CO	461	147	89	2	34	8	14	25	198	91
Grand Rapids-Wyoming, MI	2,136	717	225	7	226	117	142	169	935	315
Great Falls, MT	239	61	24	1	19	7	10	15	111	52
Greeley, CO	365	136	87	3	16	14	16	18	143	68
Green Bay, WI	694	215	73	5	66	37	34	58	324	97
Greensboro-High Point, NC	1,700	595	207	12	202	76	98	129	710	266
Greenville-Mauldin-Easley, SC	1,866	733	253	12	206	111	151	139	732	262

Table 4.14

Physicians by Metropolitan Statistical Area and Self-Designated Primary Care Specialty, 2010, continued

			Primary Care							
Metropolitan Areas	Total Physicians	Total Primary Care	Family Medicine	General Practice	Internal Medicine	OB/Gyn	Pediatrics	Primary Care Sub-specialties	All Other Specialties	Not Classi-fied/ Inactive
Greenville, NC	1,106	315	89	5	114	37	70	130	488	173
Guayama, PR	99	48	5	19	14	2	8	1	34	16
Gulfport-Biloxi, MS	549	164	37	7	65	26	29	20	269	96
Hagerstown-Martinsburg, MD-WV	521	178	62	3	59	23	31	34	206	103
Hanford-Corcoran, CA	157	77	35	9	14	7	12	3	51	26
Harrisburg-Carlisle, PA	2,366	633	180	10	241	82	120	236	1,084	413
Harrisonburg, VA	306	97	51	1	15	10	20	15	126	68
Hartford-West Hartford-East Hartford, CT	4,808	1,474	253	13	654	245	309	399	2,063	872
Hattiesburg, MS	470	135	52	2	35	22	24	37	233	65
Hickory-Lenoir-Morganton, NC	744	237	120	2	51	34	30	41	338	128
Hinesville-Fort Stewart, GA	56	27	8	1	6	6	6	3	18	8
Holland-Grand Haven, MI	414	146	62	1	35	20	28	15	148	105
Honolulu, HI	3,857	1,232	238	45	510	183	256	263	1,592	770
Hot Springs, AR	299	77	34	2	20	11	10	22	124	76
Houma-Bayou Cane-Thibodaux, LA	373	127	42	5	31	27	22	20	179	47
Houston-Sugar Land-Baytown, TX	17,871	5,008	1,345	147	1,598	788	1,130	1,796	7,947	3,120
Huntington-Ashland, WV-KY-OH	1,087	359	130	12	121	39	57	86	473	169
Huntsville, AL	1,049	382	181	3	99	41	58	65	440	162
Idaho Falls, ID	223	54	23	1	13	7	10	10	123	36
Indianapolis-Carmel, IN	7,267	2,161	698	37	695	286	445	802	3,264	1,040
Iowa City, IA	1,983	425	113	3	162	52	95	177	965	416
Ithaca, NY	307	103	41	1	34	11	16	14	128	62
Jackson, MI	220	76	32	2	23	7	12	16	84	44
Jackson, MS	2,446	691	221	18	203	107	142	207	1,139	409
Jackson, TN	471	175	70	1	53	29	22	38	192	66
Jacksonville, FL	4,591	1,361	482	46	409	168	256	384	1,998	848
Jacksonville, NC	239	92	45	3	13	18	13	11	84	52
Janesville, WI	339	145	72	2	34	18	19	17	122	55
Jefferson City, MO	220	69	28	2	13	12	14	11	102	38
Johnson City, TN	1,047	381	123	8	166	39	45	80	410	176
Johnstown, PA	416	144	72	2	50	9	11	18	167	87
Jonesboro, AR	331	127	75	3	21	16	12	25	139	40
Joplin, MO	327	93	26	1	36	14	16	29	149	56
Kalamazoo-Portage, MI	1,161	364	112	4	139	32	77	90	494	213
Kankakee-Bradley, IL	181	62	16	1	26	9	10	13	73	33
Kansas City, MO-KS	6,377	1,796	609	19	511	242	415	576	2,919	1,086
Kennewick-Pasco-Richland, WA	473	172	61	4	49	25	33	39	185	77
Killeen-Temple-Fort Hood, TX	1,352	400	127	5	150	48	70	113	650	189
Kingsport-Bristol-Bristol, TN-VA	895	335	172	5	94	34	30	57	362	141
Kingston, NY	387	164	98	9	30	8	19	14	136	73
Knoxville, TN	2,568	805	273	11	285	109	127	209	1,142	412
Kokomo, IN	173	67	33	2	14	10	8	10	68	28
La Crosse, WI-MN	679	219	90	2	86	17	24	54	291	115
Lafayette, IN	465	147	58	3	39	21	26	37	202	79
Lafayette, LA	876	331	101	13	121	44	52	51	375	119

Table 4.14

Physicians by Metropolitan Statistical Area and Self-Designated Primary Care Specialty, 2009, continued

			Primary Care							
Metropolitan Areas	Total Physicians	Total Primary Care	Family Medicine	General Practice	Internal Medicine	OB/Gyn	Pediatrics	Primary Care Sub-specialties	All Other Specialties	Not Classified/ Inactive
Lake Charles, LA	436	163	81	5	34	22	21	29	169	75
Lake Havasu City-Kingman, AZ	272	97	25	4	43	11	14	16	129	30
Lakeland-Winter Haven, FL	1,070	334	80	20	143	34	57	78	399	259
Lancaster, PA	1,085	405	253	2	70	35	45	69	387	224
Lansing-East Lansing, MI	1,137	387	127	6	127	51	76	89	438	223
Laredo, TX	261	102	38	4	20	18	22	18	88	53
Las Cruces, NM	374	141	75	8	28	15	15	20	140	73
Las Vegas-Paradise, NV	4,088	1,322	306	34	576	183	223	288	1,638	840
Lawrence, KS	262	94	37	3	36	8	10	10	93	65
Lawton, OK	263	102	53	5	20	11	13	12	99	50
Lebanon, PA	333	105	66	1	16	10	12	19	131	78
Lewiston-Auburn, ME	294	98	54		32	7	5	23	125	48
Lewiston, ID-WA	159	52	20	5	16	5	6	7	68	32
Lexington-Fayette, KY	2,605	637	176	12	257	81	111	233	1,284	451
Lima, OH	291	82	35	2	17	12	16	20	137	52
Lincoln, NE	793	275	136	2	66	26	45	48	324	146
Little Rock-North Little Rock-Conway, AR	3,220	835	294	25	194	99	223	325	1,548	512
Logan, UT-ID	198	66	28	2	13	10	13	4	89	39
Longview, TX	396	145	55	5	46	22	17	28	172	51
Longview, WA	217	70	29	1	21	7	12	13	77	57
Los Angeles-Long Beach-Santa Ana, CA	43,309	12,958	2,974	665	4,987	1,707	2,625	3,218	18,265	8,868
Louisville/Jefferson County, KY-IN	4,585	1,294	339	25	458	174	298	412	2,140	739
Lubbock, TX	1,144	320	109	7	93	46	65	94	530	200
Lynchburg, VA	570	199	113	5	41	17	23	36	208	127
Macon, GA	871	317	113	2	101	55	46	64	343	147
Madera-Chowchilla, CA	190	93	17	5	17	9	45	20	51	26
Madison, WI	3,249	949	356	11	327	90	165	293	1,482	525
Manchester-Nashua, NH	1,078	391	104	6	152	55	74	80	431	176
Manhattan, KS	218	84	35	6	15	14	14	9	84	41
Mankato-North Mankato, MN	252	88	52	1	17	9	9	12	102	50
Mansfield, OH	231	63	19	1	27	7	9	21	92	55
Mayagüez, PR	601	218	27	61	63	30	37	28	223	132
McAllen-Edinburg-Mission, TX	913	434	170	8	101	52	103	77	294	108
Medford, OR	692	200	77	8	72	21	22	50	270	172
Memphis, TN-MS-AR	4,046	1,271	267	30	488	194	292	448	1,678	649
Merced, CA	285	151	95	8	22	13	13	15	79	40
Miami-Fort Lauderdale-Pompano Beach, FL	20,317	5,501	907	411	2,276	691	1,216	1,515	8,245	5,056
Michigan City-La Porte, IN	181	57	27		14	9	7	4	79	41
Midland, TX	307	112	22	2	48	19	21	29	135	31
Milwaukee-Waukesha-West Allis, WI	6,497	1,911	576	28	687	255	365	581	2,937	1,068
Minneapolis-St. Paul-Bloomington, MN-WI	11,041	3,848	1,655	36	1,096	403	658	968	4,469	1,756
Missoula, MT	431	104	46	1	30	12	15	30	203	94
Mobile, AL	1,249	393	75	8	153	67	90	114	580	162
Modesto, CA	999	389	173	3	124	39	50	45	393	172
Monroe, LA	454	164	78	7	35	19	25	27	197	66
Monroe, MI	145	52	20	4	13	8	7	12	58	23
Montgomery, AL	811	319	105	6	129	34	45	55	319	118
Morgantown, WV	1,037	224	72	1	79	33	39	101	529	183

Table 4.14

Physicians by Metropolitan Statistical Area and Self-Designated Primary Care Specialty, 2010, continued

			Primary Care							
Metropolitan Areas	Total Physicians	Total Primary Care	Family Medicine	General Practice	Internal Medicine	OB/Gyn	Pediatrics	Primary Care Sub-specialties	All Other Specialties	Not Classified/ Inactive
Morristown, TN	193	78	29	2	20	11	16	16	59	40
Mount Vernon-Anacortes, WA	357	121	71		22	9	19	10	140	86
Muncie, IN	342	137	61	3	53	6	14	19	126	60
Muskegon-Norton Shores, MI	286	98	50	1	35	6	6	10	114	64
Myrtle Beach-North Myrtle Beach-Conway, SC	532	179	57	6	60	29	27	34	243	76
Napa, CA	569	140	44	5	53	16	22	22	256	151
Naples-Marco Island, FL	1,333	246	53	8	114	33	38	67	470	550
Nashville-Davidson-Murfreesboro-Franklin, TN	6,404	1,757	348	42	733	250	384	609	2,950	1,088
New Haven-Milford, CT	5,121	1,363	78	12	827	171	275	494	2,261	1,003
New Orleans-Metairie-Kenner, LA	5,764	1,501	260	41	578	269	353	501	2,772	990
New York-Northern New Jersey-Long Island, NY-NJ-PA	89,234	25,544	2,519	334	13,103	3,430	6,158	7,528	37,808	18,354
Niles-Benton Harbor, MI	354	137	57	6	38	16	20	20	126	71
North Port-Bradenton-Sarasota, FL	2,532	554	160	18	216	73	87	139	976	863
Norwich-New London, CT	756	209	57	1	88	25	38	70	307	170
Ocala, FL	633	187	55	8	85	13	26	53	271	122
Ocean City, NJ	148	31	10	4	9	4	4	8	56	53
Odessa, TX	255	118	42	1	48	20	7	20	78	39
Ogden-Clearfield, UT	950	308	148		57	46	57	42	427	173
Oklahoma City, OK	3,820	1,069	417	30	302	135	185	331	1,828	592
Olympia, WA	793	291	151	7	68	25	40	34	310	158
Omaha-Council Bluffs, NE-IA	3,402	1,074	376	13	351	136	198	277	1,480	571
Orlando-Kissimmee-Sanford, FL	5,313	1,803	511	80	605	243	364	401	2,209	900
Oshkosh-Neenah, WI	483	156	55	2	46	23	30	24	217	86
Owensboro, KY	231	63	16	1	23	10	13	16	114	38
Oxnard-Thousand Oaks-Ventura, CA	2,166	715	297	26	193	81	118	133	837	481
Palm Bay-Melbourne-Titusville, FL	1,418	440	127	17	184	52	60	87	627	264
Palm Coast, FL	170	43	21	3	14	2	3	5	51	71
Panama City-Lynn Haven-Panama City Beach, FL	403	109	31	7	42	16	13	28	194	72
Parkersburg-Marietta-Vienna, WV-OH	322	99	48	3	32	9	7	16	142	65
Pascagoula, MS	335	92	27	5	30	11	19	30	157	56
Pensacola-Ferry Pass-Brent, FL	1,348	406	178	10	88	47	83	104	609	229
Peoria, IL	1,237	404	170	3	127	39	65	132	504	197
Philadelphia-Camden-Wilmington, PA-NJ-DE-MD	25,667	6,700	1,323	127	2,861	859	1,530	2,441	11,319	5,207
Phoenix-Mesa-Glendale, AZ	10,938	3,200	850	69	1,214	447	620	838	4,676	2,224
Pine Bluff, AR	176	77	48	1	12	8	8	8	59	32
Pittsburgh, PA	10,137	2,679	746	47	1,127	306	453	930	4,474	2,054
Pittsfield, MA	631	181	25	2	113	12	29	24	267	159
Pocatello, ID	206	75	45	3	14	6	7	7	82	42
Ponce, PR	967	368	55	63	128	51	71	52	332	215
Port St. Lucie, FL	901	228	63	8	90	33	34	48	380	245
Portland-South Portland-Biddeford, ME	2,126	648	198	6	242	81	121	162	916	400

Table 4.14

Physicians by Metropolitan Statistical Area and Self-Designated Primary Care Specialty, 2010, continued

Metropolitan Areas	Total Physicians	Total Primary Care	Primary Care: Family Medicine	General Practice	Internal Medicine	OB/Gyn	Pediatrics	Primary Care Sub-specialties	All Other Specialties	Not Classified/ Inactive
Portland-Vancouver-Hillsboro, OR-WA	8,712	2,740	733	32	1,176	339	460	593	3,640	1,739
Poughkeepsie-Newburgh-Middletown, NY	1,837	546	90	9	249	69	129	129	822	340
Prescott, AZ	532	147	48	10	60	12	17	16	205	164
Providence-New Bedford-Fall River, RI-MA	5,627	1,737	287	23	830	215	382	488	2,305	1,097
Provo-Orem, UT	752	279	133	7	41	43	55	32	323	118
Pueblo, CO	440	140	73	1	39	12	15	19	205	76
Punta Gorda, FL	429	100	25	4	50	9	12	30	179	120
Racine, WI	332	119	48	4	31	16	20	16	148	49
Raleigh-Cary, NC	2,888	991	300	9	324	136	222	197	1,209	491
Rapid City, SD	422	130	66	6	34	11	13	27	177	88
Reading, PA	886	298	115	4	97	44	38	48	350	190
Redding, CA	494	160	83	5	46	11	15	27	214	93
Reno-Sparks, NV	1,383	382	143	4	139	47	49	92	642	267
Richmond, VA	4,712	1,442	432	38	510	191	271	368	1,973	929
Riverside-San Bernardino-Ontario, CA	7,301	2,451	800	102	799	289	461	420	2,873	1,557
Roanoke, VA	1,331	397	145	4	149	49	50	108	589	237
Rochester, MN	3,577	621	122	4	348	59	88	423	1,913	620
Rochester, NY	4,439	1,375	251	8	633	189	294	379	1,806	879
Rockford, IL	924	312	144	5	83	36	44	67	364	181
Rocky Mount, NC	209	92	28		37	18	9	12	76	29
Rome, GA	380	143	76	1	40	14	12	16	158	63
Sacramento--Arden-Arcade--Roseville, CA	7,116	2,345	717	74	843	299	412	429	3,015	1,327
Saginaw-Saginaw Township North, MI	607	231	103	2	82	29	15	38	259	79
Salem, OR	823	290	143	11	72	26	38	34	338	161
Salinas, CA	1,019	325	150	14	71	39	51	55	398	241
Salisbury, MD	341	96	10	5	43	15	23	18	165	62
Salt Lake City, UT	4,389	1,195	325	10	385	158	317	351	2,061	782
San Angelo, TX	264	84	27	3	27	13	14	12	124	44
San Antonio-New Braunfels, TX	7,171	1,982	667	43	576	275	421	629	3,330	1,230
San Diego-Carlsbad-San Marcos, CA	11,602	3,165	905	111	1,126	401	622	854	5,109	2,474
San Francisco-Oakland-Fremont, CA	21,424	6,484	1,068	169	3,016	791	1,440	1,419	8,745	4,776
San Germán-Cabo Rojo, PR	333	173	29	54	57	17	16	7	73	80
San Jose-Sunnyvale-Santa Clara, CA	7,996	2,445	429	43	1,038	357	578	613	3,291	1,647
San Juan-Caguas-Guaynabo, PR	8,903	3,286	508	915	793	359	711	440	3,335	1,842
San Luis Obispo-Paso Robles, CA	930	241	90	6	86	28	31	24	448	217
Sandusky, OH	141	33	9	2	13	3	6	8	72	28
Santa Barbara-Santa Maria-Goleta, CA	1,431	414	117	14	182	38	63	72	566	379
Santa Cruz-Watsonville, CA	838	286	121	13	73	32	47	34	341	177
Santa Fe, NM	660	179	87	5	50	13	24	34	255	192
Santa Rosa-Petaluma, CA	1,573	542	283	13	122	51	73	64	569	398

Table 4.14

Physicians by Metropolitan Statistical Area and Self-Designated Primary Care Specialty, 2010, continued

			Primary Care							
Metropolitan Areas	Total Physicians	Total Primary Care	Family Medicine	General Practice	Internal Medicine	OB/Gyn	Pediatrics	Primary Care Sub-specialties	All Other Specialties	Not Classi-fied/ Inactive
Savannah, GA	1,177	390	109	9	128	66	78	65	510	212
Scranton--Wilkes-Barre, PA	1,397	442	123	10	215	37	57	94	569	292
Seattle-Tacoma-Bellevue, WA	13,935	4,167	1,554	76	1,388	438	711	1,139	5,892	2,737
Sebastian-Vero Beach, FL	469	104	27	5	45	11	16	25	210	130
Sheboygan, WI	224	76	35	2	20	10	9	12	89	47
Sherman-Denison, TX	244	75	27	2	18	15	13	17	114	38
Shreveport-Bossier City, LA	1,961	563	145	12	207	91	108	197	896	305
Sioux City, IA-NE-SD	288	87	62		11	7	7	20	137	44
Sioux Falls, SD	934	308	142	2	98	37	29	85	422	119
South Bend-Mishawaka, IN-MI	770	281	156	4	61	27	33	53	334	102
Spartanburg, SC	680	250	130	4	54	34	28	51	289	90
Spokane, WA	1,585	476	210	14	143	50	59	105	687	317
Springfield, IL	1,210	364	127	3	129	47	58	107	560	179
Springfield, MA	2,383	784	117	17	382	83	185	239	958	402
Springfield, MO	1,064	332	135	6	102	44	45	75	498	159
Springfield, OH	221	72	31		25	6	10	16	96	37
St. Cloud, MN	506	196	91	2	55	22	26	28	222	60
St. George, UT	299	77	33	2	23	13	6	17	129	76
St. Joseph, MO-KS	209	61	20	4	22	10	5	17	103	28
St. Louis, MO-IL	10,228	2,948	537	39	1,307	409	656	939	4,482	1,859
State College, PA	358	112	38	2	31	17	24	22	156	68
Steubenville-Weirton, OH-WV	167	58	16	5	26	7	4	5	66	38
Stockton, CA	1,237	512	163	26	170	65	88	54	473	198
Sumter, SC	178	66	22	2	18	10	14	11	69	32
Syracuse, NY	2,657	745	247	8	245	96	149	223	1,225	464
Tallahassee, FL	922	336	182	10	76	32	36	49	342	195
Tampa-St. Petersburg-Clearwater, FL	8,856	2,594	628	90	1,079	304	493	744	3,808	1,710
Terre Haute, IN	367	148	85	4	35	14	10	19	148	52
Texarkana, TX-Texarkana, AR	340	127	64	4	31	17	11	16	137	60
Toledo, OH	2,286	706	298	15	187	76	130	158	989	433
Topeka, KS	582	168	64	7	56	16	25	41	245	128
Trenton-Ewing, NJ	1,622	500	66	6	258	60	110	143	665	314
Tucson, AZ	4,049	1,090	300	25	421	127	217	282	1,823	854
Tulsa, OK	2,101	707	238	17	255	86	111	152	879	363
Tuscaloosa, AL	562	214	105	5	60	24	20	29	239	80
Tyler, TX	861	255	114	4	73	31	33	80	412	114
Utica-Rome, NY	664	230	106	4	72	20	28	44	247	143
Valdosta, GA	226	81	22	4	33	13	9	11	100	34
Vallejo-Fairfield, CA	964	384	130	14	128	38	74	48	383	149
Victoria, TX	243	87	28	2	32	11	14	7	104	45
Vineland-Millville-Bridgeton, NJ	211	73	12	7	28	7	19	12	89	37
Virginia Beach-Norfolk-Newport News, VA-NC	5,493	1,800	611	55	494	244	396	366	2,387	940
Visalia-Porterville, CA	538	236	70	9	69	31	57	30	181	91
Waco, TX	549	215	130	5	35	26	19	18	238	78
Warner Robins, GA	219	89	22	2	34	10	21	14	79	37
Washington-Arlington-Alexandria, DC-VA-MD-WV	25,483	7,546	1,462	142	3,091	1,074	1,777	2,394	10,673	4,870
Waterloo-Cedar Falls, IA	360	146	91		31	15	9	17	136	61
Wausau, WI	402	129	69	2	32	7	19	24	191	58
Wenatchee-East Wenatchee, WA	317	111	56		35	12	8	20	128	58

Table 4.14

Physicians by Metropolitan Statistical Area and Self-Designated Primary Care Specialty, 2010, continued

			Primary Care							
Metropolitan Areas	Total Physicians	Total Primary Care	Family Medicine	General Practice	Internal Medicine	OB/Gyn	Pediatrics	Primary Care Sub-specialties	All Other Specialties	Not Classified/ Inactive
Wheeling, WV-OH	390	124	62	6	30	12	14	24	166	76
Wichita Falls, TX	361	138	78	3	27	14	16	16	139	68
Wichita, KS	1,633	605	311	7	148	63	76	112	646	270
Williamsport, PA	272	93	59	3	23	5	3	18	103	58
Wilmington, NC	1,026	321	92	7	133	50	39	72	422	211
Winchester, VA-WV	410	130	39	1	49	19	22	24	201	55
Winston-Salem, NC	2,441	623	174	9	240	65	135	207	1,183	428
Worcester, MA	3,083	1,079	260	7	520	94	198	277	1,187	540
Yakima, WA	470	194	101	5	46	19	23	24	172	80
Yauco, PR	286	135	27	45	34	9	20	6	72	73
York-Hanover, PA	921	336	156	2	109	27	42	67	357	161
Youngstown-Warren-Boardman, OH-PA	1,268	431	107	10	214	42	58	63	497	277
Yuba City, CA	265	111	43	3	29	13	23	13	97	44
Yuma, AZ	267	98	24	2	44	12	16	23	99	47

Notes:

FM subspecialties include FPG and FSM.

IM subspecialties include AMI, CCM, DIA, END, HEM, HEP, HO, ICE, ID, ILI, IMG, ISM, NEP, NTR, ON, PCC, and RHU.

OBG subspecialties include GO, GYN, MFM, OBS, OCC, and REN.

PD subspecialties include ADL, CCP, MPD, NPM, PDA, PDC, PDE, PDI, PDP, PDT, PEM, PG, PHO, PLI, PN, PPR, and PSM.

Table 4.15

Physicians by Micropolitan Statistical Area and Self-Designated Primary Care Specialty, 2010

			Primary Care							
Micropolitan Areas	Total Physicians	Total Primary Care	Family Medicine	General Practice	Internal Medicine	OB/Gyn	Pediatrics	Primary Care Sub-specialties	All Other Specialties	Not Classified/ Inactive
Total Micropolitan Physicians	54,313	20,487	8,848	680	5,800	2,371	2,788	2,385	20,203	11,238
Abbeville, LA	49	27	9	2	6	5	5	2	11	9
Aberdeen, SD	95	31	16	3	8	4		2	46	16
Aberdeen, WA	80	31	16	1	7	2	5	1	29	19
Ada, OK	82	25	10		6	5	4	7	34	16
Adjuntas, PR	24	13	1	6	6				7	4
Adrian, MI	107	36	14		13	5	4	5	33	33
Alamogordo, NM	86	35	19	1	10	1	4	3	30	18
Albany-Lebanon, OR	171	87	55	1	17	8	6	4	39	41
Albemarle, NC	76	29	12		6	4	7	4	27	16
Albert Lea, MN	54	22	11	1	4	3	3	1	18	13
Albertville, AL	107	57	33	1	9	5	9	3	35	12
Alexander City, AL	60	25	10	2	5	5	3	4	21	10
Alexandria, MN	90	45	26		11	4	4	6	19	20
Alice, TX	30	20	7	3	4	1	5		8	2
Allegan, MI	74	25	14		8		3	3	28	18
Alma, MI	58	24	10	1	5	4	4	4	22	8
Alpena, MI	78	22	11	1	6	4		4	35	17
Altus, OK	33	16	7		3	2	4		9	8
Americus, GA	55	20	6		7	3	4	4	14	17
Amsterdam, NY	86	33	12	1	9	4	7	4	29	20
Andrews, TX	11	8	5		2	1			2	1
Angola, IN	28	14	13			1			7	7
Arcadia, FL	32	13	4	1	2	3	3	2	6	11
Ardmore, OK	85	27	4	3	13	3	4	1	43	14
Arkadelphia, AR	24	16	7		3	2	4		6	2
Ashland, OH	63	28	13		5	4	6	1	19	15
Ashtabula, OH	89	37	13	3	15	1	5	1	22	29
Astoria, OR	71	31	15		8	5	3		22	18
Atchison, KS	19	9	8		1				6	4
Athens, OH	60	17	7	3	6		1	7	23	13
Athens, TN	57	26	12	1	6	4	3	3	19	9
Athens, TX	74	30	22		2	4	2	4	26	14
Auburn, IN	43	25	19	1	2	2	1		7	11
Auburn, NY	94	22	2		12	4	4	7	37	28
Augusta-Waterville, ME	415	155	97		36	9	13	23	157	80
Austin, MN	51	22	12		4	2	4		18	11
Bainbridge, GA	30	13	3		4	3	3	2	10	5
Baraboo, WI	99	62	46	2	8	2	4	1	27	9
Barre, VT	188	69	33		25	5	6	4	74	41
Bartlesville, OK	89	27	16		4	3	4	2	41	19
Bastrop, LA	25	14	8	3		2	1		5	6
Batavia, NY	80	26	8		6	3	9		34	20
Batesville, AR	82	37	19	3	6	7	2	1	32	12
Bay City, TX	35	19	5	1	6	4	3	2	8	6
Beatrice, NE	29	19	12	1	3	1	2	1	2	7
Beaver Dam, WI	102	53	31		10	9	3	1	29	19
Beckley, WV	223	73	9	5	36	13	10	10	101	39
Bedford, IN	61	21	9		8	1	3	5	20	15
Beeville, TX	22	13	9			3	1	2	5	2
Bellefontaine, OH	53	26	15	2	3	2	4		18	9

Table 4.15

Physicians by Micropolitan Statistical Area and Self-Designated Primary Care Specialty, 2010, continued

			Primary Care							
Micropolitan Areas	Total Physicians	Total Primary Care	Family Medicine	General Practice	Internal Medicine	OB/Gyn	Pediatrics	Primary Care Sub-specialties	All Other Specialties	Not Classified/ Inactive
Bemidji, MN	93	41	23	1	7	4	6	5	32	15
Bennettsville, SC	17	9	5	2		1	1	1	5	2
Bennington, VT	150	52	21		19	8	4	9	65	24
Berlin, NH-VT	91	41	24	2	11	2	2	1	30	19
Big Rapids, MI	43	23	8		5	5	5	3	11	6
Big Spring, TX	50	16	5	1	5	2	3		24	10
Bishop, CA	50	23	9	3	5	4	2		12	15
Blackfoot, ID	32	8	6		1		1		13	11
Bloomsburg-Berwick, PA	719	172	40	4	80	19	29	86	337	124
Bluefield, WV-VA	250	78	29	4	26	8	11	15	110	47
Blytheville, AR	34	20	9	2	5	1	3	1	7	6
Bogalusa, LA	47	24	15	2	4	2	1	2	12	9
Bonham, TX	20	11	5		6				5	4
Boone, IA	22	9	8		1				3	10
Boone, NC	174	50	18	2	12	8	10	7	71	46
Borger, TX	15	10	5		1	2	2		3	2
Bozeman, MT	291	88	44		15	16	13	12	100	91
Bradford, PA	62	22	8	1	7	2	4	2	21	17
Brainerd, MN	202	77	54	1	16	3	3	6	74	45
Branson, MO	107	50	28	3	11	4	4	5	34	18
Brenham, TX	54	22	10		4	2	6	1	18	13
Brevard, NC	84	30	10	1	11	3	5	2	21	31
Brigham City, UT	40	22	11	2	3	4	2	1	10	7
Brookhaven, MS	46	16	3		7	4	2	5	18	7
Brookings, OR	31	12	7	1	3	1		1	8	10
Brookings, SD	35	17	10		4	2	1	1	9	8
Brownsville, TN	12	8	4		3	1				4
Brownwood, TX	61	23	7	1	8	4	3	3	28	7
Bucyrus, OH	36	11	3		2	3	3	2	11	12
Burley, ID	39	17	10		5	2			11	11
Burlington, IA-IL	92	29	13	3	3	5	5	4	41	18
Butte-Silver Bow, MT	81	27	9		10	2	6	3	34	17
Cadillac, MI	77	38	18	1	10	4	5	2	19	18
Calhoun, GA	61	35	15		11	5	4	2	16	8
Cambridge, MD	61	22	5		10	2	5	5	22	12
Cambridge, OH	64	24	7		8	5	4	4	20	16
Camden, AR	24	16	10		5	1			4	4
Campbellsville, KY	38	19	5	1	5	4	4		16	3
Cañon City, CO	46	21	14	1	5	1		1	13	11
Canton, IL	32	14	8	1	2	2	1	2	7	9
Carbondale, IL	199	86	52	2	16	11	5	15	57	41
Carlsbad-Artesia, NM	70	28	7	1	10	5	5		26	16
Cedar City, UT	47	18	6	1	6	2	3	1	17	11
Cedartown, GA	27	10	8		2				6	11
Celina, OH	37	18	8	1	4	3	2	2	9	8
Central City, KY	28	13	4	1	4	2	2	1	11	3
Centralia, IL	66	22	6	1	8	1	6	3	30	11
Centralia, WA	105	42	19	3	7	3	10	1	33	29
Chambersburg, PA	247	91	46	2	20	10	13	9	93	54
Charleston-Mattoon, IL	87	32	16	1	5	3	7	5	37	13
Chester, SC	23	11	4		4	1	2	1	7	4
Chillicothe, OH	135	62	25	1	19	6	11	7	48	18
Claremont, NH	118	40	16		14	6	4	7	44	27

Table 4.15

Physicians by Micropolitan Statistical Area and Self-Designated Primary Care Specialty, 2010, continued

			Primary Care							
Micropolitan Areas	Total Physicians	Total Primary Care	Family Medicine	General Practice	Internal Medicine	OB/Gyn	Pediatrics	Primary Care Sub-specialties	All Other Specialties	Not Classified/ Inactive
Clarksburg, WV	199	81	44	5	18	5	9	12	66	40
Clarksdale, MS	46	21	3	2	7	5	4	3	16	6
Clearlake, CA	93	40	13	6	16	1	4	1	36	16
Cleveland, MS	44	25	10	1	6	5	3	1	12	6
Clewiston, FL	21	10	3		4		3	1	2	8
Clinton, IA	71	31	11	2	11	3	4	1	31	8
Clovis, NM	63	28	9		8	2	9	7	18	10
Coamo, PR	59	29	3	11	9	1	5	1	16	13
Coffeyville, KS	40	18	7	3	5	2	1	2	15	5
Coldwater, MI	54	19	2	2	7	3	5	2	15	18
Columbia, TN	213	62	27		15	8	12	25	93	33
Columbus, MS	123	40	13	1	14	8	4	6	58	19
Columbus, NE	36	17	11		1	3	2	1	13	5
Concord, NH	558	204	98	2	54	24	26	24	213	117
Connersville, IN	24	10	4		4	1	1	2	10	2
Cookeville, TN	229	73	25	3	28	8	9	12	102	42
Coos Bay, OR	172	62	20	2	24	6	10	7	54	49
Corbin, KY	84	29	12		7	3	7	2	35	18
Cordele, GA	38	19	5		6	3	5	3	6	10
Corinth, MS	66	20	10		5	3	2	4	36	6
Cornelia, GA	44	26	9		10	3	4		10	8
Corning, NY	165	66	23		26	7	10	4	62	33
Corsicana, TX	56	22	9	1	4	4	4	1	18	15
Cortland, NY	71	30	13		10	3	4		26	15
Coshocton, OH	27	15	4		6	3	2		8	4
Crawfordsville, IN	44	22	10	2	4	3	3		14	8
Crescent City, CA	49	21	9		7	2	3	1	16	11
Crossville, TN	110	40	10	1	22	4	3	7	35	28
Crowley, LA	53	28	12	3	4	3	6	3	11	11
Cullman, AL	114	50	22		16	7	5	6	47	11
Culpeper, VA	61	21	8	1	5	3	4	1	25	14
Danville, KY	129	50	24	1	11	8	6	7	54	18
Daphne-Fairhope-Foley, AL	461	163	73	6	40	21	23	18	181	99
Decatur, IN	20	12	11		1				6	2
Defiance, OH	50	24	14		8	1	1		16	10
Del Rio, TX	46	21	8	3	3	3	4	3	17	5
Deming, NM	27	10	3	2	2	2	1	2	12	3
DeRidder, LA	41	24	11		6	5	2	2	9	6
Dickinson, ND	34	17	8		5	2	2		10	7
Dillon, SC	22	16	10		4	1	1		4	2
Dixon, IL	68	33	18		9	2	4	1	24	10
Dodge City, KS	47	23	11	1	6	2	3	2	14	8
Douglas, GA	62	26	6	3	8	5	4	1	22	13
Dublin, GA	154	73	23	2	34	9	5	4	50	27
DuBois, PA	137	34	11	1	13	2	7	12	69	22
Dumas, TX	11	7	4	1	1	1			2	2
Duncan, OK	44	25	18		3	3	1	2	11	6
Dunn, NC	85	42	15	2	14	6	5	3	31	9
Durango, CO	261	64	35		7	9	13	15	117	65
Durant, OK	33	14	3		6	3	2	3	10	6
Dyersburg, TN	66	29	9		11	4	5	2	18	17
Eagle Pass, TX	32	18	3	2	5	2	6	1	7	6

Table 4.15

Physicians by Micropolitan Statistical Area and Self-Designated Primary Care Specialty, 2010, continued

			Primary Care							
Micropolitan Areas	Total Physicians	Total Primary Care	Family Medicine	General Practice	Internal Medicine	OB/Gyn	Pediatrics	Primary Care Sub-specialties	All Other Specialties	Not Classi-fied/ Inactive
East Liverpool-Salem, OH	102	45	17		14	5	9	1	33	23
East Stroudsburg, PA	248	79	21	1	30	8	19	13	106	50
Easton, MD	229	46	9	1	18	9	9	11	94	78
Edwards, CO	193	49	20	2	10	7	10	7	89	48
Effingham, IL	83	30	15	1	9	3	2	7	36	10
El Campo, TX	54	20	9		3	4	4	3	20	11
El Dorado, AR	103	44	33		4	2	5	5	36	18
Elizabeth City, NC	110	36	13	1	9	9	4	7	45	22
Elk City, OK	32	14	10		1	2	1	1	14	3
Elko, NV	58	28	10	2	6	5	5	1	19	10
Ellensburg, WA	46	23	15	3	1	1	3	1	10	12
Emporia, KS	51	22	10		5	2	5	4	14	11
Enid, OK	115	35	19		6	4	6	5	50	25
Enterprise-Ozark, AL	88	39	14	1	10	7	7		34	15
Escanaba, MI	53	25	18		5	1	1	2	15	11
Espanola, NM	45	20	13		3	2	2	1	15	9
Eufaula, AL-GA	15	10	5	1	4			1	2	2
Eureka-Arcata-Fortuna, CA	331	122	58	10	28	13	13	8	133	68
Evanston, WY	33	12	4		4	2	2	1	15	5
Fairmont, MN	42	24	14		6	3	1		13	5
Fairmont, WV	96	41	14	1	15	4	7	4	34	17
Fallon, NV	26	16	9	1	3	2	1		5	5
Faribault-Northfield, MN	120	68	46		8	9	5	5	31	16
Farmington, MO	76	30	13		12	1	4	5	23	18
Fergus Falls, MN	88	36	24		8	2	2	3	26	23
Fernley, NV	17	10	5	2	3				2	5
Findlay, OH	151	39	13	1	12	4	9	14	69	29
Fitzgerald, GA	20	12	3	2	3	1	3	1	3	4
Forest City, NC	101	44	21	1	11	4	7	4	36	17
Forrest City, AR	18	12	5	1	4	1	1	2	4	
Fort Dodge, IA	69	21	10	1	5	3	2	2	30	16
Fort Leonard Wood, MO	28	13	9	2			2		11	4
Fort Madison-Keokuk, IA-MO	55	24	7	1	8	4	4	1	21	9
Fort Morgan, CO	28	18	12		3	2	1	1	6	3
Fort Payne, AL	57	30	8	5	7	5	5	1	14	12
Fort Polk South, LA	50	20	8	1	4	3	4	4	18	8
Fort Valley, GA	12	7	4		3				2	3
Frankfort, IN	27	16	8	1	2	3	2		6	5
Frankfort, KY	96	37	16		8	5	8	6	32	21
Fredericksburg, TX	104	33	17	1	12	2	1	5	38	28
Freeport, IL	78	30	13		8	4	5	5	31	12
Fremont, NE	58	26	13		5	4	4	4	18	10
Fremont, OH	72	37	25	4	5	1	2	4	19	12
Gaffney, SC	46	24	16		3	2	3	1	12	9
Gainesville, TX	25	14	5	1	4	2	2		6	5
Galesburg, IL	120	45	23	3	10	3	6	4	49	22
Gallup, NM	167	87	42	1	17	9	18	5	45	30
Garden City, KS	45	14	5	2	3	1	3	4	19	8
Gardnerville Ranchos, NV	107	32	16	1	10	1	4	1	44	30
Georgetown, SC	146	42	21	2	9	6	4	11	54	39
Gettysburg, PA	129	52	27	2	15	2	6	6	45	26
Gillette, WY	67	32	13	1	8	6	4	3	28	4

Table 4.15

Physicians by Micropolitan Statistical Area and Self-Designated Primary Care Specialty, 2010, continued

			Primary Care							
Micropolitan Areas	Total Physicians	Total Primary Care	Family Medicine	General Practice	Internal Medicine	OB/Gyn	Pediatrics	Primary Care Sub-specialties	All Other Specialties	Not Classified/Inactive
Glasgow, KY	96	47	29	1	6	7	4	3	34	12
Gloversville, NY	70	30	11	1	10	3	5	3	20	17
Granbury, TX	76	27	12		4	6	5	4	25	20
Grand Island, NE	130	54	28	1	16	4	5	4	52	20
Grants Pass, OR	146	60	27	1	23	6	3	2	47	37
Grants, NM	28	19	11		7	1			4	5
Great Bend, KS	35	17	6	2	5	2	2		10	8
Greeneville, TN	118	52	21	4	15	6	6	3	44	19
Greensburg, IN	23	13	7		4	1	1	1	3	6
Greenville, MS	97	33	11	1	14	5	2	6	39	19
Greenville, OH	39	26	19	1	3	3		4	2	7
Greenwood, MS	67	23	5		10	4	4	5	28	11
Greenwood, SC	256	116	79	1	17	10	9	11	96	33
Grenada, MS	31	15	3		5	5	2	1	11	4
Guymon, OK	13	8	2		4	1	1		5	
Hammond, LA	149	69	18	1	24	15	11	9	49	22
Hannibal, MO	75	25	7		8	5	5	7	30	13
Harriman, TN	39	19	11	4	4			5	8	7
Harrisburg, IL	39	21	13	2	5	1		1	11	6
Harrison, AR	74	33	20	3	5	2	3	3	26	12
Hastings, NE	86	34	17		8	4	5	3	30	19
Havre, MT	29	9	5		2	2		2	10	8
Hays, KS	81	18	5		9	3	1	7	37	19
Heber, UT	31	11	8		1	1	1	1	10	9
Helena-West Helena, AR	23	7	4	1	1	1		2	4	10
Helena, MT	226	79	28	1	32	8	10	6	99	42
Henderson, NC	60	23	12	1	3	1	6	3	23	11
Hereford, TX	7	3	2	1					2	2
Hilo, HI	427	158	51	17	47	18	25	12	156	101
Hilton Head Island-Beaufort, SC	635	144	49		34	28	33	17	209	265
Hobbs, NM	58	27	5	2	12	4	4	2	18	11
Homosassa Springs, FL	329	80	26	4	34	9	7	18	127	104
Hood River, OR	104	50	30	1	8	7	4	1	37	16
Hope, AR	22	12	6	1		2	3	2	5	3
Houghton, MI	62	27	17		2	2	6	3	18	14
Hudson, NY	120	31	16	1	8	3	3	6	52	31
Humboldt, TN	44	30	20		6	1	3		8	6
Huntingdon, PA	45	19	11		6	1	1		15	11
Huntington, IN	41	20	11		2	2	5	3	12	6
Huntsville, TX	68	22	9	2	7	3	1	8	24	14
Huron, SD	22	11	5	1	4	1			8	3
Hutchinson, KS	146	49	21	1	11	6	10	8	57	32
Hutchinson, MN	51	31	25		3		3	1	14	5
Indiana, PA	128	48	19	3	14	4	8	3	50	27
Indianola, MS	18	10	8	2					3	5
Iron Mountain, MI-WI	78	31	16		8	4	3	3	32	12
Jackson, WY-ID	141	43	13	1	11	9	9	1	56	41
Jacksonville, IL	52	18	8		4	4	2		22	12
Jacksonville, TX	67	18	8	1	4	3	2	1	36	12
Jamestown-Dunkirk-Fredonia, NY	197	70	22	3	29	8	8	6	71	50
Jamestown, ND	29	15	13		1		1		12	2

Table 4.15

Physicians by Micropolitan Statistical Area and Self-Designated Primary Care Specialty, 2010, continued

			Primary Care							
Micropolitan Areas	Total Physicians	Total Primary Care	Family Medicine	General Practice	Internal Medicine	OB/Gyn	Pediatrics	Primary Care Sub-specialties	All Other Specialties	Not Classified/ Inactive
Jasper, IN	86	39	17		11	7	4	5	30	12
Jayuya, PR	19	12	1	7	2		2	1	3	3
Jennings, LA	33	19	8	2	4	3	2	1	6	7
Jesup, GA	28	14	5		4	2	3	1	9	4
Juneau, AK	93	39	27		7	1	4		43	11
Kahului-Wailuku, HI	394	138	40	8	52	15	23	18	153	85
Kalispell, MT	309	82	39	2	24	12	5	9	135	83
Kapaa, HI	188	72	27	5	20	6	14	3	77	36
Kearney, NE	142	52	24	1	12	7	8	4	70	16
Keene, NH	197	58	32		11	7	8	12	66	61
Kendallville, IN	28	17	12		3	1	1	1	7	3
Kennett, MO	39	22	6	5	5	4	2	2	9	6
Kerrville, TX	189	53	12	1	29	6	5	4	66	66
Ketchikan, AK	32	15	7	1	4		3		10	7
Key West, FL	247	55	17	5	21	6	6	5	100	87
Kill Devil Hills, NC	62	24	14	2	2	2	4	3	19	16
Kingsville, TX	27	16	7		3	1	5	1	3	7
Kinston, NC	107	36	12		15	4	5	6	39	26
Kirksville, MO	14	7	3		1	2	1		7	
Klamath Falls, OR	167	73	55		8	5	5	4	50	40
Kodiak, AK	29	19	16	1	2				6	4
La Follette, TN	40	19	7		11	1		4	9	8
La Grande, OR	54	22	7		8	2	5	1	23	8
Laconia, NH	170	46	9		20	7	10	7	74	43
LaGrange, GA	120	40	4		17	9	10	6	56	18
Lake City, FL	125	43	14	3	16	3	7	6	48	28
Lamesa, TX	7	4	2			1	1			3
Lancaster, SC	91	38	15		10	5	8	3	34	16
Laramie, WY	87	35	15	2	8	6	4	3	36	13
Las Vegas, NM	46	25	7	2	11	1	4	2	14	5
Laurel, MS	110	44	16	1	8	9	10	5	40	21
Laurinburg, NC	65	33	13	1	8	3	8	6	20	6
Lawrenceburg, TN	33	19	9		5	2	3		6	8
Lebanon, MO	27	24	11	1	4	4	4		3	
Lebanon, NH-VT	1,597	404	78	3	184	49	90	135	723	335
Levelland, TX	13	9	5		1		3		3	1
Lewisburg, PA	146	42	12	1	15	7	7	2	79	23
Lewisburg, TN	16	7	6		1			2	6	1
Lewistown, PA	54	21	11		3	4	3	2	24	7
Lexington Park, MD	129	47	14	4	13	7	9	6	49	27
Lexington, NE	21	14	13		1				6	1
Liberal, KS	37	13	3		5	2	3		16	8
Lincoln, IL	20	12	9	1		2		2	3	3
Lincolnton, NC	77	41	20	1	8	4	8	4	22	10
Lock Haven, PA	41	23	8	1	10	3	1		7	11
Logansport, IN	48	20	10		2	4	4	1	18	9
London, KY	85	34	11	2	10	7	4	7	33	11
Los Alamos, NM	66	30	13		8	3	6	3	17	16
Lufkin, TX	155	61	19	1	29	5	7	9	66	19
Lumberton, NC	149	69	23	2	26	8	10	9	48	23
Macomb, IL	42	21	10		6	1	4		11	10
Madison, IN	65	26	14	1	4	4	3		25	14

Table 4.15

Physicians by Micropolitan Statistical Area and Self-Designated Primary Care Specialty, 2010, continued

			Primary Care							
Micropolitan Areas	Total Physicians	Total Primary Care	Family Medicine	General Practice	Internal Medicine	OB/Gyn	Pediatrics	Primary Care Sub-specialties	All Other Specialties	Not Classified/ Inactive
Madisonville, KY	157	73	54	1	6	7	5	8	51	25
Magnolia, AR	26	16	10	1	2	2	1		1	9
Malone, NY	103	40	17	2	14	1	6	2	32	29
Manitowoc, WI	166	61	26		19	6	10	7	64	34
Marble Falls, TX	59	24	14	1	3	1	5	5	17	13
Marinette, WI-MI	98	43	14	1	17	6	5	5	35	15
Marion-Herrin, IL	164	53	25	2	14	4	8	9	73	29
Marion, IN	101	38	14	3	11	6	4	5	37	21
Marion, OH	123	35	11		14	5	5	7	61	20
Marquette, MI	279	96	63		18	8	7	17	115	51
Marshall, MN	25	13	10			2	1	1	8	3
Marshall, MO	19	11	9		1	1			4	4
Marshall, TX	53	22	7		5	5	5	1	21	9
Marshalltown, IA	60	24	15		5	1	3	1	19	16
Marshfield-Wisconsin Rapids, WI	552	170	29		100	11	30	66	237	79
Martin, TN	37	22	8		11	1	2		10	5
Martinsville, VA	114	41	14		15	6	6	5	43	25
Maryville, MO	29	14	6	2	3	2	1	1	13	1
Mason City, IA	171	69	45		16	2	6	6	63	33
Mayfield, KY	40	18	6	1	7	2	2	1	14	7
Maysville, KY	54	22	11	1	4	2	4	3	24	5
McAlester, OK	67	27	9		8	6	4	1	20	19
McComb, MS	86	29	10		6	8	5	4	37	16
McMinnville, TN	40	20	10		5	2	3		13	7
McPherson, KS	35	21	19	1	1				6	8
Meadville, PA	140	51	19	4	16	5	7	8	57	24
Menomonie, WI	45	24	14	1	6	1	2		11	10
Meridian, MS	264	86	26	6	28	12	14	10	129	39
Merrill, WI	38	17	13		4			1	10	10
Mexico, MO	37	18	8	1	4	2	3	1	13	5
Miami, OK	26	12	4		5	2	1		9	5
Middlesborough, KY	46	20	3	2	10	3	2	1	14	11
Midland, MI	236	101	64		20	11	6	8	88	39
Milledgeville, GA	123	44	8	5	16	6	9	2	47	30
Minden, LA	48	26	15	2	4	2	3	1	11	10
Mineral Wells, TX	21	13	6		3	2	2		4	4
Minot, ND	190	77	43	3	14	7	10	9	80	24
Mitchell, SD	41	20	7		7	2	4	1	15	5
Moberly, MO	16	4			2		2		5	7
Monroe, WI	86	31	9		9	9	4	3	29	23
Montrose, CO	102	30	12		8	3	7	1	48	23
Morehead City, NC	183	64	24	3	13	15	9	6	69	44
Morgan City, LA	67	37	16		10	5	6	1	16	13
Moscow, ID	58	27	20	1	5	1		1	22	8
Moses Lake, WA	82	48	28	1	9	4	6	2	20	12
Moultrie, GA	58	24	12		8	1	3	1	25	8
Mount Airy, NC	98	57	26		15	7	9		28	13
Mount Pleasant, MI	77	26	5		13	3	5	6	36	9
Mount Pleasant, TX	46	19	3	2	3	5	6	1	21	5
Mount Sterling, KY	32	17	6		8	2	1	3	8	4
Mount Vernon, IL	111	31	6		18	4	3	8	57	15
Mount Vernon, OH	70	30	12		11	4	3	2	21	17

Table 4.15

Physicians by Micropolitan Statistical Area and Self-Designated Primary Care Specialty, 2010, continued

			Primary Care							
Micropolitan Areas	Total Physicians	Total Primary Care	Family Medicine	General Practice	Internal Medicine	OB/Gyn	Pediatrics	Primary Care Sub-specialties	All Other Specialties	Not Classified/ Inactive
Mountain Home, AR	114	37	19		12	4	2	7	55	15
Mountain Home, ID	33	22	11	1	1	7	2		7	4
Murray, KY	70	26	9		5	8	4	5	27	12
Muscatine, IA	40	24	9		7	4	4	1	11	4
Muskogee, OK	124	37	11		17	4	5	5	53	29
Nacogdoches, TX	146	55	23	3	15	9	5	6	68	17
Natchez, MS-LA	87	34	14	2	10	3	5	3	31	19
Natchitoches, LA	46	26	11	2	5	3	5	2	11	7
New Bern, NC	293	103	25	1	46	12	19	21	121	48
New Castle, IN	56	24	10	1	7	2	4	1	18	13
New Castle, PA	113	43	14	4	12	9	4	3	43	24
New Iberia, LA	122	50	19	3	10	7	11	4	42	26
New Philadelphia-Dover, OH	111	47	19		13	7	8	2	34	28
New Ulm, MN	47	27	22		3	1	1	2	15	3
Newberry, SC	42	26	16	1	5	2	2		13	3
Newport, TN	24	20	12		5		3		3	1
Newton, IA	19	10	9	1					6	3
Nogales, AZ	52	22	11		6	2	3	1	10	19
Norfolk, NE	93	39	23	2	5	5	4	3	39	12
North Platte, NE	89	27	15	1	5	4	2	5	37	20
North Vernon, IN	13	10	6	1	2		1	1		2
North Wilkesboro, NC	71	34	14		14	4	2	4	20	13
Norwalk, OH	57	26	17		3	3	3	1	19	11
Oak Harbor, WA	176	46	18		11	7	10	4	66	60
Oak Hill, WV	40	20	7	5	5		3		9	11
Ocean Pines, MD	97	35	17	1	15	2		5	29	28
Ogdensburg-Massena, NY	183	65	18	2	25	9	11	8	77	33
Oil City, PA	95	30	11		13	3	3	8	41	16
Okeechobee, FL	44	21	5	1	10	1	4	5	16	2
Olean, NY	134	43	18	1	15	4	5	10	50	31
Oneonta, NY	348	88	9	1	55	10	13	25	180	55
Ontario, OR-ID	57	20	8	2	7	1	2		28	9
Opelousas-Eunice, LA	148	69	30	2	12	12	13	3	58	18
Orangeburg, SC	130	51	20	3	11	5	12	13	45	21
Oskaloosa, IA	22	12	11				1		6	4
Ottawa-Streator, IL	190	77	32	4	26	10	5	5	68	40
Ottumwa, IA	66	22	3		10	2	7	3	30	11
Owatonna, MN	67	39	27		7	3	2	1	14	13
Owosso, MI	58	17	7		5	2	3	2	22	17
Oxford, MS	128	34	10	2	11	5	6	5	53	36
Paducah, KY-IL	283	73	27	2	28	9	7	21	139	50
Pahrump, NV	31	11	7	1	2		1	1	8	11
Palatka, FL	84	28	7	2	12	3	4	3	30	23
Palestine, TX	60	21	4	2	6	5	4	3	23	13
Pampa, TX	23	10	3		4	1	2	1	7	5
Paragould, AR	45	25	17		3	2	3	1	12	7
Paris, TN	58	22	6	1	8	2	5		21	15
Paris, TX	114	27	5	1	11	4	6	8	58	21
Parsons, KS	43	19	8	4	1	3	3	1	17	6
Payson, AZ	88	40	19	4	10	3	4	1	21	26
Pecos, TX	3	1			1				1	1
Pella, IA	37	21	14	1	3	2	1	2	7	7

Table 4.15

Physicians by Micropolitan Statistical Area and Self-Designated Primary Care Specialty, 2010, continued

			Primary Care							
Micropolitan Areas	Total Physicians	Total Primary Care	Family Medicine	General Practice	Internal Medicine	OB/Gyn	Pediatrics	Primary Care Sub-specialties	All Other Specialties	Not Classified/ Inactive
Pendleton-Hermiston, OR	101	40	18	2	11	5	4		35	26
Peru, IN	24	10	3	1	1	3	2		7	7
Phoenix Lake-Cedar Ridge, CA	140	55	18	5	23	2	7	2	54	29
Picayune, MS	44	21	8	3	5	3	2		8	15
Pierre Part, LA	9	5	3	1	1			1	2	1
Pierre, SD	31	17	6	1	6	2	2		8	6
Pittsburg, KS	54	21	11		5	2	3	5	16	12
Plainview, TX	23	12	6		2		4		6	5
Platteville, WI	42	21	17	2		1	1	1	11	9
Plattsburgh, NY	222	64	15	1	25	11	12	11	106	41
Plymouth, IN	47	33	25	1	3	3	1	1	5	8
Point Pleasant, WV-OH	129	55	7	4	23	8	13	5	54	15
Ponca City, OK	60	25	11	4	4	3	3	1	21	13
Pontiac, IL	29	17	8	1	4	2	2	3	8	1
Poplar Bluff, MO	127	58	14	3	23	8	10	5	43	21
Port Angeles, WA	214	70	41	2	15	3	9	4	70	70
Portales, NM	13	8	4		3	1		1	3	1
Portsmouth, OH	125	33	14	2	8	2	7	8	60	24
Pottsville, PA	181	64	15	1	36	3	9	2	78	37
Price, UT	25	11	5		3	1	2	1	11	2
Prineville, OR	14	6	6						4	4
Pullman, WA	65	32	15	1	8	2	6		14	19
Quincy, IL-MO	191	51	26		15	6	4	22	81	37
Raymondville, TX	7	7	4	1	1		1			
Red Bluff, CA	70	29	9	3	9	2	6		27	14
Red Wing, MN	98	44	22	1	11	6	4	2	31	21
Rexburg, ID	45	23	10	1	4	5	3	1	13	8
Richmond-Berea, KY	144	65	27	4	18	6	10	8	43	28
Richmond, IN	169	47	20	1	19	3	4	12	82	28
Rio Grande City-Roma, TX	23	16	8	2	2		4		4	3
Riverton, WY	107	42	23		8	6	5	2	35	28
Roanoke Rapids, NC	86	34	10	3	14	2	5	5	30	17
Rochelle, IL	40	30	26		3		1		6	4
Rock Springs, WY	37	16	7	1	3	3	2		16	5
Rockingham, NC	44	21	7		8	3	3		12	11
Rockland, ME	171	44	16		14	4	10	6	64	57
Rolla, MO	76	35	10	1	12	4	8	5	26	10
Roseburg, OR	216	66	22	1	32	5	6	10	83	57
Roswell, NM	134	57	36	1	5	5	10	9	46	22
Ruidoso, NM	36	13	5	1	5	2		1	10	12
Russellville, AR	118	59	31	1	10	9	8	2	37	20
Ruston, LA	98	43	15	2	13	5	8	3	40	12
Rutland, VT	191	57	28	1	17	5	6	10	68	56
Safford, AZ	36	19	13	1	3	1	1	1	5	11
Salina, KS	174	63	43		5	8	7	8	72	31
Salisbury, NC	245	75	24	2	32	8	9	13	104	53
Sanford, NC	88	31	14		7	4	6	4	35	18
Santa Isabel, PR	23	9	2	4	2		1		5	9
Sault Ste. Marie, MI	43	16	12		2	1	1	2	15	10
Sayre, PA	276	92	38		44	7	3	15	117	52
Scottsbluff, NE	100	36	20		10	5	1	1	44	19
Scottsboro, AL	54	31	18	2	4	4	3	1	15	7

Table 4.15

Physicians by Micropolitan Statistical Area and Self-Designated Primary Care Specialty, 2010, continued

			Primary Care							
Micropolitan Areas	Total Physicians	Total Primary Care	Family Medicine	General Practice	Internal Medicine	OB/Gyn	Pediatrics	Primary Care Sub-specialties	All Other Specialties	Not Classi-fied/ Inactive
Scottsburg, IN	18	13	10		1	2		1	3	1
Seaford, DE	392	120	43	5	43	11	18	32	161	79
Searcy, AR	117	47	28		7	5	7	6	46	18
Sebring, FL	207	64	15	2	26	12	9	13	78	52
Sedalia, MO	48	17	6		3	3	5	2	20	9
Selinsgrove, PA	39	17	14		2		1	3	11	8
Selma, AL	80	32	15		7	5	5	3	24	21
Seneca Falls, NY	22	8	4		4				7	7
Seneca, SC	161	47	30	2	6	4	5	9	66	39
Sevierville, TN	79	40	26	1	4	5	4	1	22	16
Seymour, IN	58	28	20		2	4	2	2	21	7
Shawnee, OK	79	35	15		10	6	4	3	22	19
Shelby, NC	165	61	20		21	7	13	9	61	34
Shelbyville, TN	33	14	9		2		3	3	10	6
Shelton, WA	50	17	7		2	5	3		14	19
Sheridan, WY	83	27	6	1	13	4	3	2	38	16
Show Low, AZ	119	59	37	3	9	3	7	4	37	19
Sidney, OH	47	28	13		8	5	2		12	7
Sierra Vista-Douglas, AZ	136	54	18	3	20	6	7	7	52	23
Sikeston, MO	55	22	10	1	6	3	2	3	19	11
Silver City, NM	79	29	10	2	10	3	4	4	30	16
Silverthorne, CO	108	29	17		5	5	2	2	38	39
Snyder, TX	12	8	6		1		1		2	2
Somerset, KY	146	50	14	1	20	7	8	10	60	26
Somerset, PA	102	36	16	2	11	5	2	1	38	27
Southern Pines-Pinehurst, NC	407	94	18	3	43	18	12	26	210	77
Spearfish, SD	54	25	15		5	2	3		12	17
Spencer, IA	27	9	9						18	
Spirit Lake, IA	30	8	8						12	10
St. Marys, GA	55	26	9		9	3	5	3	11	15
St. Marys, PA	48	14	10			2	2		20	14
Starkville, MS	62	26	11	2	2	6	5	3	23	10
Statesboro, GA	109	46	17		12	8	9	5	43	15
Statesville-Mooresville, NC	340	133	45	1	41	22	24	23	145	39
Staunton-Waynesboro, VA	279	89	37	2	22	15	13	9	111	70
Stephenville, TX	47	23	10		7	3	3	1	16	7
Sterling, CO	23	11	7		2	2			9	3
Sterling, IL	85	34	16	4	10	1	3	5	28	18
Stevens Point, WI	136	57	21	2	20	7	7	3	53	23
Stillwater, OK	115	45	18		16	5	6	3	37	30
Storm Lake, IA	19	11	10		1				2	6
Sturgis, MI	64	32	17	2	5	4	4	1	18	13
Sulphur Springs, TX	36	19	10		2	4	3	1	11	5
Summerville, GA	11	6	3	1	1	1			3	2
Sunbury, PA	78	31	14		13	2	2	1	24	22
Susanville, CA	39	20	11	3	3	1	2	2	8	9
Sweetwater, TX	10	4	1	1	1	1		1	3	2
Tahlequah, OK	64	31	12		8	5	6	2	22	9
Talladega-Sylacauga, AL	62	29	8	1	12	2	6	2	19	12
Tallulah, LA	8	7	2	2	1		2	1		
Taos, NM	103	40	19	1	10	4	6	1	36	26
Taylorville, IL	24	15	5	3	5	1	1	1	4	4

Table 4.15

Physicians by Micropolitan Statistical Area and Self-Designated Primary Care Specialty, 2010, continued

			Primary Care							
Micropolitan Areas	Total Physicians	Total Primary Care	Family Medicine	General Practice	Internal Medicine	OB/Gyn	Pediatrics	Primary Care Sub-specialties	All Other Specialties	Not Classified/Inactive
The Dalles, OR	61	21	7	1	7	4	2	1	25	14
The Villages, FL	125	27	5	2	12	3	5	3	22	73
Thomaston, GA	42	18	7	1	4	3	3	1	15	8
Thomasville-Lexington, NC	115	60	19	3	16	9	13	2	29	24
Thomasville, GA	167	45	11	3	14	6	11	10	82	30
Tiffin, OH	56	23	8		8	4	3	1	22	10
Tifton, GA	109	42	10	1	13	6	12	4	52	11
Toccoa, GA	46	19	8		3	2	6	1	15	11
Torrington, CT	458	139	25	3	69	17	25	25	182	112
Traverse City, MI	484	129	50	2	49	12	16	24	212	119
Troy, AL	31	16	7		2		7	1	10	4
Truckee-Grass Valley, CA	288	80	32	4	21	11	12	8	129	71
Tullahoma, TN	173	71	33	2	17	9	10	7	67	28
Tupelo, MS	361	111	52	3	32	14	10	32	159	59
Tuskegee, AL	22	10	5	1	3	1		1	6	5
Twin Falls, ID	178	59	33	3	10	7	6	10	79	30
Ukiah, CA	236	95	41	3	28	10	13	8	74	59
Union City, TN-KY	60	26	11	2	6	3	4		22	12
Union, SC	32	20	9	1	6	2	2		5	7
Urbana, OH	17	9	5	1	3			1	3	4
Utuado, PR	34	20	3	10	5		2		9	5
Uvalde, TX	25	13	10		1	1	1	1	8	3
Valley, AL	29	15	4		8	1	2		9	5
Van Wert, OH	27	16	10		3	2	1		7	4
Vermillion, SD	17	10	5	2			3		6	1
Vernal, UT	25	15	8		2	3	2		9	1
Vernon, TX	20	9	5		3		1		8	3
Vicksburg, MS	89	34	14	1	9	4	6	1	32	22
Vidalia, GA	53	23	2	3	10	5	3	2	20	8
Vincennes, IN	81	30	10	1	11	3	5	3	35	13
Wabash, IN	27	14	12		2				8	5
Wahpeton, ND-MN	30	13	11		2				8	9
Walla Walla, WA	250	84	34	3	26	8	13	9	87	70
Walterboro, SC	53	21	9		8	2	2	2	16	14
Wapakoneta, OH	47	25	15	1	4	3	2	2	10	10
Warren, PA	84	26	11	2	8	2	3	2	33	23
Warrensburg, MO	46	32	18		4	5	5	2	12	
Warsaw, IN	77	30	21	3	2	3	1	1	22	24
Washington Court House, OH	19	11	8		2	1			3	5
Washington, IN	19	9	6		2		1	2	3	5
Washington, NC	85	29	12		9	3	5	3	22	31
Watertown-Fort Atkinson, WI	78	41	21	1	10	5	4	3	21	13
Watertown-Fort Drum, NY	233	67	27		16	11	13	10	96	60
Watertown, SD	70	31	15		10	4	2	1	25	13
Wauchula, FL	12	7	1	1	3	1	1	2	1	2
Waycross, GA	119	46	18	1	16	5	6	9	42	22
Weatherford, OK	32	19	11	1	2	3	2		6	7
West Plains, MO	68	26	17	2	4	1	2	4	28	10
West Point, MS	23	10	2		2	4	2	1	6	6
Whitewater, WI	122	43	24		8	7	4	3	43	33
Willimantic, CT	165	70	23	2	25	9	11	8	62	25
Williston, ND	48	20	13	1	2	3	1		18	10

Table 4.15

Physicians by Micropolitan Statistical Area and Self-Designated Primary Care Specialty, 2010, continued

			Primary Care							
Micropolitan Areas	Total Physicians	Total Primary Care	Family Medicine	General Practice	Internal Medicine	OB/Gyn	Pediatrics	Primary Care Sub-specialties	All Other Specialties	Not Classified/ Inactive
Willmar, MN	126	56	36		10	4	6	3	40	27
Wilmington, OH	83	46	28		11	3	4	2	22	13
Wilson, NC	119	39	9		18	4	8	9	50	21
Winfield, KS	32	20	13		5	2			4	8
Winona, MN	69	26	15		8	2	1	2	24	17
Woodward, OK	25	12	8		2	1	1		5	8
Wooster, OH	160	67	28	1	12	15	11	6	58	29
Worthington, MN	29	17	9		4	2	2		6	6
Yankton, SD	100	27	12		8	4	3	3	49	21
Yazoo City, MS	16	8	4	1	2	1			4	4
Zanesville, OH	162	55	19	1	17	8	10	7	68	32

Notes:

FM subspecialties include FPG and FSM.

IM subspecialties include AMI, CCM, DIA, END, HEM, HEP, HO, ICE, ID, ILI, IMG, ISM, NEP, NTR, ON, PCC, and RHU.

OBG subspecialties include GO, GYN, MFM, OBS, OCC, and REN.

PD subspecialties include ADL, CCP, MPD, NPM, PDA, PDC, PDE, PDI, PDP, PDT, PEM, PG, PHO, PLI, PN, PPR, and PSM.

Table 4.16

Non-Metropolitan Physicians by State and Self-Designated Primary Care Specialty, 2010

		Major Professional Activity								
		Patient Care								
			Office-Based Practice							
State	Total Physicians	Total Patient Care	Family Medicine	General Practice	Internal Medicine	OB/Gyn	Pediatrics	Primary Care Sub-specialties	All other Specialties	Not Classified/ Inactive
Total Non-Metropolitan Physicians	21,117	9,982	5,955	613	1,889	686	839	542	5,311	4,850
Alabama	333	204	113	18	41	16	16	4	61	64
Alaska	233	145	105	8	16	5	11	2	53	33
Arizona	79	37	13	1	12	4	7	5	21	16
Arkansas	449	269	187	31	25	14	12	6	71	103
California	345	128	74	8	26	8	12	9	111	97
Colorado	788	303	189	11	58	25	20	19	256	210
District Of Columbia	1									1
Florida	328	136	61	19	37	13	6	14	86	92
Georgia	765	385	187	23	96	36	43	23	174	183
Idaho	346	119	77	11	16	8	7	5	112	110
Illinois	455	251	144	16	55	17	19	11	98	95
Indiana	184	123	96	9	12	1	5	5	25	31
Iowa	590	313	254	19	23	8	9	6	121	150
Kansas	349	196	151	14	21	4	6	4	62	87
Kentucky	989	480	223	36	127	31	63	49	280	180
Louisiana	235	132	66	16	33	6	11	8	49	46
Maine	864	339	173	12	83	38	33	22	282	221
Maryland	123	41	25	2	7	2	5	1	38	43
Massachusetts	99	34	11	1	13	6	3	1	22	42
Michigan	865	326	151	18	89	31	37	39	271	229
Minnesota	664	407	333	8	40	15	11	9	98	150
Mississippi	401	235	140	15	48	15	17	15	62	89
Missouri	463	242	148	15	47	16	16	18	105	98
Montana	439	225	154	12	32	15	12	8	100	106
Nebraska	304	204	183	10	8		3	2	30	68
Nevada	37	26	17	2	6	1			6	5
New Hampshire	134	36	17		10	6	3	4	46	48
New Mexico	84	41	19	5	11	3	3	2	16	25
New York	507	211	101	6	63	20	21	17	146	133
North Carolina	891	411	211	18	102	39	41	16	255	209
North Dakota	159	100	62	12	20	2	4	4	21	34
Ohio	294	168	104	8	32	10	14	5	56	65
Oklahoma	288	164	101	22	27	6	8	4	50	70
Oregon	240	111	75	3	19	10	4	1	61	67
Pennsylvania	354	137	62	9	39	12	15	10	105	102
South Carolina	187	114	67	9	16	8	14	2	40	31
South Dakota	194	127	87	13	15	4	8	2	28	37
Tennessee	413	238	134	21	48	15	20	9	84	82
Texas	836	467	310	42	68	24	23	17	148	204
Utah	115	61	46	5	4	3	3	2	28	24
Vermont	449	181	83	7	46	17	28	13	144	111
Virginia	1,122	492	238	24	129	35	66	40	339	251
Washington	365	164	117	12	20	7	8	7	80	114
West Virginia	462	186	85	16	40	19	26	12	143	121
Wisconsin	1,147	560	405	13	90	24	28	24	303	260
Wyoming	219	104	79	6	10	6	3	5	62	48
Possessions	457	201	61	18	48	35	39	24	154	78
APOs and FPOs	1,040	408	216	9	61	46	76	37	408	187

Notes:

Does not include Address Unknown.

FM subspecialties include FPG and FSM.

IM subspecialties include AMI, CCM, DIA, END, HEM, HEP, HO, ICE, ID, ILI, IMG, ISM, NEP, NTR, ON, PCC, and RHU.

OBG subspecialties include GO, GYN, MFM, OBS, OCC, and REN.

PD subspecialties include ADL, CCP, MPD, NPM, PDA, PDC, PDE, PDI, PDP, PDT, PEM, PG, PHO, PLI, PN, PPR, and PSM.

Chapter 5

Osteopathic Physicians

This chapter provides statistics on several key characteristics of the Osteopathic physician population in the US as of December 31, 2010, mirroring similar tables on the Allopathic physician population in Chapters 1-4. These include information regarding major professional activity, primary specialty, age and sex, ethnicity, state of location, metropolitan areas, and primary care activities.

Activity by Age and Sex

Table 5.1 indicates that in 2010, nearly half of DOs were younger than 45 years of age (47.7%). The 35 to 44 age interval accounted for the highest percentage of total DOs (28.5%). DOs 65 and older numbered 7,961 or 12.1% of the DOs in the US. In general, the DO population trends young, and especially so when compared to the MD population as they are in Figure 5.1.

The youth trend among DOs is especially prevalent among females. Of total female DOs (19,452), the highest percent (33.2%) were 35 to 44 years of age, with 64.1% younger than 45 years of age. It's no surprise, then, that a mere 4.6% were 65 or older. While male DOs have a higher ratio of DOs under 45 than the overall MD population (40.8% to 31.2%), they are still clearly outpaced by their female counterparts in this category.

Self-Designated Specialty by Age and Sex

An analysis of Table 5.2 indicates that at the end of 2010, more than three fifths (62.8%) of all DOs (65,565) were in the following ten specialty fields:

- Family Medicine (15,341)
- Internal Medicine (7,186)
- Emergency Medicine (3,839)
- Pediatrics (2,924)
- Anesthesiology (2,718)
- General Practice (2,709)
- Obstetrics/Gynecology (2,358)
- Psychiatry (1,531)
- Orthopedic Surgery (1,325)
- Physical Medicine & Rehabilitation (1,255)

These same specialties were also highest for all male DOs (Table 5.3), with only General Surgery replacing Physical Medicine & Rehabilitation, representing 61.5% of the male population. The five disciplines with the most male DOs younger than 35 were Family Medicine (14.6% of males younger than 35), Internal Medicine (12.4%), Emergency Medicine (6.3%), Anesthesiology (5.5%), and Pediatrics (4.1%).

For female DOs, the specialties demonstrating the highest numbers differed from the male and overall DO populations. The top 10 disciplines for female DOs (Table 5.4) consisted of the following:

- Family Medicine (4,983)
- Internal Medicine (2,283)
- Pediatrics (1,704)
- Obstetrics/Gynecology (1,130)
- Emergency Medicine (827)

Figure 5.1

Percent Distribution of Total US Physicians by Age and Degree, 2010

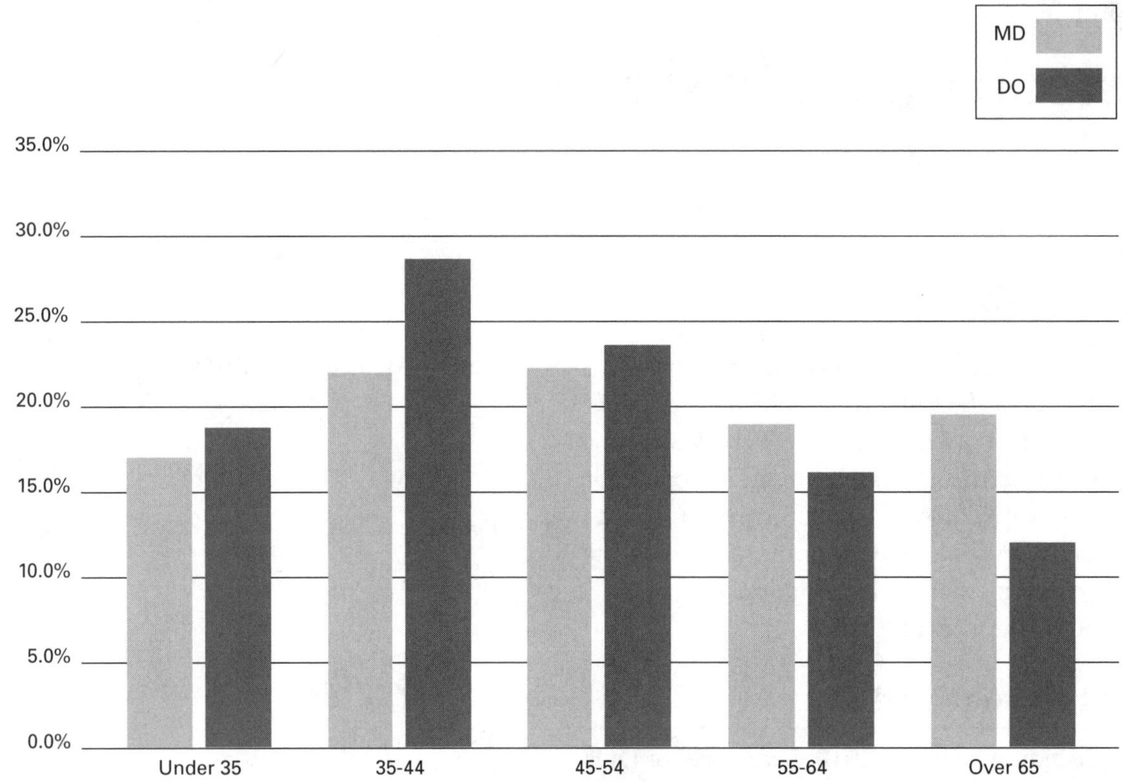

Source: Tables 1.1 & 5.1

Psychiatry (575)

Anesthesiology (513)

General Practice (434)

Physical Medicine & Rehabilitation (335)

Neurology (240)

These 10 specialties accounted for 67.0% of the female DO population, and among female DOs younger than 35, the highest percentages were found in Family Medicine (20.5% of those females younger than 35), Pediatrics (11.4%), Internal Medicine (11.4%), Obstetrics/Gynecology (5.9%), and Emergency Medicine (3.6%).

Distribution of Detail Specialties by Activity

The 10 specialties showing highest counts of DOs in 2010, in the detail specialties in Table 5.6, included: Family Medicine (15,090), Internal Medicine (5,525), Emergency Medicine (3,770), General Practice (2,709), Anesthesiology (2,502), Obstetrics/Gynecology (2,234), Pediatrics (2,219), Psychiatry (1,463), Physical Medicine and Rehabilitation (1,102), and General Surgery (975). Of these ten specialties, eight were among those in the top 10 for MDs, with General Practice and Physical Medicine and Rehabilitation for the DO population taking the place of Diagnostic Radiology and Orthopedic Surgery among the MD population.

Mean Age by Detail Specialty and Activity

Table 5.5 shows the mean age of DOs in the detail specialties. The 10 specialties with the highest mean ages include the following:

Legal Medicine (81.7)

Psychoanalysis (68.0)

Allergy (66.5)

Neurotology (Otolaryngology) (64.0)

Table J

Percent Distribution of DOs by Age and Sex, 2010

Sex	*Total*	*< 35*	*35-44*	*45-54*	*55-64*	*≥ 65*
Both	100.0	19.2	28.5	24.0	16.2	12.1
Male	100.0	14.2	26.5	24.7	19.2	15.3
Female	100.0	31.0	33.2	22.2	9.1	4.6

Source: Tables 5.13, 5.14, and 5.15

Chemical Pathology (63.0)

Immunology (62.3)

Pediatric Allergy (61.0)

Nutrition (60.7)

Radiology (59.7)

Aerospace Medicine (59.5)

MDs and DOs shared only three specialties — Psychoanalysis, Allergy, and Immunology — among their lists of 10 specialties with the highest average ages.

DOs by Self-Designated Specialty and Activity

Patient Care accounted for 84.0% of all DOs in 2010 (Table 5.7), significantly higher than the 76.4% of MDs in that category. Of the total number of DOs in Patient Care (55,091), more than three fourths (78.5%) were in Office-Based practice. Of a total of 6,354 Residents/Fellows, nearly one half (45.9%) were specialists in the disciplines of Internal Medicine, Family Medicine, Pediatrics, Emergency Medicine, and Anesthesiology. Percentages of total DOs in residency/fellowship training in these specialties are as follows: Family Medicine (13.8%), Internal Medicine (13.5%), Pediatrics (8.6%), Emergency Medicine (5.5%), and Anesthesiology (4.5%).

State of Location, Age, and Activity by Sex

Table 5.13 demonstrates that of the total 2010 US DO population (65,565), over three fifths (62.6%) were located in 10 states, a much higher concentration than the 55.0% of MDs in their top 10 most populous states. These 10 leading states for DOs were Pennsylvania (6,417), Michigan (5,629), Florida (4,708), Ohio (4,644), California (4,207), Texas (4,158), New York (3,501), New Jersey (3,015), Illinois (2,560), and Missouri (2,228).

Table 5.15 indicates that there were more female DOs in Pennsylvania in 2010 than in any other state (1,894 or 9.7% of total female DOs). Michigan followed with 1,513 female DOs, and then California with 1,438. These three states, in addition to New York (1,346), Ohio (1,281), Texas (1,194), and Florida (1,183), accounted for more than one half (50.6%) of all female DOs in 2010.

The distribution of DOs by age categories reveals a higher proportion of female DOs than male DOs younger than 35. Table J demonstrates the percent distributions by age groups and sex.

Male DOs younger than 35 (Table 5.14) showed the highest concentrations in Pennsylvania (629), Ohio (547), Michigan (492), California (462), and New York (395). Nearly two fifths (38.5%) of all male DOs younger than 35 were located in these states. Table 5.15 reveals that female DOs younger than 35 demonstrated the highest counts in Pennsylvania (637), Ohio (489), California (438), New York (390), and Michigan (384). Cumulatively, these five states accounted for 38.8% of all female DOs younger than 35.

State of Location and Activity

Tables 5.16 through 5.18 distribute total DOs, male DOs, and female DOs among the states and major professional activity. Patient Care DOs were in largest number in Pennsylvania (5,234), followed by Michigan (4,637), Florida (3,849), Ohio

(3,785), and California (3,591). Together, these states represented almost two fifths (38.3%) of all Patient-Care DOs.

For male DOs, Table 5.17 shows that Patient Care had the highest percentage representation in Utah (92.7%), North Dakota (91.8%), Montana (90.8%), and Idaho (90.7%). Lowest representation among male DOs in Patient Care was in the District of Columbia (65.7%) and Vermont (73.6%). Among female DOs (Table 5.18), Patient Care had highest proportional representation in Minnesota (94.4%), and Nebraska (93.0%). Lowest was the Rhode Island (77.9%).

Metropolitan Data

In 2010, the 366 Metropolitan Statistical Areas listed in Table 5.20 contained 86.8% of the total DO population of 65,565. In those Metropolitan Statistical Areas, Office-Based Family/General Practice represented 26.0% of the Patient Care population, while the same category in Other Specialties was 25.1%, Medical Specialties was 17.9%, and Surgical Specialties was 8.8% (Table 5.20).

Activity and Gender for Primary Care

Office-Based practice represented a higher percentage of primary care DOs (82.4%) than DOs in the primary care subspecialties (69.5%), with All Other Specialties appearing in between (71.7%).

A larger percentage of female DOs compared to male DOs were in primary care (49.2% and 39.5%, respectively). In each of the primary care specialties except for General Practice, the percentages of female DOs surpassed those of male DOs. This difference was especially apparent for Pediatrics, which represented 7.1% of all female DOs but only 1.7% of male DOs.

Age and Gender for Primary Care

The largest percentage of active DOs was in the age group 35 to 44 years (30.2%), with the age groups 45 to 54 years and Under 35 years having the next largest percentages (25.0% and 20.4%, respectively).

Among primary care DOs, the largest percentage (28.7%) were in the age group 45 to 54 years, whereas the next largest group was 35 to 44 (28.6%). The age group 55 to 64 years included only 19.1% of primary care DOs.

Primary care accounted for nearly half (43.3%) of female DOs in the age group younger than 35. The comparable percentage for male DOs was 27.2%. A similar gender gap existed for the age group 35 to 44 years. However, for the age group 65 years and older, the gender gap is actually reversed, with primary care including 27.7% of male DOs and 24.9% of female DOs.

Table 5.1

DOs by Age, Activity, and Sex, 2010

Activity	Total Physicians	< 35	35-44	45-54	55-64	≥ 65
			Both Sexes			
Total Physicians	65,565	12,578	18,693	15,712	10,621	7,961
Patient Care	55,091	9,907	16,633	14,707	9,516	4,328
Office-Based Practice	43,245	4,399	14,144	12,829	8,303	3,570
Hospital-Based Practice	11,846	5,508	2,489	1,878	1,213	758
Residents	6,354	5,119	765	88	14	368
Full-Time Staff	5,492	389	1,724	1,790	1,199	390
Other Professional Activity	1,167	32	159	366	432	178
Administration	478	4	38	153	189	94
Medical Teaching	425	20	77	148	128	52
Research	134	1	17	38	72	6
Other	130	7	27	27	43	26
Inactive	3,999	12	94	329	590	2,974
Not Classified	5,307	2,627	1,807	310	82	481
Address Unknown	1				1	
			Male			
Total Physicians	46,113	6,552	12,241	11,391	8,858	7,071
Patient Care	38,526	5,086	10,941	10,746	7,969	3,784
Office-Based Practice	31,042	2,305	9,222	9,356	6,955	3,204
Hospital-Based Practice	7,484	2,781	1,719	1,390	1,014	580
Residents	3,354	2,573	483	52	7	239
Full-Time Staff	4,130	208	1,236	1,338	1,007	341
Other Professional Activity	905	12	94	272	365	162
Administration	397	2	26	121	162	86
Medical Teaching	312	9	42	105	109	47
Research	102		11	28	58	5
Other	94	1	15	18	36	24
Inactive	3,516	3	38	196	473	2,806
Not Classified	3,165	1,451	1,168	177	50	319
Address Unknown	1				1	
			Female			
Total Physicians	19,452	6,026	6,452	4,321	1,763	890
Patient Care	16,565	4,821	5,692	3,961	1,547	544
Office-Based Practice	12,203	2,094	4,922	3,473	1,348	366
Hospital-Based Practice	4,362	2,727	770	488	199	178
Residents	3,000	2,546	282	36	7	129
Full-Time Staff	1,362	181	488	452	192	49
Other Professional Activity	262	20	65	94	67	16
Administration	81	2	12	32	27	8
Medical Teaching	113	11	35	43	19	5
Research	32	1	6	10	14	1
Other	36	6	12	9	7	2
Inactive	483	9	56	133	117	168
Not Classified	2,142	1,176	639	133	32	162

Table 5.2

DOs by Age and Self-Designated Specialty, 2010

Specialty	Total Physicians	< 35	35-44	45-54	55-64	≥ 65
Total Physicians	65,565	12,578	18,693	15,712	10,621	7,961
Aerospace Medicine	80	5	2	17	35	21
Allergy/Immunology	130	16	39	31	28	16
Anesthesiology	2,718	496	803	874	430	115
Cardiovascular Disease	784	107	194	281	176	26
Child Psychiatry	334	74	105	90	47	18
Colon/Rectal Surgery	32	6	11	7	5	3
Dermatology	550	113	169	141	91	36
Diagnostic Radiology	774	139	251	185	145	54
Emergency Medicine	3,839	628	1,167	1,134	774	136
Family Medicine	15,341	2,187	4,647	4,551	2,833	1,123
Forensic Pathology	28	6	11	8	2	1
Gastroenterology	468	79	135	151	85	18
General Practice	2,709	3	99	826	1,129	652
General Preventive Medicine	229	19	60	69	57	24
General Surgery	1,182	184	413	346	156	83
Internal Medicine	7,186	1,502	2,415	1,977	1,002	290
Medical Genetics	10	3	5	2		
Neurological Surgery	85	9	25	30	16	5
Neurology	732	141	226	216	120	29
Nuclear Medicine	49	4	9	8	15	13
Obstetrics/Gynecology	2,358	465	779	629	373	112
Occupational Medicine	228		18	97	87	26
Ophthalmology	408	25	122	130	98	33
Orthopedic Surgery	1,325	86	397	437	298	107
Otolaryngology	377	22	94	146	78	37
Pathology-Anatomic/Clinical	450	108	112	104	78	48
Pediatric Cardiology	33	15	10	6	2	
Pediatrics	2,924	957	1,003	563	302	99
Physical Medicine & Rehabilitation	1,255	338	424	327	130	36
Plastic Surgery	101	7	32	37	20	5
Psychiatry	1,531	294	339	412	356	130
Public Health & General Preventive Medicine	37	3	5	11	11	7
Pulmonary Diseases	497	102	143	141	91	20
Radiation Oncology	78	5	19	27	23	4
Radiology	447	36	124	98	98	91
Thoracic Surgery	76	7	18	19	23	9
Transplant Surgery	1	1				
Urological Surgery	212	17	45	67	65	18
Vascular Medicine	5		1	3	1	
Other Specialty	349	48	72	84	93	52
Unspecified	6,306	1,682	2,249	791	575	1,009
Inactive	3,999	12	94	329	590	2,974
Not Classified	5,307	2,627	1,807	310	82	481
Address Unknown	1				1	

Table 5.3

Male DOs by Age and Self-Designated Specialty, 2010

Specialty	Total Physicians	< 35	35-44	45-54	55-64	≥ 65
Total Physicians	46,113	6,552	12,241	11,391	8,858	7,071
Aerospace Medicine	76	4	2	16	34	20
Allergy/Immunology	95	9	29	18	24	15
Anesthesiology	2,205	358	651	706	380	110
Cardiovascular Disease	667	78	156	243	165	25
Child Psychiatry	188	33	59	54	28	14
Colon/Rectal Surgery	27	4	9	6	5	3
Dermatology	356	41	99	102	78	36
Diagnostic Radiology	604	92	195	137	126	54
Emergency Medicine	3,012	414	892	918	671	117
Family Medicine	10,358	954	2,876	3,193	2,334	1,001
Forensic Pathology	21	4	7	7	2	1
Gastroenterology	405	55	118	134	80	18
General Practice	2,275	3	68	622	967	615
General Preventive Medicine	156	7	41	44	44	20
General Surgery	973	119	330	301	146	77
Internal Medicine	4,903	815	1,585	1,424	834	245
Medical Genetics	5	1	4			
Neurological Surgery	81	8	23	29	16	5
Neurology	492	73	139	155	102	23
Nuclear Medicine	40	2	9	4	12	13
Obstetrics/Gynecology	1,228	108	326	389	306	99
Occupational Medicine	184		13	79	70	22
Ophthalmology	354	21	101	106	93	33
Orthopedic Surgery	1,207	72	362	396	273	104
Otolaryngology	339	17	80	134	73	35
Pathology-Anatomic/Clinical	307	57	76	68	61	45
Pediatric Cardiology	19	8	7	2	2	
Pediatrics	1,220	268	403	256	218	75
Physical Medicine & Rehabilitation	920	224	308	252	103	33
Plastic Surgery	89	6	27	32	19	5
Psychiatry	956	150	195	264	235	112
Public Health & General Preventive Medicine	21	1	1	7	6	6
Pulmonary Diseases	396	59	106	124	87	20
Radiation Oncology	63	3	13	23	21	3
Radiology	384	29	97	83	84	91
Thoracic Surgery	71	5	15	19	23	9
Transplant Surgery	1	1				
Urological Surgery	192	12	40	58	64	18
Vascular Medicine	5		1	3	1	
Other Specialty	251	24	47	59	78	43
Unspecified	4,285	959	1,525	551	469	781
Inactive	3,516	3	38	196	473	2,806
Not Classified	3,165	1,451	1,168	177	50	319
Address Unknown	1				1	

Table 5.4

Female DOs by Age and Self-Designated Specialty, 2010

Specialty	Total Physicians	< 35	35-44	45-54	55-64	≥ 65
Total Physicians	19,452	6,026	6,452	4,321	1,763	890
Aerospace Medicine	4	1		1	1	1
Allergy/Immunology	35	7	10	13	4	1
Anesthesiology	513	138	152	168	50	5
Cardiovascular Disease	117	29	38	38	11	1
Child Psychiatry	146	41	46	36	19	4
Colon/Rectal Surgery	5	2	2	1		
Dermatology	194	72	70	39	13	
Diagnostic Radiology	170	47	56	48	19	
Emergency Medicine	827	214	275	216	103	19
Family Medicine	4,983	1,233	1,771	1,358	499	122
Forensic Pathology	7	2	4	1		
Gastroenterology	63	24	17	17	5	
General Practice	434		31	204	162	37
General Preventive Medicine	73	12	19	25	13	4
General Surgery	209	65	83	45	10	6
Internal Medicine	2,283	687	830	553	168	45
Medical Genetics	5	2	1	2		
Neurological Surgery	4	1	2	1		
Neurology	240	68	87	61	18	6
Nuclear Medicine	9	2		4	3	
Obstetrics/Gynecology	1,130	357	453	240	67	13
Occupational Medicine	44		5	18	17	4
Ophthalmology	54	4	21	24	5	
Orthopedic Surgery	118	14	35	41	25	3
Otolaryngology	38	5	14	12	5	2
Pathology-Anatomic/Clinical	143	51	36	36	17	3
Pediatric Cardiology	14	7	3	4		
Pediatrics	1,704	689	600	307	84	24
Physical Medicine & Rehabilitation	335	114	116	75	27	3
Plastic Surgery	12	1	5	5	1	
Psychiatry	575	144	144	148	121	18
Public Health & General Preventive Medicine	16	2	4	4	5	1
Pulmonary Diseases	101	43	37	17	4	
Radiation Oncology	15	2	6	4	2	1
Radiology	63	7	27	15	14	
Thoracic Surgery	5	2	3			
Urological Surgery	20	5	5	9	1	
Other Specialty	98	24	25	25	15	9
Unspecified	2,021	723	724	240	106	228
Inactive	483	9	56	133	117	168
Not Classified	2,142	1,176	639	133	32	162

Table 5.5

DOs Mean Age by Self-Designated Specialty and Activity (177 Specialties), 2010

		Patient Care				Other Professional Activity			
				Hospital Based					
Specialty	Total Physicians	Total Patient Care	Office Based	Resid./ Fellows	Phys. Staff	Admin.	Med. Teach.	Research	Other
All Physicians	48.4	47.1	48.6	35.2	49.2	56.8	52.8	54.3	55.3
A	66.5	66.4	66.4			67.0			
ACA	35.2	35.2	37.4	31.7	36.0				
ADL	45.5	43.1	49.5	31.8	52.0	66.0	57.0		
ADM	59.1	60.0	60.3		59.0	56.5	53.0	54.0	
ADP	42.9	41.4	45.5	33.0	40.0	56.0	55.0		
AI	47.1	47.1	48.9	34.4	46.5	56.0	45.5		
ALI	48.0	48.0			48.0				
AM	59.5	59.3	60.5		58.0	60.4	53.0	56.5	64.7
AN	45.4	45.3	46.7	30.9	49.3	58.4	51.6	53.5	69.5
APM	42.6	42.6	42.2		46.2				
AR	36.0	36.0	36.0	34.7	38.0				
AS	55.7	55.7	49.0		59.0				
ATP	56.7	57.4	63.4		42.5	58.0	50.0		
BBK	42.2	42.2	47.8	29.5	38.0				
CCA	40.3	40.3	42.6	34.4	42.0				
CCM	43.1	42.7	44.3	33.0	47.0	52.0	59.0	50.0	
CCP	39.6	39.6	42.8	31.6	52.7				
CCS	42.2	41.8	45.8	36.8	39.0	58.0			
CD	47.4	47.2	49.4	33.4	46.7	57.0	57.7	59.5	76.0
CHN	42.2	41.4	48.1	31.5	42.0			56.5	
CHP	44.9	44.5	46.0	36.4	48.2	55.2	53.8	46.3	
CLP	43.7	48.5	39.0		58.0				34.0
CN	37.3	37.2	38.1	31.9	46.3	50.0	38.0		
CPP	28.0	28.0		28.0					
CRS	47.1	47.1	49.2	32.0	50.5				
CS	46.4	46.4	46.4						
D	45.5	45.4	48.7	31.4	45.3	59.0	63.0	46.0	49.0
DBP	37.3	37.3	50.7	30.5	38.0				
DIA	50.7	53.0	53.0				42.0	57.0	
DMP	41.8	42.3	42.7	33.0	45.0				35.0
DR	46.2	46.0	48.9	31.8	50.1	79.0	57.0		53.3
DS	47.2	46.5	46.5				50.0		
EFM	47.2	47.2	51.0		46.3				
EM	46.5	46.4	47.3	32.7	49.1	53.6	49.7	57.8	43.5
EMP	31.5	31.5		31.5					
END	40.7	40.5	42.3	31.5	41.7	48.0	57.0	43.0	
EP	52.0							52.0	
ESM	37.0	37.0	34.3		39.7				

A	Allergy
ACA	Adult Cardiothoracic Anesthesiology (Anesthesiology)
ADL	Adolescent Medicine (Pediatrics)
ADM	Addiction Medicine
ADP	Addiction Psychiatry
AI	Allergy And Immunology
ALI	Clinical Laboratory Immunology (Allergy & Immunology)
AM	Aerospace Medicine
AN	Anesthesiology
APM	Pain Medicine (Anesthesiology)
AR	Abdominal Radiology
AS	Abdominal Surgery
ATP	Anatomic Pathology
BBK	Blood Banking/Transfusion Medicine
CCA	Critical Care Medicine (Anesthesiology)
CCM	Critical Care Medicine (Internal Medicine)
CCP	Pediatric Critical Care Medicine
CCS	Surgical Critical Care (Surgery)
CD	Cardiovascular Disease
CHN	Child Neurology
CHP	Child & Adolescent Psychiatry
CLP	Clinical Pathology
CN	Clinical Neurophysiology
CPP	Pediatrics/Psychiatry/Child & Adolescent Psychiatry
CRS	Colon And Rectal Surgery
CS	Cosmetic Surgery
D	Dermatology
DBP	Developmental-Behavioral Pediatrics
DIA	Diabetes
DMP	Dermatopathology (Pathology)
DR	Diagnostic Radiology
DS	Dermatologic Surgery
EFM	Emergency Medicine/Family Medicine
EM	Emergency Medicine
EMP	Pediatrics/Emergency Medicine
END	Endocrinology, Diabetes & Metabolism
EP	Epidemiology
ESM	Sports Medicine (Emergency Medicine)

Table 5.5

DOs Mean Age by Self-Designated Specialty and Activity (177 Specialties), 2010, continued

		Patient Care				Other Professional Activity			
				Hospital Based					
Specialty	Total Physicians	Total Patient Care	Office Based	Resid./ Fellows	Phys. Staff	Admin.	Med. Teach.	Research	Other
ETX	33.9	33.9	36.5	31.7	39.0				
FM	47.7	47.6	48.5	31.1	49.4	54.2	51.2	52.1	63.1
FOP	43.0	41.0	41.8	31.5	42.3	55.0			54.7
FPG	51.0	50.9	51.4	34.5	55.2	53.3			
FPP	38.6	38.6	41.5	34.3					
FPS	46.3	46.3	46.3						
FSM	39.4	39.1	40.7	31.8	39.0	54.0	54.0		
GE	45.9	45.7	47.6	33.5	46.8	61.0	54.0	62.7	
GO	50.9	50.9	50.9		51.0				
GP	59.4	59.4	59.6		57.3	62.1	60.8		
GPM	50.3	50.0	52.6	35.9	52.0	56.0	52.5	51.0	38.0
GS	46.1	45.9	48.0	33.7	48.8	75.0	63.8		
GYN	58.9	58.0	58.2		57.0	69.7	55.0	62.7	71.0
HEM	52.5	51.9	53.8	29.0				58.0	
HMP	44.2	44.2	41.1	50.0					
HNS	50.0	50.0			50.0				
HO	40.1	39.9	42.3	32.2	44.1	56.0		38.0	64.0
HOS	43.1	43.1	41.1		46.6				
HPM	35.7	35.7	38.8	34.5					
HS	48.2	48.2	48.1		50.0				
HSO	36.8	36.8	37.3	35.9	35.0				
IC	39.8	39.8	40.9	33.6	43.3				
ICE	41.4	41.1	42.9	35.3	38.0		43.5	51.0	
ID	43.2	42.7	44.5	31.9	49.4	50.3	63.5	52.3	
IEC	42.0	42.0			42.0				
IFP	39.0	39.0	43.4	28.0					
IG	62.3	64.0	64.0				59.0		
IM	44.9	44.7	46.8	29.8	45.5	54.6	52.2	55.7	47.1
IMD	33.0	33.0		33.0					
IMG	43.3	42.8	44.0	34.1	48.6	54.0	35.0	46.5	
IPM	30.0	30.0	30.0						
ISM	41.1	41.1	41.1						
LM	81.7	92.5	92.5			63.0			59.4
MDM	54.9					54.9			
MEM	33.5	33.5	37.0	32.6					
MFM	52.7	52.7	52.6		52.9				
MG	38.2	38.2	39.4	35.5	43.0				
MGP	35.0	35.0		35.0					

ETX Medical Toxicology (Emergency Medicine)
FM Family Medicine
FOP Forensic Pathology
FPG Geriatric Medicine (Family Medicine)
FPP Psychiatry/Family Medicine
FPS Facial Plastic Surgery
FSM Sports Medicine (Family Practice)
GE Gastroenterology
GO Gynecological Oncology
GP General Practice
GPM General Preventive Medicine
GS General Surgery
GYN Gynecology
HEM Hematology (Internal Medicine)
HMP Hematology (Pathology)
HNS Head And Neck Surgery
HO Hematology/Oncology
HOS Hospitalist
HPM Hospice & Palliative Medicine
HS Hand Surgery
HSO Hand Surgery (Orthopedics)
IC Interventional Cardiology
ICE Clinical Cardiac Electrophysiology
ID Infectious Disease
IEC Internal Medicine/Emergency Medicine/Critical Care Medicine
IFP Internal Medicine/Family Practice
IG Immunology
IM Internal Medicine
IMD Internal Medicine/Dermatology
IMG Geriatric Medicine (Internal Medicine)
IPM Internal Medicine/Preventive Medicine
ISM Sports Medicine (Internal Medicine)
LM Legal Medicine
MDM Medical Management
MEM Internal Medicine/Emergency Medicine
MFM Maternal And Fetal Medicine
MG Medical Genetics
MGP Molecular Genetic Pathology (Pathology And Medical Genetics)

Table 5.5

DOs Mean Age by Self-Designated Specialty and Activity (177 Specialties), 2010, continued

		Patient Care				Other Professional Activity			
				Hospital Based					
Specialty	Total Physicians	Total Patient Care	Office Based	Resid./ Fellows	Phys. Staff	Admin.	Med. Teach.	Research	Other
MM	47.3	47.3	51.0		40.0				
MP	32.3	32.3		31.7	36.0				
MPD	37.4	37.3	40.6	30.2	37.2	40.0	41.0		
MSR	33.9	33.9	36.3	32.5	32.0				
N	46.8	46.6	49.3	32.0	49.6	51.5	62.8	51.6	49.7
NEP	42.9	42.5	43.5	34.8	43.8	62.3	64.0	55.0	
NM	54.7	55.3	56.7	29.7	58.2	58.0	39.0	62.0	34.0
NMN	35.5	35.5	36.4	31.0					
NMP	36.0	36.0	36.0						
NO	64.0						64.0		
NP	51.3	52.0	52.0						50.0
NPM	44.1	43.9	46.2	33.9	49.4	55.0	52.0		
NR	47.4	47.4	47.7		45.0				
NRN	53.0	53.0	53.0						
NS	48.1	48.1	49.3	30.8	46.9				
NSP	46.5	46.5	34.0		59.0				
NTR	60.7	62.5	62.5				57.0		
OAR	46.9	46.9	48.3	38.0	40.0				
OBG	44.4	44.3	45.9	30.7	48.4	56.0	52.4		57.3
OBS	48.0	47.9	47.2		52.0		49.0		
OCC	55.3	55.3	55.3						
OFA	44.4	44.4	44.4						
OM	55.4	54.8	54.9		54.5	56.8	57.4	55.0	71.8
OMM	54.0	54.3	54.8		44.6	45.0	50.5	39.0	
OMO	48.0	48.0	48.0						
ON	52.2	51.8	52.3	32.8	53.5	72.0		60.3	49.0
OP	46.4	46.4	48.2	31.5	50.0				
OPH	49.7	49.6	49.7	31.6	54.0		64.3	59.0	
ORS	50.3	50.2	50.9	32.3	50.7	55.0	54.0	63.0	58.5
OS	53.5	51.7	53.4	30.9	50.5	63.4	61.6	45.0	49.0
OSM	40.6	40.6	41.3	32.4	45.5				
OSS	42.6	42.6	42.9	34.0					
OTO	50.2	50.2	50.7	29.4	46.8		73.0		
OTR	39.3	39.3	40.3	35.0	37.0				
P	48.0	47.7	50.6	32.4	52.9	58.7	53.2	61.0	50.0
PA	58.5						67.0	50.0	
PAN	38.8	38.8	40.0	34.5	39.0		39.0		
PCC	38.6	38.6	41.0	31.9	44.9	56.0	37.0	41.0	

MM Medical Microbiology
MP Internal Med/Psychiatry
MPD Internal Medicine/Pediatrics
MSR Musculoskeletal Radiology
N Neurology
NEP Nephrology
NM Nuclear Medicine
NMN Neuromuscular Medicine (Neurology)
NMP Neonatal Perinatal Medicine
NO Neurotology (Otolaryngology)
NP Neuropathology
NPM Neonatal-Perinatal Medicine
NR Nuclear Radiology
NRN Neurology/Diagnostic Radiology/Neuroradiology
NS Neurological Surgery
NSP Pediatric Surgery (Neurology)
NTR Nutrition
OAR Adult Reconstructive Orthopedics
OBG Obstetrics & Gynecology
OBS Obstetrics
OCC Critical Care Medicine (Obstetrics & Gynecology)
OFA Foot And Ankle Orthopedics
OM Occupational Medicine
OMM Osteopathic Manipulative Medicine
OMO Musculoskeletal Oncology
ON Medical Oncology
OP Pediatric Orthopedics
OPH Ophthalmology
ORS Orthopedic Surgery
OS Other Specialty
OSM Sports Medicine (Orthopedic Surgery)
OSS Orthopedic Surgery Of The Spine
OTO Otolaryngology
OTR Orthopedic Trauma
P Psychiatry
PA Clinical Pharmacology
PAN Pediatric Anesthesiology (Anesthesiology)
PCC Pulmonary & Critical Care Medicine

Table 5.5

DOs Mean Age by Self-Designated Specialty and Activity (177 Specialties), 2010, continued

		Patient Care				Other Professional Activity			
				Hospital Based					
Specialty	Total Physicians	Total Patient Care	Office Based	Resid./ Fellows	Phys. Staff	Admin.	Med. Teach.	Research	Other
PCH	63.0	57.0	57.0						69.0
PCP	40.4	40.4	42.1	35.4	45.7				
PD	42.2	41.9	44.0	28.5	45.1	62.0	51.3	56.8	50.1
PDA	61.0	61.0	59.0		62.0				
PDC	37.6	37.6	42.9	32.0	48.0				
PDE	37.7	36.5	48.2	30.6	38.0			60.0	
PDI	36.4	35.5	43.5	30.3	38.0			47.0	
PDO	47.3	51.0	51.0				38.0		
PDP	38.5	37.7	42.3	30.2	53.0			53.0	
PDR	44.8	44.6	44.8	30.0	47.8				46.5
PDS	46.5	46.5	55.0	38.0					
PE	33.2	33.2	38.3	29.8					
PEM	38.7	38.7	45.1	32.2	49.6			38.0	
PFP	41.6	40.8	42.8	33.5	41.0	58.0			
PG	35.0	35.0	37.9	30.4	42.0				
PHL	50.8	50.8	50.8						
PHM	49.5	50.0			50.0			49.3	
PHO	36.0	35.7	40.9	30.7	46.5			47.0	
PHP	53.3	52.8	52.6		53.3	55.8	55.0	50.5	47.7
PLM	46.1	45.4	46.5		34.0	63.0	38.0		
PM	43.2	43.0	45.0	31.4	48.9	58.7	54.5	58.0	53.0
PME	55.2	55.2	55.2		54.3				
PMM	38.2	38.2	40.0	32.4	49.0				
PMP	41.0	41.0	41.0						
PN	41.4	41.9	46.8	35.0	39.0		38.0		
PO	46.0	46.0	46.0						
PP	42.2	42.2	44.5	33.0					
PPM	33.0	33.0		33.0					
PPR	31.5	31.5		31.5					
PRO	56.3	56.3	56.3						
PRS	47.6	47.6	46.8		51.0				
PS	48.4	47.9	49.6	34.4	43.8	61.0		65.0	
PSM	40.5	40.5	47.3	30.3					
PTH	47.5	46.6	52.8	31.4	53.3	59.5	62.3	54.5	59.5
PTX	41.0	41.0	41.0						
PUD	54.6	54.3	54.5	32.0	55.3	60.0	61.5	61.7	
PYA	68.0	68.0	68.0						
PYG	46.0	46.1	45.5	49.0	44.3		44.0		

PCH Chemical Pathology
PCP Cytopathology
PD Pediatrics
PDA Pediatric Allergy
PDC Pediatric Cardiology
PDE Pediatric Endocrinology
PDI Pediatric Infectious Disease
PDO Pediatric Otolaryngology
PDP Pediatric Pulmonology
PDR Pediatric Radiology
PDS Pediatric Surgery (Surgery)
PE Pediatric Emergency Med (Emergency Med)
PEM Pediatric Emergency Medicine (Pediatrics)
PFP Forensic Psychiatry
PG Pediatric Gastroenterology
PHL Phlebology
PHM Pharmaceutical Medicine
PHO Pediatric Hematology/Oncology
PHP Public Health And General Preventive Medicine
PLM Palliative Medicine
PM Physical Medicine And Rehabilitation
PME Pain Management
PMM Pain Medicine
PMP Pain Medicine (Physical Medicine & Rehabilitation)
PN Pediatric Nephrology
PO Pediatric Opthalmology
PP Pediatric Pathology
PPM Pediatrics/Physical Medicine And Rehabilitation
PPR Pediatric Rheumatology
PRO Proctology
PRS Sports Medicine (Physical Medicine & Rehabilitation)
PS Plastic Surgery
PSM Sports Medicine (Pediatrics)
PTH Anatomic/Clinical Pathology
PTX Medical Toxicology (Preventive Medicine)
PUD Pulmonary Disease
PYA Psychoanalysis
PYG Geriatric Psychiatry

Table 5.5

DOs Mean Age by Self-Designated Specialty and Activity (177 Specialties), 2010, continued

		Patient Care				Other Professional Activity			
				Hospital Based					
Specialty	Total Physicians	Total Patient Care	Office Based	Resid./ Fellows	Phys. Staff	Admin.	Med. Teach.	Research	Other
PYM	37.0	37.0	40.0	32.5					
PYN	48.3	48.3	56.0	33.0	56.0				
R	59.7	59.4	57.8	32.0	65.5	69.2	58.5		66.5
REN	57.8	57.8	57.7		59.0				
RHU	43.7	43.5	44.8	31.6	50.1	60.0	51.0	43.0	50.0
RNR	42.2	42.0	42.7	35.5	44.9				59.0
RO	49.4	49.2	50.0	31.2	52.5	67.0	48.0		
RPM	41.8	41.8	56.7	32.8					
SCI	39.4	39.4	39.4						
SME	42.1	42.1	46.9	32.0	31.0				
SO	40.0	40.0	41.6	35.0	34.0				
SP	37.6	37.6	38.8	34.5	39.0				
TRS	48.5	48.5	51.3		45.7				
TS	50.7	50.2	52.4	32.1	50.1	59.5		69.0	
TSI	29.0	29.0		29.0					
TTS	33.0	33.0			33.0				
U	51.3	50.9	52.7	30.9	49.3	76.0	53.0	38.0	71.0
UCM	48.6	48.6	48.2		51.6				
UM	49.0	49.0	47.3		51.3				
UP	36.5	36.5	40.0	35.0	31.0				
US	48.8	48.8	49.4	47.4	47.4	63.6	43.7	43.5	36.0
VIR	41.3	41.3	41.5	34.9	44.8				
VM	47.6	46.8	51.0		42.5	51.0			
VN	33.8	33.8	35.0	30.0	40.0				
VS	46.2	46.2	48.0	34.7	44.4		48.0		41.0
Inactive	73.0								
Not Classified	41.7								
Address Unknown	56.0								

PYM Psychosomatic Medicine
PYN Psychiatry/Neurology
R Radiology
REN Reproductive Endocrinology And Infertility
RHU Rheumatology
RNR Neuroradiology
RO Radiation Oncology
RPM Pediatric Rehabilitation Medicine
SCI Spinal Cord Injury Medicine
SME Sleep Medicine
SO Surgical Oncology
SP Selective Pathology
TRS Traumatic Surgery
TS Thoracic Surgery
TSI Thoracic Surgery-Integrated
TTS Transplant Surgery
U Urology
UCM Urgent Care Medicine
UM Underseas Medicine (Preventive Medicine)
UP Pediatric Urology
US Unspecified
VIR Vascular And Interventional Radiology
VM Vascular Medicine
VN Vascular Neurology
VS Vascular Surgery

Table 5.6

DOs by Self-Designated Specialty and Activity (177 Specialties), 2010

		Patient Care				Other Professional Activity			
				Hospital Based					
Specialty	Total Physicians	Total Patient Care	Office Based	Resid./ Fellows	Phys. Staff	Admin.	Med. Teach.	Research	Other
Total Physicians	65,565	55,091	43,245	6,354	5,492	478	425	134	130
A	6	5	5			1			
ACA	21	21	10	7	4				
ADL	15	13	6	5	2	1	1		
ADM	23	19	15		4	2	1	1	
ADP	20	18	11	5	2	1	1		
AI	120	117	99	14	4	1	2		
ALI	1	1			1				
AM	80	64	34		30	10	1	2	3
AN	2,502	2,474	1,913	272	289	11	11	4	2
APM	104	104	93		11				
AR	8	8	3	3	2				
AS	3	3	1		2				
ATP	9	7	5		2	1	1		
BBK	10	10	6	2	2				
CCA	30	30	16	8	6				
CCM	85	82	53	15	14	1	1	1	
CCP	55	55	28	21	6				
CCS	39	38	20	13	5	1			
CD	784	767	617	100	50	2	6	8	1
CHN	35	33	19	13	1			2	
CHP	334	320	231	57	32	6	5	3	
CLP	3	2	1		1				1
CN	75	73	55	15	3	1	1		
CPP	3	3		3					
CRS	23	23	18	3	2				
CS	12	12	12						
D	550	545	421	98	26	1	1	2	1
DBP	10	10	3	6	1				
DIA	3	1	1				1	1	
DMP	14	13	10	1	2				1
DR	774	758	514	135	109	1	6		9
DS	5	4	4				1		
EFM	5	5	1		4				
EM	3,770	3,677	2,435	335	907	52	29	8	4
EMP	2	2		2					
END	138	135	107	22	6	1	1	1	
EP	2							2	
ESM	6	6	3		3				

A Allergy
ACA Adult Cardiothoracic Anesthesiology (Anesthesiology)
ADL Adolescent Medicine (Pediatrics)
ADM Addiction Medicine
ADP Addiction Psychiatry
AI Allergy And Immunology
ALI Clinical Laboratory Immunology (Allergy & Immunology)
AM Aerospace Medicine
AN Anesthesiology
APM Pain Medicine (Anesthesiology)
AR Abdominal Radiology
AS Abdominal Surgery
ATP Anatomic Pathology
BBK Blood Banking/Transfusion Medicine
CCA Critical Care Medicine (Anesthesiology)
CCM Critical Care Medicine (Internal Medicine)
CCP Pediatric Critical Care Medicine
CCS Surgical Critical Care (Surgery)
CD Cardiovascular Disease
CHN Child Neurology
CHP Child & Adolescent Psychiatry
CLP Clinical Pathology
CN Clinical Neurophysiology
CPP Pediatrics/Psychiatry/Child & Adolescent Psychiatry
CRS Colon And Rectal Surgery
CS Cosmetic Surgery
D Dermatology
DBP Developmental-Behavioral Pediatrics
DIA Diabetes
DMP Dermatopathology (Pathology)
DR Diagnostic Radiology
DS Dermatologic Surgery
EFM Emergency Medicine/Family Medicine
EM Emergency Medicine
EMP Pediatrics/Emergency Medicine
END Endocrinology, Diabetes & Metabolism
EP Epidemiology
ESM Sports Medicine (Emergency Medicine)

Table 5.6

DOs by Self-Designated Specialty and Activity (177 Specialties), 2010, continued

		Patient Care				Other Professional Activity			
				Hospital Based					
Specialty	Total Physicians	Total Patient Care	Office Based	Resid./ Fellows	Phys. Staff	Admin.	Med. Teach.	Research	Other
ETX	12	12	4	7	1				
FM	15,090	14,777	12,714	847	1,216	123	146	15	29
FOP	28	24	19	2	3	1			3
FPG	73	70	57	4	9	3			
FPP	10	10	6	4					
FPS	6	6	6						
FSM	178	175	139	29	7	1	2		
GE	468	461	372	61	28	2	2	3	
GO	13	13	10		3				
GP	2,709	2,672	2,421		251	26	11		
GPM	221	205	144	31	30	11	2	2	1
GS	975	964	699	149	116	3	8		
GYN	67	59	53		6	3	1	3	1
HEM	29	26	24	2				3	
HMP	17	17	11	6					
HNS	1	1			1				
HO	218	215	152	53	10	1		1	1
HOS	22	22	14		8				
HPM	14	14	4	10					
HS	38	38	36		2				
HSO	26	26	17	8	1				
IC	76	76	60	13	3				
ICE	40	37	27	7	3		2	1	
ID	227	216	153	40	23	3	2	6	
IEC	1	1			1				
IFP	7	7	5	2					
IG	3	2	2				1		
IM	5,525	5,429	4,264	620	545	39	37	12	8
IMD	1	1		1					
IMG	113	105	85	15	5	5	1	2	
IPM	1	1	1						
ISM	7	7	7						
LM	18	12	12			1			5
MDM	8					8			
MEM	10	10	2	8					
MFM	22	22	14		8				
MG	10	10	5	4	1				
MGP	1	1		1					

ETX Medical Toxicology (Emergency Medicine)
FM Family Medicine
FOP Forensic Pathology
FPG Geriatric Medicine (Family Medicine)
FPP Psychiatry/Family Medicine
FPS Facial Plastic Surgery
FSM Sports Medicine (Family Practice)
GE Gastroenterology
GO Gynecological Oncology
GP General Practice
GPM General Preventive Medicine
GS General Surgery
GYN Gynecology
HEM Hematology (Internal Medicine)
HMP Hematology (Pathology)
HNS Head And Neck Surgery
HO Hematology/Oncology
HOS Hospitalist
HPM Hospice & Palliative Medicine
HS Hand Surgery
HSO Hand Surgery (Orthopedics)
IC Interventional Cardiology
ICE Clinical Cardiac Electrophysiology
ID Infectious Disease
IEC Internal Medicine/Emergency Medicine/Critical Care Medicine
IFP Internal Medicine/Family Practice
IG Immunology
IM Internal Medicine
IMD Internal Medicine/Dermatology
IMG Geriatric Medicine (Internal Medicine)
IPM Internal Medicine/Preventive Medicine
ISM Sports Medicine (Internal Medicine)
LM Legal Medicine
MDM Medical Management
MEM Internal Medicine/Emergency Medicine
MFM Maternal And Fetal Medicine
MG Medical Genetics
MGP Molecular Genetic Pathology (Pathology And Medical Genetics)

Table 5.6

DOs by Self-Designated Specialty and Activity (177 Specialties), 2010, continued

		Patient Care				Other Professional Activity			
				Hospital Based					
Specialty	Total Physicians	Total Patient Care	Office Based	Resid./ Fellows	Phys. Staff	Admin.	Med. Teach.	Research	Other
MM	3	3	2		1				
MP	7	7		6	1				
MPD	220	217	143	65	9	2	1		
MSR	8	8	3	4	1				
N	618	603	458	97	48	2	5	5	3
NEP	347	340	284	38	18	4	1	2	
NM	49	45	30	3	12	1	1	1	1
NMN	6	6	5	1					
NMP	1	1	1						
NO	1						1		
NP	3	2	2						1
NPM	146	142	90	32	20	1	3		
NR	10	10	9		1				
NRN	1	1	1						
NS	83	83	68	4	11				
NSP	2	2	1		1				
NTR	3	2	2				1		
OAR	20	20	17	2	1				
OBG	2,234	2,213	1,781	256	176	8	10		3
OBS	8	7	6		1		1		
OCC	3	3	3						
OFA	5	5	5						
OM	228	189	149		40	29	5	1	4
OMM	213	199	189		10	2	11	1	
OMO	2	2	2						
ON	122	116	99	4	13	1		4	1
OP	17	17	13	2	2				
OPH	404	400	368	9	23		3	1	
ORS	927	912	776	32	104	3	7	1	4
OS	188	155	124	9	22	17	14	1	1
OSM	70	70	61	7	2				
OSS	33	33	32	1					
OTO	369	368	336	5	27		1		
OTR	12	12	9	1	2				
P	1,463	1,423	976	251	196	22	9	5	4
PA	2						1	1	
PAN	56	55	36	10	9		1		
PCC	282	279	185	80	14	1	1	1	

MM Medical Microbiology
MP Internal Med/Psychiatry
MPD Internal Medicine/Pediatrics
MSR Musculoskeletal Radiology
N Neurology
NEP Nephrology
NM Nuclear Medicine
NMN Neuromuscular Medicine (Neurology)
NMP Neonatal Perinatal Medicine
NO Neurotology (Otolaryngology)
NP Neuropathology
NPM Neonatal-Perinatal Medicine
NR Nuclear Radiology
NRN Neurology/Diagnostic Radiology/Neuroradiology
NS Neurological Surgery
NSP Pediatric Surgery (Neurology)
NTR Nutrition
OAR Adult Reconstructive Orthopedics
OBG Obstetrics & Gynecology
OBS Obstetrics
OCC Critical Care Medicine (Obstetrics & Gynecology)
OFA Foot And Ankle Orthopedics
OM Occupational Medicine
OMM Osteopathic Manipulative Medicine
OMO Musculoskeletal Oncology
ON Medical Oncology
OP Pediatric Orthopedics
OPH Ophthalmology
ORS Orthopedic Surgery
OS Other Specialty
OSM Sports Medicine (Orthopedic Surgery)
OSS Orthopedic Surgery Of The Spine
OTO Otolaryngology
OTR Orthopedic Trauma
P Psychiatry
PA Clinical Pharmacology
PAN Pediatric Anesthesiology (Anesthesiology)
PCC Pulmonary & Critical Care Medicine

Table 5.6

DOs by Self-Designated Specialty and Activity (177 Specialties), 2010, continued

		Patient Care				Other Professional Activity			
				Hospital Based					
Specialty	Total Physicians	Total Patient Care	Office Based	Resid./ Fellows	Phys. Staff	Admin.	Med. Teach.	Research	Other
PCH	2	1	1						1
PCP	25	25	14	8	3				
PD	2,219	2,175	1,699	306	170	9	24	4	7
PDA	3	3	1		2				
PDC	33	33	14	17	2				
PDE	20	19	6	12	1			1	
PDI	14	13	4	7	2			1	
PDO	7	5	5				2		
PDP	20	19	8	9	2			1	
PDR	27	25	20	1	4				2
PDS	2	2	1	1					
PE	10	10	4	6					
PEM	40	39	9	22	8			1	
PFP	21	20	14	4	2	1			
PG	36	36	16	16	4				
PHL	5	5	5						
PHM	4	1			1			3	
PHO	36	35	14	19	2			1	
PHP	37	19	13		6	12	1	2	3
PLM	14	12	11		1	1	1		
PM	1,102	1,086	835	177	74	7	6	1	2
PME	61	61	58		3				
PMM	133	133	88	39	6				
PMP	3	3	3						
PN	9	8	4	2	2		1		
PO	4	4	4						
PP	5	5	4	1					
PPM	1	1		1					
PPR	4	4		4					
PRO	9	9	9						
PRS	5	5	4		1				
PS	83	80	68	7	5	1		2	
PSM	10	10	6	4					
PTH	344	322	172	94	56	8	6	2	6
PTX	1	1	1						
PUD	215	207	186	2	19	1	4	3	
PYA	1	1	1						
PYG	21	20	11	5	4		1		

PCH Chemical Pathology
PCP Cytopathology
PD Pediatrics
PDA Pediatric Allergy
PDC Pediatric Cardiology
PDE Pediatric Endocrinology
PDI Pediatric Infectious Disease
PDO Pediatric Otolaryngology
PDP Pediatric Pulmonology
PDR Pediatric Radiology
PDS Pediatric Surgery (Surgery)
PE Pediatric Emergency Med (Emergency Med)
PEM Pediatric Emergency Medicine (Pediatrics)
PFP Forensic Psychiatry
PG Pediatric Gastroenterology
PHL Phlebology
PHM Pharmaceutical Medicine
PHO Pediatric Hematology/Oncology
PHP Public Health And General Preventive Medicine
PLM Palliative Medicine
PM Physical Medicine And Rehabilitation
PME Pain Management
PMM Pain Medicine
PMP Pain Medicine (Physical Medicine & Rehabilitation)
PN Pediatric Nephrology
PO Pediatric Opthalmology
PP Pediatric Pathology
PPM Pediatrics/Physical Medicine And Rehabilitation
PPR Pediatric Rheumatology
PRO Proctology
PRS Sports Medicine (Physical Medicine & Rehabilitation)
PS Plastic Surgery
PSM Sports Medicine (Pediatrics)
PTH Anatomic/Clinical Pathology
PTX Medical Toxicology (Preventive Medicine)
PUD Pulmonary Disease
PYA Psychoanalysis
PYG Geriatric Psychiatry

Table 5.6

DOs by Self-Designated Specialty and Activity (177 Specialties), 2010, continued

		Patient Care				Other Professional Activity			
				Hospital Based					
Specialty	Total Physicians	Total Patient Care	Office Based	Resid./ Fellows	Phys. Staff	Admin.	Med. Teach.	Research	Other
PYM	5	5	3	2					
PYN	3	3	1	1	1				
R	252	241	185	1	55	5	4		2
REN	11	11	10		1				
RHU	231	226	181	28	17	2	1	1	1
RNR	93	92	74	11	7				1
RO	78	76	59	5	12	1	1		
RPM	8	8	3	5					
SCI	8	8	8						
SME	28	28	19	8	1				
SO	9	9	7	1	1				
SP	14	14	9	4	1				
TRS	12	12	6		6				
TS	75	72	58	7	7	2		1	
TSI	1	1		1					
TTS	1	1			1				
U	208	202	170	14	18	1	1	1	3
UCM	41	41	36		5				
UM	7	7	4		3				
UP	4	4	2	1	1				
US	6,297	6,268	4,412	1,484	372	9	9	2	9
VIR	49	49	31	7	11				
VM	5	4	2		2	1			
VN	4	4	1	2	1				
VS	98	96	76	10	10		1		1
Inactive	3,999								
Not Classified	5,307								
Address Unknown	1								

PYM Psychosomatic Medicine
PYN Psychiatry/Neurology
R Radiology
REN Reproductive Endocrinology And Infertility
RHU Rheumatology
RNR Neuroradiology
RO Radiation Oncology
RPM Pediatric Rehabilitation Medicine
SCI Spinal Cord Injury Medicine
SME Sleep Medicine
SO Surgical Oncology
SP Selective Pathology
TRS Traumatic Surgery
TS Thoracic Surgery
TSI Thoracic Surgery-Integrated
TTS Transplant Surgery
U Urology
UCM Urgent Care Medicine
UM Underseas Medicine (Preventive Medicine)
UP Pediatric Urology
US Unspecified
VIR Vascular And Interventional Radiology
VM Vascular Medicine
VN Vascular Neurology
VS Vascular Surgery

Table 5.7

DOs by Self-Designated Specialty and Activity, 2010

Specialty	Total Physicians	Patient Care				Other Professional Activity			
				Hospital Based					
		Total Patient Care	Office Based	Resid./ Fellows	Phys. Staff	Admin.	Med. Teach.	Research	Other
Total Physicians	65,565	55,091	43,245	6,354	5,492	478	425	134	130
FM/GP	18,050	17,694	15,331	880	1,483	153	159	15	29
Family Medicine	15,341	15,022	12,910	880	1,232	127	148	15	29
General Practice	2,709	2,672	2,421		251	26	11		
Medical Specialties	12,572	12,316	9,493	1,774	1,049	79	96	61	20
Allergy and Immunology	130	125	106	14	5	2	3		
Cardiovascular Disease	784	767	617	100	50	2	6	8	1
Dermatology	550	545	421	98	26	1	1	2	1
Gastroenterology	468	461	372	61	28	2	2	3	
Internal Medicine	7,186	7,035	5,513	857	665	57	48	35	11
Pediatric Cardiology	33	33	14	17	2				
Pediatrics	2,924	2,864	2,079	545	240	13	31	9	7
Pulmonary Disease	497	486	371	82	33	2	5	4	
Surgical Specialties	6,156	6,062	4,973	534	555	24	48	10	12
Colon and Rectal Surgery	32	32	27	3	2				
General Surgery	1,182	1,167	850	174	143	4	10		1
Neurological Surgery	85	85	69	4	12				
Obstetrics & Gynecology	2,358	2,328	1,877	256	195	11	12	3	4
Ophthalmology	408	404	372	9	23		3	1	
Orthopedic Surgery	1,325	1,296	1,121	53	122	5	18	2	4
Otolaryngology	377	373	341	5	27		4		
Plastic Surgery	101	98	86	7	5	1		2	
Thoracic Surgery	76	73	58	8	7	2		1	
Urology	212	206	172	15	19	1	1	1	3
Other Specialties	19,480	19,019	13,448	3,166	2,405	222	122	48	69
Aerospace Medicine	80	64	34		30	10	1	2	3
Anatomic/Clinical Pathology	450	422	237	117	68	9	7	2	10
Anesthesiology	2,718	2,690	2,090	287	313	11	11	4	2
Child & Adolescent Psychiatry	334	320	231	57	32	6	5	3	
Diagnostic Radiology	774	758	514	135	109	1	6		9
Emergency Medicine	3,839	3,746	2,482	348	916	52	29	8	4
Forensic Pathology	28	24	19	2	3	1			3
General Preventive Medicine	229	213	149	31	33	11	2	2	1
Medical Genetics	10	10	5	4	1				
Neurology	732	713	533	127	53	3	6	7	3
Nuclear Medicine	49	45	30	3	12	1	1	1	1
Occupational Medicine	228	189	149		40	29	5	1	4
Other Specialty	349	289	207	46	36	29	17	8	6
Physical Medicine and Rehabilitation	1,255	1,239	941	217	81	7	6	1	2
Psychiatry	1,531	1,487	1,016	267	204	24	11	5	4
Public Health and General Preventive Medicine	37	19	13		6	12	1	2	3
Radiation Oncology	78	76	59	5	12	1	1		
Radiology	447	433	325	27	81	5	4		5
Transplant Surgery	1	1			1				
Unspecified	6,306	6,277	4,412	1,493	372	9	9	2	9
Vascular Medicine	5	4	2		2	1			
Inactive	3,999								
Not Classified	5,307								
Address Unknown	1								

Subspecialties in this table are condensed into major specialties. See Appendix A.

Table 5.8

Male DOs by Self-Designated Specialty and Activity, 2010

Specialty	Total Physicians	Patient Care: Total Patient Care	Patient Care: Office Based	Patient Care: Hospital Based: Resid./Fellows	Patient Care: Hospital Based: Phys. Staff	Other Professional Activity: Admin.	Other Professional Activity: Med. Teach.	Other Professional Activity: Research	Other Professional Activity: Other
Total Physicians	46,113	38,526	31,042	3,354	4,130	397	312	102	94
FM/GP	12,633	12,365	10,865	373	1,127	131	107	10	20
Family Medicine	10,358	10,122	8,823	373	926	108	98	10	20
General Practice	2,275	2,243	2,042		201	23	9		
Medical Specialties	8,061	7,869	6,354	823	692	64	67	46	15
Allergy and Immunology	95	90	81	8	1	2	3		
Cardiovascular Disease	667	652	539	72	41	2	4	8	1
Dermatology	356	352	300	35	17	1	1	1	1
Gastroenterology	405	398	338	36	24	2	2	3	
Internal Medicine	4,903	4,787	3,877	455	455	46	35	26	9
Pediatric Cardiology	19	19	10	9					
Pediatrics	1,220	1,184	895	162	127	11	17	4	4
Pulmonary Disease	396	387	314	46	27		5	4	
Surgical Specialties	4,561	4,485	3,783	249	453	21	40	6	9
Colon and Rectal Surgery	27	27	24	1	2				
General Surgery	973	959	726	108	125	4	9		1
Neurological Surgery	81	81	66	4	11				
Obstetrics & Gynecology	1,228	1,207	1,019	58	130	9	9	1	2
Ophthalmology	354	352	323	7	22		2		
Orthopedic Surgery	1,207	1,184	1,025	44	115	4	15	1	3
Otolaryngology	339	335	310	3	22		4		
Plastic Surgery	89	86	75	7	4	1		2	
Thoracic Surgery	71	68	55	6	7	2		1	
Urology	192	186	160	11	15	1	1	1	3
Other Specialties	14,176	13,807	10,040	1,909	1,858	181	98	40	50
Aerospace Medicine	76	62	32		30	8	1	2	3
Anatomic/Clinical Pathology	307	284	170	62	52	9	7		7
Anesthesiology	2,205	2,178	1,721	201	256	10	11	4	2
Child & Adolescent Psychiatry	188	178	130	29	19	4	4	2	
Diagnostic Radiology	604	589	406	95	88	1	5		9
Emergency Medicine	3,012	2,932	1,966	240	726	47	23	7	3
Forensic Pathology	21	17	14	1	2	1			3
General Preventive Medicine	156	143	105	16	22	9	1	2	1
Medical Genetics	5	5	3	1	1				
Neurology	492	475	386	62	27	3	5	7	2
Nuclear Medicine	40	37	23	2	12	1	1	1	
Occupational Medicine	184	157	124		33	22	4		1
Other Specialty	251	205	153	24	28	23	10	7	6
Physical Medicine and Rehabilitation	920	909	699	154	56	5	4	1	1
Psychiatry	956	923	660	123	140	17	10	4	2
Public Health and General Preventive Medicine	21	11	9		2	8		1	1
Radiation Oncology	63	61	48	3	10	1	1		
Radiology	384	371	276	21	74	4	4		5
Transplant Surgery	1	1			1				
Unspecified	4,285	4,265	3,113	875	277	7	7	2	4
Vascular Medicine	5	4	2		2	1			
Inactive	3,516								
Not Classified	3,165								
Address Unknown	1								

Subspecialties in this table are condensed into major specialties. See Appendix A.

Table 5.9

Female DOs by Self-Designated Specialty and Activity, 2010

		Patient Care				Other Professional Activity			
				Hospital Based					
Specialty	Total Physicians	Total Patient Care	Office Based	Resid./ Fellows	Phys. Staff	Admin.	Med. Teach.	Research	Other
Total Physicians	19,452	16,565	12,203	3,000	1,362	81	113	32	36
FM/GP	5,417	5,329	4,466	507	356	22	52	5	9
Family Medicine	4,983	4,900	4,087	507	306	19	50	5	9
General Practice	434	429	379		50	3	2		
Medical Specialties	4,511	4,447	3,139	951	357	15	29	15	5
Allergy and Immunology	35	35	25	6	4				
Cardiovascular Disease	117	115	78	28	9		2		
Dermatology	194	193	121	63	9			1	
Gastroenterology	63	63	34	25	4				
Internal Medicine	2,283	2,248	1,636	402	210	11	13	9	2
Pediatric Cardiology	14	14	4	8	2				
Pediatrics	1,704	1,680	1,184	383	113	2	14	5	3
Pulmonary Disease	101	99	57	36	6	2			
Surgical Specialties	1,595	1,577	1,190	285	102	3	8	4	3
Colon and Rectal Surgery	5	5	3	2					
General Surgery	209	208	124	66	18		1		
Neurological Surgery	4	4	3		1				
Obstetrics & Gynecology	1,130	1,121	858	198	65	2	3	2	2
Ophthalmology	54	52	49	2	1		1	1	
Orthopedic Surgery	118	112	96	9	7	1	3	1	1
Otolaryngology	38	38	31	2	5				
Plastic Surgery	12	12	11		1				
Thoracic Surgery	5	5	3	2					
Urology	20	20	12	4	4				
Other Specialties	5,304	5,212	3,408	1,257	547	41	24	8	19
Aerospace Medicine	4	2	2			2			
Anatomic/Clinical Pathology	143	138	67	55	16			2	3
Anesthesiology	513	512	369	86	57	1			
Child & Adolescent Psychiatry	146	142	101	28	13	2	1	1	
Diagnostic Radiology	170	169	108	40	21		1		
Emergency Medicine	827	814	516	108	190	5	6	1	1
Forensic Pathology	7	7	5	1	1				
General Preventive Medicine	73	70	44	15	11	2	1		
Medical Genetics	5	5	2	3					
Neurology	240	238	147	65	26		1		1
Nuclear Medicine	9	8	7	1					1
Occupational Medicine	44	32	25		7	7	1	1	3
Other Specialty	98	84	54	22	8	6	7	1	
Physical Medicine and Rehabilitation	335	330	242	63	25	2	2		1
Psychiatry	575	564	356	144	64	7	1	1	2
Public Health and General Preventive Medicine	16	8	4		4	4	1	1	2
Radiation Oncology	15	15	11	2	2				
Radiology	63	62	49	6	7	1			
Unspecified	2,021	2,012	1,299	618	95	2	2		5
Inactive	483								
Not Classified	2,142								

Subspecialties in this table are condensed into major specialties. See Appendix A.

Table 5.10

DOs by Race/Ethnicity, 2010

Specialty	Total Physicians	White	Black	Hispanic	Asian	Other	American Indian/ Alaskan Native	Unknown
Total Physicians	65,565	22,044	479	805	2,161	247	46	39,783
Aerospace Medicine	80	31				1		48
Allergy/Immunology	130	70	1	1	11			47
Anesthesiology	2,718	1,228	17	30	125	16		1,302
Cardiovascular Disease	784	450	6	4	40	6		278
Child Psychiatry	334	201	9	9	29		2	84
Colon/Rectal Surgery	32	19						13
Dermatology	550	159	2	5	8	3		373
Diagnostic Radiology	774	348	9	9	28	4		376
Emergency Medicine	3,839	1,514	19	37	78	16	3	2,172
Family Medicine	15,341	5,674	103	199	468	64	15	8,818
Forensic Pathology	28	21	1					6
Gastroenterology	468	257	4	6	37	6		158
General Practice	2,709	540	5	12	11	4	1	2,136
General Preventive Medicine	229	115	5		11	1	1	96
General Surgery	1,182	374	10	11	26	2		759
Internal Medicine	7,186	2,902	83	126	461	51	5	3,558
Medical Genetics	10	6	1					3
Neurological Surgery	85	27		1	1			56
Neurology	732	376	8	10	48	3	1	286
Nuclear Medicine	49	20			3			26
Obstetrics/Gynecology	2,358	958	32	37	59	6		1,266
Occupational Medicine	228	113	2		5	2		106
Ophthalmology	408	175		4	9	3		217
Orthopedic Surgery	1,325	361	1	3	8	1		951
Otolaryngology	377	135		1	1	1		239
Pathology-Anatomic/Clinical	450	237	2	4	12	1	1	193
Pediatric Cardiology	33	22			3			8
Pediatrics	2,924	1,297	39	101	150	12	3	1,322
Physical Medicine & Rehabilitation	1,255	558	13	21	78	6	3	576
Plastic Surgery	101	45		2	4	1		49
Psychiatry	1,531	804	26	31	73	9	1	587
Public Health & General Preventive Medicine	37	20	1		2			14
Pulmonary Diseases	497	278	1	9	34	2		173
Radiation Oncology	78	41			4	1	1	31
Radiology	447	175	2	5	23	4	1	237
Thoracic Surgery	76	37		2	1			36
Transplant Surgery	1							1
Urological Surgery	212	78	1	4	4	1		124
Vascular Medicine	5	3						2
Other Specialty	349	146	1	1	10	2	2	187
Unspecified	6,306	75	7	6	8			6,210
Inactive	3,999	1,412	16	16	22	4	1	2,528
Not Classified	5,307	742	52	98	266	14	5	4,130
Address Unknown	1							1

Table 5.11

Male DOs by Race/Ethnicity, 2010

Specialty	Total Physicians	White	Black	Hispanic	Asian	Other	American Indian/ Alaskan Native	Unknown
Total Physicians	46,113	15,910	250	483	1,345	174	30	27,921
Aerospace Medicine	76	30				1		45
Allergy/Immunology	95	51			8			36
Anesthesiology	2,205	980	11	24	100	11		1,079
Cardiovascular Disease	667	385	3	4	33	4		238
Child Psychiatry	188	120	4	3	12		1	48
Colon/Rectal Surgery	27	16						11
Dermatology	356	137	2	1	4	3		209
Diagnostic Radiology	604	278	7	7	14	3		295
Emergency Medicine	3,012	1,207	16	32	53	12	3	1,689
Family Medicine	10,358	3,925	38	121	283	44	11	5,936
Forensic Pathology	21	16	1					4
Gastroenterology	405	226	4	5	29	4		137
General Practice	2,275	446	4	10	8	3	1	1,803
General Preventive Medicine	156	74	2		9	1	1	69
General Surgery	973	315	6	9	21	2		620
Internal Medicine	4,903	2,041	54	79	291	35	5	2,398
Medical Genetics	5	3						2
Neurological Surgery	81	26		1	1			53
Neurology	492	265	4	8	31	3		181
Nuclear Medicine	40	17			2			21
Obstetrics/Gynecology	1,228	569	16	18	31	4		590
Occupational Medicine	184	94	1		4	2		83
Ophthalmology	354	157		2	8	2		185
Orthopedic Surgery	1,207	330	1	2	8	1		865
Otolaryngology	339	127		1	1	1		209
Pathology-Anatomic/Clinical	307	173		1	7		1	125
Pediatric Cardiology	19	10			3			6
Pediatrics	1,220	573	14	39	46	5	1	542
Physical Medicine & Rehabilitation	920	428	9	14	53	5	2	409
Plastic Surgery	89	41		2	4			42
Psychiatry	956	522	11	12	39	9		363
Public Health & General Preventive Medicine	21	13						8
Pulmonary Diseases	396	231		6	20	1		138
Radiation Oncology	63	33			3	1	1	25
Radiology	384	149	1	4	18	3		209
Thoracic Surgery	71	34		2	1			34
Transplant Surgery	1							1
Urological Surgery	192	73	1	4	2	1		111
Vascular Medicine	5	3						2
Other Specialty	251	106		1	3			141
Unspecified	4,285	60	4	5	6			4,210
Inactive	3,516	1,217	14	11	15	4		2,255
Not Classified	3,165	409	22	55	174	9	3	2,493
Address Unknown	1							1

Table 5.12

Female DOs by Race/Ethnicity, 2010

Specialty	Total Physicians	White	Black	Hispanic	Asian	Other	American Indian/ Alaskan Native	Unknown
Total Physicians	19,452	6,134	229	322	816	73	16	11,862
Aerospace Medicine	4	1						3
Allergy/Immunology	35	19	1	1	3			11
Anesthesiology	513	248	6	6	25	5		223
Cardiovascular Disease	117	65	3		7	2		40
Child Psychiatry	146	81	5	6	17		1	36
Colon/Rectal Surgery	5	3						2
Dermatology	194	22		4	4			164
Diagnostic Radiology	170	70	2	2	14	1		81
Emergency Medicine	827	307	3	5	25	4		483
Family Medicine	4,983	1,749	65	78	185	20	4	2,882
Forensic Pathology	7	5						2
Gastroenterology	63	31		1	8	2		21
General Practice	434	94	1	2	3	1		333
General Preventive Medicine	73	41	3		2			27
General Surgery	209	59	4	2	5			139
Internal Medicine	2,283	861	29	47	170	16		1,160
Medical Genetics	5	3	1					1
Neurological Surgery	4	1						3
Neurology	240	111	4	2	17		1	105
Nuclear Medicine	9	3			1			5
Obstetrics/Gynecology	1,130	389	16	19	28	2		676
Occupational Medicine	44	19	1		1			23
Ophthalmology	54	18		2	1	1		32
Orthopedic Surgery	118	31		1				86
Otolaryngology	38	8						30
Pathology-Anatomic/Clinical	143	64	2	3	5	1		68
Pediatric Cardiology	14	12						2
Pediatrics	1,704	724	25	62	104	7	2	780
Physical Medicine & Rehabilitation	335	130	4	7	25	1	1	167
Plastic Surgery	12	4				1		7
Psychiatry	575	282	15	19	34		1	224
Public Health & General Preventive Medicine	16	7	1		2			6
Pulmonary Diseases	101	47	1	3	14	1		35
Radiation Oncology	15	8			1			6
Radiology	63	26	1	1	5	1	1	28
Thoracic Surgery	5	3						2
Urological Surgery	20	5			2			13
Other Specialty	98	40	1		7	2	2	46
Unspecified	2,021	15	3	1	2			2,000
Inactive	483	195	2	5	7		1	273
Not Classified	2,142	333	30	43	92	5	2	1,637

Table 5.13

DOs by Age and State of Location, 2010

State	Total Physicians	< 35	35-44	45-54	55-64	≥ 65
Total Physicians	65,565	12,578	18,693	15,712	10,621	7,961
Alabama	438	74	120	138	84	22
Alaska	167	20	38	54	42	13
Arizona	1,962	252	554	433	358	365
Arkansas	289	41	81	82	62	23
California	4,207	900	1,540	917	573	277
Colorado	1,192	156	360	291	240	145
Connecticut	477	125	184	119	29	20
Delaware	308	65	86	78	47	32
District Of Columbia	120	52	35	25	4	4
Florida	4,708	589	1,273	1,193	760	893
Georgia	947	142	295	245	177	88
Hawaii	221	40	76	52	39	14
Idaho	289	34	114	76	50	15
Illinois	2,560	671	808	602	321	158
Indiana	952	164	239	283	170	96
Iowa	1,289	255	311	292	291	140
Kansas	763	171	170	187	156	79
Kentucky	542	178	155	114	62	33
Louisiana	180	66	45	35	25	9
Maine	738	116	192	221	140	69
Maryland	741	159	291	173	76	42
Massachusetts	794	228	272	177	75	42
Michigan	5,629	876	1,232	1,336	991	1,194
Minnesota	578	155	172	141	79	31
Mississippi	362	79	107	90	66	20
Missouri	2,228	428	441	517	506	336
Montana	159	18	43	50	41	7
Nebraska	197	61	63	34	26	13
Nevada	608	88	171	161	100	88
New Hampshire	275	40	107	89	29	10
New Jersey	3,015	445	902	850	425	393
New Mexico	311	32	72	68	80	59
New York	3,501	785	1,234	913	309	260
North Carolina	949	247	380	189	83	50
North Dakota	67	13	18	21	12	3
Ohio	4,644	1,036	1,135	1,002	758	713
Oklahoma	1,736	246	451	435	395	209
Oregon	748	118	213	173	165	79
Pennsylvania	6,417	1,266	1,672	1,567	1,005	907
Rhode Island	247	53	57	78	40	19
South Carolina	534	144	174	125	62	29
South Dakota	146	29	45	37	22	13
Tennessee	700	136	213	167	123	61
Texas	4,158	865	1,138	851	803	501
Utah	359	79	157	72	36	15
Vermont	77	8	20	24	14	11
Virginia	1,006	232	320	253	130	71
Washington	1,035	194	282	219	225	115
West Virginia	768	147	207	201	149	64
Wisconsin	940	206	301	201	139	93
Wyoming	98	12	34	29	15	8
Possessions	18	3	5	4	4	2
APO's and FPO's	170	39	88	28	7	8
Address Unknown	1				1	

Table 5.14

Male DOs by Age and State of Location, 2010

State	Total Physicians	< 35	35-44	45-54	55-64	≥ 65
Total Physicians	46,113	6,552	12,241	11,391	8,858	7,071
Alabama	343	43	90	114	76	20
Alaska	109	10	21	33	34	11
Arizona	1,471	129	387	316	305	334
Arkansas	222	23	61	65	56	17
California	2,769	462	974	645	455	233
Colorado	848	75	220	205	214	134
Connecticut	297	55	119	88	17	18
Delaware	208	28	51	58	41	30
District Of Columbia	70	25	21	17	3	4
Florida	3,525	311	858	888	648	820
Georgia	680	78	191	177	153	81
Hawaii	153	25	59	30	28	11
Idaho	237	22	99	61	42	13
Illinois	1,649	322	513	422	258	134
Indiana	705	93	168	203	152	89
Iowa	921	136	205	214	241	125
Kansas	544	88	112	144	133	67
Kentucky	377	103	112	87	49	26
Louisiana	119	37	31	23	21	7
Maine	468	49	104	145	108	62
Maryland	466	97	172	111	52	34
Massachusetts	502	99	177	121	67	38
Michigan	4,116	492	810	953	804	1,057
Minnesota	365	74	111	98	56	26
Mississippi	275	47	76	72	62	18
Missouri	1,675	221	311	398	435	310
Montana	120	10	31	41	34	4
Nebraska	140	41	43	25	21	10
Nevada	464	57	126	122	88	71
New Hampshire	171	18	66	58	22	7
New Jersey	2,120	228	554	597	369	372
New Mexico	219	16	40	46	66	51
New York	2,155	395	732	585	227	216
North Carolina	649	133	273	135	68	40
North Dakota	49	5	11	19	11	3
Ohio	3,363	547	735	803	667	611
Oklahoma	1,268	140	310	311	316	191
Oregon 504	54	137	110	135	68	
Pennsylvania	4,523	629	1,067	1,152	855	820
Rhode Island	170	24	33	59	36	18
South Carolina	362	77	121	90	49	25
South Dakota	104	22	27	27	20	8
Tennessee	508	66	157	135	100	50
Texas	2,964	457	751	630	670	456
Utah	300	56	141	59	31	13
Vermont	53	3	10	19	10	11
Virginia 669	115	215	186	102	51	
Washington	741	115	194	144	181	107
West Virginia	532	64	136	153	129	50
Wisconsin	636	97	185	150	119	85
Wyoming	74	7	25	22	12	8
Possessions	15	3	4	3	3	2
APO's and FPO's	125	29	64	22	6	4
Address Unknown	1				1	

Table 5.15

Female DOs by Age and State of Location, 2010

State	Total Physicians	< 35	35-44	45-54	55-64	≥ 65
Total Physicians	19,452	6,026	6,452	4,321	1,763	890
Alabama	95	31	30	24	8	2
Alaska	58	10	17	21	8	2
Arizona	491	123	167	117	53	31
Arkansas	67	18	20	17	6	6
California	1,438	438	566	272	118	44
Colorado	344	81	140	86	26	11
Connecticut	180	70	65	31	12	2
Delaware	100	37	35	20	6	2
District Of Columbia	50	27	14	8	1	
Florida	1,183	278	415	305	112	73
Georgia	267	64	104	68	24	7
Hawaii	68	15	17	22	11	3
Idaho	52	12	15	15	8	2
Illinois	911	349	295	180	63	24
Indiana	247	71	71	80	18	7
Iowa	368	119	106	78	50	15
Kansas	219	83	58	43	23	12
Kentucky	165	75	43	27	13	7
Louisiana	61	29	14	12	4	2
Maine	270	67	88	76	32	7
Maryland	275	62	119	62	24	8
Massachusetts	292	129	95	56	8	4
Michigan	1,513	384	422	383	187	137
Minnesota	213	81	61	43	23	5
Mississippi	87	32	31	18	4	2
Missouri	553	207	130	119	71	26
Montana	39	8	12	9	7	3
Nebraska	57	20	20	9	5	3
Nevada	144	31	45	39	12	17
New Hampshire	104	22	41	31	7	3
New Jersey	895	217	348	253	56	21
New Mexico	92	16	32	22	14	8
New York	1,346	390	502	328	82	44
North Carolina	300	114	107	54	15	10
North Dakota	18	8	7	2	1	
Ohio	1,281	489	400	199	91	102
Oklahoma	468	106	141	124	79	18
Oregon	244	64	76	63	30	11
Pennsylvania	1,894	637	605	415	150	87
Rhode Island	77	29	24	19	4	1
South Carolina	172	67	53	35	13	4
South Dakota	42	7	18	10	2	5
Tennessee	192	70	56	32	23	11
Texas	1,194	408	387	221	133	45
Utah	59	23	16	13	5	2
Vermont	24	5	10	5	4	
Virginia	337	117	105	67	28	20
Washington	294	79	88	75	44	8
West Virginia	236	83	71	48	20	14
Wisconsin	304	109	116	51	20	8
Wyoming	24	5	9	7	3	
Possessions	3		1	1	1	
APO's and FPO's	45	10	24	6	1	4

Table 5.16

DOs by State of Location and Major Professional Activity, 2010

		Patient Care				Other Professional Activity			
				Hospital Based					
State	Total Physicians	Total Patient Care	Office Based	Resid./ Fellows	Phys. Staff	Admin.	Med. Teach.	Research	Other*
Total Physicians	65,565	55,091	43,245	6,354	5,492	478	425	134	130
Alabama	438	388	316	46	26	1	6	1	
Alaska	167	149	113	5	31	2	1		2
Arizona	1,962	1,608	1,326	127	155	17	8	2	8
Arkansas	289	252	202	23	27	2			
California	4,207	3,591	2,914	397	280	27	20	4	12
Colorado	1,192	1,046	892	58	96	15	5	1	
Connecticut	477	400	315	51	34	2	3	1	1
Delaware	308	256	192	48	16	3			1
District Of Columbia	120	87	49	26	12	4		1	
Florida	4,708	3,849	3,211	285	353	37	35	9	9
Georgia	947	780	633	59	88	6	13	6	1
Hawaii	221	184	129	23	32	3	1		1
Idaho	289	261	229	8	24		1	1	1
Illinois	2,560	2,146	1,616	296	234	25	18	9	7
Indiana	952	844	663	81	100	6	6	4	
Iowa	1,289	1,155	907	134	114	9	5	1	2
Kansas	763	665	506	98	61	4	2	1	
Kentucky	542	450	315	86	49	5	4		
Louisiana	180	152	78	56	18		1		
Maine	738	634	470	76	88	4	4		
Maryland	741	598	434	79	85	11	2	4	4
Massachusetts	794	664	461	148	55	4	1	3	3
Michigan	5,629	4,637	3,701	464	472	44	40	7	12
Minnesota	578	528	373	91	64	4	1		
Mississippi	362	318	227	39	52	2	3		
Missouri	2,228	1,898	1,438	227	233	16	16	2	5
Montana	159	144	126	2	16				1
Nebraska	197	177	118	42	17	1	2		
Nevada	608	530	389	90	51	5	5		1
New Hampshire	275	243	195	12	36	3	1		1
New Jersey	3,015	2,508	2,169	144	195	16	20	15	10
New Mexico	311	260	208	18	34	3	1	1	
New York	3,501	2,858	2,243	348	267	29	24	5	10
North Carolina	949	813	586	108	119	5	3	4	1
North Dakota	67	60	46	4	10				
Ohio	4,644	3,785	2,787	721	277	22	42	10	5
Oklahoma	1,736	1,481	1,201	90	190	11	12	2	2
Oregon	748	641	525	56	60	4	5		2
Pennsylvania	6,417	5,234	4,149	578	507	48	47	24	14
Rhode Island	247	202	154	25	23	2		2	
South Carolina	534	468	336	70	62	4	3		
South Dakota	146	129	104	17	8	2			
Tennessee	700	604	466	70	68	7	8		
Texas	4,158	3,523	2,745	479	299	34	30	11	4
Utah	359	330	264	29	37				
Vermont	77	59	45	6	8		1	1	
Virginia1,006	882	603	136	143	10	10		4	
Washington	1,035	903	725	98	80	6	4		2
West Virginia	768	650	532	52	66	3	8		1
Wisconsin	940	838	663	110	65	6	1	2	2
Wyoming	98	82	59	9	14		2		
Possessions	18	12	9	1	2				
APO's and FPO's	170	135	88	8	39	4			1
Address Unknown	1								

** Includes Other, Inactive and Not Classified Physicians*

Table 5.17

Male DOs by State of Location and Major Professional Activity, 2010

		Patient Care				Other Professional Activity			
				Hospital Based					
State	Total Physicians	Total Patient Care	Office Based	Resid./ Fellows	Phys. Staff	Admin.	Med. Teach.	Research	Other*
Total Physicians	46,113	38,526	31,042	3,354	4,130	397	312	102	94
Alabama	343	308	258	26	24	1	5		
Alaska	109	97	75	3	19	1			2
Arizona	1,471	1,185	1,007	62	116	15	7	2	4
Arkansas	222	196	162	11	23	1			
California	2,769	2,356	1,949	202	205	22	12	3	8
Colorado	848	733	638	24	71	12	3	1	
Connecticut	297	253	205	24	24		2	1	1
Delaware	208	169	137	21	11	3			
District Of Columbia	70	46	27	10	9	2		1	
Florida	3,525	2,837	2,404	148	285	29	28	8	7
Georgia	680	554	455	34	65	5	12	3	1
Hawaii	153	125	85	15	25	3	1		1
Idaho	237	215	188	7	20		1	1	
Illinois	1,649	1,381	1,077	138	166	19	16	6	5
Indiana	705	624	498	52	74	4	3	4	
Iowa	921	815	655	71	89	6	4	1	2
Kansas	544	474	373	54	47	3	1		
Kentucky	377	311	218	52	41	4	2		
Louisiana	119	99	59	26	14		1		
Maine	468	401	296	37	68	3	2		
Maryland	466	378	271	51	56	8	2	2	3
Massachusetts	502	422	312	71	39	4		2	3
Michigan	4,116	3,339	2,740	254	345	41	29	6	7
Minnesota	365	327	236	44	47	4	1		
Mississippi	275	243	185	21	37	1	2		
Missouri	1,675	1,428	1,123	111	194	12	10	1	5
Montana	120	109	96	1	12				1
Nebraska	140	124	81	28	15	1	2		
Nevada	464	406	301	61	44	5	3		1
New Hampshire	171	151	119	6	26	1			1
New Jersey	2,120	1,761	1,548	80	133	14	13	12	6
New Mexico	219	186	151	11	24	3	1		
New York	2,155	1,747	1,407	166	174	20	16	5	5
North Carolina	649	564	416	67	81	5	2	3	1
North Dakota	49	45	37		8				
Ohio	3,363	2,709	2,071	412	226	20	34	10	5
Oklahoma	1,268	1,070	882	45	143	10	8	2	2
Oregon	504	423	357	26	40	3	3		2
Pennsylvania	4,523	3,686	3,002	301	383	40	35	15	11
Rhode Island	170	142	116	11	15	2		2	
South Carolina	362	315	233	37	45	3	2		
South Dakota	104	93	76	12	5	2			
Tennessee	508	440	358	30	52	6	6		
Texas	2,964	2,509	2,008	262	239	32	21	10	2
Utah	300	278	228	19	31				
Vermont	53	39	30	2	7			1	
Virginia	669	579	409	69	101	10	9		4
Washington	741	649	519	60	70	5	3		
West Virginia	532	453	379	22	52	3	8		1
Wisconsin	636	561	462	50	49	6			2
Wyoming	74	61	45	3	13		2		
Possessions	15	10	7	1	2				
APO's and FPO's	125	100	71	3	26	3			1
Address Unknown	1								

** Includes Other, Inactive and Not Classified Physicians*

Table 5.18

Female DOs by State of Location and Major Professional Activity, 2010

		Patient Care				Other Professional Activity			
				Hospital Based					
State	Total Physicians	Total Patient Care	Office Based	Resid./ Fellows	Phys. Staff	Admin.	Med. Teach.	Research	Other*
Total Physicians	19,452	16,565	12,203	3,000	1,362	81	113	32	36
Alabama	95	80	58	20	2		1	1	
Alaska	58	52	38	2	12	1	1		
Arizona	491	423	319	65	39	2	1		4
Arkansas	67	56	40	12	4	1			
California	1,438	1,235	965	195	75	5	8	1	4
Colorado	344	313	254	34	25	3	2		
Connecticut	180	147	110	27	10	2	1		
Delaware	100	87	55	27	5				1
District Of Columbia	50	41	22	16	3	2			
Florida	1,183	1,012	807	137	68	8	7	1	2
Georgia	267	226	178	25	23	1	1	3	
Hawaii	68	59	44	8	7				
Idaho	52	46	41	1	4				1
Illinois	911	765	539	158	68	6	2	3	2
Indiana	247	220	165	29	26	2	3		
Iowa	368	340	252	63	25	3	1		
Kansas	219	191	133	44	14	1	1	1	
Kentucky	165	139	97	34	8	1	2		
Louisiana	61	53	19	30	4				
Maine	270	233	174	39	20	1	2		
Maryland	275	220	163	28	29	3		2	1
Massachusetts	292	242	149	77	16		1	1	
Michigan	1,513	1,298	961	210	127	3	11	1	5
Minnesota	213	201	137	47	17				
Mississippi	87	75	42	18	15	1	1		
Missouri	553	470	315	116	39	4	6	1	
Montana	39	35	30	1	4				
Nebraska	57	53	37	14	2				
Nevada	144	124	88	29	7		2		
New Hampshire	104	92	76	6	10	2	1		
New Jersey	895	747	621	64	62	2	7	3	4
New Mexico	92	74	57	7	10			1	
New York	1,346	1,111	836	182	93	9	8		5
North Carolina	300	249	170	41	38		1	1	
North Dakota	18	15	9	4	2				
Ohio	1,281	1,076	716	309	51	2	8		
Oklahoma	468	411	319	45	47	1	4		
Oregon	244	218	168	30	20	1	2		
Pennsylvania	1,894	1,548	1,147	277	124	8	12	9	3
Rhode Island	77	60	38	14	8				
South Carolina	172	153	103	33	17	1	1		
South Dakota	42	36	28	5	3				
Tennessee	192	164	108	40	16	1	2		
Texas	1,194	1,014	737	217	60	2	9	1	2
Utah	59	52	36	10	6				
Vermont	24	20	15	4	1		1		
Virginia	337	303	194	67	42		1		
Washington	294	254	206	38	10	1	1		2
West Virginia	236	197	153	30	14				
Wisconsin	304	277	201	60	16		1	2	
Wyoming	24	21	14	6	1				
Possessions	3	2	2						
APO's and FPO's	45	35	17	5	13	1			

** Includes Other, Inactive and Not Classified Physicians*

Table 5.19

DOs by State, Self-Designated Specialty, and Activity, 2010
Alabama

		Patient Care				Other Professional Activity			
				Hospital Based					
Specialty	Total Physicians	Total Patient Care	Office Based	Resid./ Fellows	Phys. Staff	Admin.	Med. Teach.	Research	Other
Total Physicians	438	388	316	46	26	1	6	1	
FM/GP	148	145	124	12	9		3		
Family Medicine	134	131	111	12	8		3		
General Practice	14	14	13		1				
Medical Specialties	82	80	65	13	2		1	1	
Allergy and Immunology	2	2	2						
Cardiovascular Disease	6	6	5	1					
Dermatology	2	2	2						
Gastroenterology	4	4	3	1					
Internal Medicine	54	52	42	8	2		1	1	
Pediatrics	13	13	11	2					
Pulmonary Disease	1	1		1					
Surgical Specialties	39	39	32	5	2				
General Surgery	11	11	8	2	1				
Obstetrics & Gynecology	12	12	10	2					
Ophthalmology	5	5	5						
Orthopedic Surgery	5	5	5						
Otolaryngology	4	4	2	1	1				
Urology	2	2	2						
Other Specialties	127	124	95	16	13	1	2		
Aerospace Medicine	1	1			1				
Anatomic/Clinical Pathology	5	5	4	1					
Anesthesiology	19	19	17		2				
Child & Adolescent Psychiatry	4	3	2	1		1			
Diagnostic Radiology	4	4	3	1					
Emergency Medicine	24	24	16	2	6				
General Preventive Medicine	2	2	2						
Neurology	9	8	6	2			1		
Nuclear Medicine	1						1		
Physical Medicine and Rehabilitation	14	14	12	1	1				
Psychiatry	12	12	7	4	1				
Radiology	2	2	2						
Unspecified	30	30	24	4	2				
Inactive	15								
Not Classified	27								

Note: Excludes Address Unknown.

Subspecialties in this table are condensed into major specialties. See Appendix A.

Table 5.19

DOs by State, Self-Designated Specialty, and Activity, 2010, continued
Alaska

		Patient Care				Other Professional Activity			
				Hospital Based					
Specialty	Total Physicians	Total Patient Care	Office Based	Resid./ Fellows	Phys. Staff	Admin.	Med. Teach.	Research	Other
Total Physicians	167	149	113	5	31	2	1		2
FM/GP	68	66	50	4	12	1	1		
Family Medicine	58	56	41	4	11	1	1		
General Practice	10	10	9		1				
Medical Specialties	28	27	21		6				1
Cardiovascular Disease	2	2	2						
Dermatology	3	3	2		1				
Gastroenterology	2	2	1		1				
Internal Medicine	11	11	9		2				
Pediatric Cardiology	2	2	2						
Pediatrics	8	7	5		2				1
Surgical Specialties	16	16	13		3				
General Surgery	2	2	2						
Obstetrics & Gynecology	6	6	5		1				
Orthopedic Surgery	6	6	5		1				
Otolaryngology	1	1	1						
Urology	1	1			1				
Other Specialties	42	40	29	1	10	1			1
Anesthesiology	4	4	4						
Child & Adolescent Psychiatry	2	2	2						
Diagnostic Radiology	4	3	2		1				1
Emergency Medicine	6	6	3		3				
Neurology	1	1	1						
Other Specialty	1					1			
Physical Medicine and Rehabilitation	2	2	2						
Psychiatry	8	8	5		3				
Radiology	2	2	1		1				
Unspecified	12	12	9	1	2				
Inactive	4								
Not Classified	9								

Note: Excludes Address Unknown.

Subspecialties in this table are condensed into major specialties. See Appendix A.

Table 5.19

DOs by State, Self-Designated Specialty, and Activity, 2010, continued
Arizona

		Patient Care				Other Professional Activity			
				Hospital Based					
Specialty	Total Physicians	Total Patient Care	Office Based	Resid./ Fellows	Phys. Staff	Admin.	Med. Teach.	Research	Other
Total Physicians	1,962	1,608	1,326	127	155	17	8	2	8
FM/GP	515	507	439	16	52	3	1	1	3
Family Medicine	428	420	365	16	39	3	1	1	3
General Practice	87	87	74		13				
Medical Specialties	387	382	306	52	24	2	2		1
Allergy and Immunology	1	1	1						
Cardiovascular Disease	32	32	27	4	1				
Dermatology	32	32	27	5					
Gastroenterology	15	15	11	4					
Internal Medicine	204	201	165	22	14	2			1
Pediatrics	80	80	58	14	8				
Pulmonary Disease	23	21	17	3	1		2		
Surgical Specialties	183	178	154	10	14	2	2		1
Colon and Rectal Surgery	2	2	2						
General Surgery	38	35	27	4	4	2	1		
Obstetrics & Gynecology	63	63	54	4	5				
Ophthalmology	8	8	7		1				
Orthopedic Surgery	41	39	34	2	3		1		1
Otolaryngology	14	14	13		1				
Plastic Surgery	7	7	7						
Thoracic Surgery	2	2	2						
Urology	8	8	8						
Other Specialties	558	541	427	49	65	10	3	1	3
Aerospace Medicine	2	2	1		1				
Anatomic/Clinical Pathology	14	14	10	1	3				
Anesthesiology	79	78	69	3	6				1
Child & Adolescent Psychiatry	18	17	11	4	2	1			
Diagnostic Radiology	19	19	14	3	2				
Emergency Medicine	95	93	69		24	1	1		
Forensic Pathology	2	1	1						1
General Preventive Medicine	8	7	7			1			
Neurology	26	26	19	6	1				
Nuclear Medicine	3	3	2		1				
Occupational Medicine	7	6	4		2	1			
Other Specialty	6	2	2			3	1		
Physical Medicine and Rehabilitation	25	23	20	1	2		1	1	
Psychiatry	39	36	29	4	3	2			1
Radiation Oncology	3	3	3						
Radiology	15	15	11		4				
Unspecified	197	196	155	27	14	1			
Inactive	181								
Not Classified	138								

Note: Excludes Address Unknown.

Subspecialties in this table are condensed into major specialties. See Appendix A.

Table 5.19

DOs by State, Self-Designated Specialty, and Activity, 2010, continued
Arkansas

		Patient Care				Other Professional Activity			
				Hospital Based					
Specialty	Total Physicians	Total Patient Care	Office Based	Resid./ Fellows	Phys. Staff	Admin.	Med. Teach.	Research	Other
Total Physicians	289	252	202	23	27	2			
FM/GP	111	111	100	4	7				
Family Medicine	94	94	85	4	5				
General Practice	17	17	15		2				
Medical Specialties	51	49	34	7	8	2			
Cardiovascular Disease	7	7	7						
Dermatology	1	1	1						
Gastroenterology	1	1	1						
Internal Medicine	31	29	20	3	6	2			
Pediatrics	11	11	5	4	2				
Surgical Specialties	21	21	19	1	1				
General Surgery	5	5	4	1					
Neurological Surgery	3	3	2		1				
Obstetrics & Gynecology	6	6	6						
Ophthalmology	3	3	3						
Orthopedic Surgery	4	4	4						
Other Specialties	71	71	49	11	11				
Aerospace Medicine	2	2	1		1				
Anatomic/Clinical Pathology	1	1		1					
Anesthesiology	14	14	6	6	2				
Diagnostic Radiology	4	4	1	3					
Emergency Medicine	15	15	9	1	5				
Neurology	3	3	3						
Nuclear Medicine	1	1	1						
Occupational Medicine	1	1	1						
Other Specialty	3	3	3						
Physical Medicine and Rehabilitation	6	6	5		1				
Psychiatry	3	3	2		1				
Radiation Oncology	1	1	1						
Radiology	1	1	1						
Unspecified	16	16	15		1				
Inactive	14								
Not Classified	21								

Note: Excludes Address Unknown.

Subspecialties in this table are condensed into major specialties. See Appendix A.

Table 5.19

DOs by State, Self-Designated Specialty, and Activity, 2010, continued
California

		Patient Care				Other Professional Activity			
				Hospital Based					
Specialty	Total Physicians	Total Patient Care	Office Based	Resid./ Fellows	Phys. Staff	Admin.	Med. Teach.	Research	Other
Total Physicians	4,207	3,591	2,914	397	280	27	20	4	12
FM/GP	1,313	1,296	1,167	65	64	8	6		3
Family Medicine	1,186	1,171	1,053	65	53	7	5		3
General Practice	127	125	114		11	1	1		
Medical Specialties	834	822	649	115	58	6	3	2	1
Allergy and Immunology	4	4	2	1	1				
Cardiovascular Disease	24	23	17	5	1		1		
Dermatology	39	39	31	4	4				
Gastroenterology	17	17	13	2	2				
Internal Medicine	525	515	420	61	34	6	2	2	
Pediatric Cardiology	2	2		2					
Pediatrics	198	197	146	36	15				1
Pulmonary Disease	25	25	20	4	1				
Surgical Specialties	336	329	264	36	29	2	3		2
Colon and Rectal Surgery	1	1	1						
General Surgery	64	63	37	18	8				1
Neurological Surgery	6	6	5		1				
Obstetrics & Gynecology	140	139	109	16	14				1
Ophthalmology	21	21	19		2				
Orthopedic Surgery	71	68	63	2	3	1	2		
Otolaryngology	16	15	14		1		1		
Plastic Surgery	9	9	9						
Thoracic Surgery	2	1	1			1			
Urology	6	6	6						
Other Specialties	1,171	1,144	834	181	129	11	8	2	6
Aerospace Medicine	2	2	1		1				
Anatomic/Clinical Pathology	35	34	21	11	2	1			
Anesthesiology	156	156	134	7	15				
Child & Adolescent Psychiatry	23	22	18	1	3			1	
Diagnostic Radiology	38	37	24	7	6				1
Emergency Medicine	225	220	152	20	48	3	2		
Forensic Pathology	2	1	1						1
General Preventive Medicine	24	24	18	2	4				
Neurology	49	48	41	6	1			1	
Nuclear Medicine	4	3	2		1				1
Occupational Medicine	19	15	11		4	2	1		1
Other Specialty	15	13	11		2	1	1		
Physical Medicine and Rehabilitation	81	80	64	13	3				1
Psychiatry	123	120	87	18	15	3			
Public Health and General Preventive Medicine	10	7	3		4	1	1		1
Radiation Oncology	5	5	3	1	1				
Radiology	17	16	15		1		1		
Unspecified	343	341	228	95	18		2		
Inactive	118								
Not Classified	435								

Note: Excludes Address Unknown.

Subspecialties in this table are condensed into major specialties. See Appendix A.

Table 5.19

DOs by State, Self-Designated Specialty, and Activity, 2010, continued
Colorado

		Patient Care				Other Professional Activity			
				Hospital Based					
Specialty	Total Physicians	Total Patient Care	Office Based	Resid./ Fellows	Phys. Staff	Admin.	Med. Teach.	Research	Other
Total Physicians	1,192	1,046	892	58	96	15	5	1	
FM/GP	443	437	381	26	30	5	1		
Family Medicine	388	382	328	26	28	5	1		
General Practice	55	55	53		2				
Medical Specialties	169	164	139	13	12	1	3	1	
Allergy and Immunology	1	1	1						
Cardiovascular Disease	4	4	4						
Dermatology	9	9	6	1	2				
Gastroenterology	5	5	4		1				
Internal Medicine	100	96	86	4	6	1	2	1	
Pediatric Cardiology	1	1		1					
Pediatrics	41	40	30	7	3		1		
Pulmonary Disease	8	8	8						
Surgical Specialties	104	104	84	3	17				
General Surgery	16	16	7	3	6				
Obstetrics & Gynecology	37	37	30		7				
Ophthalmology	7	7	7						
Orthopedic Surgery	29	29	26		3				
Otolaryngology	6	6	6						
Plastic Surgery	2	2	2						
Thoracic Surgery	3	3	2		1				
Urology	4	4	4						
Other Specialties	351	341	288	16	37	9	1		
Aerospace Medicine	6	5	4		1	1			
Anatomic/Clinical Pathology	11	11	6	4	1				
Anesthesiology	58	57	51	1	5	1			
Child & Adolescent Psychiatry	12	12	9	2	1				
Diagnostic Radiology	12	11	9		2		1		
Emergency Medicine	71	70	60		10	1			
Forensic Pathology	3	3	2	1					
General Preventive Medicine	7	5	3	1	1	2			
Neurology	10	9	9			1			
Occupational Medicine	7	6	6			1			
Other Specialty	3	3	3						
Physical Medicine and Rehabilitation	24	24	22	1	1				
Psychiatry	21	21	14	2	5				
Public Health and General Preventive Medicine	3	1	1			2			
Radiology	7	7	4		3				
Unspecified	96	96	85	4	7				
Inactive	81								
Not Classified	44								

Note: Excludes Address Unknown.

Subspecialties in this table are condensed into major specialties. See Appendix A.

Table 5.19

DOs by State, Self-Designated Specialty, and Activity, 2010, continued
Connecticut

		Patient Care				Other Professional Activity			
				Hospital Based					
Specialty	Total Physicians	Total Patient Care	Office Based	Resid./ Fellows	Phys. Staff	Admin.	Med. Teach.	Research	Other
Total Physicians	477	400	315	51	34	2	3	1	1
FM/GP	56	55	51	1	3	1			
Family Medicine	55	54	50	1	3	1			
General Practice	1	1	1						
Medical Specialties	140	137	115	13	9		1	1	1
Allergy and Immunology	2	2	2						
Cardiovascular Disease	5	5	4	1					
Dermatology	4	4	4						
Gastroenterology	4	4	3	1					
Internal Medicine	86	84	71	6	7			1	1
Pediatrics	31	30	25	4	1		1		
Pulmonary Disease	8	8	6	1	1				
Surgical Specialties	55	55	41	12	2				
Colon and Rectal Surgery	2	2	2						
General Surgery	6	6	2	3	1				
Obstetrics & Gynecology	37	37	27	9	1				
Ophthalmology	2	2	2						
Orthopedic Surgery	7	7	7						
Plastic Surgery	1	1	1						
Other Specialties	156	153	108	25	20	1	2		
Anatomic/Clinical Pathology	6	6	3	2	1				
Anesthesiology	29	28	25	3			1		
Child & Adolescent Psychiatry	3	3	2	1					
Diagnostic Radiology	9	9	6	3					
Emergency Medicine	45	44	27	4	13		1		
General Preventive Medicine	2	2	1	1					
Neurology	7	7	4	2	1				
Occupational Medicine	3	2	2			1			
Other Specialty	6	6	5	1					
Physical Medicine and Rehabilitation	9	9	8		1				
Psychiatry	11	11	5	4	2				
Radiology	4	4	4						
Unspecified	22	22	16	4	2				
Inactive	13								
Not Classified	57								

Note: Excludes Address Unknown.

Subspecialties in this table are condensed into major specialties. See Appendix A.

Table 5.19

DOs by State, Self-Designated Specialty, and Activity, 2010, continued
Delaware

		Patient Care				Other Professional Activity			
				Hospital Based					
Specialty	Total Physicians	Total Patient Care	Office Based	Resid./ Fellows	Phys. Staff	Admin.	Med. Teach.	Research	Other
Total Physicians	308	256	192	48	16	3			1
FM/GP	87	86	76	6	4	1			
Family Medicine	82	81	71	6	4	1			
General Practice	5	5	5						
Medical Specialties	71	70	50	17	3	1			
Allergy and Immunology	1	1	1						
Cardiovascular Disease	11	11	9	2					
Dermatology	1	1	1						
Gastroenterology	1	1	1						
Internal Medicine	26	26	21	4	1				
Pediatric Cardiology	1	1	1						
Pediatrics	28	27	14	11	2	1			
Pulmonary Disease	2	2	2						
Surgical Specialties	40	39	29	8	2				1
General Surgery	7	7	1	6					
Obstetrics & Gynecology	19	18	15	2	1				1
Ophthalmology	1	1	1						
Orthopedic Surgery	9	9	8		1				
Otolaryngology	3	3	3						
Thoracic Surgery	1	1	1						
Other Specialties	62	61	37	17	7	1			
Anesthesiology	9	9	8		1				
Diagnostic Radiology	6	6	1	5					
Emergency Medicine	13	13	8	3	2				
Neurology	4	4	4						
Occupational Medicine	1					1			
Other Specialty	3	3	1	2					
Physical Medicine and Rehabilitation	8	8	5	3					
Psychiatry	3	3	2		1				
Radiology	2	2	1		1				
Unspecified	13	13	7	4	2				
Inactive	23								
Not Classified	25								

Note: Excludes Address Unknown.

Subspecialties in this table are condensed into major specialties. See Appendix A.

Table 5.19

DOs by State, Self-Designated Specialty, and Activity, 2010, continued
District of Columbia

		Patient Care				Other Professional Activity			
				Hospital Based					
Specialty	Total Physicians	Total Patient Care	Office Based	Resid./ Fellows	Phys. Staff	Admin.	Med. Teach.	Research	Other
Total Physicians	120	87	49	26	12	4		1	
FM/GP	13	13	10	1	2				
Family Medicine	13	13	10	1	2				
Medical Specialties	33	33	15	13	5				
Allergy and Immunology	1	1			1				
Internal Medicine	18	18	11	5	2				
Pediatrics	11	11	3	6	2				
Pulmonary Disease	3	3	1	2					
Surgical Specialties	2	2	2						
General Surgery	1	1	1						
Obstetrics & Gynecology	1	1	1						
Other Specialties	44	39	22	12	5	4		1	
Aerospace Medicine	1	1			1				
Anatomic/Clinical Pathology	2	2	1	1					
Anesthesiology	5	5	4	1					
Child & Adolescent Psychiatry	1	1	1						
Diagnostic Radiology	1	1		1					
Emergency Medicine	1					1			
General Preventive Medicine	5	5	2	1	2				
Neurology	3	3	1	2					
Other Specialty	2	1		1		1			
Physical Medicine and Rehabilitation	10	10	7	1	2				
Psychiatry	10	8	4	4		2			
Public Health and General Preventive Medicine	1							1	
Unspecified	2	2	2						
Inactive	2								
Not Classified	26								

Note: Excludes Address Unknown.

Subspecialties in this table are condensed into major specialties. See Appendix A.

Table 5.19

DOs by State, Self-Designated Specialty, and Activity, 2010, continued
Florida

		Patient Care				Other Professional Activity			
				Hospital Based					
Specialty	Total Physicians	Total Patient Care	Office Based	Resid./ Fellows	Phys. Staff	Admin.	Med. Teach.	Research	Other
Total Physicians	4,708	3,849	3,211	285	353	37	35	9	9
FM/GP	1,212	1,184	1,060	16	108	14	12	1	1
Family Medicine	991	968	868	16	84	11	10	1	1
General Practice	221	216	192		24	3	2		
Medical Specialties	836	817	664	100	53	4	10	4	1
Allergy and Immunology	7	7	6	1					
Cardiovascular Disease	46	44	38	4	2		2		
Dermatology	89	88	65	19	4			1	
Gastroenterology	32	32	30	1	1				
Internal Medicine	467	459	392	38	29	3	2	3	
Pediatric Cardiology	2	2	2						
Pediatrics	161	153	106	32	15	1	6		1
Pulmonary Disease	32	32	25	5	2				
Surgical Specialties	430	423	385	11	27	1	5		1
Colon and Rectal Surgery	4	4	4						
General Surgery	73	71	58	4	9		2		
Neurological Surgery	8	8	7		1				
Obstetrics & Gynecology	130	129	119	3	7		1		
Ophthalmology	38	38	36		2				
Orthopedic Surgery	104	101	94	4	3	1	2		
Otolaryngology	35	35	34		1				
Plastic Surgery	11	11	11						
Thoracic Surgery	5	5	5						
Urology	22	21	17		4				1
Other Specialties	1,461	1,425	1,102	158	165	18	8	4	6
Aerospace Medicine	8	6	4		2	1			1
Anatomic/Clinical Pathology	26	25	15	3	7	1			
Anesthesiology	173	173	150	8	15				
Child & Adolescent Psychiatry	10	10	8		2				
Diagnostic Radiology	46	46	33	4	9				
Emergency Medicine	290	281	200	13	68	4	1	3	1
Forensic Pathology	1	1	1						
General Preventive Medicine	19	18	10	3	5		1		
Medical Genetics	1	1		1					
Neurology	59	57	47	8	2		2		
Nuclear Medicine	2	2	1		1				
Occupational Medicine	11	8	7		1	3			
Other Specialty	27	23	17	2	4	1	2		1
Physical Medicine and Rehabilitation	83	83	69	12	2				
Psychiatry	82	79	58	7	14	1		1	1
Public Health and General Preventive Medicine	2					2			
Radiation Oncology	5	4	3		1		1		
Radiology	47	43	35		8	3			1
Unspecified	568	564	443	97	24	2	1		1
Vascular Medicine	1	1	1						
Inactive	485								
Not Classified	284								

Note: Excludes Address Unknown.

Subspecialties in this table are condensed into major specialties. See Appendix A.

Table 5.19

DOs by State, Self-Designated Specialty, and Activity, 2010, continued
Georgia

		Patient Care				Other Professional Activity			
				Hospital Based					
Specialty	Total Physicians	Total Patient Care	Office Based	Resid./ Fellows	Phys. Staff	Admin.	Med. Teach.	Research	Other
Total Physicians	947	780	633	59	88	6	13	6	1
FM/GP	292	282	247	9	26	2	5	2	1
Family Medicine	252	243	212	9	22	1	5	2	1
General Practice	40	39	35		4	1			
Medical Specialties	154	148	119	12	17	2	3	1	
Allergy and Immunology	1	1	1						
Cardiovascular Disease	8	8	5	2	1				
Dermatology	6	6	6						
Gastroenterology	9	9	8		1				
Internal Medicine	90	86	69	5	12	2	2		
Pediatric Cardiology	2	2	1		1				
Pediatrics	31	29	24	4	1		1	1	
Pulmonary Disease	7	7	5	1	1				
Surgical Specialties	108	106	85	11	10		2		
General Surgery	16	15	12	2	1		1		
Obstetrics & Gynecology	39	39	34	3	2				
Ophthalmology	4	4	2		2				
Orthopedic Surgery	37	36	27	6	3		1		
Otolaryngology	7	7	6		1				
Urology	5	5	4		1				
Other Specialties	252	244	182	27	35	2	3	3	
Aerospace Medicine	2	1	1					1	
Anatomic/Clinical Pathology	10	9	6	1	2		1		
Anesthesiology	41	40	30	3	7		1		
Child & Adolescent Psychiatry	7	7	5	1	1				
Diagnostic Radiology	14	14	10	3	1				
Emergency Medicine	59	57	42	7	8		1	1	
General Preventive Medicine	7	7	6		1				
Neurology	2	2	2						
Nuclear Medicine	2	2			2				
Occupational Medicine	3	2	1		1	1			
Other Specialty	3	2	2			1			
Physical Medicine and Rehabilitation	21	21	18	1	2				
Psychiatry	24	24	21	1	2				
Public Health and General Preventive Medicine	2	1	1					1	
Radiation Oncology	1	1			1				
Radiology	3	3		2	1				
Unspecified	51	51	37	8	6				
Inactive	59								
Not Classified	82								

Note: Excludes Address Unknown.

Subspecialties in this table are condensed into major specialties. See Appendix A.

Table 5.19

DOs by State, Self-Designated Specialty, and Activity, 2010, continued
Hawaii

		Patient Care				Other Professional Activity			
				Hospital Based					
Specialty	Total Physicians	Total Patient Care	Office Based	Resid./ Fellows	Phys. Staff	Admin.	Med. Teach.	Research	Other
Total Physicians	221	184	129	23	32	3	1		1
FM/GP	53	51	38	2	11	2			
Family Medicine	43	41	29	2	10	2			
General Practice	10	10	9		1				
Medical Specialties	48	47	37	3	7				1
Cardiovascular Disease	4	4	3		1				
Gastroenterology	3	3	2	1					
Internal Medicine	30	29	23	2	4				1
Pediatrics	10	10	8		2				
Pulmonary Disease	1	1	1						
Surgical Specialties	19	19	10	6	3				
General Surgery	5	5	1	4					
Obstetrics & Gynecology	6	6	3	1	2				
Ophthalmology	3	3	2		1				
Orthopedic Surgery	2	2	1	1					
Otolaryngology	2	2	2						
Plastic Surgery	1	1	1						
Other Specialties	69	67	44	12	11	1	1		
Anatomic/Clinical Pathology	1	1	1						
Anesthesiology	5	5	3		2				
Child & Adolescent Psychiatry	3	3	1	2					
Diagnostic Radiology	5	5	1	3	1				
Emergency Medicine	17	17	12		5				
Neurology	1	1			1				
Occupational Medicine	2	2	2						
Other Specialty	5	3	2	1		1	1		
Physical Medicine and Rehabilitation	6	6	6						
Psychiatry	8	8	4	4					
Radiation Oncology	1	1	1						
Radiology	1	1	1						
Unspecified	14	14	10	2	2				
Inactive	12								
Not Classified	20								

Note: Excludes Address Unknown.

Subspecialties in this table are condensed into major specialties. See Appendix A.

Table 5.19

DOs by State, Self-Designated Specialty, and Activity, 2010, continued
Idaho

		Patient Care				Other Professional Activity			
				Hospital Based					
Specialty	Total Physicians	Total Patient Care	Office Based	Resid./ Fellows	Phys. Staff	Admin.	Med. Teach.	Research	Other
Total Physicians	289	261	229	8	24		1	1	1
FM/GP	115	114	103	6	5		1		
Family Medicine	109	108	97	6	5		1		
General Practice	6	6	6						
Medical Specialties	39	39	35	1	3				
Cardiovascular Disease	4	4	4						
Dermatology	3	3	2	1					
Gastroenterology	3	3	3						
Internal Medicine	16	16	13		3				
Pediatrics	11	11	11						
Pulmonary Disease	2	2	2						
Surgical Specialties	21	21	21						
General Surgery	2	2	2						
Obstetrics & Gynecology	9	9	9						
Orthopedic Surgery	4	4	4						
Otolaryngology	4	4	4						
Thoracic Surgery	1	1	1						
Urology	1	1	1						
Other Specialties	89	87	70	1	16			1	1
Anatomic/Clinical Pathology	2	1	1						1
Anesthesiology	12	12	10		2				
Child & Adolescent Psychiatry	3	3			3				
Diagnostic Radiology	7	7	6		1				
Emergency Medicine	15	15	10		5				
General Preventive Medicine	3	3	3						
Neurology	3	3	3						
Other Specialty	5	5	4		1				
Physical Medicine and Rehabilitation	3	3	3						
Psychiatry	6	6	6						
Radiology	2	2	2						
Unspecified	28	27	22	1	4			1	
Inactive	13								
Not Classified	12								

Note: Excludes Address Unknown.

Subspecialties in this table are condensed into major specialties. See Appendix A.

Table 5.19

DOs by State, Self-Designated Specialty, and Activity, 2010, continued
Illinois

		Patient Care				Other Professional Activity			
				Hospital Based					
Specialty	Total Physicians	Total Patient Care	Office Based	Resid./ Fellows	Phys. Staff	Admin.	Med. Teach.	Research	Other
Total Physicians	2,560	2,146	1,616	296	234	25	18	9	7
FM/GP	663	649	547	42	60	7	6	1	
Family Medicine	606	593	499	42	52	7	5	1	
General Practice	57	56	48		8		1		
Medical Specialties	527	508	386	80	42	7	5	5	2
Allergy and Immunology	5	5	5						
Cardiovascular Disease	36	36	28	5	3				
Dermatology	9	9	8	1					
Gastroenterology	21	21	15	6					
Internal Medicine	292	275	204	42	29	6	4	5	2
Pediatric Cardiology	1	1			1				
Pediatrics	148	146	111	26	9	1	1		
Pulmonary Disease	15	15	15						
Surgical Specialties	246	242	198	25	19		2	1	1
General Surgery	42	41	28	9	4		1		
Neurological Surgery	1	1	1						
Obstetrics & Gynecology	121	119	99	11	9			1	1
Ophthalmology	21	21	19	2					
Orthopedic Surgery	38	37	32	2	3		1		
Otolaryngology	10	10	9		1				
Plastic Surgery	3	3	3						
Thoracic Surgery	2	2	2						
Urology	8	8	5	1	2				
Other Specialties	769	747	485	149	113	11	5	2	4
Anatomic/Clinical Pathology	23	21	10	8	3		1	1	
Anesthesiology	110	109	79	18	12	1			
Child & Adolescent Psychiatry	11	10	7	1	2	1			
Diagnostic Radiology	41	40	19	14	7				1
Emergency Medicine	216	208	142	17	49	5	2		1
General Preventive Medicine	3	2	1	1		1			
Neurology	23	23	18	2	3				
Nuclear Medicine	2	2	1		1				
Occupational Medicine	17	17	11		6				
Other Specialty	8	6	3	2	1	1	1		
Physical Medicine and Rehabilitation	56	54	29	17	8	1			1
Psychiatry	48	46	29	10	7		1	1	
Radiation Oncology	5	5	4		1				
Radiology	18	16	12		4	1			1
Unspecified	188	188	120	59	9				
Inactive	72								
Not Classified	283								

Note: Excludes Address Unknown.

Subspecialties in this table are condensed into major specialties. See Appendix A.

Table 5.19

DOs by State, Self-Designated Specialty, and Activity, 2010, continued
Indiana

		Patient Care				Other Professional Activity			
				Hospital Based					
Specialty	Total Physicians	Total Patient Care	Office Based	Resid./ Fellows	Phys. Staff	Admin.	Med. Teach.	Research	Other
Total Physicians	952	844	663	81	100	6	6	4	
FM/GP	312	306	245	25	36	3	2	1	
Family Medicine	259	256	201	25	30	1	1	1	
General Practice	53	50	44		6	2	1		
Medical Specialties	154	152	117	22	13		1	1	
Allergy and Immunology	4	4	4						
Cardiovascular Disease	22	22	20	1	1				
Dermatology	1	1	1						
Gastroenterology	5	5	5						
Internal Medicine	89	87	69	10	8		1	1	
Pediatric Cardiology	1	1		1					
Pediatrics	28	28	15	9	4				
Pulmonary Disease	4	4	3	1					
Surgical Specialties	113	112	99	3	10			1	
Colon and Rectal Surgery	2	2	2						
General Surgery	13	13	11		2				
Obstetrics & Gynecology	47	47	39	2	6				
Ophthalmology	6	6	6						
Orthopedic Surgery	32	31	29		2			1	
Otolaryngology	9	9	9						
Plastic Surgery	1	1		1					
Urology	3	3	3						
Other Specialties	281	274	202	31	41	3	3	1	
Aerospace Medicine	2	2	1		1				
Anatomic/Clinical Pathology	8	8	1	6	1				
Anesthesiology	50	48	37	5	6		2		
Child & Adolescent Psychiatry	2	2	1	1					
Diagnostic Radiology	11	10	7		3		1		
Emergency Medicine	65	64	45	5	14	1			
General Preventive Medicine	3	3	3						
Neurology	7	7	6	1					
Nuclear Medicine	1	1	1						
Occupational Medicine	6	6	6						
Other Specialty	13	11	6	4	1	1		1	
Physical Medicine and Rehabilitation	12	12	10	2					
Psychiatry	10	10	6	1	3				
Public Health and General Preventive Medicine	1					1			
Radiation Oncology	2	2	1		1				
Radiology	10	10	9		1				
Unspecified	78	78	62	6	10				
Inactive	49								
Not Classified	43								

Note: Excludes Address Unknown.

Subspecialties in this table are condensed into major specialties. See Appendix A.

Table 5.19

DOs by State, Self-Designated Specialty, and Activity, 2010, continued
Iowa

		Patient Care				Other Professional Activity			
				Hospital Based					
Specialty	Total Physicians	Total Patient Care	Office Based	Resid./ Fellows	Phys. Staff	Admin.	Med. Teach.	Research	Other
Total Physicians	1,289	1,155	907	134	114	9	5	1	2
FM/GP	551	545	451	58	36	3	3		
Family Medicine	496	490	400	58	32	3	3		
General Practice	55	55	51		4				
Medical Specialties	231	229	170	36	23	1	1		
Cardiovascular Disease	15	15	12	1	2				
Dermatology	5	5	5						
Gastroenterology	9	9	7	1	1				
Internal Medicine	131	130	95	18	17		1		
Pediatric Cardiology	2	2		2					
Pediatrics	60	59	44	12	3	1			
Pulmonary Disease	9	9	7	2					
Surgical Specialties	105	102	86	1	15	2	1		
General Surgery	23	23	17		6				
Obstetrics & Gynecology	40	38	34	1	3	1	1		
Ophthalmology	5	5	4		1				
Orthopedic Surgery	23	23	19		4				
Otolaryngology	5	5	5						
Plastic Surgery	3	3	3						
Thoracic Surgery	2	1	1			1			
Urology	4	4	3		1				
Other Specialties	285	279	200	39	40	3		1	2
Aerospace Medicine	1					1			
Anatomic/Clinical Pathology	7	6	5		1				1
Anesthesiology	55	53	42	7	4	1		1	
Child & Adolescent Psychiatry	6	6	5	1					
Diagnostic Radiology	14	14	10	1	3				
Emergency Medicine	52	51	33	2	16	1			
General Preventive Medicine	4	4	3	1					
Medical Genetics	1	1		1					
Neurology	11	11	5	4	2				
Occupational Medicine	4	4	4						
Other Specialty	3	2	2						1
Physical Medicine and Rehabilitation	11	11	8	1	2				
Psychiatry	31	31	24	2	5				
Radiology	5	5	4		1				
Transplant Surgery	1	1			1				
Unspecified	79	79	55	19	5				
Inactive	75								
Not Classified	42								

Note: Excludes Address Unknown.

Subspecialties in this table are condensed into major specialties. See Appendix A.

Table 5.19

DOs by State, Self-Designated Specialty, and Activity, 2010, continued
Kansas

		Patient Care				Other Professional Activity			
				Hospital Based					
Specialty	Total Physicians	Total Patient Care	Office Based	Resid./ Fellows	Phys. Staff	Admin.	Med. Teach.	Research	Other
Total Physicians	763	665	506	98	61	4	2	1	
FM/GP	279	278	241	18	19	1			
Family Medicine	222	222	187	18	17				
General Practice	57	56	54		2	1			
Medical Specialties	116	114	81	22	11	2			
Allergy and Immunology	4	3	2		1	1			
Cardiovascular Disease	11	11	8	3					
Dermatology	3	3	2	1					
Gastroenterology	5	5	3	1	1				
Internal Medicine	59	59	42	11	6				
Pediatrics	29	29	22	4	3				
Pulmonary Disease	5	4	2	2		1			
Surgical Specialties	70	70	52	10	8				
General Surgery	21	21	16	4	1				
Neurological Surgery	2	2	1	1					
Obstetrics & Gynecology	29	29	22	4	3				
Ophthalmology	5	5	5						
Orthopedic Surgery	5	5	4		1				
Otolaryngology	4	4	2		2				
Plastic Surgery	1	1			1				
Urology	3	3	2	1					
Other Specialties	207	203	132	48	23	1	2	1	
Anatomic/Clinical Pathology	7	6	5	1				1	
Anesthesiology	31	31	17	11	3				
Child & Adolescent Psychiatry	9	8	4	1	3		1		
Diagnostic Radiology	10	10	7	3					
Emergency Medicine	28	28	16	3	9				
Forensic Pathology	1	1	1						
General Preventive Medicine	4	4	4						
Neurology	10	10	6	4					
Occupational Medicine	1	1	1						
Other Specialty	2	2		2					
Physical Medicine and Rehabilitation	13	13	10	2	1				
Psychiatry	24	23	16	5	2		1		
Radiology	3	2	1		1	1			
Unspecified	64	64	44	16	4				
Inactive	38								
Not Classified	53								

Note: Excludes Address Unknown.

Subspecialties in this table are condensed into major specialties. See Appendix A.

Table 5.19

DOs by State, Self-Designated Specialty, and Activity, 2010, continued
Kentucky

		Patient Care				Other Professional Activity			
				Hospital Based					
Specialty	Total Physicians	Total Patient Care	Office Based	Resid./ Fellows	Phys. Staff	Admin.	Med. Teach.	Research	Other
Total Physicians	542	450	315	86	49	5	4		
FM/GP	131	127	105	11	11	3	1		
Family Medicine	116	112	94	11	7	3	1		
General Practice	15	15	11		4				
Medical Specialties	110	110	66	36	8				
Cardiovascular Disease	4	4	3	1					
Dermatology	2	2	2						
Gastroenterology	9	9	5	4					
Internal Medicine	59	59	39	14	6				
Pediatrics	33	33	15	16	2				
Pulmonary Disease	3	3	2	1					
Surgical Specialties	49	48	37	3	8	1			
General Surgery	8	8	6		2				
Obstetrics & Gynecology	27	27	22	3	2				
Ophthalmology	1	1			1				
Orthopedic Surgery	4	3	2		1	1			
Otolaryngology	5	5	3		2				
Thoracic Surgery	1	1	1						
Urology	3	3	3						
Other Specialties	169	165	107	36	22	1	3		
Anatomic/Clinical Pathology	8	8	3	5					
Anesthesiology	27	27	19	3	5				
Child & Adolescent Psychiatry	5	4	1	1	2	1			
Diagnostic Radiology	6	6	4	1	1				
Emergency Medicine	19	18	13	3	2		1		
Forensic Pathology	2	2	2						
Neurology	7	6	3	3			1		
Occupational Medicine	4	4	3		1				
Other Specialty	5	4	3	1			1		
Physical Medicine and Rehabilitation	10	10	5	4	1				
Psychiatry	12	12	11	1					
Radiation Oncology	1	1	1						
Radiology	3	3	2	1					
Unspecified	60	60	37	13	10				
Inactive	15								
Not Classified	68								

Note: Excludes Address Unknown.

Subspecialties in this table are condensed into major specialties. See Appendix A.

Table 5.19

DOs by State, Self-Designated Specialty, and Activity, 2010, continued
Louisiana

		Patient Care				Other Professional Activity			
				Hospital Based					
Specialty	Total Physicians	Total Patient Care	Office Based	Resid./ Fellows	Phys. Staff	Admin.	Med. Teach.	Research	Other
Total Physicians	180	152	78	56	18		1		
FM/GP	26	25	17	3	5		1		
Family Medicine	22	21	13	3	5		1		
General Practice	4	4	4						
Medical Specialties	41	41	23	14	4				
Allergy and Immunology	3	3		3					
Cardiovascular Disease	4	4	1	2	1				
Dermatology	1	1	1						
Internal Medicine	16	16	12	2	2				
Pediatrics	14	14	7	6	1				
Pulmonary Disease	3	3	2	1					
Surgical Specialties	21	21	10	10	1				
General Surgery	2	2		2					
Neurological Surgery	1	1		1					
Obstetrics & Gynecology	12	12	6	6					
Orthopedic Surgery	3	3	2	1					
Otolaryngology	2	2	2						
Urology	1	1			1				
Other Specialties	65	65	28	29	8				
Anatomic/Clinical Pathology	3	3	1	2					
Anesthesiology	7	7	4	1	2				
Child & Adolescent Psychiatry	2	2		2					
Diagnostic Radiology	2	2		1	1				
Emergency Medicine	19	19	7	9	3				
General Preventive Medicine	2	2	1	1					
Neurology	1	1	1						
Other Specialty	5	5	1	4					
Physical Medicine and Rehabilitation	6	6	2	4					
Psychiatry	4	4	3	1					
Radiology	1	1			1				
Unspecified	13	13	8	4	1				
Inactive	11								
Not Classified	16								

Note: Excludes Address Unknown.

Subspecialties in this table are condensed into major specialties. See Appendix A.

Table 5.19

DOs by State, Self-Designated Specialty, and Activity, 2010, continued
Maine

		Patient Care				Other Professional Activity			
				Hospital Based					
Specialty	Total Physicians	Total Patient Care	Office Based	Resid./ Fellows	Phys. Staff	Admin.	Med. Teach.	Research	Other
Total Physicians	738	634	470	76	88	4	4		
FM/GP	287	283	219	34	30	1	3		
Family Medicine	257	253	193	34	26	1	3		
General Practice	30	30	26		4				
Medical Specialties	129	129	95	21	13				
Allergy and Immunology	1	1	1						
Cardiovascular Disease	6	6	6						
Dermatology	2	2	2						
Gastroenterology	3	3	3						
Internal Medicine	76	76	52	14	10				
Pediatrics	32	32	26	4	2				
Pulmonary Disease	9	9	5	3	1				
Surgical Specialties	56	55	42	2	11		1		
General Surgery	12	12	8	1	3				
Obstetrics & Gynecology	20	20	15	1	4				
Ophthalmology	1	1			1				
Orthopedic Surgery	20	19	18		1		1		
Otolaryngology	2	2	1		1				
Urology	1	1			1				
Other Specialties	170	167	114	19	34	3			
Anatomic/Clinical Pathology	2	2	1		1				
Anesthesiology	19	18	15	1	2	1			
Child & Adolescent Psychiatry	7	7	6		1				
Diagnostic Radiology	4	4	2	1	1				
Emergency Medicine	39	39	23	1	15				
General Preventive Medicine	3	3	2		1				
Neurology	4	4	3		1				
Occupational Medicine	4	3	2		1	1			
Other Specialty	6	6	6						
Physical Medicine and Rehabilitation	12	11	10	1		1			
Psychiatry	24	24	12	4	8				
Radiology	2	2	1		1				
Unspecified	44	44	31	11	2				
Inactive	41								
Not Classified	55								

Note: Excludes Address Unknown.

Subspecialties in this table are condensed into major specialties. See Appendix A.

Table 5.19

DOs by State, Self-Designated Specialty, and Activity, 2010, continued
Maryland

		Patient Care				Other Professional Activity			
				Hospital Based					
Specialty	Total Physicians	Total Patient Care	Office Based	Resid./ Fellows	Phys. Staff	Admin.	Med. Teach.	Research	Other
Total Physicians	741	598	434	79	85	11	2	4	4
FM/GP	119	117	99	3	15	2			
Family Medicine	107	105	89	3	13	2			
General Practice	12	12	10		2				
Medical Specialties	171	166	126	17	23	2	2	1	
Allergy and Immunology	5	5	5						
Cardiovascular Disease	10	9	7		2	1			
Dermatology	4	4	2	1	1				
Gastroenterology	7	7	4	1	2				
Internal Medicine	101	98	73	12	13	1	1	1	
Pediatric Cardiology	1	1	1						
Pediatrics	37	36	28	3	5		1		
Pulmonary Disease	6	6	6						
Surgical Specialties	79	78	48	17	13			1	
General Surgery	18	18	9	7	2				
Obstetrics & Gynecology	28	27	19	6	2			1	
Ophthalmology	6	6	4		2				
Orthopedic Surgery	20	20	11	3	6				
Otolaryngology	4	4	3		1				
Plastic Surgery	2	2	1	1					
Urology	1	1	1						
Other Specialties	250	237	161	42	34	7		2	4
Aerospace Medicine	1	1	1						
Anatomic/Clinical Pathology	2	2	1	1					
Anesthesiology	39	39	28	8	3				
Child & Adolescent Psychiatry	8	8	7		1				
Diagnostic Radiology	8	8	3	4	1				
Emergency Medicine	40	39	30	2	7	1			
Forensic Pathology	2	2	1		1				
General Preventive Medicine	18	16	5	6	5	1		1	
Medical Genetics	1	1	1						
Neurology	9	9	5	3	1				
Occupational Medicine	7	3	2		1	3			1
Other Specialty	7	5	3	1	1			1	1
Physical Medicine and Rehabilitation	31	31	24	3	4				
Psychiatry	26	25	16	2	7	1			
Public Health and General Preventive Medicine	1								1
Radiation Oncology	1					1			
Radiology	3	3	2		1				
Unspecified	46	45	32	12	1				1
Inactive	15								
Not Classified	107								

Note: Excludes Address Unknown.

Subspecialties in this table are condensed into major specialties. See Appendix A.

Table 5.19

DOs by State, Self-Designated Specialty, and Activity, 2010, continued
Massachusetts

		Patient Care				Other Professional Activity			
				Hospital Based					
Specialty	Total Physicians	Total Patient Care	Office Based	Resid./ Fellows	Phys. Staff	Admin.	Med. Teach.	Research	Other
Total Physicians	794	664	461	148	55	4	1	3	3
FM/GP	128	125	109	10	6			1	2
Family Medicine	116	113	100	10	3			1	2
General Practice	12	12	9		3				
Medical Specialties	266	261	172	61	28	2	1	1	1
Allergy and Immunology	2	2	2						
Cardiovascular Disease	11	11	7	3	1				
Dermatology	5	5	3	1	1				
Gastroenterology	6	6	4	2					
Internal Medicine	180	176	115	41	20	2	1		1
Pediatrics	54	53	38	9	6			1	
Pulmonary Disease	8	8	3	5					
Surgical Specialties	69	69	52	13	4				
General Surgery	13	13	7	5	1				
Obstetrics & Gynecology	34	34	28	5	1				
Ophthalmology	2	2	2						
Orthopedic Surgery	15	15	13	1	1				
Otolaryngology	2	2	1		1				
Plastic Surgery	2	2		2					
Urology	1	1	1						
Other Specialties	212	209	128	64	17	2		1	
Anatomic/Clinical Pathology	6	6	2	4					
Anesthesiology	48	48	30	16	2				
Child & Adolescent Psychiatry	3	3	2	1					
Diagnostic Radiology	8	8	4	3	1				
Emergency Medicine	46	44	28	7	9	1		1	
Forensic Pathology	1	1	1						
General Preventive Medicine	2	2		2					
Neurology	9	9	5	4					
Occupational Medicine	3	3	2		1				
Other Specialty	5	5	4	1					
Physical Medicine and Rehabilitation	25	25	15	9	1				
Psychiatry	25	25	10	13	2				
Radiation Oncology	1	1	1						
Radiology	2	2	2						
Unspecified	27	27	22	4	1				
Vascular Medicine	1					1			
Inactive	21								
Not Classified	98								

Note: Excludes Address Unknown.

Subspecialties in this table are condensed into major specialties. See Appendix A.

Table 5.19

DOs by State, Self-Designated Specialty, and Activity, 2010, continued
Michigan

		Patient Care				Other Professional Activity			
				Hospital Based					
Specialty	Total Physicians	Total Patient Care	Office Based	Resid./ Fellows	Phys. Staff	Admin.	Med. Teach.	Research	Other
Total Physicians	5,629	4,637	3,701	464	472	44	40	7	12
FM/GP	1,333	1,308	1,165	24	119	14	8	2	1
Family Medicine	1,059	1,039	926	24	89	9	8	2	1
General Practice	274	269	239		30	5			
Medical Specialties	848	820	661	84	75	8	15	3	2
Allergy and Immunology	9	8	8				1		
Cardiovascular Disease	67	63	59	3	1		1	2	1
Dermatology	61	59	40	19			1		1
Gastroenterology	25	24	21	2	1	1			
Internal Medicine	495	481	388	37	56	5	8	1	
Pediatric Cardiology	3	3	2	1					
Pediatrics	152	146	115	19	12	2	4		
Pulmonary Disease	36	36	28	3	5				
Surgical Specialties	598	591	508	26	57	1	4	1	1
Colon and Rectal Surgery	1	1	1						
General Surgery	125	125	112	5	8				
Neurological Surgery	8	8	4	1	3				
Obstetrics & Gynecology	186	184	152	11	21	1	1		
Ophthalmology	43	42	37	2	3		1		
Orthopedic Surgery	155	153	129	4	20		1		1
Otolaryngology	39	39	37	1	1				
Plastic Surgery	4	4	4						
Thoracic Surgery	10	9	8		1			1	
Urology	27	26	24	2			1		
Other Specialties	1,961	1,918	1,367	330	221	21	13	1	8
Aerospace Medicine	1	1	1						
Anatomic/Clinical Pathology	25	22	16	2	4	2			1
Anesthesiology	204	200	156	19	25	3	1		
Child & Adolescent Psychiatry	23	22	19	3			1		
Diagnostic Radiology	74	73	56	7	10				1
Emergency Medicine	352	348	237	32	79	3	1		
General Preventive Medicine	11	11	11						
Neurology	64	63	50	8	5			1	
Nuclear Medicine	3	3	2	1					
Occupational Medicine	24	21	18		3	2			1
Other Specialty	28	21	17	1	3	3	3		1
Physical Medicine and Rehabilitation	90	87	62	23	2	1	2		
Psychiatry	114	110	87	11	12	3	1		
Public Health and General Preventive Medicine	3	1	1			2			
Radiation Oncology	10	10	8	1	1				
Radiology	53	50	38	2	10		1		2
Unspecified	882	875	588	220	67	2	3		2
Inactive	511								
Not Classified	378								

Note: Excludes Address Unknown.

Subspecialties in this table are condensed into major specialties. See Appendix A.

Table 5.19

DOs by State, Self-Designated Specialty, and Activity, 2010, continued
Minnesota

		Patient Care				Other Professional Activity			
				Hospital Based					
Specialty	Total Physicians	Total Patient Care	Office Based	Resid./ Fellows	Phys. Staff	Admin.	Med. Teach.	Research	Other
Total Physicians	578	528	373	91	64	4	1		
FM/GP	176	173	137	20	16	3			
Family Medicine	160	158	126	20	12	2			
General Practice	16	15	11		4	1			
Medical Specialties	104	104	69	20	15				
Cardiovascular Disease	4	4	3	1					
Dermatology	2	2	2						
Gastroenterology	2	2	1	1					
Internal Medicine	61	61	39	10	12				
Pediatric Cardiology	1	1		1					
Pediatrics	30	30	20	7	3				
Pulmonary Disease	4	4	4						
Surgical Specialties	69	69	50	10	9				
General Surgery	14	14	8	1	5				
Neurological Surgery	1	1	1						
Obstetrics & Gynecology	28	28	19	6	3				
Ophthalmology	3	3	3						
Orthopedic Surgery	19	19	15	3	1				
Otolaryngology	1	1	1						
Plastic Surgery	1	1	1						
Urology	2	2	2						
Other Specialties	184	182	117	41	24	1	1		
Anatomic/Clinical Pathology	4	3	1	2		1			
Anesthesiology	22	22	14	4	4				
Child & Adolescent Psychiatry	10	10	9	1					
Diagnostic Radiology	9	9	6	1	2				
Emergency Medicine	20	19	11	1	7		1		
General Preventive Medicine	2	2	1	1					
Neurology	12	12	8	4					
Occupational Medicine	3	3	1		2				
Other Specialty	4	4	4						
Physical Medicine and Rehabilitation	23	23	17	5	1				
Psychiatry	24	24	16	5	3				
Radiation Oncology	2	2	2						
Radiology	6	6	3	1	2				
Unspecified	43	43	24	16	3				
Inactive	21								
Not Classified	24								

Note: Excludes Address Unknown.

Subspecialties in this table are condensed into major specialties. See Appendix A.

Table 5.19

DOs by State, Self-Designated Specialty, and Activity, 2010, continued
Mississippi

Specialty	Total Physicians	Patient Care: Total Patient Care	Patient Care: Office Based	Hospital Based: Resid./Fellows	Hospital Based: Phys. Staff	Other Professional Activity: Admin.	Other Professional Activity: Med. Teach.	Other Professional Activity: Research	Other Professional Activity: Other
Total Physicians	362	318	227	39	52	2	3		
FM/GP	135	131	106	4	21	1	3		
Family Medicine	117	113	92	4	17	1	3		
General Practice	18	18	14		4				
Medical Specialties	71	70	46	15	9	1			
Allergy and Immunology	1	1		1					
Cardiovascular Disease	2	2	2						
Dermatology	1	1	1						
Gastroenterology	5	5	4	1					
Internal Medicine	40	39	23	10	6	1			
Pediatrics	17	17	13	2	2				
Pulmonary Disease	5	5	3	1	1				
Surgical Specialties	35	35	26	4	5				
General Surgery	14	14	8	4	2				
Obstetrics & Gynecology	13	13	11		2				
Ophthalmology	3	3	3						
Orthopedic Surgery	1	1			1				
Otolaryngology	2	2	2						
Thoracic Surgery	2	2	2						
Other Specialties	82	82	49	16	17				
Aerospace Medicine	1	1			1				
Anatomic/Clinical Pathology	1	1			1				
Anesthesiology	10	10	9		1				
Child & Adolescent Psychiatry	1	1			1				
Diagnostic Radiology	7	7	4	3					
Emergency Medicine	31	31	18	6	7				
Neurology	4	4	2	1	1				
Occupational Medicine	1	1	1						
Other Specialty	2	2	2						
Physical Medicine and Rehabilitation	5	5	5						
Psychiatry	4	4	1		3				
Radiology	2	2	1		1				
Unspecified	13	13	6	6	1				
Inactive	11								
Not Classified	28								

Note: Excludes Address Unknown.

Subspecialties in this table are condensed into major specialties. See Appendix A.

Table 5.19

DOs by State, Self-Designated Specialty, and Activity, 2010, continued
Missouri

		Patient Care				Other Professional Activity			
				Hospital Based					
Specialty	Total Physicians	Total Patient Care	Office Based	Resid./ Fellows	Phys. Staff	Admin.	Med. Teach.	Research	Other
Total Physicians	2,228	1,898	1,438	227	233	16	16	2	5
FM/GP	701	692	575	39	78	4	3	1	1
Family Medicine	516	508	413	39	56	3	3	1	1
General Practice	185	184	162		22	1			
Medical Specialties	349	338	242	61	35	4	5		2
Allergy and Immunology	4	3	2	1		1			
Cardiovascular Disease	15	15	11	3	1				
Dermatology	10	10	8	2					
Gastroenterology	13	13	13						
Internal Medicine	200	194	147	24	23	2	2		2
Pediatrics	97	95	57	28	10	1	1		
Pulmonary Disease	10	8	4	3	1		2		
Surgical Specialties	217	209	175	17	17	1	6		1
General Surgery	45	44	33	4	7		1		
Neurological Surgery	4	4	4						
Obstetrics & Gynecology	75	73	56	12	5		2		
Ophthalmology	14	14	14						
Orthopedic Surgery	55	52	46	1	5	1	2		
Otolaryngology	14	13	13				1		
Thoracic Surgery	3	3	3						
Urology	7	6	6						1
Other Specialties	670	659	446	110	103	7	2	1	1
Aerospace Medicine	2	2	1		1				
Anatomic/Clinical Pathology	22	21	12	9					1
Anesthesiology	99	98	73	14	11	1			
Child & Adolescent Psychiatry	9	8	7	1				1	
Diagnostic Radiology	28	28	16	7	5				
Emergency Medicine	107	106	58	2	46	1			
General Preventive Medicine	8	6	6			2			
Neurology	19	19	17	1	1				
Nuclear Medicine	4	4	3	1					
Occupational Medicine	10	9	6		3	1			
Other Specialty	9	9	8		1				
Physical Medicine and Rehabilitation	25	25	19	5	1				
Psychiatry	47	45	30	6	9	1	1		
Public Health and General Preventive Medicine	1	1	1						
Radiology	19	19	14		5				
Unspecified	261	259	175	64	20	1	1		
Inactive	166								
Not Classified	125								

Note: Excludes Address Unknown.

Subspecialties in this table are condensed into major specialties. See Appendix A.

Table 5.19

DOs by State, Self-Designated Specialty, and Activity, 2010, continued
Montana

		Patient Care				Other Professional Activity			
				Hospital Based					
Specialty	Total Physicians	Total Patient Care	Office Based	Resid./ Fellows	Phys. Staff	Admin.	Med. Teach.	Research	Other
Total Physicians	159	144	126	2	16				1
FM/GP	64	63	56	1	6				1
Family Medicine	58	57	52	1	4				1
General Practice	6	6	4		2				
Medical Specialties	22	22	20		2				
Allergy and Immunology	1	1	1						
Cardiovascular Disease	5	5	4		1				
Gastroenterology	1	1	1						
Internal Medicine	13	13	12		1				
Pediatric Cardiology	1	1	1						
Pediatrics	1	1	1						
Surgical Specialties	17	17	16	1					
General Surgery	7	7	7						
Obstetrics & Gynecology	6	6	5	1					
Ophthalmology	1	1	1						
Orthopedic Surgery	1	1	1						
Otolaryngology	2	2	2						
Other Specialties	42	42	34		8				
Anesthesiology	9	9	8		1				
Child & Adolescent Psychiatry	1	1	1						
Emergency Medicine	6	6	4		2				
General Preventive Medicine	1	1	1						
Neurology	4	4	4						
Physical Medicine and Rehabilitation	3	3	3						
Psychiatry	8	8	4		4				
Radiation Oncology	1	1	1						
Radiology	1	1	1						
Unspecified	8	8	7		1				
Inactive	7								
Not Classified	7								

Note: Excludes Address Unknown.

Subspecialties in this table are condensed into major specialties. See Appendix A.

Table 5.19

DOs by State, Self-Designated Specialty, and Activity, 2010, continued
Nebraska

		Patient Care				Other Professional Activity			
				Hospital Based					
Specialty	Total Physicians	Total Patient Care	Office Based	Resid./ Fellows	Phys. Staff	Admin.	Med. Teach.	Research	Other
Total Physicians	197	177	118	42	17	1	2		
FM/GP	71	69	52	13	4	1	1		
Family Medicine	65	63	48	13	2	1	1		
General Practice	6	6	4		2				
Medical Specialties	42	42	20	18	4				
Allergy and Immunology	2	2	2						
Cardiovascular Disease	1	1		1					
Gastroenterology	2	2	1	1					
Internal Medicine	15	15	9	4	2				
Pediatrics	15	15	7	7	1				
Pulmonary Disease	7	7	1	5	1				
Surgical Specialties	20	20	17	1	2				
General Surgery	4	4	4						
Obstetrics & Gynecology	9	9	8		1				
Ophthalmology	1	1	1						
Orthopedic Surgery	4	4	3	1					
Otolaryngology	1	1	1						
Thoracic Surgery	1	1			1				
Other Specialties	47	46	29	10	7		1		
Anatomic/Clinical Pathology	3	3	2	1					
Anesthesiology	7	6	5		1		1		
Diagnostic Radiology	3	3	2	1					
Emergency Medicine	10	10	5	3	2				
Neurology	1	1	1						
Other Specialty	1	1	1						
Physical Medicine and Rehabilitation	3	3	2		1				
Psychiatry	5	5	2	2	1				
Radiology	1	1	1						
Unspecified	13	13	8	3	2				
Inactive	4								
Not Classified	13								

Note: Excludes Address Unknown.

Subspecialties in this table are condensed into major specialties. See Appendix A.

Table 5.19

DOs by State, Self-Designated Specialty, and Activity, 2010, continued
Nevada

		Patient Care				Other Professional Activity			
				Hospital Based					
Specialty	Total Physicians	Total Patient Care	Office Based	Resid./ Fellows	Phys. Staff	Admin.	Med. Teach.	Research	Other
Total Physicians	608	530	389	90	51	5	5		1
FM/GP	154	150	124	9	17	3	1		
Family Medicine	119	116	96	9	11	2	1		
General Practice	35	34	28		6	1			
Medical Specialties	95	95	71	12	12				
Cardiovascular Disease	3	3	2		1				
Dermatology	13	13	8	4	1				
Gastroenterology	1	1	1						
Internal Medicine	63	63	50	4	9				
Pediatrics	15	15	10	4	1				
Surgical Specialties	51	49	41	4	4		2		
General Surgery	7	7	4	2	1				
Neurological Surgery	1	1	1						
Obstetrics & Gynecology	15	14	12	2			1		
Ophthalmology	8	8	7		1				
Orthopedic Surgery	11	10	8		2		1		
Otolaryngology	7	7	7						
Plastic Surgery	2	2	2						
Other Specialties	241	236	153	65	18	2	2		1
Aerospace Medicine	1								1
Anatomic/Clinical Pathology	3	3	3						
Anesthesiology	38	37	34	1	2		1		
Child & Adolescent Psychiatry	2	2	1	1					
Diagnostic Radiology	4	4	4						
Emergency Medicine	42	41	26	6	9		1		
Forensic Pathology	2	2	2						
General Preventive Medicine	1					1			
Neurology	5	5	5						
Occupational Medicine	3	3	3						
Other Specialty	2	2	2						
Physical Medicine and Rehabilitation	5	5	5						
Psychiatry	20	20	10	8	2				
Public Health and General Preventive Medicine	1					1			
Radiation Oncology	1	1			1				
Radiology	4	4	4						
Unspecified	107	107	54	49	4				
Inactive	28								
Not Classified	39								

Note: Excludes Address Unknown.

Subspecialties in this table are condensed into major specialties. See Appendix A.

Table 5.19

DOs by State, Self-Designated Specialty, and Activity, 2010, continued
New Hampshire

		Patient Care				Other Professional Activity			
				Hospital Based					
Specialty	Total Physicians	Total Patient Care	Office Based	Resid./ Fellows	Phys. Staff	Admin.	Med. Teach.	Research	Other
Total Physicians	275	243	195	12	36	3	1		1
FM/GP	84	83	69	2	12		1		
Family Medicine	82	81	67	2	12		1		
General Practice	2	2	2						
Medical Specialties	66	65	53	1	11	1			
Allergy and Immunology	2	2	2						
Cardiovascular Disease	2	2	2						
Dermatology	3	3	2		1				
Gastroenterology	2	2	2						
Internal Medicine	46	45	35	1	9	1			
Pediatrics	11	11	10		1				
Surgical Specialties	24	23	22		1	1			
General Surgery	3	3	3						
Obstetrics & Gynecology	6	6	6						
Ophthalmology	1	1	1						
Orthopedic Surgery	13	12	11		1	1			
Otolaryngology	1	1	1						
Other Specialties	74	72	51	9	12	1			1
Anatomic/Clinical Pathology	3	3	2		1				
Anesthesiology	14	14	11		3				
Child & Adolescent Psychiatry	1	1		1					
Diagnostic Radiology	2	2	2						
Emergency Medicine	10	10	7		3				
General Preventive Medicine	1	1		1					
Neurology	7	6	4	1	1				1
Physical Medicine and Rehabilitation	10	10	8	1	1				
Psychiatry	6	5	4	1		1			
Radiology	1	1		1					
Unspecified	19	19	13	3	3				
Inactive	10								
Not Classified	17								

Note: Excludes Address Unknown.

Subspecialties in this table are condensed into major specialties. See Appendix A.

Table 5.19

DOs by State, Self-Designated Specialty, and Activity, 2010, continued
New Jersey

		Patient Care				Other Professional Activity			
				Hospital Based					
Specialty	Total Physicians	Total Patient Care	Office Based	Resid./ Fellows	Phys. Staff	Admin.	Med. Teach.	Research	Other
Total Physicians	3,015	2,508	2,169	144	195	16	20	15	10
FM/GP	617	602	570	6	26	2	10		3
Family Medicine	527	513	483	6	24	1	10		3
General Practice	90	89	87		2	1			
Medical Specialties	789	773	670	47	56	2	3	10	1
Allergy and Immunology	7	7	7						
Cardiovascular Disease	75	71	60	9	2		1	3	
Dermatology	24	24	23		1				
Gastroenterology	43	42	38	4			1		
Internal Medicine	415	408	365	15	28	1	1	5	
Pediatrics	175	172	139	15	18	1		1	1
Pulmonary Disease	50	49	38	4	7			1	
Surgical Specialties	305	298	256	20	22	3	1	1	2
Colon and Rectal Surgery	2	2	2						
General Surgery	39	39	28	5	6				
Neurological Surgery	1	1			1				
Obstetrics & Gynecology	135	132	112	11	9	3			
Ophthalmology	21	21	21						
Orthopedic Surgery	58	56	48	3	5		1		1
Otolaryngology	22	22	21	1					
Plastic Surgery	10	10	9		1				
Thoracic Surgery	5	5	5						
Urology	12	10	10					1	1
Other Specialties	858	835	673	71	91	9	6	4	4
Aerospace Medicine	1	1	1						
Anatomic/Clinical Pathology	15	13	6	2	5	1			1
Anesthesiology	140	139	120	8	11			1	
Child & Adolescent Psychiatry	17	16	14	2			1		
Diagnostic Radiology	36	36	22	7	7				
Emergency Medicine	170	162	120	6	36	6	2		
Forensic Pathology	1	1	1						
General Preventive Medicine	3	3	2	1					
Medical Genetics	1	1	1						
Neurology	39	35	31	3	1			3	1
Nuclear Medicine	3	2			2	1			
Occupational Medicine	2	2	2						
Other Specialty	17	16	14		2		1		
Physical Medicine and Rehabilitation	74	74	63	7	4				
Psychiatry	62	60	49	3	8	1	1		
Radiation Oncology	4	4	4						
Radiology	30	29	19	3	7		1		
Unspecified	243	241	204	29	8				2
Inactive	211								
Not Classified	235								

Note: Excludes Address Unknown.

Subspecialties in this table are condensed into major specialties. See Appendix A.

Table 5.19

DOs by State, Self-Designated Specialty, and Activity, 2010, continued
New Mexico

		Patient Care				Other Professional Activity			
				Hospital Based					
Specialty	Total Physicians	Total Patient Care	Office Based	Resid./ Fellows	Phys. Staff	Admin.	Med. Teach.	Research	Other
Total Physicians	311	260	208	18	34	3	1	1	
FM/GP	106	104	91	1	12	2			
Family Medicine	86	84	73	1	10	2			
General Practice	20	20	18		2				
Medical Specialties	40	39	27	9	3			1	
Allergy and Immunology	1	1	1						
Cardiovascular Disease	2	2	1	1					
Dermatology	3	2	1	1				1	
Internal Medicine	25	25	16	7	2				
Pediatrics	8	8	7		1				
Pulmonary Disease	1	1	1						
Surgical Specialties	28	28	25	1	2				
General Surgery	7	7	6	1					
Obstetrics & Gynecology	6	6	6						
Ophthalmology	3	3	3						
Orthopedic Surgery	9	9	8		1				
Otolaryngology	1	1			1				
Urology	2	2	2						
Other Specialties	91	89	65	7	17	1	1		
Anatomic/Clinical Pathology	1	1			1				
Anesthesiology	12	12	10		2				
Child & Adolescent Psychiatry	4	4	3	1					
Diagnostic Radiology	5	5	4		1				
Emergency Medicine	13	13	7		6				
General Preventive Medicine	4	4	2	1	1				
Neurology	2	2	2						
Occupational Medicine	1	1	1						
Other Specialty	2	1			1	1			
Physical Medicine and Rehabilitation	8	8	7		1				
Psychiatry	11	10	5	5			1		
Radiation Oncology	1	1	1						
Radiology	2	2	1		1				
Unspecified	25	25	22		3				
Inactive	25								
Not Classified	21								

Note: Excludes Address Unknown.

Subspecialties in this table are condensed into major specialties. See Appendix A.

Table 5.19

DOs by State, Self-Designated Specialty, and Activity, 2010, continued
New York

Specialty	Total Physicians	Patient Care		Hospital Based		Other Professional Activity			
		Total Patient Care	Office Based	Resid./ Fellows	Phys. Staff	Admin.	Med. Teach.	Research	Other
Total Physicians	3,501	2,858	2,243	348	267	29	24	5	10
FM/GP	691	673	612	14	47	8	9		1
Family Medicine	621	606	551	14	41	7	7		1
General Practice	70	67	61		6	1	2		
Medical Specialties	967	948	743	140	65	8	4	3	4
Allergy and Immunology	12	11	10	1			1		
Cardiovascular Disease	54	54	36	16	2				
Dermatology	35	35	27	8					
Gastroenterology	33	33	28	5					
Internal Medicine	528	516	418	59	39	6	1	3	2
Pediatric Cardiology	2	2	1	1					
Pediatrics	257	251	185	43	23	2	2		2
Pulmonary Disease	46	46	38	7	1				
Surgical Specialties	273	267	218	29	20	2	4		
Colon and Rectal Surgery	1	1	1						
General Surgery	52	51	35	9	7	1			
Neurological Surgery	5	5	4	1					
Obstetrics & Gynecology	127	125	107	10	8	1	1		
Ophthalmology	14	13	12		1		1		
Orthopedic Surgery	51	49	40	5	4		2		
Otolaryngology	6	6	6						
Plastic Surgery	5	5	5						
Thoracic Surgery	2	2	1	1					
Urology	10	10	7	3					
Other Specialties	995	970	670	165	135	11	7	2	5
Anatomic/Clinical Pathology	23	22	14	4	4				1
Anesthesiology	144	142	113	15	14		1		1
Child & Adolescent Psychiatry	33	32	20	8	4			1	
Diagnostic Radiology	27	27	20	2	5				
Emergency Medicine	195	190	110	27	53	2	2		1
Forensic Pathology	1	1		1					
General Preventive Medicine	11	11	8	2	1				
Medical Genetics	2	2	1	1					
Neurology	68	66	49	11	6	1		1	
Nuclear Medicine	2	2	1		1				
Occupational Medicine	1	1	1						
Other Specialty	13	9	4	4	1	3	1		
Physical Medicine and Rehabilitation	134	131	97	21	13	2	1		
Psychiatry	95	90	55	18	17	3	2		
Public Health and General Preventive Medicine	3	3	2		1				
Radiation Oncology	3	3	2		1				
Radiology	20	19	12	2	5				1
Unspecified	220	219	161	49	9				1
Inactive	143								
Not Classified	432								

Note: Excludes Address Unknown.

Subspecialties in this table are condensed into major specialties. See Appendix A.

Table 5.19

DOs by State, Self-Designated Specialty, and Activity, 2010, continued
North Carolina

		Patient Care				Other Professional Activity			
				Hospital Based					
Specialty	Total Physicians	Total Patient Care	Office Based	Resid./ Fellows	Phys. Staff	Admin.	Med. Teach.	Research	Other
Total Physicians	949	813	586	108	119	5	3	4	1
FM/GP	261	257	188	29	40	1	2	1	
Family Medicine	253	249	182	29	38	1	2	1	
General Practice	8	8	6		2				
Medical Specialties	199	196	137	27	32	2		1	
Allergy and Immunology	1	1			1				
Cardiovascular Disease	13	13	10	1	2				
Dermatology	15	14	11		3	1			
Gastroenterology	4	4	3		1				
Internal Medicine	111	110	77	14	19			1	
Pediatrics	49	48	32	10	6	1			
Pulmonary Disease	6	6	4	2					
Surgical Specialties	83	83	61	11	11				
Colon and Rectal Surgery	1	1	1						
General Surgery	13	13	8	3	2				
Neurological Surgery	1	1	1						
Obstetrics & Gynecology	36	36	25	8	3				
Ophthalmology	5	5	5						
Orthopedic Surgery	14	14	11		3				
Otolaryngology	8	8	6		2				
Urology	5	5	4		1				
Other Specialties	283	277	200	41	36	2	1	2	1
Aerospace Medicine	2	1			1	1			
Anatomic/Clinical Pathology	3	3	2		1				
Anesthesiology	40	40	25	5	10				
Child & Adolescent Psychiatry	11	10	9		1	1			
Diagnostic Radiology	14	14	11	2	1				
Emergency Medicine	66	66	53	4	9				
General Preventive Medicine	5	5	4	1					
Neurology	15	14	11	2	1				1
Nuclear Medicine	1	1		1					
Occupational Medicine	2	2	1		1				
Other Specialty	6	4	2	2				2	
Physical Medicine and Rehabilitation	28	28	20	6	2				
Psychiatry	24	23	15	3	5		1		
Radiation Oncology	1	1		1					
Radiology	7	7	6	1					
Unspecified	58	58	41	13	4				
Inactive	29								
Not Classified	94								

Note: Excludes Address Unknown.

Subspecialties in this table are condensed into major specialties. See Appendix A.

Table 5.19

DOs by State, Self-Designated Specialty, and Activity, 2010, continued
North Dakota

		Patient Care				Other Professional Activity			
				Hospital Based					
Specialty	Total Physicians	Total Patient Care	Office Based	Resid./ Fellows	Phys. Staff	Admin.	Med. Teach.	Research	Other
Total Physicians	67	60	46	4	10				
FM/GP	20	20	14	1	5				
Family Medicine	18	18	12	1	5				
General Practice	2	2	2						
Medical Specialties	15	15	13	2					
Cardiovascular Disease	1	1	1						
Internal Medicine	10	10	8	2					
Pediatrics	4	4	4						
Surgical Specialties	8	8	6	1	1				
General Surgery	5	5	4		1				
Neurological Surgery	1	1	1						
Obstetrics & Gynecology	1	1		1					
Orthopedic Surgery	1	1	1						
Other Specialties	17	17	13		4				
Anesthesiology	4	4	3		1				
Child & Adolescent Psychiatry	1	1			1				
Emergency Medicine	4	4	3		1				
Occupational Medicine	1	1	1						
Physical Medicine and Rehabilitation	1	1	1						
Psychiatry	3	3	3						
Radiology	1	1	1						
Unspecified	2	2	1		1				
Inactive	2								
Not Classified	5								

Note: Excludes Address Unknown.

Subspecialties in this table are condensed into major specialties. See Appendix A.

Table 5.19

DOs by State, Self-Designated Specialty, and Activity, 2010, continued
Ohio

		Patient Care				Other Professional Activity			
				Hospital Based					
Specialty	Total Physicians	Total Patient Care	Office Based	Resid./ Fellows	Phys. Staff	Admin.	Med. Teach.	Research	Other
Total Physicians	4,644	3,785	2,787	721	277	22	42	10	5
FM/GP	998	967	869	39	59	8	20	1	2
Family Medicine	793	765	680	39	46	7	18	1	2
General Practice	205	202	189		13	1	2		
Medical Specialties	804	791	581	161	49	1	5	7	
Allergy and Immunology	7	6	5	1			1		
Cardiovascular Disease	57	56	46	5	5			1	
Dermatology	46	46	32	13	1				
Gastroenterology	28	27	21	3	3			1	
Internal Medicine	452	446	346	69	31	1	3	2	
Pediatrics	180	177	108	61	8		1	2	
Pulmonary Disease	34	33	23	9	1			1	
Surgical Specialties	479	471	377	57	37		7	1	
Colon and Rectal Surgery	5	5	3	2					
General Surgery	100	99	72	14	13		1		
Neurological Surgery	13	13	13						
Obstetrics & Gynecology	158	156	121	29	6		2		
Ophthalmology	37	36	33	1	2		1		
Orthopedic Surgery	102	99	85	4	10		3		
Otolaryngology	26	26	24		2				
Plastic Surgery	10	9	7	2				1	
Thoracic Surgery	10	10	7	2	1				
Urology	18	18	12	3	3				
Other Specialties	1,583	1,556	960	464	132	13	10	1	3
Aerospace Medicine	2	2	2						
Anatomic/Clinical Pathology	36	33	20	9	4	1	1		1
Anesthesiology	179	177	130	23	24	1	1		
Child & Adolescent Psychiatry	20	19	14	5			1		
Diagnostic Radiology	57	56	41	7	8		1		
Emergency Medicine	310	303	202	51	50	3	4		
Forensic Pathology	2	1	1						1
General Preventive Medicine	10	10	6	2	2				
Neurology	40	39	21	11	7			1	
Nuclear Medicine	5	5	5						
Occupational Medicine	15	12	8		4	3			
Other Specialty	22	20	11	8	1	1			1
Physical Medicine and Rehabilitation	43	43	35	6	2				
Psychiatry	102	100	64	28	8	1	1		
Public Health and General Preventive Medicine	1					1			
Radiation Oncology	2	2	2						
Radiology	30	30	25	2	3				
Unspecified	705	702	373	312	17	2	1		
Vascular Medicine	2	2			2				
Inactive	316								
Not Classified	464								

Note: Excludes Address Unknown.

Subspecialties in this table are condensed into major specialties. See Appendix A.

Table 5.19

DOs by State, Self-Designated Specialty, and Activity, 2010, continued
Oklahoma

		Patient Care				Other Professional Activity			
				Hospital Based					
Specialty	Total Physicians	Total Patient Care	Office Based	Resid./ Fellows	Phys. Staff	Admin.	Med. Teach.	Research	Other
Total Physicians	1,736	1,481	1,201	90	190	11	12	2	2
FM/GP	582	575	502	17	56	4	3		
Family Medicine	483	477	420	17	40	3	3		
General Practice	99	98	82		16	1			
Medical Specialties	222	212	170	23	19	3	6	1	
Cardiovascular Disease	8	8	8						
Dermatology	6	6	6						
Gastroenterology	12	12	9	1	2				
Internal Medicine	108	103	81	9	13	3	1	1	
Pediatrics	78	74	60	11	3		4		
Pulmonary Disease	10	9	6	2	1		1		
Surgical Specialties	164	162	138		24		2		
General Surgery	38	37	30		7		1		
Neurological Surgery	9	9	7		2				
Obstetrics & Gynecology	42	41	31		10		1		
Ophthalmology	17	17	17						
Orthopedic Surgery	40	40	37		3				
Otolaryngology	11	11	9		2				
Plastic Surgery	3	3	3						
Thoracic Surgery	1	1	1						
Urology	3	3	3						
Other Specialties	540	532	391	50	91	4	1	1	2
Aerospace Medicine	5	2	2			3			
Anatomic/Clinical Pathology	5	5	5						
Anesthesiology	78	78	62	7	9				
Child & Adolescent Psychiatry	3	3	3						
Diagnostic Radiology	26	25	14	4	7				1
Emergency Medicine	106	105	57	4	44		1		
Medical Genetics	1	1	1						
Neurology	9	9	8		1				
Nuclear Medicine	3	3	3						
Occupational Medicine	8	8	7		1				
Other Specialty	10	9	5	2	2			1	
Physical Medicine and Rehabilitation	10	9	6		3	1			
Psychiatry	37	37	28	6	3				
Public Health and General Preventive Medicine	1	1	1						
Radiation Oncology	1	1	1						
Radiology	9	9	7	1	1				
Unspecified	228	227	181	26	20				1
Inactive	109								
Not Classified	119								

Note: Excludes Address Unknown.

Subspecialties in this table are condensed into major specialties. See Appendix A.

Table 5.19

DOs by State, Self-Designated Specialty, and Activity, 2010, continued
Oregon

		Patient Care				Other Professional Activity			
				Hospital Based					
Specialty	Total Physicians	Total Patient Care	Office Based	Resid./ Fellows	Phys. Staff	Admin.	Med. Teach.	Research	Other
Total Physicians	748	641	525	56	60	4	5		2
FM/GP	238	234	212	3	19		3		1
Family Medicine	199	195	177	3	15		3		1
General Practice	39	39	35		4				
Medical Specialties	158	158	116	28	14				
Allergy and Immunology	2	2	2						
Cardiovascular Disease	4	4	3		1				
Dermatology	2	2	2						
Gastroenterology	4	4	3		1				
Internal Medicine	112	112	79	24	9				
Pediatric Cardiology	1	1		1					
Pediatrics	31	31	25	3	3				
Pulmonary Disease	2	2	2						
Surgical Specialties	60	59	52	1	6				1
General Surgery	10	10	7		3				
Neurological Surgery	1	1	1						
Obstetrics & Gynecology	20	19	18	1					1
Ophthalmology	5	5	5						
Orthopedic Surgery	19	19	16		3				
Otolaryngology	4	4	4						
Urology	1	1	1						
Other Specialties	196	190	145	24	21	4	2		
Aerospace Medicine	1	1			1				
Anatomic/Clinical Pathology	4	4	3		1				
Anesthesiology	26	26	22	3	1				
Child & Adolescent Psychiatry	3	3	3						
Diagnostic Radiology	7	7	7						
Emergency Medicine	39	37	27	1	9	1	1		
General Preventive Medicine	2	2	2						
Medical Genetics	1	1			1				
Neurology	9	9	8	1					
Other Specialty	8	5	4		1	2	1		
Physical Medicine and Rehabilitation	9	9	7	1	1				
Psychiatry	16	15	9	4	2	1			
Radiation Oncology	1	1	1						
Radiology	4	4	4						
Unspecified	66	66	48	14	4				
Inactive	58								
Not Classified	38								

Note: Excludes Address Unknown.

Subspecialties in this table are condensed into major specialties. See Appendix A.

Table 5.19

DOs by State, Self-Designated Specialty, and Activity, 2010, continued
Pennsylvania

		Patient Care				Other Professional Activity			
				Hospital Based					
Specialty	Total Physicians	Total Patient Care	Office Based	Resid./ Fellows	Phys. Staff	Admin.	Med. Teach.	Research	Other
Total Physicians	6,417	5,234	4,149	578	507	48	47	24	14
FM/GP	1,622	1,579	1,413	45	121	18	19	2	4
Family Medicine	1,381	1,340	1,183	45	112	16	19	2	4
General Practice	241	239	230		9	2			
Medical Specialties	1,366	1,334	1,049	179	106	8	14	9	1
Allergy and Immunology	11	11	9	2					
Cardiovascular Disease	110	108	86	13	9		1	1	
Dermatology	37	37	29	7	1				
Gastroenterology	75	74	62	11	1			1	
Internal Medicine	796	778	623	90	65	5	10	3	
Pediatric Cardiology	3	3		3					
Pediatrics	279	270	195	47	28	2	3	3	1
Pulmonary Disease	55	53	45	6	2	1		1	
Surgical Specialties	594	584	474	60	50	3	4	2	1
Colon and Rectal Surgery	6	6	4	1	1				
General Surgery	119	117	80	24	13		2		
Neurological Surgery	4	4	2		2				
Obstetrics & Gynecology	227	224	178	26	20	2		1	
Ophthalmology	47	47	45	2					
Orthopedic Surgery	99	98	88	2	8				1
Otolaryngology	45	43	40	2	1		2		
Plastic Surgery	12	11	8	1	2			1	
Thoracic Surgery	10	10	7	1	2				
Urology	25	24	22	1	1	1			
Other Specialties	1,785	1,737	1,213	294	230	19	10	11	8
Aerospace Medicine	3	3			3				
Anatomic/Clinical Pathology	30	29	16	5	8		1		
Anesthesiology	266	261	195	37	29	1	2	2	
Child & Adolescent Psychiatry	19	18	11	5	2	1			
Diagnostic Radiology	73	69	50	9	10		1		3
Emergency Medicine	349	345	193	54	98	2		1	1
Forensic Pathology	3	2	2			1			
General Preventive Medicine	11	9	9				1		1
Medical Genetics	1	1		1					
Neurology	63	62	44	11	7		1		
Nuclear Medicine	4	3	2		1			1	
Occupational Medicine	21	13	10		3	6	1	1	
Other Specialty	28	18	13	1	4	5	1	3	1
Physical Medicine and Rehabilitation	113	112	88	22	2	1			
Psychiatry	127	119	85	18	16	2	1	3	2
Public Health and General Preventive Medicine	2	2	2						
Radiation Oncology	10	10	8	1	1				
Radiology	49	48	35	3	10		1		
Unspecified	613	613	450	127	36				
Inactive	489								
Not Classified	561								

Note: Excludes Address Unknown.

Subspecialties in this table are condensed into major specialties. See Appendix A.

Table 5.19

DOs by State, Self-Designated Specialty, and Activity, 2010, continued
Puerto Rico

		Patient Care				Other Professional Activity			
				Hospital Based					
Specialty	Total Physicians	Total Patient Care	Office Based	Resid./ Fellows	Phys. Staff	Admin.	Med. Teach.	Research	Other
Total Physicians	2	1			1				
FM/GP	1	1			1				
Family Medicine	1	1			1				
Inactive	1								

Note: Excludes Address Unknown.

Subspecialties in this table are condensed into major specialties. See Appendix A.

Table 5.19

DOs by State, Self-Designated Specialty, and Activity, 2010, continued
Rhode Island

		Patient Care				Other Professional Activity			
				Hospital Based					
Specialty	Total Physicians	Total Patient Care	Office Based	Resid./ Fellows	Phys. Staff	Admin.	Med. Teach.	Research	Other
Total Physicians	247	202	154	25	23	2		2	
FM/GP	70	70	65	3	2				
Family Medicine	58	58	53	3	2				
General Practice	12	12	12						
Medical Specialties	61	59	49	3	7			2	
Cardiovascular Disease	3	3	3						
Dermatology	1	1	1						
Gastroenterology	5	5	4		1				
Internal Medicine	43	41	34	2	5			2	
Pediatrics	6	6	4	1	1				
Pulmonary Disease	3	3	3						
Surgical Specialties	9	9	8	1					
Obstetrics & Gynecology	5	5	5						
Otolaryngology	2	2	2						
Plastic Surgery	1	1	1						
Urology	1	1		1					
Other Specialties	66	64	32	18	14	2			
Anatomic/Clinical Pathology	2	2	2						
Anesthesiology	10	10	6		4				
Child & Adolescent Psychiatry	1	1	1						
Diagnostic Radiology	1					1			
Emergency Medicine	10	9	3	3	3	1			
Neurology	6	6	4	2					
Occupational Medicine	1	1	1						
Other Specialty	1	1			1				
Physical Medicine and Rehabilitation	3	3	3						
Psychiatry	12	12	7		5				
Unspecified	19	19	5	13	1				
Inactive	14								
Not Classified	27								

Note: Excludes Address Unknown.

Subspecialties in this table are condensed into major specialties. See Appendix A.

Table 5.19

DOs by State, Self-Designated Specialty, and Activity, 2010, continued
South Carolina

		Patient Care				Other Professional Activity			
				Hospital Based					
Specialty	Total Physicians	Total Patient Care	Office Based	Resid./ Fellows	Phys. Staff	Admin.	Med. Teach.	Research	Other
Total Physicians	534	468	336	70	62	4	3		
FM/GP	140	138	105	20	13	1	1		
Family Medicine	129	127	94	20	13	1	1		
General Practice	11	11	11						
Medical Specialties	121	120	94	16	10		1		
Allergy and Immunology	3	3	3						
Cardiovascular Disease	3	3	3						
Dermatology	1	1	1						
Gastroenterology	3	3	3						
Internal Medicine	82	82	63	11	8				
Pediatrics	21	20	15	4	1		1		
Pulmonary Disease	8	8	6	1	1				
Surgical Specialties	51	51	34	8	9				
Colon and Rectal Surgery	1	1	1						
General Surgery	9	9	6	3					
Obstetrics & Gynecology	23	23	14	4	5				
Ophthalmology	2	2	2						
Orthopedic Surgery	10	10	8		2				
Otolaryngology	2	2	1		1				
Plastic Surgery	1	1			1				
Thoracic Surgery	1	1		1					
Urology	2	2	2						
Other Specialties	163	159	103	26	30	3	1		
Aerospace Medicine	1	1	1						
Anatomic/Clinical Pathology	2	2		1	1				
Anesthesiology	18	18	13	2	3				
Child & Adolescent Psychiatry	3	3	2	1					
Diagnostic Radiology	9	8	6	1	1		1		
Emergency Medicine	47	46	25	3	18	1			
Neurology	13	13	10	3					
Other Specialty	5	4	1	3		1			
Physical Medicine and Rehabilitation	6	6	5		1				
Psychiatry	11	11	8	2	1				
Public Health and General Preventive Medicine	1					1			
Radiation Oncology	2	2	2						
Radiology	3	3	1	1	1				
Unspecified	41	41	28	9	4				
Vascular Medicine	1	1	1						
Inactive	21								
Not Classified	38								

Note: Excludes Address Unknown.

Subspecialties in this table are condensed into major specialties. See Appendix A.

Table 5.19

DOs by State, Self-Designated Specialty, and Activity, 2010, continued
South Dakota

Specialty	Total Physicians	Patient Care: Total Patient Care	Patient Care: Office Based	Hospital Based: Resid./Fellows	Hospital Based: Phys. Staff	Other Professional Activity: Admin.	Med. Teach.	Research	Other
Total Physicians	146	129	104	17	8	2			
FM/GP	47	45	35	6	4	2			
Family Medicine	43	41	31	6	4	2			
General Practice	4	4	4						
Medical Specialties	35	35	30	4	1				
Cardiovascular Disease	1	1	1						
Dermatology	2	2	2						
Gastroenterology	2	2	2						
Internal Medicine	23	23	18	4	1				
Pediatrics	5	5	5						
Pulmonary Disease	2	2	2						
Surgical Specialties	15	15	14		1				
General Surgery	3	3	3						
Obstetrics & Gynecology	5	5	4		1				
Orthopedic Surgery	3	3	3						
Otolaryngology	4	4	4						
Other Specialties	34	34	25	7	2				
Anatomic/Clinical Pathology	1	1		1					
Anesthesiology	2	2	2						
Child & Adolescent Psychiatry	1	1		1					
Diagnostic Radiology	1	1	1						
Emergency Medicine	5	5	4		1				
Neurology	3	3	3						
Physical Medicine and Rehabilitation	2	2	2						
Psychiatry	12	12	7	4	1				
Radiology	1	1	1						
Unspecified	6	6	5	1					
Inactive	9								
Not Classified	6								

Note: Excludes Address Unknown.

Subspecialties in this table are condensed into major specialties. See Appendix A.

Table 5.19

DOs by State, Self-Designated Specialty, and Activity, 2010, continued
Tennessee

		Patient Care				Other Professional Activity			
				Hospital Based					
Specialty	Total Physicians	Total Patient Care	Office Based	Resid./ Fellows	Phys. Staff	Admin.	Med. Teach.	Research	Other
Total Physicians	700	604	466	70	68	7	8		
FM/GP	225	217	185	13	19	4	4		
Family Medicine	185	177	147	13	17	4	4		
General Practice	40	40	38		2				
Medical Specialties	130	127	95	21	11	2	1		
Allergy and Immunology	2	2	2						
Cardiovascular Disease	4	4	4						
Dermatology	3	3	3						
Gastroenterology	5	4	3		1		1		
Internal Medicine	85	83	63	11	9	2			
Pediatrics	27	27	18	8	1				
Pulmonary Disease	4	4	2	2					
Surgical Specialties	79	78	60	10	8		1		
General Surgery	18	18	16	1	1				
Obstetrics & Gynecology	36	35	25	8	2		1		
Ophthalmology	3	3	1	1	1				
Orthopedic Surgery	17	17	14		3				
Otolaryngology	3	3	2		1				
Plastic Surgery	1	1	1						
Thoracic Surgery	1	1	1						
Other Specialties	185	182	126	26	30	1	2		
Aerospace Medicine	3	3			3				
Anatomic/Clinical Pathology	8	8	1	4	3				
Anesthesiology	30	30	22	3	5				
Child & Adolescent Psychiatry	2	2		2					
Diagnostic Radiology	6	6	5		1				
Emergency Medicine	44	42	29	2	11	1	1		
General Preventive Medicine	4	4	3		1				
Neurology	4	4	2	1	1				
Occupational Medicine	4	4	4						
Other Specialty	3	3	3						
Physical Medicine and Rehabilitation	10	9	9				1		
Psychiatry	19	19	9	9	1				
Radiation Oncology	1	1	1						
Radiology	2	2	1		1				
Unspecified	45	45	37	5	3				
Inactive	33								
Not Classified	48								

Note: Excludes Address Unknown.

Subspecialties in this table are condensed into major specialties. See Appendix A.

Table 5.19

DOs by State, Self-Designated Specialty, and Activity, 2010, continued
Texas

		Patient Care				Other Professional Activity			
				Hospital Based					
Specialty	Total Physicians	Total Patient Care	Office Based	Resid./ Fellows	Phys. Staff	Admin.	Med. Teach.	Research	Other
Total Physicians	4,158	3,523	2,745	479	299	34	30	11	4
FM/GP	1,289	1,265	1,083	89	93	10	12	1	1
Family Medicine	1,044	1,022	857	89	76	9	11	1	1
General Practice	245	243	226		17	1	1		
Medical Specialties	733	719	512	135	72	5	4	4	1
Allergy and Immunology	13	13	9	3	1				
Cardiovascular Disease	37	35	27	5	3	1		1	
Dermatology	28	28	20	7	1				
Gastroenterology	24	22	14	5	3	1		1	
Internal Medicine	398	390	282	67	41	3	3	1	1
Pediatric Cardiology	3	3	2	1					
Pediatrics	210	209	146	44	19		1		
Pulmonary Disease	20	19	12	3	4			1	
Surgical Specialties	376	371	300	50	21	3	1	1	
General Surgery	69	69	54	11	4				
Neurological Surgery	11	11	11						
Obstetrics & Gynecology	167	163	125	29	9	3	1		
Ophthalmology	15	15	13	1	1				
Orthopedic Surgery	72	71	61	5	5			1	
Otolaryngology	19	19	19						
Plastic Surgery	4	4	4						
Thoracic Surgery	7	7	4	3					
Urology	12	12	9	1	2				
Other Specialties	1,204	1,168	850	205	113	16	13	5	2
Aerospace Medicine	16	14	8		6	1		1	
Anatomic/Clinical Pathology	50	47	23	19	5	1	2		
Anesthesiology	179	179	134	18	27				
Child & Adolescent Psychiatry	17	16	13	2	1		1		
Diagnostic Radiology	53	52	36	13	3		1		
Emergency Medicine	236	221	166	26	29	9	4	2	
Forensic Pathology	3	3	2		1				
General Preventive Medicine	16	15	12	1	2			1	
Neurology	37	37	25	9	3				
Nuclear Medicine	3	3	2		1				
Occupational Medicine	14	9	7		2	2	2		1
Other Specialty	19	18	14	1	3		1		
Physical Medicine and Rehabilitation	79	78	56	16	6		1		
Psychiatry	106	104	66	29	9	2			
Public Health and General Preventive Medicine	2	2	1		1				
Radiation Oncology	4	4	3		1				
Radiology	27	27	25	1	1				
Unspecified	343	339	257	70	12	1	1	1	1
Inactive	239								
Not Classified	317								

Note: Excludes Address Unknown.

Subspecialties in this table are condensed into major specialties. See Appendix A.

Table 5.19

DOs by State, Self-Designated Specialty, and Activity, 2010, continued
Utah

		Patient Care				Other Professional Activity			
				Hospital Based					
Specialty	Total Physicians	Total Patient Care	Office Based	Resid./ Fellows	Phys. Staff	Admin.	Med. Teach.	Research	Other
Total Physicians	359	330	264	29	37				
FM/GP	134	134	113	9	12				
Family Medicine	128	128	107	9	12				
General Practice	6	6	6						
Medical Specialties	43	43	31	5	7				
Allergy and Immunology	2	2	2						
Cardiovascular Disease	2	2			2				
Dermatology	3	3	3						
Internal Medicine	17	17	11	2	4				
Pediatric Cardiology	1	1		1					
Pediatrics	17	17	14	2	1				
Pulmonary Disease	1	1	1						
Surgical Specialties	34	34	29		5				
General Surgery	5	5	4		1				
Obstetrics & Gynecology	20	20	17		3				
Ophthalmology	1	1			1				
Orthopedic Surgery	7	7	7						
Otolaryngology	1	1	1						
Other Specialties	119	119	91	15	13				
Aerospace Medicine	2	2	2						
Anesthesiology	21	21	18	2	1				
Child & Adolescent Psychiatry	3	3	2	1					
Diagnostic Radiology	1	1	1						
Emergency Medicine	21	21	15		6				
Neurology	3	3	1	1	1				
Other Specialty	2	2	2						
Physical Medicine and Rehabilitation	19	19	14	4	1				
Psychiatry	15	15	11	3	1				
Radiology	2	2	1		1				
Unspecified	30	30	24	4	2				
Inactive	9								
Not Classified	20								

Note: Excludes Address Unknown.

Subspecialties in this table are condensed into major specialties. See Appendix A.

Table 5.19

DOs by State, Self-Designated Specialty, and Activity, 2010, continued
Vermont

		Patient Care				Other Professional Activity			
				Hospital Based					
Specialty	Total Physicians	Total Patient Care	Office Based	Resid./ Fellows	Phys. Staff	Admin.	Med. Teach.	Research	Other
Total Physicians	77	59	45	6	8		1	1	
FM/GP	21	20	15		5		1		
Family Medicine	16	15	12		3		1		
General Practice	5	5	3		2				
Medical Specialties	10	9	8	1				1	
Cardiovascular Disease	1	1	1						
Internal Medicine	7	6	5	1				1	
Pediatrics	2	2	2						
Surgical Specialties	10	10	8	1	1				
General Surgery	2	2	1	1					
Obstetrics & Gynecology	3	3	2		1				
Ophthalmology	1	1	1						
Orthopedic Surgery	3	3	3						
Urology	1	1	1						
Other Specialties	20	20	14	4	2				
Anatomic/Clinical Pathology	1	1		1					
Anesthesiology	3	3	2	1					
Diagnostic Radiology	1	1			1				
Emergency Medicine	2	2	1		1				
Other Specialty	1	1	1						
Physical Medicine and Rehabilitation	1	1	1						
Psychiatry	3	3	1	2					
Radiology	1	1	1						
Unspecified	7	7	7						
Inactive	9								
Not Classified	7								

Note: Excludes Address Unknown.

Subspecialties in this table are condensed into major specialties. See Appendix A.

Table 5.19

DOs by State, Self-Designated Specialty, and Activity, 2010, continued
Virginia

		Patient Care				Other Professional Activity			
				Hospital Based					
Specialty	Total Physicians	Total Patient Care	Office Based	Resid./ Fellows	Phys. Staff	Admin.	Med. Teach.	Research	Other
Total Physicians	1,006	882	603	136	143	10	10		4
FM/GP	241	233	176	20	37	1	5		2
Family Medicine	223	216	161	20	35	1	4		2
General Practice	18	17	15		2		1		
Medical Specialties	213	210	150	35	25	1	2		
Cardiovascular Disease	10	10	7	1	2				
Dermatology	17	17	14	1	2				
Gastroenterology	5	5	3	1	1				
Internal Medicine	122	120	84	22	14	1	1		
Pediatric Cardiology	3	3	1	2					
Pediatrics	48	47	34	8	5		1		
Pulmonary Disease	8	8	7		1				
Surgical Specialties	85	85	61	8	16				
Colon and Rectal Surgery	2	2	1		1				
General Surgery	23	23	17	3	3				
Neurological Surgery	1	1	1						
Obstetrics & Gynecology	34	34	22	5	7				
Ophthalmology	3	3	3						
Orthopedic Surgery	17	17	14		3				
Otolaryngology	4	4	2		2				
Urology	1	1	1						
Other Specialties	367	354	216	73	65	8	3		2
Aerospace Medicine	6	3			3	2	1		
Anatomic/Clinical Pathology	11	9	1	2	6	1			1
Anesthesiology	49	49	33	3	13				
Child & Adolescent Psychiatry	2	2	1	1					
Diagnostic Radiology	11	11	8	1	2				
Emergency Medicine	77	73	42	12	19	2	2		
Forensic Pathology	1	1	1						
General Preventive Medicine	11	10	4		6	1			
Neurology	16	16	12	3	1				
Nuclear Medicine	2	2	2						
Occupational Medicine	6	5	4		1	1			
Other Specialty	13	12	9		3	1			
Physical Medicine and Rehabilitation	37	37	24	11	2				
Psychiatry	27	27	15	7	5				
Public Health and General Preventive Medicine	1								1
Radiation Oncology	2	2	1	1					
Radiology	5	5	4	1					
Unspecified	90	90	55	31	4				
Inactive	29								
Not Classified	71								

Note: Excludes Address Unknown.

Subspecialties in this table are condensed into major specialties. See Appendix A.

Table 5.19

DOs by State, Self-Designated Specialty, and Activity, 2010, continued
Virgin Islands

		Patient Care				Other Professional Activity			
				Hospital Based					
Specialty	Total Physicians	Total Patient Care	Office Based	Resid./ Fellows	Phys. Staff	Admin.	Med. Teach.	Research	Other
Total Physicians	4	4	4						
FM/GP	1	1	1						
Family Medicine	1	1	1						
Medical Specialties	2	2	2						
Internal Medicine	2	2	2						
Other Specialties	1	1	1						
Emergency Medicine	1	1	1						

Note: Excludes Address Unknown.

Subspecialties in this table are condensed into major specialties. See Appendix A.

Table 5.19

DOs by State, Self-Designated Specialty, and Activity, 2010, continued
Washington

		Patient Care				Other Professional Activity			
				Hospital Based					
Specialty	Total Physicians	Total Patient Care	Office Based	Resid./ Fellows	Phys. Staff	Admin.	Med. Teach.	Research	Other
Total Physicians	1,035	903	725	98	80	6	4		2
FM/GP	375	370	313	32	25	2	2		1
Family Medicine	321	317	264	32	21	1	2		1
General Practice	54	53	49		4	1			
Medical Specialties	124	124	96	14	14				
Allergy and Immunology	2	2	2						
Cardiovascular Disease	5	5	5						
Dermatology	5	5	4		1				
Gastroenterology	4	4	4						
Internal Medicine	78	78	55	11	12				
Pediatrics	27	27	23	3	1				
Pulmonary Disease	3	3	3						
Surgical Specialties	109	109	98	7	4				
Colon and Rectal Surgery	1	1	1						
General Surgery	15	15	12	2	1				
Neurological Surgery	1	1	1						
Obstetrics & Gynecology	38	38	34	3	1				
Ophthalmology	7	7	7						
Orthopedic Surgery	32	32	30	2					
Otolaryngology	9	9	8		1				
Plastic Surgery	2	2	2						
Urology	4	4	3		1				
Other Specialties	307	300	218	45	37	4	2		1
Aerospace Medicine	3	3	2		1				
Anatomic/Clinical Pathology	8	7	5	2					1
Anesthesiology	53	53	35	11	7				
Child & Adolescent Psychiatry	4	4	4						
Diagnostic Radiology	21	21	12	8	1				
Emergency Medicine	55	54	39	2	13	1			
Forensic Pathology	1	1			1				
General Preventive Medicine	4	2	2			2			
Medical Genetics	1	1	1						
Neurology	12	11	8	2	1		1		
Nuclear Medicine	2	2	1		1				
Occupational Medicine	4	4	3		1				
Other Specialty	9	8	4	1	3		1		
Physical Medicine and Rehabilitation	17	17	13	3	1				
Psychiatry	20	20	17	2	1				
Public Health and General Preventive Medicine	1					1			
Radiation Oncology	1	1	1						
Radiology	7	7	3	3	1				
Unspecified	84	84	68	11	5				
Inactive	63								
Not Classified	57								

Note: Excludes Address Unknown.

Subspecialties in this table are condensed into major specialties. See Appendix A.

Table 5.19

DOs by State, Self-Designated Specialty, and Activity, 2010, continued
West Virginia

		Patient Care				Other Professional Activity			
				Hospital Based					
Specialty	Total Physicians	Total Patient Care	Office Based	Resid./ Fellows	Phys. Staff	Admin.	Med. Teach.	Research	Other
Total Physicians	768	650	532	52	66	3	8		1
FM/GP	302	298	264	6	28	1	3		
Family Medicine	234	231	201	6	24		3		
General Practice	68	67	63		4	1			
Medical Specialties	117	115	100	9	6		2		
Cardiovascular Disease	5	5	5						
Dermatology	5	5	5						
Gastroenterology	3	3	2		1				
Internal Medicine	66	65	57	4	4		1		
Pediatrics	34	33	28	4	1		1		
Pulmonary Disease	4	4	3	1					
Surgical Specialties	62	61	40	11	10	1			
Colon and Rectal Surgery	1	1	1						
General Surgery	17	16	11	2	3	1			
Neurological Surgery	1	1			1				
Obstetrics & Gynecology	22	22	13	7	2				
Ophthalmology	2	2	2						
Orthopedic Surgery	14	14	10		4				
Otolaryngology	2	2	2						
Urology	3	3	1	2					
Other Specialties	181	176	128	26	22	1	3		1
Anatomic/Clinical Pathology	2	1	1				1		
Anesthesiology	22	21	18	1	2	1			
Child & Adolescent Psychiatry	1	1	1						
Diagnostic Radiology	5	4	3		1				1
Emergency Medicine	49	49	35	2	12				
General Preventive Medicine	2	2	1	1					
Occupational Medicine	1						1		
Other Specialty	4	3	3				1		
Physical Medicine and Rehabilitation	3	3	2	1					
Psychiatry	17	17	14	2	1				
Radiation Oncology	4	4	2		2				
Radiology	2	2	1		1				
Unspecified	69	69	47	19	3				
Inactive	28								
Not Classified	78								

Note: Excludes Address Unknown.

Subspecialties in this table are condensed into major specialties. See Appendix A.

Table 5.19

DOs by State, Self-Designated Specialty, and Activity, 2010, continued
Wisconsin

		Patient Care				Other Professional Activity			
				Hospital Based					
Specialty	Total Physicians	Total Patient Care	Office Based	Resid./ Fellows	Phys. Staff	Admin.	Med. Teach.	Research	Other
Total Physicians	940	838	663	110	65	6	1	2	2
FM/GP	328	324	275	33	16	3			1
Family Medicine	291	288	241	33	14	2			1
General Practice	37	36	34		2	1			
Medical Specialties	185	182	139	33	10	1	1	1	
Allergy and Immunology	4	4	4						
Cardiovascular Disease	16	16	10	6					
Dermatology	5	5	3	1	1				
Gastroenterology	5	5	3	1	1				
Internal Medicine	98	97	70	20	7	1			
Pediatrics	53	51	46	4	1		1	1	
Pulmonary Disease	4	4	3	1					
Surgical Specialties	92	90	76	7	7	1		1	
General Surgery	15	15	9	3	3				
Neurological Surgery	1	1	1						
Obstetrics & Gynecology	42	42	36	3	3				
Ophthalmology	9	8	8					1	
Orthopedic Surgery	15	15	13	1	1				
Otolaryngology	5	5	5						
Plastic Surgery	1					1			
Thoracic Surgery	3	3	3						
Urology	1	1	1						
Other Specialties	244	242	173	37	32	1			1
Anatomic/Clinical Pathology	6	5	4	1					1
Anesthesiology	36	36	25	7	4				
Child & Adolescent Psychiatry	3	3	1	1	1				
Diagnostic Radiology	12	12	9	1	2				
Emergency Medicine	46	46	31	2	13				
General Preventive Medicine	1	1	1						
Neurology	17	17	11	5	1				
Nuclear Medicine	1	1	1						
Occupational Medicine	5	5	5						
Other Specialty	6	5	4	1		1			
Physical Medicine and Rehabilitation	25	25	12	9	4				
Psychiatry	21	21	17	2	2				
Radiation Oncology	1	1	1						
Radiology	8	8	5	2	1				
Unspecified	56	56	46	6	4				
Inactive	39								
Not Classified	52								

Note: Excludes Address Unknown.

Subspecialties in this table are condensed into major specialties. See Appendix A.

Table 5.19

DOs by State, Self-Designated Specialty, and Activity, 2010, continued
Wyoming

		Patient Care				Other Professional Activity			
				Hospital Based					
Specialty	Total Physicians	Total Patient Care	Office Based	Resid./ Fellows	Phys. Staff	Admin.	Med. Teach.	Research	Other
Total Physicians	98	82	59	9	14		2		
FM/GP	34	32	21	8	3		2		
Family Medicine	32	30	19	8	3		2		
General Practice	2	2	2						
Medical Specialties	8	8	5	1	2				
Cardiovascular Disease	1	1			1				
Dermatology	1	1		1					
Internal Medicine	4	4	3		1				
Pediatrics	2	2	2						
Surgical Specialties	11	11	10		1				
General Surgery	1	1	1						
Obstetrics & Gynecology	3	3	3						
Ophthalmology	1	1	1						
Orthopedic Surgery	3	3	3						
Plastic Surgery	1	1	1						
Thoracic Surgery	1	1			1				
Urology	1	1	1						
Other Specialties	31	31	23		8				
Anesthesiology	8	8	7		1				
Diagnostic Radiology	4	4	4						
Emergency Medicine	9	9	5		4				
Other Specialty	1	1	1						
Physical Medicine and Rehabilitation	1	1	1						
Psychiatry	3	3	2		1				
Unspecified	5	5	3		2				
Inactive	5								
Not Classified	9								

Note: Excludes Address Unknown.

Subspecialties in this table are condensed into major specialties. See Appendix A.

Table 5.19

DOs by State, Self-Designated Specialty, and Activity, 2010, continued
Pacific Islands

		Patient Care				Other Professional Activity			
				Hospital Based					
Specialty	Total Physicians	Total Patient Care	Office Based	Resid./ Fellows	Phys. Staff	Admin.	Med. Teach.	Research	Other
Total Physicians	12	7	5	1	1				
FM/GP	5	5	4		1				
Family Medicine	4	4	3		1				
General Practice	1	1	1						
Other Specialties	2	2	1	1					
Anesthesiology	1	1		1					
Psychiatry	1	1	1						
Inactive	1								
Not Classified	4								

Note: Excludes Address Unknown.

Subspecialties in this table are condensed into major specialties. See Appendix A.

Table 5.20

DOs by Metropolitan Statistical Area, 2010

		Major Professional Activity								
		Patient Care								
			Office-Based Practice							
Metropolitan Statistical Area	Total Physicians	Total Patient Care	FM/GP Practice	Medical Specialties	Surgical Specialties	Other Specialties	Hospital Based Practice	Other Professional Activity	Inactive	Not Classified
Total Metropolitan Physicians	56,925	47,576	12,350	8,507	4,182	11,947	10,590	1,066	3,424	4,859
Abilene, TX	35	34	13	4	5	12				1
Akron, OH	420	346	78	52	34	80	102	7	29	38
Albany-Schenectady-Troy, NY	169	142	46	35	6	28	27	3	5	19
Albany, GA	25	23	5	6	1	5	6			2
Albuquerque, NM	152	120	40	12	9	32	27	4	12	16
Alexandria, LA	4	4				3	1			
Allentown-Bethlehem-Easton, PA-NJ	522	435	118	102	42	93	80	11	35	41
Altoona, PA	63	57	20	10	5	8	14		1	5
Amarillo, TX	29	25	9	7	2	4	3	1	3	
Ames, IA	18	17	8		2	4	3		1	
Anchorage, AK	97	87	23	18	5	21	20	4	2	4
Anderson, IN	4	3	1			2			1	
Anderson, SC	10	9	5			3	1	1		
Ann Arbor, MI	113	96	17	12	5	30	32	3	3	11
Anniston-Oxford, AL	8	8	4	1	1		2			
Appleton, WI	31	29	13	4	1	7	4		1	1
Asheville, NC	75	63	16	13	4	13	17		5	7
Athens-Clarke County, GA	14	13	3	4	1	5				1
Atlanta-Sandy Springs-Marietta, GA	387	315	106	52	33	80	44	13	29	30
Atlantic City-Hammonton, NJ	161	138	26	53	9	35	15	2	17	4
Auburn-Opelika, AL	9	9	3	2		4				
Augusta-Richmond County, GA-SC	132	112	18	17	6	21	50	2	4	14
Austin-Round Rock-San Marcos, TX	263	222	66	52	16	50	38	3	12	26
Bakersfield-Delano, CA	70	60	14	8	7	21	10	2	5	3
Baltimore-Towson, MD	343	276	40	73	18	73	72	7	4	56
Bangor, ME	78	67	31	7	2	10	17		3	8
Barnstable Town, MA	42	35	9	15	2	7	2	2	2	3
Baton Rouge, LA	23	17	2	2	1	3	9		2	4
Battle Creek, MI	38	31	13	3	5	4	6	2	4	1
Bay City, MI	56	44	20	3	2	13	6	1	6	5
Beaumont-Port Arthur, TX	47	43	22	5	2	11	3	1	1	2
Bellingham, WA	21	18	4	4	4	6			2	1
Bend, OR	36	31	10	10	3	5	3		3	2
Billings, MT	30	29	5	5	2	11	6			1
Binghamton, NY	54	48	19	7	3	8	11	2	1	3
Birmingham-Hoover, AL	104	88	22	16	6	20	24	5	1	10
Bismarck, ND	15	15	3	6		3	3			
Blacksburg-Christiansburg-Radford, VA	50	43	8	8	2	11	14	4	1	2
Bloomington-Normal, IL	41	28	5	8	1	9	5	1	2	10
Bloomington, IN	15	14	5	4	1	2	2	1		
Boise City-Nampa, ID	95	87	32	15	2	27	11	3	3	2
Boston-Cambridge-Quincy, MA-NH	489	414	80	98	28	81	127	6	12	57
Boulder, CO	72	64	22	7	6	24	5		6	2
Bowling Green, KY	10	8	1		1	4	2		1	1
Bremerton-Silverdale, WA	44	39	12	2	3	9	13		1	4
Bridgeport-Stamford-Norwalk, CT	119	104	13	38	13	28	12	3	4	8
Brownsville-Harlingen, TX	29	26	7	3	4	7	5		1	2

Table 5.20

DOs by Metropolitan Statistical Area, 2010, continued

		Major Professional Activity									
		Patient Care									
			Office-Based Practice								
Metropolitan Statistical Area	Total Physicians	Total Patient Care	FM/GP Practice	Medical Specialties	Surgical Specialties	Other Specialties	Hospital Based Practice	Other Professional Activity	Inactive	Not Classified
Brunswick, GA	15	13	4		2	6	1		1	1
Buffalo-Niagara Falls, NY	183	156	37	34	12	41	32	5	7	15
Burlington-South Burlington, VT	28	20	6	1	3	3	7	1	1	6
Canton-Massillon, OH	201	161	30	32	20	45	34	4	16	20
Cape Coral-Fort Myers, FL	204	170	61	37	25	35	12	2	26	6
Cape Girardeau-Jackson, MO-IL	51	46	8	6	7	19	6		2	3
Carson City, NV	12	11	3	3		4	1		1	
Casper, WY	15	12	2		1	2	7	1		2
Cedar Rapids, IA	39	38	14	6	2	10	6		1	
Champaign-Urbana, IL	36	33	13	4	2	5	9	3		
Charleston-North Charleston-Summerville, SC	117	102	15	24	3	28	32	3	2	10
Charleston, WV	153	127	46	31	6	22	22	2	6	18
Charlotte-Gastonia-Rock Hill, NC-SC	169	155	36	36	13	40	30	1	2	11
Charlottesville, VA	27	26	6	3	3	7	7	1		
Chattanooga, TN-GA	91	80	22	15	9	18	16	3	4	4
Cheyenne, WY	23	20	6		2	7	5	1		2
Chicago-Joliet-Naperville, IL-IN-WI	2,151	1,787	423	341	160	419	444	50	58	256
Chico, CA	24	21	9	4	2	3	3		1	2
Cincinnati-Middletown, OH-KY-IN	353	306	71	42	21	70	102	3	17	27
Clarksville, TN-KY	40	36	10	6	3	6	11	1		3
Cleveland-Elyria-Mentor, OH	831	664	107	109	23	163	262	10	47	110
Cleveland, TN	22	20	4		4	7	5	1	1	
Coeur d'Alene, ID	18	15	5	2	2	5	1		2	1
College Station-Bryan, TX	33	28	12	3		8	5		1	4
Colorado Springs, CO	201	177	59	24	11	55	28	7	8	9
Columbia, MO	90	77	9	12	6	16	34	1	5	7
Columbia, SC	55	49	7	15	2	6	19			6
Columbus, GA-AL	81	57	21	4	9	9	14	7	3	14
Columbus, IN	4	4	1		2		1			
Columbus, OH	978	786	174	125	84	211	192	18	57	117
Corpus Christi, TX	105	85	25	7	6	16	31	3	10	7
Corvallis, OR	35	31	6	2	4	9	10		1	3
Crestview-Fort Walton Beach-Destin, FL	50	35	7	4	8	11	5	3	3	9
Cumberland, MD-WV	9	9	3	2	2	2				
Dallas-Fort Worth-Arlington, TX	1,672	1,424	437	232	135	374	246	39	107	102
Dalton, GA	5	5	2	1		2				
Danville, IL	5	4	1			2	1			1
Danville, VA	11	10	1	1	3	3	2		1	
Davenport-Moline-Rock Island, IA-IL	110	92	30	11	5	31	15		10	8
Dayton, OH	533	426	75	54	60	109	128	10	44	53
Decatur, AL	6	6	2	2		1	1			
Decatur, IL	11	9	1	3	2	1	2		1	1
Deltona-Daytona Beach-Ormond Beach, FL	111	83	32	12	7	24	8	2	23	3
Denver-Aurora-Broomfield, CO	531	454	175	66	33	121	59	10	43	24
Des Moines-West Des Moines, IA	568	504	166	98	38	96	106	15	32	17

Table 5.20

DOs by Metropolitan Statistical Area, 2010, continued

		Major Professional Activity								
		Patient Care								
			Office-Based Practice							
Metropolitan Statistical Area	Total Physicians	Total Patient Care	FM/GP Practice	Medical Specialties	Surgical Specialties	Other Specialties	Hospital Based Practice	Other Professional Activity	Inactive	Not Classified
Detroit-Warren-Livonia, MI	2,863	2,313	479	375	237	680	542	50	264	236
Dothan, AL	20	19	5	2	2	9	1		1	
Dover, DE	38	36	13	10	2	9	2		1	1
Dubuque, IA	16	14	5	6	2		1		1	1
Duluth, MN-WI	39	33	6	5	5	7	10		3	3
Durham-Chapel Hill, NC	61	43	6	3	1	12	21	2	1	15
Eau Claire, WI	35	30	12	3	1	7	7	1	2	2
El Centro, CA	3	2				2				1
El Paso, TX	105	88	16	11	14	19	28	1	3	13
Elizabethtown, KY	14	13	3	1	3	2	4	1		
Elkhart-Goshen, IN	28	27	8	1	4	9	5		1	
Elmira, NY	18	18	5	5	1	2	5			
Erie, PA	294	231	77	26	23	52	53	7	19	37
Eugene-Springfield, OR	37	33	9	4	1	12	7	1	3	
Evansville, IN-KY	65	60	22	6	8	11	13		1	4
Fairbanks, AK	27	25	9		4	4	8			2
Fargo, ND-MN	17	16	3	3		4	6		1	
Farmington, NM	23	19	5	1	2	7	4	1	2	1
Fayetteville-Springdale-Rogers, AR-MO	60	54	21	8	7	7	11		4	2
Fayetteville, NC	73	59	14	6	5	11	23	3	1	10
Flagstaff, AZ	35	28	5	5	4	8	6	1	2	4
Flint, MI	320	262	84	29	35	56	58	3	28	27
Florence-Muscle Shoals, AL	24	20	6	2	4	6	2		1	3
Florence, SC	10	10	4			1	5			
Fond du Lac, WI	13	10	5	1		4			1	2
Fort Collins-Loveland, CO	75	70	19	10	5	24	12	1	1	3
Fort Smith, AR-OK	83	75	33	10	10	16	6		4	4
Fort Wayne, IN	67	64	23	10	2	16	13	1		2
Fresno, CA	103	83	15	15	2	22	29		8	12
Gadsden, AL	14	13	4	1	2	6			1	
Gainesville, FL	70	59	10	5	3	11	30		1	10
Gainesville, GA	9	8	4	1		1	2		1	
Glens Falls, NY	15	15	7	3	1	3	1			
Goldsboro, NC	16	14	4	1	4	4	1			2
Grand Forks, ND-MN	7	7	1	2	2	2				
Grand Junction, CO	96	85	26	13	11	20	15		10	1
Grand Rapids-Wyoming, MI	400	343	84	41	45	117	56	6	30	21
Great Falls, MT	24	23	5	4	6	5	3			1
Greeley, CO	34	32	12	10	1	4	5	1	1	
Green Bay, WI	55	51	13	15	5	14	4		3	1
Greensboro-High Point, NC	41	35	11	11	1	6	6	1	1	4
Greenville-Mauldin-Easley, SC	84	73	12	15	10	15	21		5	6
Greenville, NC	42	39	3	6	1	9	20		1	2
Gulfport-Biloxi, MS	66	49	4	9	6	11	19	4	5	8
Hagerstown-Martinsburg, MD-WV	32	27	5	2	4	14	2		2	3
Hanford-Corcoran, CA	15	9	1		4	2	2			6
Harrisburg-Carlisle, PA	342	281	57	50	32	69	73	8	25	28
Harrisonburg, VA	13	12	3	3	1	5			1	
Hartford-West Hartford-East Hartford, CT	207	176	25	43	19	44	45	4	6	21
Hattiesburg, MS	30	30	9	5	3	6	7			
Hickory-Lenoir-Morganton, NC	28	24	7	2	1	5	9		3	1
Hinesville-Fort Stewart, GA	4	3	2				1			1

Table 5.20

DOs by Metropolitan Statistical Area, 2010, continued

		Major Professional Activity									
		Patient Care									
			Office-Based Practice								
Metropolitan Statistical Area	Total Physicians	Total Patient Care	FM/GP Practice	Medical Specialties	Surgical Specialties	Other Specialties	Hospital Based Practice	Other Professional Activity	Inactive	Not Classified
Holland-Grand Haven, MI	100	84	27	11	10	28	8	4	9	3
Honolulu, HI	158	131	21	25	5	28	52	4	8	15
Hot Springs, AR	18	15	6			7	2	1	2	
Houma-Bayou Cane-Thibodaux, LA	4	2	1			1			2	
Houston-Sugar Land-Baytown, TX	591	481	152	53	41	120	115	10	32	68
Huntington-Ashland, WV-KY-OH	96	80	28	14	9	18	11	1	3	12
Huntsville, AL	42	39	15	3	3	14	4	1	1	1
Idaho Falls, ID	37	32	10	8	6	7	1		2	3
Indianapolis-Carmel, IN	281	242	52	41	29	48	72	5	15	19
Iowa City, IA	88	77	9	5	3	10	50		6	5
Ithaca, NY	12	12	2	3		5	2			
Jackson, MI	43	38	14	6	3	9	6		4	1
Jackson, MS	70	61	14	5	6	4	32		1	8
Jackson, TN	18	17	6	5	2	4				1
Jacksonville, FL	315	273	73	39	16	60	85	13	12	17
Jacksonville, NC	38	27	8	4	1	2	12	1		10
Janesville, WI	17	15	7	1	2	4	1		1	1
Jefferson City, MO	96	83	22	12	11	25	13	3	9	1
Johnson City, TN	51	44	9	5	3	13	14		3	4
Johnstown, PA	43	40	19	3	2	6	10	1		2
Jonesboro, AR	23	21	10	3	1	5	2			2
Joplin, MO	134	112	22	16	14	22	38		10	12
Kalamazoo-Portage, MI	115	101	22	26	6	30	17	3	5	6
Kankakee-Bradley, IL	17	16	2	5	1	2	6	1		
Kansas City, MO-KS	888	739	192	112	49	159	227	13	61	75
Kennewick-Pasco-Richland, WA	52	50	16	7	6	15	6		1	1
Killeen-Temple-Fort Hood, TX	147	131	26	21	4	27	53	1	1	14
Kingsport-Bristol-Bristol, TN-VA	54	50	16	10	8	9	7		1	3
Kingston, NY	24	23	11	5	1	3	3		1	
Knoxville, TN	103	95	17	29	8	23	18	1	3	4
Kokomo, IN	6	5	4			1				1
La Crosse, WI-MN	31	28	7	9		3	9		1	2
Lafayette, IN	20	19	5	1	1	6	6			1
Lafayette, LA	7	7		2	1	3	1			
Lake Charles, LA	7	6			2	2	2		1	
Lake Havasu City-Kingman, AZ	79	62	18	7	6	10	21	1	3	13
Lakeland-Winter Haven, FL	60	53	10	10	10	19	4		3	4
Lancaster, PA	245	192	61	35	31	34	31	3	32	18
Lansing-East Lansing, MI	537	432	90	56	51	161	74	22	40	43
Laredo, TX	9	9	2	1	4	1	1			
Las Cruces, NM	31	28	12	3	1	7	5		2	1
Las Vegas-Paradise, NV	473	410	85	50	39	122	114	8	21	34
Lawrence, KS	15	12	5		1	3	3		1	2
Lawton, OK	47	40	16	1	4	6	13		2	5
Lebanon, PA	44	34	9	8	2	9	6		6	4
Lewiston-Auburn, ME	45	40	12	4	3	5	16	1	1	3
Lewiston, ID-WA	13	12	3	2	3	3	1		1	
Lexington-Fayette, KY	98	84	13	11	6	29	25	1	3	10
Lima, OH	35	32	2	6	6	17	1			3
Lincoln, NE	29	27	9	4		5	9		1	1

Table 5.20

DOs by Metropolitan Statistical Area, 2010, continued

		Major Professional Activity									
		Patient Care									
			Office-Based Practice								
Metropollitan Statistical Area	Total Physicians	Total Patient Care	FM/GP Practice	Medical Specialties	Surgical Specialties	Other Specialties	Hospital Based Practice	Other Professional Activity	Inactive	Not Classified
Little Rock-North Little Rock-Conway, AR	63	53	11	11		10	21	1	2	7
Logan, UT-ID	20	18	1	1	3	5	8			2
Longview, TX	14	13	3	3		4	3			1
Longview, WA	11	9	4	1		3	1		1	1
Los Angeles-Long Beach-Santa Ana, CA	1,517	1,292	453	241	82	296	220	21	33	171
Louisville/Jefferson County, KY-IN	119	104	11	12	2	27	52	2	4	9
Lubbock, TX	43	35	13	5	1	10	6	2	5	1
Lynchburg, VA	21	18	8	4	1	1	4	1		2
Macon, GA	11	7	1	1		4	1		2	2
Madera-Chowchilla, CA	8	8	2	1	2	2	1			
Madison, WI	99	88	20	16	6	17	29	1	1	9
Manchester-Nashua, NH	71	64	17	18	5	18	6	3	1	3
Manhattan, KS	18	15	7	2	1	1	4	1		2
Mankato-North Mankato, MN	20	20	8	1		3	8			
Mansfield, OH	29	24	6	3	2	9	4		5	
McAllen-Edinburg -Mission, TX	22	19	4	3	3	7	2		1	2
Medford, OR	57	48	23	2	2	19	2	1	7	1
Memphis, TN-MS-AR	68	49	11	5	2	7	24	1	3	15
Merced, CA	13	11	4		2	4	1			2
Miami-Fort Lauderdale-Pompano Beach, FL	1,528	1,216	335	242	114	356	169	35	151	126
Michigan City-La Porte, IN	10	9	3	2		2	2		1	
Midland, TX	11	9		1	3	1	4		1	1
Milwaukee-Waukesha-West Allis, WI	325	280	88	41	21	59	71	6	17	22
Minneapolis-St. Paul-Bloomington, MN-WI	298	264	65	37	27	66	69	2	14	18
Missoula, MT	19	16	11	2		2	1		2	1
Mobile, AL	48	41	6	11	2	3	19	2	1	4
Modesto, CA	37	37	13	4	3	13	4			
Monroe, LA	8	7	4			1	2	1		
Monroe, MI	34	33	8	4	3	13	5		1	
Montgomery, AL	36	32	11	9		9	3		2	2
Morgantown, WV	51	39	7	8	2	10	12	2	2	8
Morristown, TN	13	12	6		1	3	2		1	
Mount Vernon-Anacortes, WA	13	10	3	1		5	1		3	
Muncie, IN	12	12	7		1	1	3			
Muskegon-Norton Shores, MI	104	84	33	6	16	15	14		16	4
Myrtle Beach-North Myrtle Beach-Conway, SC	60	54	13	10	2	20	9	1	3	2
Napa, CA	18	14	2	2	3	3	4		1	3
Naples-Marco Island, FL	93	69	17	17	7	24	4	2	19	3
Nashville-Davidson-Murfreesboro-Franklin, TN	137	114	29	10	13	26	36	2	9	12
New Haven-Milford, CT	90	69	4	19	6	20	20		3	18
New Orleans-Metairie-Kenner, LA	82	71	4	14	1	9	43		2	9
New York-Northern New Jersey-Long Island, NY-NJ-PA	4,037	3,296	640	920	285	823	628	74	190	477

Table 5.20

DOs by Metropolitan Statistical Area, 2010, continued

Metropolitan Statistical Area	Total Physicians	Major Professional Activity: Patient Care: Total Patient Care	Office-Based Practice: FM/GP Practice	Office-Based Practice: Medical Specialties	Office-Based Practice: Surgical Specialties	Office-Based Practice: Other Specialties	Hospital Based Practice	Other Professional Activity	Inactive	Not Classified
Niles-Benton Harbor, MI	48	40	13	7	4	10	6		6	2
North Port-Bradenton-Sarasota, FL	196	166	42	25	12	60	27	5	22	3
Norwich-New London, CT	29	21	2	7	1	10	1			8
Ocala, FL	54	42	13	5	6	15	3	1	9	2
Ocean City, NJ	76	64	19	20	7	16	2	1	6	5
Odessa, TX	15	14	3	1	2	3	5		1	
Ogden-Clearfield, UT	66	64	25	12	4	13	10		1	1
Oklahoma City, OK	449	392	108	37	35	117	95	4	16	37
Olympia, WA	58	48	16	4	2	11	15	1	5	4
Omaha-Council Bluffs, NE-IA	132	119	28	14	11	22	44	1	1	11
Orlando-Kissimmee-Sanford, FL	416	355	103	54	43	107	48	10	32	19
Oshkosh-Neenah, WI	30	28	8	9	4	4	3			2
Owensboro, KY	12	8	5			3		1	2	1
Oxnard-Thousand Oaks-Ventura, CA	70	64	23	13	7	14	7		3	3
Palm Bay-Melbourne-Titusville, FL	109	91	18	16	9	40	8	2	14	2
Palm Coast, FL	15	14	4	2	3	4	1		1	
Panama City-Lynn Haven-Panama City Beach, FL	31	26	9	1	4	11	1		4	1
Parkersburg-Marietta-Vienna, WV-OH	78	66	28	8	6	17	7	1	5	6
Pascagoula, MS	25	21	4	5	2	3	7		1	3
Pensacola-Ferry Pass-Brent, FL	109	92	19	3	12	31	27	2	4	11
Peoria, IL	99	89	22	10	9	24	24	3	1	6
Philadelphia-Camden-Wilmington, PA-NJ-DE-MD	3,986	3,155	820	657	253	797	628	105	369	357
Phoenix-Mesa-Glendale, AZ	1,406	1,154	301	234	115	321	183	22	132	98
Pine Bluff, AR	8	7	3		1	1	2			1
Pittsburgh, PA	699	588	136	142	45	136	129	16	18	77
Pittsfield, MA	39	29	2	8	5	5	9		2	8
Pocatello, ID	26	25	12	2	2	3	6		1	
Port St. Lucie, FL	101	80	28	16	3	22	11		14	7
Portland-South Portland-Biddeford, ME	393	340	100	59	28	74	79	5	22	26
Portland-Vancouver-Hillsboro, OR-WA	446	369	110	81	33	75	70	8	36	33
Poughkeepsie-Newburgh-Middletown, NY	103	95	22	26	17	18	12	2	2	4
Prescott, AZ	64	56	19	7	6	19	5	1	4	3
Providence-New Bedford-Fall River, RI-MA	291	241	74	58	17	40	52	4	16	30
Provo-Orem, UT	75	73	26	9	7	20	11			2
Pueblo, CO	39	38	14	2	6	4	12	1		
Punta Gorda, FL	55	48	16	6	7	17	2		6	1
Racine, WI	16	15	7	4		2	2			1
Raleigh-Cary, NC	77	63	16	5	1	24	17	3	5	6
Rapid City, SD	28	26	10	3	3	4	6		1	1
Reading, PA	145	125	41	19	8	35	22	3	6	11
Redding, CA	39	36	18	5	3	5	5			3
Reno-Sparks, NV	91	81	22	16		22	21	2	5	3
Richmond, VA	135	120	19	16	11	28	46	1	2	12

Table 5.20

DOs by Metropolitan Statistical Area, 2010, continued

		Major Professional Activity									
		Patient Care									
			Office-Based Practice								
Metropolitan Statistical Area	Total Physicians	Total Patient Care	FM/GP Practice	Medical Specialties	Surgical Specialties	Other Specialties	Hospital Based Practice	Other Professional Activity	Inactive	Not Classified
Riverside-San Bernardino-Ontario, CA	564	473	158	66	30	104	115	9	15	67
Roanoke, VA	80	68	14	10	3	9	32	2	2	8
Rochester, MN	76	71	7	6	5	10	43	2	1	2
Rochester, NY	130	109	19	23	5	36	26	1	7	13
Rockford, IL	47	42	9	5	11	10	7	2	3	
Rocky Mount, NC	10	8	2	1	2	2	1	1	1	
Rome, GA	18	15	5	3	1	2	4		3	
Sacramento-Arden-Arcade-Roseville, CA	248	212	68	35	14	53	42	3	8	25
Saginaw-Saginaw Township North, MI	77	68	22	7	5	22	12		8	1
Salem, OR	51	50	23	5	3	9	10	1		
Salinas, CA	39	37	17	9	1	7	3	1		1
Salisbury, MD	21	19	2	5	1	7	4			2
Salt Lake City, UT	132	115	26	5	7	42	35		4	13
San Angelo, TX	15	14	3	4	2	4	1	1		
San Antonio-New Braunfels, TX	436	344	53	44	16	69	162	14	20	58
San Diego-Carlsbad-San Marcos, CA	491	414	127	54	29	91	113	6	19	52
San Francisco-Oakland-Fremont, CA	376	314	67	94	29	76	48	11	4	47
San Jose-Sunnyvale-Santa Clara, CA	118	103	23	30	9	25	16	1	1	13
San Juan-Caguas-Guaynabo, PR	1	1					1			
San Luis Obispo-Paso Robles, CA	48	40	11	8	1	18	2		5	3
Sandusky, OH	90	75	26	9	11	19	10	2	8	5
Santa Barbara-Santa Maria-Goleta, CA	33	30	7	11	2	4	6	1	1	1
Santa Cruz-Watsonville, CA	45	42	16	6	4	10	6		2	1
Santa Fe, NM	19	16	5	2	2	5	2		2	1
Santa Rosa-Petaluma, CA	63	51	30	4	4	11	2	3	6	3
Savannah, GA	56	45	12	11	4	11	7		2	9
Scranton--Wilkes-Barre, PA	260	230	70	54	27	46	33	4	16	10
Seattle-Tacoma-Bellevue, WA	495	429	130	40	51	111	97	7	27	32
Sebastian-Vero Beach, FL	34	28	6	6	2	11	3	1	5	
Sheboygan, WI	12	10	3	2	1	2	2	1	1	
Sherman-Denison, TX	16	14	5	1	2	4	2			2
Shreveport-Bossier City, LA	20	16	1	1	2	3	9		2	2
Sioux City, IA-NE-SD	39	35	16	3	2	8	6		3	1
Sioux Falls, SD	60	54	10	11	5	12	16	2	1	3
South Bend-Mishawaka, IN-MI	94	70	27	5	7	16	15	2	18	4
Spartanburg, SC	43	38	10	2	1	6	19	1	1	3
Spokane, WA	89	84	34	17	3	15	15		3	2
Springfield, IL	22	20	5	1		5	9			2
Springfield, MA	107	92	10	31	2	16	33	2	2	11
Springfield, MO	179	162	56	20	12	42	32	2	11	4
Springfield, OH	25	21	5	3	4	7	2	1	2	1
St. Cloud, MN	28	27	8	4	2	8	5		1	
St. George, UT	20	17	9	2	1	4	1		3	
St. Joseph, MO-KS	37	35	13	5	4	9	4			2
St. Louis, MO-IL	514	430	118	62	45	117	88	14	28	42
State College, PA	47	44	11	6	6	14	7			3

Table 5.20

DOs by Metropolitan Statistical Area, 2010, continued

		Major Professional Activity								
		Patient Care								
			Office-Based Practice							
Metropolitan Statistical Area	Total Physicians	Total Patient Care	FM/GP Practice	Medical Specialties	Surgical Specialties	Other Specialties	Hospital Based Practice	Other Professional Activity	Inactive	Not Classified
Steubenville-Weirton, OH-WV	24	21	7	4	2	6	2	2		1
Stockton, CA	48	43	17	12	1	10	3		2	3
Sumter, SC	10	9		2	1	3	3			1
Syracuse, NY	84	68	19	14	4	13	18	3	4	9
Tallahassee, FL	28	23	7	4	3	6	3	1	4	
Tampa-St. Petersburg-Clearwater, FL	971	788	192	146	75	206	169	10	117	56
Terre Haute, IN	23	22	5	3	4	3	7			1
Texarkana, TX-Texarkana, AR	8	8	1	2	1	3	1			
Toledo, OH	246	196	34	21	23	51	67	4	14	32
Topeka, KS	48	42	21	9	2	4	6	1	3	2
Trenton-Ewing, NJ	83	68	15	17	10	16	10	1	7	7
Tucson, AZ	263	216	59	44	13	51	49	8	29	10
Tulsa, OK	826	688	208	104	73	194	109	19	59	60
Tuscaloosa, AL	13	13	4	5		2	2			
Tyler, TX	61	54	16	7	5	15	11		5	2
Utica-Rome, NY	51	44	18	6	4	8	8	2	2	3
Valdosta, GA	14	13	2	2	2	4	3			1
Vallejo-Fairfield, CA	79	63	16	10	6	13	18	3	2	11
Victoria, TX	15	14	5	3	2	2	2			1
Vineland-Millville-Bridgeton, NJ	39	31	8	9	2	9	3	2	3	3
Virginia Beach-Norfolk-Newport News, VA-NC	277	242	37	41	12	53	99	5	7	23
Visalia-Porterville, CA	27	26	6	6	6	5	3	1		
Waco, TX	40	34	10	2	2	8	12	1	3	2
Warner Robins, GA	19	14	6	1	4	2	1		2	3
Washington-Arlington-Alexandria, DC-VA-MD-WV	672	537	89	91	33	150	174	28	21	86
Waterloo-Cedar Falls, IA	55	54	16	9	5	10	14		1	
Wausau, WI	38	36	8	4	9	8	7		1	1
Wenatchee-East Wenatchee, WA	11	9	4	1		3	1		1	1
Wheeling, WV-OH	94	74	20	9	2	16	27		2	18
Wichita Falls, TX	22	19	5	2		10	2		3	
Wichita, KS	202	185	74	19	13	36	43	2	8	7
Williamsport, PA	37	33	7	5	4	8	9	2	1	1
Wilmington, NC	59	54	14	8	4	11	17		2	3
Winchester, VA-WV	21	19	4	1	2	7	5			2
Winston-Salem, NC	72	59	10	6	2	17	24			13
Worcester, MA	158	132	26	27	13	25	41	1	3	22
Yakima, WA	63	51	21	3	5	12	10	1	6	5
York-Hanover, PA	220	192	48	31	29	53	31		14	14
Youngstown-Warren-Boardman, OH-PA	383	304	101	57	30	76	40	7	40	32
Yuba City, CA	21	19	6	3	2	4	4	1	1	
Yuma, AZ	23	20	7	2		9	2		3	

Note: Does not include Address Unknown.

Table 5.21

DOs by Micropolitan Statistical Area, 2010

		Major Professional Activity								
		Patient Care								
			Office-Based Practice							
Micropolitan Statistical Area	Total Physicians	Total Patient Care	FM/GP Practice	Medical Specialties	Surgical Specialties	Other Specialties	Hospital Based Practice	Other Professional Activity	Inactive	Not Classified
Total Micropolitan Physicians	5,672	4,984	1,728	771	590	1,055	840	62	344	282
Aberdeen, SD	6	5	1	4						1
Aberdeen, WA	14	13	4	1	1	6	1		1	
Ada, OK	14	13	3	2	1	2	5	1		
Adrian, MI	20	18	5	2	3	6	2		2	
Alamogordo, NM	12	10	2	2	3	2	1		1	1
Albany-Lebanon, OR	11	9	1	2	2	2	2		2	
Albemarle, NC	4	4	2			1	1			
Albert Lea, MN	3	3		1	1		1			
Albertville, AL	8	7	1	2	1	2	1		1	
Alexander City, AL	1	1		1						
Alexandria, MN	8	8	2	1	1	3	1			
Alice, TX	5	4	1			2	1		1	
Allegan, MI	13	12	5	1	2	2	2		1	
Alma, MI	15	11	3			5	3		4	
Alpena, MI	16	13	5	2	4	2			2	1
Altus, OK	9	8	2	1		3	2	1		
Americus, GA	2	2	1	1						
Amsterdam, NY	6	5	4				1			1
Andrews, TX	2	2		1			1			
Angola, IN	2	1	1						1	
Arcadia, FL	2	2	2							
Ardmore, OK	23	22	8	2	4	4	4			1
Ashland, OH	5	5	2	2			1			
Ashtabula, OH	18	15	6	3	2	3	1	1	2	
Astoria, OR	5	5	1	1	1	2				
Atchison, KS	1	1					1			
Athens, OH	120	90	21	13	8	29	19	9	9	12
Athens, TN	3	3	2				1			
Athens, TX	9	9	6			2	1			
Auburn, IN	5	5	3	1			1			
Auburn, NY	6	5	1	2			2			1
Augusta-Waterville, ME	81	73	31	10	3	7	22	1	2	5
Austin, MN	6	6	1			2	3			
Bainbridge, GA	3	2	1			1				1
Baraboo, WI	5	5	2	1		1	1			
Barre, VT	8	8		2	2	3	1			
Bartlesville, OK	22	20	8	2	1	6	3		1	1
Batavia, NY	3	2	1			1				1
Batesville, AR	5	5	3				2			
Bay City, TX	2	2	1		1					
Beatrice, NE	1	1			1					
Beaver Dam, WI	14	14	7	2	3	1	1			
Beckley, WV	39	32	15	5	2	7	3	2	3	2
Bedford, IN	4	3	1		1	1			1	
Beeville, TX	1								1	
Bellefontaine, OH	23	22	6	2	3	6	5		1	
Bemidji, MN	5	4	2		1	1		1		
Bennettsville, SC	2	2					2			
Bennington, VT	5	4	1		1	1	1			1
Berlin, NH-VT	9	9	2	1	2		4			
Big Rapids, MI	13	10	3	1	2	3	1		2	1
Big Spring, TX	5	4	2				2			1
Bishop, CA	1	1	1							
Blackfoot, ID	17	17	6	1	2	7	1			
Bloomsburg-Berwick, PA	162	128	14	37	11	12	54	2	3	29

Table 5.21

DOs by Micropolitan Statistical Area, 2010, continued

		Major Professional Activity								
		Patient Care								
			Office-Based Practice							
Micropolitan Statistical Area	Total Physicians	Total Patient Care	FM/GP Practice	Medical Specialties	Surgical Specialties	Other Specialties	Hospital Based Practice	Other Professional Activity	Inactive	Not Classified
Bluefield, WV-VA	49	46	10	8	6	11	11			3
Blytheville, AR	1	1	1							
Bonham, TX	3	3	2				1			
Boone, IA	11	11	6		1	2	2			
Boone, NC	4	4	2			2				
Bozeman, MT	8	7	5			2			1	
Bradford, PA	8	7	1	3		2	1		1	
Brainerd, MN	9	8	1	3		2	2			1
Branson, MO	18	16	5	2	3	2	4			2
Brenham, TX	3	3	2			1				
Brevard, NC	1	1				1				
Brigham City, UT	4	4	1		1	2				
Brookings, OR	7	5	3	1		1			2	
Brookings, SD	1	1	1							
Brownsville, TN	1	1	1							
Brownwood, TX	10	9	2	2		3	2		1	
Bucyrus, OH	10	9	3	2		2	2			1
Burley, ID	11	11	5		1	3	2			
Burlington, IA-IL	15	14	4	2	2	4	2			1
Butte-Silver Bow, MT	4	4	3	1						
Cadillac, MI	19	15	6	1	4	2	2		3	1
Calhoun, GA	5	3	2			1			2	
Cambridge, MD	5	5	3	1		1				
Cambridge, OH	5	5	1	2		1	1			
Camden, AR	3	3	1		1		1			
Campbellsville, KY	4	4	2	1		1				
Cañon City, CO	7	6	2	2	1		1		1	
Canton, IL	3	2		1			1		1	
Carbondale, IL	20	17	11	1	2	2	1			3
Carlsbad-Artesia, NM	6	6	3	1	1	1				
Cedar City, UT	11	10	4	2	2	2				1
Cedartown, GA	2	2	1		1					
Celina, OH	9	7	4			2	1		1	1
Centralia, IL	3	3	1	1	1					
Centralia, WA	12	9	2	1	4	2			3	
Chambersburg, PA	26	25	10	3	3	7	2	1		
Charleston-Mattoon, IL	24	22	4	3	3	7	5		1	1
Chester, SC	2	2	1	1						
Chillicothe, OH	36	36	11	8	6	9	2			
Claremont, NH	6	5		2	1	1	1		1	
Clarksburg, WV	42	38	24	2	1	6	5			4
Clarksdale, MS	1	1	1							
Clearlake, CA	1	1	1							
Cleveland, MS	4	4			1	3				
Clewiston, FL	3	3	1	1			1			
Clinton, IA	9	7	3	2		1	1		2	
Clovis, NM	8	7	1	1	1	2	2		1	
Coffeyville, KS	11	10	3	1	3	1	2			1
Coldwater, MI	18	14	5	3	2	3	1		2	2
Columbia, TN	2	2	2							
Columbus, MS	4	4		3		1				
Columbus, NE	2	2		1			1			
Concord, NH	39	33	12	7	1	6	7	1	2	3
Connersville, IN	2	2		1			1			
Cookeville, TN	10	10	4	1	2	2	1			
Coos Bay, OR	8	8	1	4	2	1				
Corbin, KY	8	7	3		2		2			1

Table 5.21

DOs by Micropolitan Statistical Area, 2010, continued

		Major Professional Activity									
		Patient Care									
			Office-Based Practice								
Micropolitan Statistical Area	Total Physicians	Total Patient Care	FM/GP Practice	Medical Specialties	Surgical Specialties	Other Specialties	Hospital Based Practice	Other Professional Activity	Inactive	Not Classified
Cordele, GA	2	2		1		1				
Corinth, MS	5	3	1	1			1		1	1
Cornelia, GA	5	4	1	1	1	1			1	
Corning, NY	10	8	1	2	1	3	1		1	1
Corsicana, TX	3	3	1	1		1				
Cortland, NY	4	4	1	2			1			
Coshocton, OH	6	6	5		1					
Crawfordsville, IN	2	2			2					
Crescent City, CA	4	4	2	1	1					
Crossville, TN	7	3	2				1		4	
Cullman, AL	5	5	3		2					
Danville, KY	2	1		1						1
Daphne-Fairhope-Foley, AL	31	26	6	1	7	9	3		2	3
Defiance, OH	9	9	4	1	4					
Del Rio, TX	2	1				1				1
Deming, NM	2	2	1		1					
DeRidder, LA	4	4	2			1	1			
Dickinson, ND	2	2	1		1					
Dillon, SC	2	2		1	1					
Dixon, IL	4	4	1		2		1			
Dodge City, KS	2	2	1		1					
Douglas, GA	5	5	2	2		1				
Dublin, GA	11	9	1	1	2	3	2	1		1
DuBois, PA	46	40	8	13	3	4	12	1	3	2
Dumas, TX	2	2	1	1						
Duncan, OK	4	2	1	1					2	
Dunn, NC	8	8	2	1		1	4			
Durango, CO	17	15	3	1		7	4		1	1
Durant, OK	23	19	8	1	1	4	5			4
Dyersburg, TN	4	3	2		1					1
Eagle Pass, TX	4	3	2	1					1	
East Liverpool-Salem, OH	38	36	15	9	5	5	2		1	1
East Stroudsburg, PA	29	22	6	8	1	6	1	2	4	1
Easton, MD	17	16	3	4	4	4	1		1	
Edwards, CO	10	7	2			5			3	
Effingham, IL	6	5	2	1		1	1			1
El Campo, TX	5	5	3				2			
El Dorado, AR	1	1				1				
Elizabeth City, NC	8	8		3	2	2	1			
Elk City, OK	5	4	3			1			1	
Elko, NV	9	8	2	1	1	2	2			1
Ellensburg, WA	4	3	2				1			1
Emporia, KS	7	4		1	1	1	1		1	2
Enid, OK	30	26	7	2	5	8	4		3	1
Enterprise-Ozark, AL	14	13	4	2		2	5		1	
Escanaba, MI	15	15	6		2	2	5			
Espanola, NM	3	3	3							
Eufaula, AL-GA	2	2	2							
Eureka-Arcata-Fortuna, CA	14	13	6		1	3	3		1	
Evanston, WY	1	1					1			
Fairmont, MN	2	2			1	1				
Fairmont, WV	10	10	7	1		1	1			
Fallon, NV	4	3	1		1		1	1		
Faribault-Northfield, MN	5	5	3				2			
Farmington, MO	40	37	20	2	3	6	6		2	1
Fergus Falls, MN	5	5	1			1	3			
Fernley, NV	2	1	1							1
Findlay, OH	15	14	6	3	2	2	1		1	

Table 5.21

DOs by Micropolitan Statistical Area, 2010, continued

		Major Professional Activity								
		Patient Care								
			Office-Based Practice							
Micropolitan Statistical Area	Total Physicians	Total Patient Care	FM/GP Practice	Medical Specialties	Surgical Specialties	Other Specialties	Hospital Based Practice	Other Professional Activity	Inactive	Not Classified
Fitzgerald, GA	4	3	3						1	
Forest City, NC	4	3	1	1		1			1	
Fort Dodge, IA	12	12	4	6		1	1			
Fort Leonard Wood, MO	18	14	5	2	3	3	1		1	3
Fort Madison-Keokuk, IA-MO	13	13	5	1	3	3	1			
Fort Morgan, CO	3	3	2			1				
Fort Payne, AL	2	1				1				1
Fort Polk South, LA	7	6	1			1	4			1
Fort Valley, GA	1	1	1							
Frankfort, IN	1	1					1			
Frankfort, KY	3	3	2		1					
Fredericksburg, TX	8	8	4	1		2	1			
Fremont, NE	3	3	2		1					
Fremont, OH	18	17	3	2	5	4	3		1	
Gaffney, SC	6	6	4	1		1				
Gainesville, TX	4	4	3			1				
Galesburg, IL	8	8	2	2	2		2			
Gallup, NM	7	7	1		1	3	2			
Garden City, KS	6	6	4		1		1			
Gardnerville Ranchos, NV	5	5	4			1				
Georgetown, SC	9	7	2	2	1		2			2
Gettysburg, PA	22	21	9		2	7	3			1
Gillette, WY	5	4			1	2	1			1
Glasgow, KY	1	1					1			
Gloversville, NY	5	4	2				2			1
Granbury, TX	23	21	8	4	2	7			1	1
Grand Island, NE	5	3		1		2		1	1	
Grants Pass, OR	22	20	8	7	2		3		1	1
Grants, NM	1	1	1							
Great Bend, KS	3	3	1		2					
Greeneville, TN	12	12	4	4	1	1	2			
Greensburg, IN	1	1				1				
Greenville, MS	1	1	1							
Greenville, OH	6	4	2	2				1	1	
Greenwood, MS	6	5	2	1	1		1		1	
Greenwood, SC	7	7	1	2	1	2	1			
Grenada, MS	2	2	1			1				
Guymon, OK	4	3	3						1	
Hammond, LA	1								1	
Hannibal, MO	16	15	10	1	1	2	1		1	
Harriman, TN	2	2	2							
Harrisburg, IL	3	3	2				1			
Harrison, AR	6	3	2			1			2	1
Havre, MT	4	3	1	1		1			1	
Hays, KS	11	11	2	4	1	3	1			
Heber, UT	4	4	2		2					
Helena-West Helena, AR	3	2	2						1	
Helena, MT	14	14	3	2	4	4	1			
Henderson, NC	3	3	1		1	1				
Hereford, TX	3	3	1	1			1			
Hilo, HI	24	18	4	3	4	6	1	1	3	2
Hilton Head Island-Beaufort, SC	39	29	6	6	4	8	5		6	4
Hobbs, NM	10	9	6	1			2			1
Homosassa Springs, FL	40	38	15	2	10	8	3	1	1	
Hood River, OR	5	5	2	1		2				
Houghton, MI	15	14	6	1	4	2	1		1	
Hudson, NY	14	10	3	3	1	1	2		3	1

Table 5.21

DOs by Micropolitan Statistical Area, 2010, continued

		Major Professional Activity									
		Patient Care									
			Office-Based Practice								
Micropolitan Statistical Area	Total Physicians	Total Patient Care	FM/GP Practice	Medical Specialties	Surgical Specialties	Other Specialties	Hospital Based Practice	Other Professional Activity	Inactive	Not Classified
Humboldt, TN	2	2	1				1			
Huntingdon, PA	10	8	5	3					1	1
Huntington, IN	1	1				1				
Huntsville, TX	7	7	3	1	1	2				
Huron, SD	2	2		1		1				
Hutchinson, KS	3	2				1	1	1		
Hutchinson, MN	8	8	3	1	2	1	1			
Indiana, PA	25	23	7	5	2	4	5			2
Iron Mountain, MI-WI	17	16	3	1	3	5	4			1
Jackson, WY-ID	11	9	1	1	2	3	2		2	
Jacksonville, IL	3	3			1	1	1			
Jacksonville, TX	9	6	2	3	1				3	
Jamestown-Dunkirk-Fredonia, NY	13	9	3	3		2	1		4	
Jasper, IN	11	11	1	1	1	5	3			
Jesup, GA	5	5	1	1	1	2				
Juneau, AK	5	4		3		1				1
Kahului-Wailuku, HI	28	25	13	2	1	7	2		1	2
Kalispell, MT	12	11	2	1		7	1			1
Kapaa, HI	11	10		7		3				1
Kearney, NE	4	4	2		1		1			
Keene, NH	10	10		2		4	4			
Kendallville, IN	1	1	1							
Kennett, MO	6	5	1	1		1	2		1	
Kerrville, TX	9	6	1		1	2	2		2	1
Key West, FL	27	25	13	4	1	4	3		1	1
Kill Devil Hills, NC	3	3	1			1	1			
Kinston, NC	3	3			2	1				
Kirksville, MO	127	100	23	12	11	18	36	8	15	4
Klamath Falls, OR	9	7	4		2	1		2		
Kodiak, AK	4	3	1		1		1		1	
La Follette, TN	6	6	4	2						
La Grande, OR	3	1					1		1	1
Laconia, NH	9	8	5	1		2				1
LaGrange, GA	9	7	1		3	2	1		1	1
Lake City, FL	12	11	4		2	1	4			1
Lamesa, TX	1	1	1							
Lancaster, SC	6	6	2	2		2				
Laramie, WY	6	5	2	2			1			1
Las Vegas, NM	4	4	2		1		1			
Laurel, MS	11	11	6	2		3				
Laurinburg, NC	5	5	2		1	2				
Lawrenceburg, TN	1									1
Lebanon, MO	14	13	6		3	1	3		1	
Lebanon, NH-VT	44	35	5	6	4	4	16	2	3	4
Levelland, TX	1	1	1							
Lewisburg, PA	21	20	5	4	2	3	6		1	
Lewisburg, TN	2	2	1	1						
Lewistown, PA	14	8	5		2	1			6	
Lexington Park, MD	6	6	2	1		1	2			
Lexington, NE	2	2	2							
Liberal, KS	4	4	2		1	1				
Lincolnton, NC	5	4	3			1			1	
Lock Haven, PA	8	8	2		1	3	2			
Logansport, IN	3	2	1		1				1	
London, KY	2									2
Los Alamos, NM	1	1	1							

Table 5.21

DOs by Micropolitan Statistical Area, 2010, continued

		Major Professional Activity								
		Patient Care								
			Office-Based Practice							
Micropolitan Statistical Area	Total Physicians	Total Patient Care	FM/GP Practice	Medical Specialties	Surgical Specialties	Other Specialties	Hospital Based Practice	Other Professional Activity	Inactive	Not Classified
Lufkin, TX	20	20	10	2	3	2	3			
Lumberton, NC	5	5		2		2	1			
Macomb, IL	7	6		2		3	1	1		
Madison, IN	2	2				2				
Madisonville, KY	10	10	4	2		3	1			
Malone, NY	4	3	1	1		1				1
Manitowoc, WI	6	6	1			2	3			
Marble Falls, TX	4	4	1	1	1		1			
Marinette, WI-MI	8	7	3		1	3			1	
Marion-Herrin, IL	14	12	4	2	1	2	3		2	
Marion, IN	15	13	5	1	3	3	1			2
Marion, OH	10	9		4	2	2	1	1		
Marquette, MI	34	32	4	3	2	14	9		2	
Marshall, MN	4	4	2	1		1				
Marshall, MO	6	6	2	1	1		2			
Marshall, TX	6	6		2	1	2	1			
Marshalltown, IA	6	6	2	2	1		1			
Marshfield-Wisconsin Rapids, WI	29	28	5	4	6	6	7			1
Martin, TN	1	1			1					
Martinsville, VA	3	3	2				1			
Maryville, MO	3	3	2				1			
Mason City, IA	47	43	21	5	5	1	11		1	3
Mayfield, KY	4	4	1		1	1	1			
Maysville, KY	6	5	1		2	2			1	
McAlester, OK	13	13	6			2	5			
McComb, MS	6	6		2		2	2			
McMinnville, TN	6	5	2	2	1					1
McPherson, KS	3	1				1			1	1
Meadville, PA	44	37	15	4	3	12	3		3	4
Menomonie, WI	6	5	3		1		1			1
Meridian, MS	28	25	13	4	2	2	4			3
Merrill, WI	3	3	3							
Mexico, MO	9	7	2	2		1	2		2	
Miami, OK	10	7	3	1	1		2		2	1
Middlesborough, KY	1								1	
Midland, MI	31	28	3	3	3	13	6	1	2	
Milledgeville, GA	6	4	1		1	2			2	
Minden, LA	2	2			1	1				
Mineral Wells, TX	5	4	1	2		1			1	
Minot, ND	14	11	2	2	2	2	3			3
Mitchell, SD	4	4	1		2	1				
Moberly, MO	16	14	7	2	1	2	2		2	
Monroe, WI	6	6	2	1		2	1			
Montrose, CO	14	11	7	1	2	1			3	
Morehead City, NC	9	7	1	1	1	2	2			2
Moscow, ID	3	3	1			1	1			
Moses Lake, WA	7	6	4			1	1	1		
Moultrie, GA	2	2	2							
Mount Airy, NC	10	8	3	3	2					2
Mount Pleasant, MI	30	28	14	2	1	10	1	1	1	
Mount Pleasant, TX	9	7	2	2	1	1	1		2	
Mount Sterling, KY	4	3	2				1			1
Mount Vernon, IL	7	6	3	1		2				1
Mount Vernon, OH	9	8	5		1	2			1	
Mountain Home, AR	7	5	1	1		1	2			2
Mountain Home, ID	10	7	5	1		1			2	1
Murray, KY	6	6	2	3		1				

Table 5.21

DOs by Micropolitan Statistical Area, 2010, continued

		Major Professional Activity								
		Patient Care								
			Office-Based Practice							
Micropolitan Statistical Area	Total Physicians	Total Patient Care	FM/GP Practice	Medical Specialties	Surgical Specialties	Other Specialties	Hospital Based Practice	Other Professional Activity	Inactive	Not Classified
Muscatine, IA	9	7	4	1			2		2	
Muskogee, OK	19	17	6	3	1	6	1		1	1
Nacogdoches, TX	7	6	2	1	2		1		1	
Natchez, MS-LA	1	1	1							
Natchitoches, LA	2	2		1	1					
New Bern, NC	20	16	2	2	1	6	5		1	3
New Castle, IN	3	3		1			2			
New Castle, PA	31	28	8	2	6	4	8		2	1
New Iberia, LA	2	2	1	1						
New Philadelphia-Dover, OH	24	21	4	5	2	7	3		3	
New Ulm, MN	2	1		1					1	
Newberry, SC	3	3		1	2					
Newton, IA	10	10	4	2		3	1			
Nogales, AZ	2	2				1	1			
Norfolk, NE	5	3	1		1		1		1	1
North Platte, NE	2	2					2			
North Vernon, IN	2	2	2							
North Wilkesboro, NC	5	5	2		1	2				
Norwalk, OH	19	16	3	3	7	3			2	1
Oak Harbor, WA	11	10	4		2	3	1		1	
Oak Hill, WV	16	15	10	1		2	2			1
Ocean Pines, MD	18	16	5	1	5	2	3			2
Ogdensburg-Massena, NY	19	16	6	1	6	1	2		2	1
Oil City, PA	14	14	1	3		8	2			
Okeechobee, FL	1	1				1				
Olean, NY	5	4		1	2		1			1
Oneonta, NY	22	20		7	4	4	5			2
Ontario, OR-ID	5	4	1	1	1		1			1
Orangeburg, SC	14	12	3	1	1	3	4		2	
Oskaloosa, IA	5	5	1	1			3			
Ottawa-Streator, IL	22	19	6		4	3	6		2	1
Ottumwa, IA	10	10	3	2	1	4				
Owatonna, MN	5	4	1			2	1			1
Owosso, MI	29	27	10	5	3	5	4		2	
Oxford, MS	12	10	2	2	2	3	1			2
Paducah, KY-IL	10	9	1	4	3	1				1
Pahrump, NV	8	7	3	1		1	2		1	
Palatka, FL	8	8	3	2		2	1			
Palestine, TX	13	11	7		3		1		2	
Pampa, TX	6	6	2		1	2	1			
Paragould, AR	2	2	1				1			
Paris, TN	2	1		1					1	
Paris, TX	7	6	4			2				1
Parsons, KS	7	7	3		1	1	2			
Payson, AZ	20	11	8	1	1	1			5	4
Pecos, TX	2	2	1	1						
Pella, IA	20	17	10	2	3	2			3	
Pendleton-Hermiston, OR	15	15	7	3		4	1			
Peru, IN	8	7		2	2	3				1
Phoenix Lake-Cedar Ridge, CA	7	6	5			1				1
Picayune, MS	1								1	
Pierre, SD	3	3	1	1	1					
Pittsburg, KS	15	15	4	2	1	6	2			
Plainview, TX	7	7	4		1	1	1			
Platteville, WI	4	4	2				2			

Table 5.21

DOs by Micropolitan Statistical Area, 2010, continued

Micropolitan Statistical Area	Total Physicians	Major Professional Activity								
		Patient Care								
			Office-Based Practice							
		Total Patient Care	FM/GP Practice	Medical Specialties	Surgical Specialties	Other Specialties	Hospital Based Practice	Other Professional Activity	Inactive	Not Classified
Plattsburgh, NY	9	9	5	2	1	1				
Plymouth, IN	12	11	2	3	4	1	1		1	
Point Pleasant, WV-OH	21	19	9	1	2	6	1		1	1
Ponca City, OK	6	4	2	1		1				2
Pontiac, IL	10	10	5	1	1	3				
Poplar Bluff, MO	16	15	2	2	2	8	1		1	
Port Angeles, WA	13	11	9		1	1			2	
Portales, NM	5	4	2			2			1	
Portsmouth, OH	53	43	13	5	4	8	13		4	6
Pottsville, PA	64	60	24	16	11	7	2	1	2	1
Price, UT	3	3	2				1			
Pullman, WA	7	7	3		2	2				
Quincy, IL-MO	38	35	16	6	4	3	6	1		2
Red Bluff, CA	9	9	4	1	2	1	1			
Red Wing, MN	5	5	4				1			
Rexburg, ID	10	9	4		2	3				1
Richmond-Berea, KY	9	6	1	3		1	1		2	1
Richmond, IN	15	15	6		2	7				
Riverton, WY	8	6	1	1	1	3				2
Roanoke Rapids, NC	1	1	1							
Rochelle, IL	4	3	2	1					1	
Rock Springs, WY	3	3	1		1	1				
Rockingham, NC	1	1				1				
Rockland, ME	12	10	1	5		2	2		1	1
Rolla, MO	33	28	5	7	3	7	6		2	3
Roseburg, OR	34	28	13	3	3	4	5		6	
Roswell, NM	9	8	3	2	1	1	1		1	
Ruidoso, NM	7	6	1	1	2		2		1	
Russellville, AR	3	3	3							
Ruston, LA	3	3		1	1		1			
Rutland, VT	5	4	2	2					1	
Safford, AZ	5	5	3			1	1			
Salina, KS	15	14	4	1	1	6	2		1	
Salisbury, NC	5	5	1	1		1	2			
Sanford, NC	6	6	2	2	1		1			
Sault Ste. Marie, MI	16	14	9	2	1	1	1		1	1
Sayre, PA	18	15	6	5		2	2		3	
Scottsbluff, NE	4	4		1	1	2				
Scottsboro, AL	2	2				1	1			
Scottsburg, IN	1	1					1			
Seaford, DE	47	42	16	7	10	4	5		2	3
Searcy, AR	3	3	1				2			
Sebring, FL	15	14	4	1	2	5	2		1	
Sedalia, MO	10	9	3	1	2	3			1	
Selinsgrove, PA	13	11	6			4	1		1	1
Selma, AL	5	4	2		1	1				1
Seneca Falls, NY	1	1					1			
Seneca, SC	10	9	5	1	1	1	1	1		
Sevierville, TN	5	5	4			1				
Seymour, IN	2	2	2							
Shawnee, OK	14	13	5	2		4	2			1
Shelby, NC	6	6		1		4	1			
Shelbyville, TN	3	2	1				1	1		
Shelton, WA	4	3	1	1			1		1	
Sheridan, WY	6	6	2			1	3			
Show Low, AZ	25	22	11	2	5	2	2		2	1
Sidney, OH	9	8	2		4	2				1

Table 5.21

DOs by Micropolitan Statistical Area, 2010, continued

		Major Professional Activity									
		Patient Care									
			Office-Based Practice								
Micropolitan Statistical Area	Total Physicians	Total Patient Care	FM/GP Practice	Medical Specialties	Surgical Specialties	Other Specialties	Hospital Based Practice	Other Professional Activity	Inactive	Not Classified
Sierra Vista-Douglas, AZ	28	24	5	3	3	4	9	1	1	2
Sikeston, MO	6	6	3			1	2			
Silver City, NM	3	3	1	1		1				
Silverthorne, CO	6	4	2			2		1	1	
Somerset, KY	6	6	1	2		3				
Somerset, PA	20	14	4		2	4	4		4	2
Southern Pines-Pinehurst, NC	26	22	5	8	1	4	4		2	2
Spearfish, SD	8	5	2	3					3	
Spencer, IA	7	7	2		2	3				
Spirit Lake, IA	8	7	4	1			2		1	
St. Marys, GA	3	2					2		1	
St. Marys, PA	8	7	2	1		2	2			1
Starkville, MS	2	2				2				
Statesboro, GA	4	3	1		1	1				1
Statesville-Mooresville, NC	16	16	2	7	1	3	3			
Staunton-Waynesboro, VA	8	8	2		1	4	1			
Stephenville, TX	6	6	1	2	1	1	1			
Sterling, CO	6	6	4	1			1			
Sterling, IL	6	6	4	1		1				
Stevens Point, WI	26	24	8	3	3	4	6		1	1
Stillwater, OK	21	21	11	3	2	3	2			
Storm Lake, IA	3	3	2		1					
Sturgis, MI	7	5	1			2	2		1	1
Sulphur Springs, TX	2	2				2				
Sunbury, PA	18	15	6	2	1	5	1			3
Susanville, CA	1	1	1							
Sweetwater, TX	6	5	4		1				1	
Tahlequah, OK	34	31	10	4	3	9	5	1	2	
Talladega-Sylacauga, AL	2	1	1							1
Tallulah, LA	1	1					1			
Taos, NM	3	3				2	1			
Taylorville, IL	1	1					1			
The Dalles, OR	6	5			1	2	2		1	
The Villages, FL	10	3	1			1	1		6	1
Thomaston, GA	2	2	1		1					
Thomasville-Lexington, NC	3	3		1			2			
Thomasville, GA	9	8	3		1	4				1
Tiffin, OH	3	3	2				1			
Tifton, GA	3	3					3			
Toccoa, GA	2	2			2					
Torrington, CT	18	17	1	7	2	3	4			1
Traverse City, MI	126	107	44	18	7	26	12	4	14	1
Troy, AL	3	3	2			1				
Truckee-Grass Valley, CA	17	17	6	2	3	6				
Tullahoma, TN	20	18	10	1	3	4		1	1	
Tupelo, MS	27	26	8	3		5	10			1
Twin Falls, ID	21	18	3	4	1	8	2			3
Ukiah, CA	14	14	6	2	2	2	2			
Union City, TN-KY	4	4	3		1					
Union, SC	1									1
Uvalde, TX	3	2	2						1	
Valley, AL	1	1		1						
Van Wert, OH	3	1				1			1	1
Vermillion, SD	1	1	1							
Vernal, UT	3	3	2			1				
Vernon, TX	2	2		1			1			
Vicksburg, MS	4	4	3				1			

Table 5.21

DOs by Micropolitan Statistical Area, 2010, continued

		Major Professional Activity									
		Patient Care									
			Office-Based Practice								
Micropolitan Statistical Area	Total Physicians	Total Patient Care	FM/GP Practice	Medical Specialties	Surgical Specialties	Other Specialties	Hospital Based Practice	Other Professional Activity	Inactive	Not Classified
Vidalia, GA	4	4	1	2			1			
Vincennes, IN	17	16	5	4		6	1		1	
Wabash, IN	3	3	2	1						
Wahpeton, ND-MN	1	1	1							
Walla Walla, WA	9	9	5		1	2	1			
Walterboro, SC	2	2	1				1			
Wapakoneta, OH	8	7		1	3	3			1	
Warren, PA	5	4	1			2	1			1
Warrensburg, MO	11	10	2	1	1	3	3	1		
Warsaw, IN	11	11	3	4	2	1	1			
Washington Court House, OH	3	3	1	1		1				
Washington, IN	12	10		1	3	4	2		1	1
Washington, NC	2	2	1			1				
Watertown-Fort Atkinson, WI	8	6	4		1	1			2	
Watertown-Fort Drum, NY	26	20	3	5		8	4		1	5
Watertown, SD	3	3		1	1	1				
Waycross, GA	7	6	1	3	1	1		1		
Weatherford, OK	5	4	3				1		1	
West Plains, MO	17	15	4		1	6	4		1	1
West Point, MS	4	4	4							
Whitewater, WI	7	7	2	2	2	1				
Willimantic, CT	14	13	6	1		3	3			1
Willmar, MN	9	9	1	3	2	2	1			
Wilmington, OH	8	8	2	1	4		1			
Wilson, NC	7	6	2	2	1	1		1		
Winfield, KS	6	4	3			1			1	1
Winona, MN	8	8	2	2	1	2	1			
Woodward, OK	3	3	1	1	1					
Wooster, OH	26	22	10	5		5	2		4	
Worthington, MN	2	2		1	1					
Yankton, SD	2	1		1					1	
Zanesville, OH	30	25	6	4	2	10	3		3	2
Zanesville, OH	30	25	6	4	2	10	3		3	2

Note: Does not include Address Unknown.

Table 5.22

Non-Metropolitan DOs by State, 2010

		Major Professional Activity									
		Patient Care									
			Office-Based Practice								
State	Total Physicians	Total Patient Care	FM/GP Practice	Medical Specialties	Surgical Specialties	Other Specialties	Hospital Based Practice	Other Professional Activity	Inactive	Not Classified
Total Non-Metropolitan Physicians	2,968	2,531	1,253	215	201	446	416	39	231	166
Alabama	37	33	21	4	1	4	3		3	1
Alaska	34	30	17		3	3	7	1	1	2
Arizona	12	8	3	1	1		3	1		3
Arkansas	31	27	21	1	2	3			2	2
California	22	21	12	2		3	4			1
Colorado	81	74	32	2	8	20	12		3	4
Florida	40	33	15	4	1	10	3		6	1
Georgia	61	54	28	7	5	9	5	2	5	
Idaho	33	30	19	1	2	4	4		2	1
Illinois	42	38	17	4	3	8	6	1	2	1
Indiana	23	21	9	1	1	5	5		2	
Iowa	193	172	121	8	8	14	21	2	13	6
Kansas	77	72	51		5	6	10		4	1
Kentucky	132	98	29	14	10	19	26	3	2	29
Louisiana	3	2	1	1					1	
Maine	129	104	44	10	6	16	28	1	12	12
Maryland	10	9	5	1		3			1	
Michigan	339	284	103	28	38	76	39	3	44	8
Minnesota	40	37	20	2	3	7	5		3	
Mississippi	43	40	27	3	2	2	6	1	1	1
Missouri	242	203	103	13	16	42	29	2	30	7
Montana	44	37	21	4	4	2	6	1	3	3
Nebraska	16	15	11		2		2	1		
Nevada	4	4	3			1				
New Hampshire	12	9	3	2	2	2			3	
New Mexico	5	3	1				2		2	
New York	27	24	9	5	2	3	5		2	1
North Carolina	34	31	10	4	7	4	6		1	2
North Dakota	12	9	3	1	1	2	2		1	2
Ohio	49	42	28	2	1	4	7		6	1
Oklahoma	125	104	62	2	3	18	19	1	15	5
Oregon	15	15	6	1		4	4			
Pennsylvania	104	87	32	12	11	13	19		11	6
South Carolina	13	12	7		3	1	1			1
South Dakota	21	17	8	2	1	3	3		3	1
Tennessee	50	42	24	2	3	9	4	4	3	1
Texas	149	133	87	5	7	23	11	2	11	3
Utah	23	21	15		2	2	2		1	1
Vermont	21	16	4	1	2	7	2		5	
Virginia	87	76	22	18	4	19	13	1	4	6
Washington	31	30	17		3	2	8			1
West Virginia	207	173	87	24	12	26	24	5	13	16
Wisconsin	87	79	42	11	4	14	8	2	3	3
Wyoming	20	16	6	1	2	4	3		3	1
Possessions	17	11	5	2		2	2		2	4
APOs and FPOs	170	135	42	9	10	27	47	5	2	28

Note: Does not include Address Unknown.

Table 5.23

DOs by Self-Designated Primary Care Specialty, Activity, and Sex, 2010

		Patient Care				Other Professional Activity			
				Hospital Based					
Specialty	Total Physicians	Total Patient Care	Office Based	Resid./ Fellows	Phys. Staff	Admin.	Med. Teach.	Research	Other
				Both Sexes					
Total Physicians	65,565	55,091	43,245	6,354	5,492	478	425	134	130
Active Physicians	61,565	55,091	43,245	6,354	5,492	478	425	134	130
Primary Care	27,777	27,266	22,879	2,029	2,358	205	228	31	47
Family Medicine	15,090	14,777	12,714	847	1,216	123	146	15	29
General Practice	2,709	2,672	2,421		251	26	11		
Internal Medicine	5,525	5,429	4,264	620	545	39	37	12	8
Obstetrics/Gynecology	2,234	2,213	1,781	256	176	8	10		3
Pediatrics	2,219	2,175	1,699	306	170	9	24	4	7
Prim. Care Subspec.	2,881	2,793	2,001	572	220	30	22	32	4
FM Subspecialties	251	245	196	33	16	4	2		
IM Subspecialties	1,845	1,787	1,360	304	123	19	12	24	3
OBG Subspecialties	124	115	96		19	3	2	3	1
PD Subspecialties	661	646	349	235	62	4	6	5	
All Other Specialties	25,600	25,032	18,365	3,753	2,914	243	175	71	79
Inactive	3,999								
Not Classified	5,307								
Address Unknown	1								
				Male					
Total Physicians	46,113	38,526	31,042	3,354	4,130	397	312	102	94
Active Physicians	42,596	38,526	31,042	3,354	4,130	397	312	102	94
Primary Care	18,214	17,832	15,341	808	1,683	176	151	23	32
Family Medicine	10,171	9,940	8,674	352	914	105	96	10	20
General Practice	2,275	2,243	2,042		201	23	9		
Internal Medicine	3,776	3,700	2,998	331	371	33	25	11	7
Obstetrics/Gynecology	1,145	1,129	955	58	116	7	8		1
Pediatrics	847	820	672	67	81	8	13	2	4
Prim. Care Subspec.	1,849	1,789	1,366	272	151	21	17	19	3
FM Subspecialties	187	182	149	21	12	3	2		
IM Subspecialties	1,235	1,193	950	157	86	13	11	16	2
OBG Subspecialties	83	78	64		14	2	1	1	1
PD Subspecialties	344	336	203	94	39	3	3	2	
All Other Specialties	19,368	18,905	14,335	2,274	2,296	200	144	60	59
Inactive	3,516								
Not Classified	3,165								
Address Unknown	1								
				Female					
Total Physicians	19,452	16,565	12,203	3,000	1,362	81	113	32	36
Active Physicians	18,969	16,565	12,203	3,000	1,362	81	113	32	36
Primary Care	9,563	9,434	7,538	1,221	675	29	77	8	15
Family Medicine	4,919	4,837	4,040	495	302	18	50	5	9
General Practice	434	429	379		50	3	2		
Internal Medicine	1,749	1,729	1,266	289	174	6	12	1	1
Obstetrics/Gynecology	1,089	1,084	826	198	60	1	2		2
Pediatrics	1,372	1,355	1,027	239	89	1	11	2	3
Prim. Care Subspec.	1,032	1,004	635	300	69	9	5	13	1
FM Subspecialties	64	63	47	12	4	1			
IM Subspecialties	610	594	410	147	37	6	1	8	1
OBG Subspecialties	41	37	32		5	1	1	2	
PD Subspecialties	317	310	146	141	23	1	3	3	
All Other Specialties	6,232	6,127	4,030	1,479	618	43	31	11	20
Inactive	483								
Not Classified	2,142								

Table 5.24

DOs by Self-Designated Primary Care Specialty, Age, and Sex, 2010

Activity	Total Physicians	< 35	35-44	45-54	55-64	≥ 65
			Both Sexes			
Total Physicians	65,565	12,578	18,693	15,712	10,621	7,961
Active Physicians	61,565	12,566	18,599	15,383	10,030	4,987
Primary Care	27,777	4,388	7,947	7,969	5,295	2,178
Family Medicine	15,090	2,106	4,559	4,513	2,804	1,108
General Practice	2,709	3	99	826	1,129	652
Internal Medicine	5,525	1,135	1,768	1,599	782	241
Obstetrics/Gynecology	2,234	464	767	584	330	89
Pediatrics	2,219	680	754	447	250	88
Prim. Care Subspec.	2,881	796	1,040	604	342	99
FM Subspecialties	251	81	88	38	29	15
IM Subspecialties	1,845	449	717	407	222	50
OBG Subspecialties	124	1	12	45	43	23
PD Subspecialties	661	265	223	114	48	11
All Other Specialties	25,600	4,755	7,805	6,500	4,311	2,229
Inactive	3,999	12	94	329	590	2,974
Not Classified	5,307	2,627	1,807	310	82	481
Address Unknown	1				1	
			Male			
Total Physicians	46,113	6,552	12,241	11,391	8,858	7,071
Active Physicians	42,596	6,549	12,203	11,195	8,384	4,265
Primary Care	18,214	1,781	4,613	5,485	4,379	1,956
Family Medicine	10,171	899	2,809	3,165	2,308	990
General Practice	2,275	3	68	622	967	615
Internal Medicine	3,776	614	1,150	1,155	652	205
Obstetrics/Gynecology	1,145	107	321	364	273	80
Pediatrics	847	158	265	179	179	66
Prim. Care Subspec.	1,849	407	667	417	278	80
FM Subspecialties	187	55	67	28	26	11
IM Subspecialties	1,235	246	476	290	182	41
OBG Subspecialties	83	1	5	25	33	19
PD Subspecialties	344	105	119	74	37	9
All Other Specialties	19,368	2,910	5,755	5,116	3,677	1,910
Inactive	3,516	3	38	196	473	2,806
Not Classified	3,165	1,451	1,168	177	50	319
Address Unknown	1				1	
			Female			
Total Physicians	19,452	6,026	6,452	4,321	1,763	890
Active Physicians	18,969	6,017	6,396	4,188	1,646	722
Primary Care	9,563	2,607	3,334	2,484	916	222
Family Medicine	4,919	1,207	1,750	1,348	496	118
General Practice	434		31	204	162	37
Internal Medicine	1,749	521	618	444	130	36
Obstetrics/Gynecology	1,089	357	446	220	57	9
Pediatrics	1,372	522	489	268	71	22
Prim. Care Subspec.	1,032	389	373	187	64	19
FM Subspecialties	64	26	21	10	3	4
IM Subspecialties	610	203	241	117	40	9
OBG Subspecialties	41		7	20	10	4
PD Subspecialties	317	160	104	40	11	2
All Other Specialties	6,232	1,845	2,050	1,384	634	319
Inactive	483	9	56	133	117	168
Not Classified	2,142	1,176	639	133	32	162

Table 5.25

DOs by Self Designated Primary Care Specialty and State of Location, 2010

State	Total Physicians	Total Primary Care	Family Medicine	General Practice	Internal Medicine	OB/Gyn	Pediatrics	Primary Care Sub-specialties	All Other Specialties	Not Classi-fied	Inactive/ Address Unknown
Total Physicians	65,565	27,777	15,090	2,709	5,525	2,234	2,219	2,881	25,600	5,307	3,999
Alabama	438	209	134	14	38	12	11	19	168	27	15
Alaska	167	90	58	10	9	6	7	5	59	9	4
Arizona	1,962	782	420	87	157	60	58	86	775	138	181
Arkansas	289	146	94	17	22	6	7	10	98	21	14
California	4,207	2,028	1,165	127	442	136	158	159	1,467	435	118
Colorado	1,192	578	380	55	78	35	30	48	441	44	81
Connecticut	477	174	54	1	60	36	23	36	197	57	13
Delaware	308	137	78	5	22	17	15	23	100	25	23
District Of Columbia	120	33	13		12	1	7	13	46	26	2
Florida	4,708	1,814	978	221	364	123	128	168	1,957	284	485
Georgia	947	416	249	40	65	36	26	38	352	82	59
Hawaii	221	84	43	10	21	4	6	14	91	20	12
Idaho	289	143	106	6	14	9	8	8	113	12	13
Illinois	2,560	1,090	592	57	222	110	109	133	982	283	72
Indiana	952	429	254	53	58	45	19	48	383	43	49
Iowa	1,289	748	493	55	110	37	53	37	387	42	75
Kansas	763	373	218	57	49	27	22	27	272	53	38
Kentucky	542	226	114	15	48	27	22	24	209	68	15
Louisiana	180	60	22	4	12	12	10	10	83	16	11
Maine	738	391	255	30	61	19	26	30	221	55	41
Maryland	741	243	105	12	74	26	26	42	334	107	15
Massachusetts	794	334	107	12	142	32	41	65	276	98	21
Michigan	5,629	2,004	1,041	274	385	179	125	167	2,569	378	511
Minnesota	578	259	156	16	40	27	20	39	235	24	21
Mississippi	362	186	117	18	29	13	9	22	115	28	11
Missouri	2,228	980	507	185	151	71	66	98	859	125	166
Montana	159	82	58	6	12	5	1	3	60	7	7
Nebraska	197	105	64	6	13	9	13	11	64	13	4
Nevada	608	234	115	35	55	14	15	12	295	39	28
New Hampshire	275	135	82	2	35	5	11	12	101	17	10
New Jersey	3,015	1,165	514	90	299	122	140	190	1,214	235	211
New Mexico	311	144	86	20	24	6	8	1	120	21	25
New York	3,501	1,372	616	70	363	123	200	257	1,297	432	143
North Carolina	949	398	245	8	79	35	31	59	369	94	29
North Dakota	67	29	18	2	6	1	2	5	26	5	2
Ohio	4,644	1,629	776	205	367	151	130	174	2,061	464	316
Oklahoma	1,736	760	478	99	87	40	56	52	696	119	109
Oregon	748	365	198	39	91	17	20	38	249	38	58
Pennsylvania	6,417	2,629	1,348	241	605	211	224	304	2,434	561	489
Rhode Island	247	115	58	12	36	5	4	8	83	27	14
South Carolina	534	238	125	11	64	22	16	31	206	38	21
South Dakota	146	73	43	4	17	5	4	9	49	6	9
Tennessee	700	337	182	40	68	35	12	35	247	48	33
Texas	4,158	1,894	1,033	245	291	161	164	165	1,543	317	239
Utah	359	179	126	6	15	18	14	9	142	20	9
Vermont	77	31	16	5	6	3	1	1	29	7	9
Virginia	1,006	403	220	18	96	33	36	45	458	71	29
Washington	1,035	487	318	54	63	33	19	28	400	57	63
West Virginia	768	401	233	68	54	22	24	24	237	78	28
Wisconsin	940	485	288	37	80	42	38	34	330	52	39
Wyoming	98	42	32	2	4	3	1	1	41	9	5
Possessions	188	88	65	3	10	7	3	4	60	32	4
Address Unknown	1										

Notes:

Total Physicians include Active, Inactive, and Address Unknown.

FM subspecialties include FPG and FSM.

IM subspecialties include AMI, CCM, DIA, END, HEM, HEP, HO, ICE, ID, ILI, IMG, ISM, NEP, NTR, ON, PCC, and RHU.

OBG subspecialties include GO, GYN, MFM, OBS, OCC, and REN.

PD subspecialties include ADL, CCP, MPD, NPM, PDA, PDC, PDE, PDI, PDP, PDT, PEM, PG, PHO, PLI, PN, PPR, and PSM.

Chapter 6

Physician Trends

Increased demand for health services in the last two decades, along with forecasts of health care resources and the number of physicians per capita through the year 2000, resulted in concern throughout the medical community that the physician workforce would prove inadequate to meet the emerging health needs of the nation. To ensure the supply of physicians, a variety of measures were implemented. Complicated immigration regulations were modified to more readily allow the entry of foreign physicians into US medicine. Earlier exchange programs were extended to allow aliens to waive the two-year foreign residence requirement in the home or third country after studying in the US if their admission was in the public interest,[1] and medical schools received additional funding to expand capacities and accommodate larger enrollments. Government at the state and federal levels authorized financing procedures and programs to achieve new health care objectives, and private foundations and medical associations undertook measures to parallel these efforts.

The 1970s and, in some cases, the early 1980s witnessed additional environmental developments that promised to have important effects on organized medicine. Some of these included a change in the demographic characteristics and growth rate of the US population, a shift in migration patterns, and an overall change in the composition of the physician supply.[2]

An examination of the historical physician profile reflects some of these general trends. Although these historical data should be useful to workforce planners and health policy analysts, readers should not interpret these data as indicative of misdistribution, oversupply, or undersupply.

Collection and Classification Systems

The *Re-Classification of Physicians' Professional Activities* project was initiated in 1967.[3] The purpose of the project was to increase the validity and reliability of physicians' records and to facilitate the classification of the physician workforce in functional categories.

Traditionally, the physician population was distributed between the two categories of Private Practice and Not in Private Practice, a classification scheme affected more by the type of employer and fee-for-service vs. salary forms of remuneration than by the actual activity of individual physicians. The new system introduced the functional categories Patient Care and Other Professional Activity. This classification concept is based on the extent to which a physician is engaged in direct care of patients and is, therefore, more meaningful than a concept based on the financial characteristics of a practice.

A good example of how the earlier system was based on employment rather than activity was the category Medical School Faculty. Most physicians who were employed by medical schools were placed in this category, even though many of them spent more time in Research, Administration, or even in Patient Care than in actual teaching. In the new system, Medical Teaching replaced Medical School Faculty to emphasize that only physicians who are actively teaching are included in this category.

Under the new system, the Not Classified category was introduced as a contingency category for physicians for whom no information is available. Physicians are temporarily assigned to this category until additional follow-up information can be obtained that can ensure proper classification. Also in 1968, as part of the reclassification effort, Fellows were classified in Research rather than in Residency programs to reflect the assessment that a majority of Fellows were engaged in medical research at that time. In 1986, a separate category was added for Clinical Fellows, which previously had been included in Research. (See the "Definitions" section in the Introduction for more information on physician classifications.) In 1994, the separate category of Fellows was discontinued; Fellows were tabulated as Residents/Fellows.

Total US Physicians

Major Categories

Table K demonstrates the total population of physicians in the US, with a numeric distribution of physicians in such major categories as Patient Care, the primary care specialties, school of graduation, and sex from 1970 to 2010. An analysis of the table reveals that the vast majority of US physicians have remained in Patient Care: 83.4% (1970), 80.5% (1980), and 76.4 (2010). The proportion of female physicians to total physicians has nearly quadrupled between 1970 and 2010, from 7.6% to 30.1%.

Although physicians in the primary care specialties showed a fairly steady decline as a percentage of the total physician population in the 39-year period — 40.2% (1970), 36.5% (1980), 34.7% (1990), 30.9% (2010) — they demonstrated a percentage growth of 126.8% from 134,354 physicians in 1970 to 304,687 physicians in 2010.

Table K also suggests some striking distribution patterns for international and US medical graduates. International Medical Graduates (IMGs), for example, comprised 17.1% of total physicians in 1970, but in 2010, they constituted 25.8%. US medical graduates accounted for 81.0% of all physicians in 1970 and 73.0% four decades later.

Activity

The major professional activity classification of physicians indicates whether a physician is engaged

Table K

Total US Physicians by Major Categories, 1970-2010

Category	*1970*	*1980*	*1990*	*2010*
Total Physicians*	**334,028**	**467,679**	**615,421**	**985,375**
Patient Care	278,535	376,512	503,870	752,572
Non-patient Care	32,310	38,404	43,440	42,290
Primary Care†	134,354	170,705	213,514	304,687
Primary Care Subspecialties‡	25,401	16,642	30,911	76,122
Male	308,627	413,395	511,227	688,468
Female	25,401	54,284	104,194	296,907
US Graduates§	270,637	362,307	475,394	719,122
International Med. Graduates	57,217	97,726	131,764	254,396
Canadian Graduates	6,174	7,646	8,263	11,857

**Address Unknown is excluded from all Federal/Nonfederal categories, and Not-Classified, Inactive, and Address Unknown are excluded from Patient Care/Non-patient Care categories.*

†Includes General Specialties of Family Practice, General Practice, Internal Medicine, Obstetrics/Gynecology, and Pediatrics.

‡Includes primary care subspecialties as listed in footnote for Family Practice, General Practice, Internal Medicine, Obstetrics/Gynecology, and Pediatrics on Table 4.7,

§Includes graduates from Inactive Schools.

Source: Tables 1.1 and 1.17, and Table 4.1

in direct care of patients or in Other Professional Activity. Patient Care is further subcategorized into Office-Based and Hospital-Based practice, which includes Residents/Fellows and full-time Hospital Staff. Other Professional Activity includes Medical Teaching, Administration, Research, and the category of Other. Other was introduced in 1968 for physicians engaged in such activities as journalism, law, or sales or employed by pharmaceutical companies, medical societies, and so on. (The "Definitions" section of the Introduction explains the categories in Major Professional Activity.)

During the 10-year period from 1975 to 1985 (Table 6.1), the number of physicians in Patient Care increased by 136,883 for a gain of 43.9%. Between 1980 and 2010, 376,060 physicians were added to the Patient Care physician population for an increase of 99.9%. Within the Patient Care category between 1975 and 1985 there were increases of 53.3% in Office-Based practice and 22.9% in Hospital-Based practice. Since 1980, the complement of Office-Based physicians grew by 107.7%, and that in Hospital-Based practice did so by 79.5%.

Proportionate percentages of physicians in residency/fellowship training since 1975 showed little fluctuation until recently: 14.7% (1975), 13.3% (1980), 13.6% (1985), 15.0% (1990), and 11.0% (2010). However, the total number of Residents/Fellows since 1975 grew by 50,340, or 87.1%. Figure 6.1 displays the distribution of the total physician population between 1975 and 2010 and the distribution of physicians in Patient Care, Office-Based, and Hospital-Based practice.

Table L displays a profile of country and year of graduation for physicians as of 2010. Of the 254,396 IMGs included in the US physician workforce in 2010, nearly one quarter (20.8%), or 53,075, received their MD degrees before 1970, whereas one fifth (16.7%) of the graduates from US active schools, or 119,663 physicians, did so in the same time period. Table L shows that one fifth of physicians graduated from medical schools before 1970 (17.9%). This percentage is greater for graduates of Canadian medical schools. For Canadian graduates, nearly one third (28.3%) graduated before 1970.

Specialty

Tables 6.2 through 6.4 demonstrate the relationship between specialization and physician supply between 1975 and 2010. The number of physicians in General Practice greatly diminished in the 35-year period, decreasing by 33,783. The decline may be explained in part by the establishment in 1975 of the discipline of Family Medicine. Between 1975 and 2010, Family Medicine showed an increase of 75,435 physicians.

Between 1975 and 1985, the total physician population increased by 40.4% (Table 6.4). However, the number of physicians in General Practice decreased by 36.2% in this same interval. By contrast, in absolute numbers, Internal Medicine demonstrated a dramatic increase of 63.6% from 1975 (54,331) to 1985 (88,862). Between 1980 and 2010, Internal Medicine increased by 125.5% for a gain of 89,745 physicians. In 1975, Diagnostic Radiology account-

Table L

Physicians by Year and Country of Graduation, 2010

	Number				Percent			
Country of Graduation	*Total*	*Prior to 1970*	*1970-1989*	*1990 & Later*	*Total*	*Prior to 1970*	*1970-1989*	*1990 & Later*
Total Physicians	**985,375**	**176,341**	**375,814**	**433,220**	**100.0**	**17.9**	**38.1**	**44.0**
US Medical Schools								
Active Schools	718,521	119,663	267,446	331,412	100.0	16.7	37.2	46.1
Inactive Schools	601	251	305	45	100.0	41.8	50.7	7.5
Canadian Schools	11,857	3,352	5,065	3,440	100.0	28.3	42.7	29.0
International Schools	254,396	53,075	102,998	98,323	100.0	20.9	40.5	38.6

Source: Table 1.17

Figure 6.1

Physicians by Major Professional Activity, 1975-2010

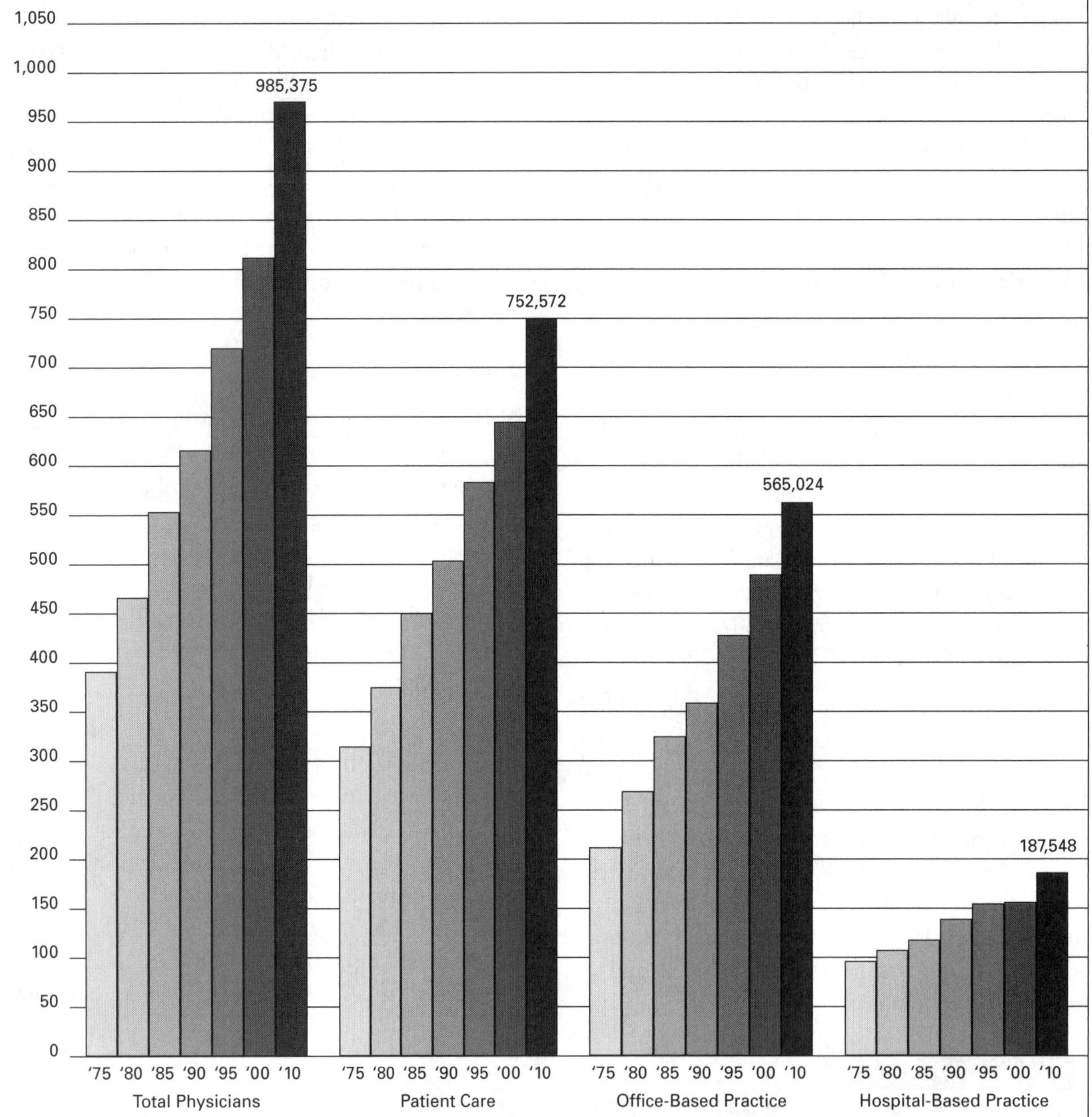

Source: Table 6.1

ed for only 3,544 physicians of a total physician workforce of 393,742 or 0.9%. In 2010, however, Diagnostic Radiologists numbered 26,054, representing 2.6% of all physicians for the year. Figure 6.2 demonstrates trends in the five largest specialties in 2010 for selected years 1975 to 2010.

Age and Sex

An age and sex profile of all physicians in the US (Table 6.5) indicated that a little more than half were younger than 45 years in each of the selected years 1975 to 1990. In 2010, this proportion was 38.6%. This trend was also true of the male physician population, but the female physician population consistently showed higher percentages in the young age groups compared with the male population. In 1975, 62.3% of female physicians were younger than 45 years compared with 72.9% in

Figure 6.2

Trends in the Distribution of Physicians by Self-Designated Specialty for Selected Years, 1975-2010

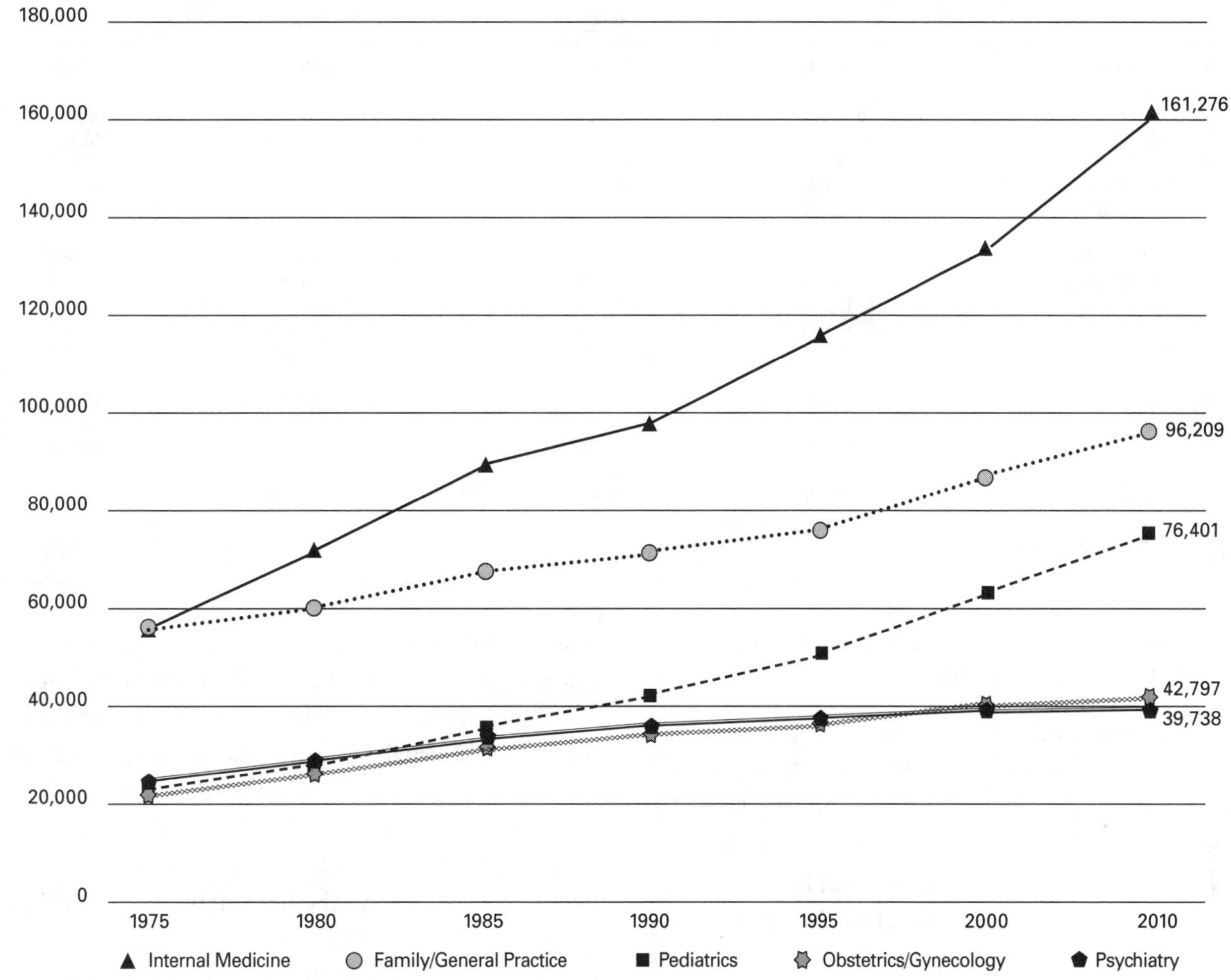

Source: Table 6.2

1985 and 55.6% in 2010. Between 1975 and 2010, the number of female physicians younger than 45 years showed a more than sixfold increase.

The total number of physicians 65 years and older more than tripled from 50,993 in 1975 to 194,857 in 2010, and the percentage of total physicians increased from 13.0% to 19.8%. The male/female distribution in this group has shown little change during the period, with physicians 65 years or older being 92.8% male and 7.2% female in 1975 and 88.4% male and 11.6% female in 2010.

International Medical Graduates (IMGs)

Activity

A trend analysis of Tables 6.6 through 6.8 compared with Table 6.1 reveals that the total number of physicians increased by 591,633 between 1975 and 2010, or 150.3%; IMGs accounted for more than one fourth (29.0%) of this increase by gaining 171,548 physicians. In the 35-year period, the number of non-IMGs grew by 133.6%, whereas the number of IMGs increased by 214.7%. Table M further reveals that in 1980, IMGs accounted for 20.9% of the total physician count of 467,679. The

Table M

Total Physicians and International Medical Graduates by Activity for 1980 and 2010

	1980		2010	
Activity	*Total*	*IMGs*	*Total*	*IMGs*
Total Physicians	**467,679**	**97,726**	**985,375**	**254,396**
Patient Care	376,512	72,935	752,572	192,046
Office-Based Practice	272,000	45,764	565,024	140,246
Hospital-Based Practice	104,512	27,171	187,548	51,800
Residents/Fellows	62,042	11,424	108,142	28,434
Full-Time Staff	42,470	15,747	79,406	23,366
Other Prof. Activity	38,404	8,656	42,290	6,908
Medical Teaching	7,942	1,569	14,009	1,812
Administration	12,209	1,533	9,909	1,654
Research	15,377	4,918	13,755	2,462
Other	2,876	636	4,617	980
Not Classified	20,629	10,235	64,153	25,748
Inactive	25,744	2,731	125,928	29,608
Address Unknown	6,390	3,169	432	86

Source: Tables 6.1 and 6.9

percentage climbed to 25.8% of the total count of 985,375 physicians in 2010.

As a study of Table M and Table 6.9 indicates, however, the percentage of IMGs in full-time staff positions decreased from 16.1% in 1980 to 9.2% 30 years later. This decrease may be attributed in large part to the variety of questions raised in the 1970s regarding the escalating number of alien physicians in the US and the enactment of federal legislation in 1976 that placed limitations on the immigration of foreign nationals.* Figure 6.3 depicts the percentage change of IMGs and total physicians by major professional activity categories from 1980 to 2010.

Specialty

All specialties listed in Table 6.6 except Aerospace Medicine, General Practice, Public Health, and Radiology had a larger number of IMGs in 2010 than in 1975. The following specialties increased more than 100% from 1975 to 2010: Allergy and Immunology, Anesthesiology, Cardiovascular Diseases, Child Psychiatry, Colon and Rectal Surgery, Diagnostic Radiology, Family Medicine, Forensic Pathology, Gastroenterology, General Preventive Medicine, Internal Medicine, Neurology, Pediatrics, Pediatric Cardiology, Physical Medicine and Rehabilitation, Plastic Surgery, Psychiatry, Pulmonary Diseases, Radiation Oncology, and Thoracic Surgery. Table N displays the percentage of total IMGs among the largest IMG specialties, ranked by size, in 2010. The table also provides percentages and ranks for 1980.

* Health Professions Educational Assistance Act of 1976 (P.L. 94 484). Title VI of P.L. 94 484 "Limitation of Foreign Medical Graduates" as amended by the Health Services Extension Act of 1977 further required IMGs emigrating to the US for Graduate Medical Education to take and pass the VISA Qualifying Examination (VQE).

Table N

Percentage of IMGs in Highest IMG Self-Designated Specialties Ranked by Size, 2010

	Percentage of Total IMGs		Rank	
Specialty	*1980*	*2010*	*1980*	*2010*
Internal Medicine	**13.4%**	**24.0%**	**1**	**1**
General/Family Practice	**9.4%**	**9.6%**	**2**	**2**
Pediatrics	**6.8%**	**8.0%**	**5**	**3**
Psychaitry	**7.0%**	**4.9%**	**3**	**4**
Anesthesiology	**6.0%**	**4.5%**	**6**	**5**
Cardiovascular Disease	**2.3%**	**2.8%**	**9**	**6**
Obstetrics/Gynecology	**5.4%**	**2.7%**	**7**	**7**
General Surgery	**6.9%**	**2.6%**	**4**	**8**
Pathology	**4.0%**	**2.4%**	**8**	**9**

Source: Table 6.7

Figure 6.3

Percentage Change in Total Physicians and International Medical Graduates by Major Professional Activity, 1980-2010

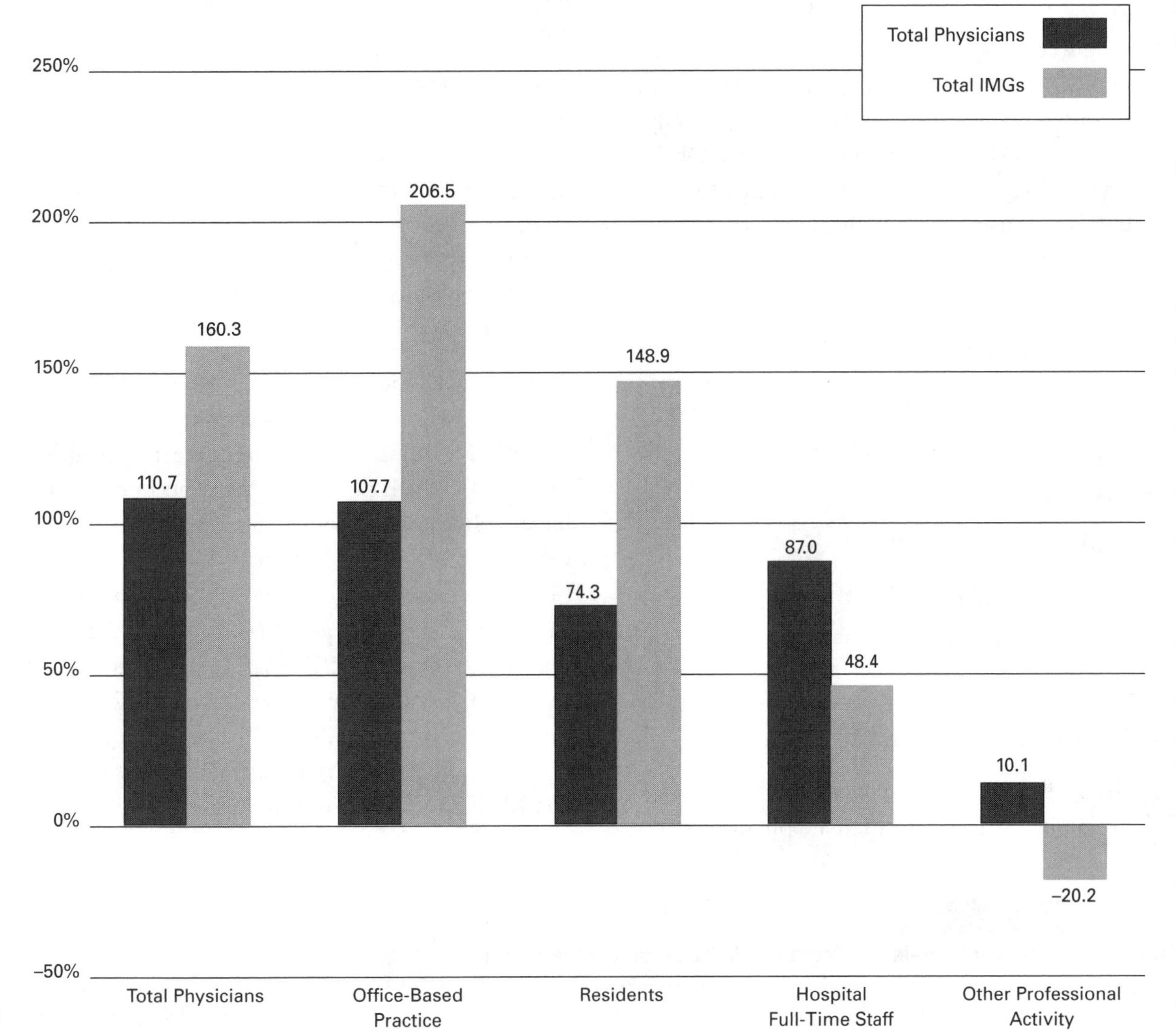

Source: Tables 6.1 and 6.9

Table 6.9 shows changes in major professional activity for IMGs from 1975 to 2010. Although most IMGs were in Patient Care for the years surveyed, the percentage in Patient Care has remained about the same. However, Office-Based practice increased from 1975 to 2010 (40.6% and 55.1%).

Female Physicians

Activity

Between 1980 and 2010, the total number of physicians in the US grew by 110.7% (Table O), whereas the total number of female physicians increased 447.0%. Female physicians in Patient Care increased by 498.0%, which was largely accounted for by the high increase in the number of female physicians in Office-Based practice (703.5%). The next largest increase was in female Full-Time Staff (303.0%).

Table O also indicates increased representation of women in residency programs, growing from 21.5% of total Resident physicians in 1980 to 45.4% in 2010. Women also demonstrated considerable percentage increases in Patient Care, from 10.6% of all physicians in the category in 1980 to 31.8% in 2010 (see also Table 6.13).

Specialty

The total number of female physicians increased more than six-fold between 1975 and 2010 from 35,626 to 296,907 physicians (Table 6.10). In 1975, only seven specialties had more than 1,000 female physicians: Pediatrics (5,135), Internal Medicine (4,006), Psychiatry (3,144), General/Family Medicine (2,866), Anesthesiology (1,819), Obstetrics/Gynecology (1,777), and Pathology (1,674). By 2010, there were 10 specialties with more than 5,000 female physicians:

Internal Medicine (54,182)

Pediatrics (43,079)

General/Family Medicine (32,376)

Obstetrics/Gynecology (20,820)

Psychiatry (14,264)

Anesthesiology (10,437)

Emergency Medicine (8,300)

Pathology (7,013)

General Surgery (6,660)

Diagnostic Radiology (6,135)

Although rankings changed over time, all seven of the specialties with the most female physicians in 1975 remained among the top ranking in 2010. Pediatrics had the highest count of female physicians in 1975 and 1980, but Internal Medicine had the most female physicians in 1985, 1990, 1995, 2000, and 2010.

The total number of female physicians more than doubled between 1975 and 1985 (Table 6.12). In that decade, 10 specialties grew four times or more in the numbers of female physicians: Family Medicine, Diagnostic Radiology, Thoracic Surgery, Urological Surgery, Forensic Pathology, Gastroenterology, Neurological Surgery, Orthopedic Surgery, Aerospace Medicine, and Otolaryngology.

As Table 6.12 indicates, from 1990 to 2010, the total number of female physicians increased by 185.0%. During these 20 years, sixteen specialties exhibited growth of 200% or more in numbers of female physicians: Thoracic Surgery (784.0%), Colon & Rectal Surgery (693.5%), Urological Surgery (489.6%), Gastroenterology (305.9%), Emergency Medicine (303.3%), Family Medicine (292.5%), Pulmonary Diseases (274.9%), Otolaryngology (263.1%), General Preventive Medicine (258.6%), Orthopedic Surgery (241.3%), Plastic Surgery (233.0%), Pediatric Cardiology (223.1%), Neurology (210.2%), Neurological Surgery (209.4%),

Table O

Total Physicians and Female Physicians by Activity for 1980 and 2010

	1980		2010	
Activity	*Total*	*Female*	*Total*	*Female*
Total Physicians	**467,679**	**54,284**	**985,375**	**296,907**
Patient Care	376,512	39,969	752,572	238,980
Office-Based Practice	272,000	20,609	565,024	165,595
Hospital-Based Practice	104,512	19,360	187,548	73,385
Residents/Fellows	62,042	13,322	108,142	49,053
Full-Time Staff	42,470	6,038	79,406	24,332
Other Prof. Activity	38,404	4,737	42,290	10,280
Medical Teaching	7,942	1,090	14,009	2,973
Administration	12,209	1,178	9,909	2,775
Research	15,377	2,077	13,755	3,094
Other	2,876	392	4,617	1,438
Not Classified	20,629	4,030	64,153	28,655
Inactive	25,744	3,773	125,928	18,856
Address Unknown	6,390	1,775	432	136

Source: Tables 6.1 and 6.9

Cardiovascular Disease (209.2%), and Dermatology (200.5%).

Table 6.13 shows that although the number of women in each of the activities increased from 1975 to 2010, the percentage distributions decreased for most of the activities. Prominent among the few activities seeing distributional increases, Patient Care accounted for 68.3% of female physicians' activity in 1975 and 80.5% in 2010. Office-Based practice represented 35.1% of female physicians' activity in 1975 and more than half (55.8%) in 2010.

Physician-Population Ratios

The physician-population ratios and rank by state in Chapter 6 should not be interpreted as indicative of oversupply, misdistribution, or undersupply. Although some have used aggregate physician-population ratios to suggest availability or shortage, the ratios alone should not be construed as constituting an adequate measure of the quantity or quality of health care received by the American public. An analysis of health care requirements, ancillary medical resources, demographic and socioeconomic factors, and geographic location, among other factors, is required to assess equitable or optimal access to services. The ratios are provided, therefore, as general guidelines to allow comparisons of the distribution of physicians over time and among the states, as well as of selected specialties.

National Ratios

An analysis of Table 6.14 indicates that the number of physicians increased by 237.4% between 1965 and 2010, whereas the US population did so by only 56.8%. The ratios of Patient Care physicians per 100,000 civilians between 1965 and 2010 showed similar patterns. Physicians in Patient Care totaled 259,418 in 1965 and 752,572 in 2010, a 190.1% gain. As a result, in 1965 there were 132 Patient Care physicians per 100,000 people, but by 2010 there were 244, an increase of 84.8%. The number of people per physician in Patient Care steadily declined between 1965 and 2010 from 760 (1965) to 411 (2010).

State Ratios

Although the number of physicians per 100,000 population averaged 314 in 2010 (Table 6.15), one state in 2010 had a ratio of 205: Oklahoma. However, no state, the District of Columbia, or Possessions have seen a decrease in this ratio since 1975.

In 2010, 20 states (including the District of Columbia) demonstrated physician-population ratios in Patient Care at or above the national average of 240 physicians per 100,000 people (Table 6.17). In this group, the District of Columbia (674), Massachusetts (390), Maryland (339), Rhode Island (333), and New York (327) had the highest Patient Care ratios. Mississippi (166), Idaho (163), and Oklahoma (162) had the lowest.

Specialty Ratios

As Table 6.19 indicates, ratios between 1980 and 2010 showed increases of 55.0% for Office-Based physicians, from 120.6 per 100,000 (1980) to 186.9 per 100,000 (2010), and more than 57.6% for total physicians: 207.3 (1980) to 326.7 (2010). As General Practice ratios in Office-Based practice declined in the 1980s, Family Medicine ratios demonstrated continuous increases: 8.1 (1980), 15.2 (1990), and 23.1 (2010).

The ratio spread was small between total physicians and Office-Based physicians in General Practice in 1980 (14.4 per 100,000 vs 13.1 per 100,000) and 2010 (2.8 vs. 2.4). Pathology, conversely, illustrates that physicians in this discipline are not Office Based in as large numbers as are General Practitioners: 6.0 vs 2.7 (1980) and 6.5 vs. 3.7 (2010).

References

1. *Foreign Medical Graduates in the US 1970.* Chicago, IL: Center for Health Services Research and Development, American Medical Association; 1971.

2. *The Environment of Medicine: Report of the Council on Long Range Planning and Development.* Chicago, IL: American Medical Association; December 1983.

3. *Reclassification of Physicians, 1968.* Chicago, IL: Center for Health Services Research and Development, American Medical Association; 1971.

Table 6.1

Physicians by Activity, 1975-2010

	1975	1980	1985	1990	1995	2000	2010
			Number				
Total Physicians	393,742	467,679	552,716	615,421	720,325	813,770	985,375
Patient Care	311,937	376,512	448,820	503,870	582,131	647,430	752,572
Office-Based Practice	215,429	272,000	330,197	360,995	427,275	490,398	565,024
Hospital-Based Practice	96,508	104,512	118,623	142,875	154,856	157,032	187,548
Residents/Fellows*	57,802	62,042	75,411	92,080	96,352	95,725	108,142
Full-Time Staff	38,706	42,470	43,212	50,795	58,504	61,307	79,406
Other Prof. Activity	28,343	38,404	48,320	43,440	43,312	44,938	42,290
Administration	11,161	12,209	13,810	14,819	16,345	16,210	14,009
Medical Teaching	6,445	7,942	7,832	8,090	9,469	10,214	9,909
Research**	7,944	15,377	23,268	16,930	14,340	14,598	13,755
Other	2,793	2,876	3,410	3,601	3,158	3,916	4,617
Inactive	21,449	25,744	38,646	52,653	72,326	75,168	125,928
Not Classified	26,145	20,629	13,950	12,678	20,579	45,136	64,153
Address Unknown	5,868	6,390	2,980	2,780	1,977	1,098	432
			Percent Distribution				
Total Physicians	100.0	100.0	100.0	100.0	100.0	100.0	100.0
Patient Care	79.2	80.5	81.2	81.9	80.8	79.6	76.4
Office-Based Practice	54.7	58.2	59.7	58.7	59.3	60.3	57.3
Hospital-Based Practice	24.5	22.3	21.5	23.2	21.5	19.3	19.0
Residents/Fellows*	14.7	13.3	13.6	15.0	13.4	11.8	11.0
Full-Time Staff	9.8	9.1	7.8	8.3	8.1	7.5	8.1
Other Prof. Activity	7.2	8.2	8.7	7.1	6.0	5.5	4.3
Administration	2.8	2.6	2.5	2.4	2.3	2.0	1.4
Medical Teaching	1.6	1.7	1.4	1.3	1.3	1.3	1.0
Research**	2.0	3.3	4.2	2.8	2.0	1.8	1.4
Other	0.7	0.6	0.6	0.6	0.4	0.5	0.5
Inactive	5.4	5.5	7.0	8.6	10.0	9.2	12.8
Not Classified	6.6	4.4	2.5	2.1	2.9	5.5	6.5
Address Unknown	1.5	1.4	0.5	0.5	0.3	0.1	0.0
			Percent Change				
	1975-2010	1975-1985	1985-1995	1975-1980	1980-1985	1985-1990	1990-2010
Total Physicians	150.3	40.4	30.3	18.8	18.2	11.3	60.1
Patient Care	141.3	43.9	29.7	20.7	19.2	12.3	49.4
Office-Based Practice	162.3	53.3	29.4	26.3	21.4	9.3	56.5
Hospital-Based Practice	94.3	22.9	30.5	8.3	13.5	20.4	31.3
Residents/Fellows*	87.1	30.5	27.8	7.3	21.5	22.1	17.4
Full-Time Staff	105.2	11.6	35.4	9.7	1.7	17.5	56.3
Other Prof. Activity	49.2	70.5	–10.4	35.5	25.8	–10.1	-2.6
Administration	117.4	23.7	18.4	9.4	13.1	7.3	73.2
Medical Teaching	–11.2	21.5	20.9	23.2	-1.4	3.3	-33.1
Research**	73.1	192.9	–38.4	93.6	51.3	–27.2	–18.8
Other	65.3	22.1	-7.4	3.0	18.6	5.6	28.2
Inactive	487.1	80.2	87.2	20.0	50.1	36.2	139.2
Not Classified	145.4	–46.6	47.5	–21.1	–32.4	–9.1	406.0
Address Unknown	–92.6	–49.2	–33.7	8.9	–53.4	–6.7	–84.5

Note: Data for 1990 through 1994 are as of January 1; data prior to 1990 and for 1995-2010 are as of December 31.

**Includes all years of residency.*

***Includes physicians in research activities and Research Fellows.*

Table 6.2

Physicians by Self Designated Specialty, 1975-2010

Specialty	1975	1980	1985	1990	1995	2000	2010
Total Physicians	393,742	467,679	552,716	615,421	720,325	813,770	985,375
Aerospace Medicine	684	587	674	687	575	473	413
Allergy/Immunology	1,716	1,518	3,060	3,388	3,775	3,998	4,312
Anesthesiology	12,861	15,958	22,021	25,981	32,853	35,715	43,359
Cardiovascular Dis.	6,933	9,823	13,224	15,862	18,998	21,025	22,888
Child Psychiatry	2,581	3,271	3,783	4,343	5,542	6,158	7,438
Colon/Rectal Surgery	661	719	817	882	990	1,127	1,491
Dermatology	4,661	5,660	6,582	7,557	8,563	9,675	11,316
Diagnostic Radiology	3,544	7,048	12,887	15,412	19,808	21,104	26,054
Emergency Medicine*		5,699	11,283	14,243	19,112	23,064	33,278
Family Medicine	12,183	27,530	40,021	47,639	59,345	71,635	87,618
Forensic Pathology	190	240	311	414	496	577	670
Gastroenterology	2,381	4,046	5,917	7,493	9,551	10,627	13,210
General Practice	42,374	32,519	27,030	22,841	16,867	15,213	8,591
Gen. Preventive Med.	789	810	933	1,036	1,269	1,718	2,227
General Surgery	31,562	34,034	38,169	38,376	37,569	36,716	37,291
Internal Medicine	54,331	71,531	88,862	98,349	115,168	134,539	161,276
Medical Genetics**					179	361	597
Neurological Surgery	2,926	3,341	4,019	4,358	4,888	4,997	5,781
Neurology	4,131	5,685	7,776	9,237	11,397	12,333	15,850
Nuclear Medicine*			1,352	1,340	1,435	1,448	1,456
Obstetrics/Gynecology	21,731	26,305	30,867	33,697	37,652	40,241	42,797
Occupational Medicine	2,355	2,358	2,640	2,744	3,031	2,990	2,426
Ophthalmology	11,129	12,974	14,881	16,073	17,464	18,126	18,457
Orthopedic Surgery	11,379	13,996	17,166	19,138	22,037	22,287	25,241
Otolaryngology	5,745	6,553	7,267	8,138	9,086	9,417	10,326
Path.-Anatomic/Clin.	11,720	13,402	15,456	16,170	17,824	18,220	19,027
Pediatric Cardiology	538	659	813	1,006	1,336	1,536	2,101
Pediatrics	22,192	28,803	36,026	40,893	50,620	62,386	76,401
Physical Med./Rehab.	1,664	2,146	3,258	4,105	5,565	6,512	9,045
Plastic Surgery	2,236	2,980	3,951	4,590	5,493	6,200	7,418
Psychiatry	23,922	27,481	32,255	35,163	38,098	39,457	39,738
Public Health	2,665	2,316	2,060	2,015	1,760	1,830	1,283
Pulmonary Diseases	2,335	3,715	5,083	6,080	7,453	8,706	11,126
Radiation Oncology	1,169	1,581	2,272	2,821	3,630	3,904	4,698
Radiology	11,527	11,653	8,757	8,492	8,038	8,661	9,386
Thoracic Surgery	1,979	2,133	2,183	2,063	2,310	4,953	4,605
Urological Surgery	6,667	7,743	8,836	9,372	9,886	10,302	10,701
Other Specialty	7,277	5,810	6,398	7,254	7,307	5,810	5,512
Unspecified	7,542	12,289	8,250	8,058	8,473	8,327	9,458
Inactive	21,449	25,744	38,646	52,653	72,326	75,168	125,928
Not Classified	26,145	20,629	13,950	12,678	20,579	45,136	64,153
Address Unknown	5,868	6,390	2,980	2,780	1,977	1,098	432

Note: Data for 1990 are as of January 1; data for all other years, December 31.

**Data were not available for Emergency Medicine prior to 1980 and Nuclear Medicine prior to 1985.*

***Data on Medical Genetics were not available prior to 1994.*

Table 6.3

Percent Distribution of Physicians by Self-Designated Specialty, 1975-2010

Specialty	1975	1980	1985	1990	1995	2000	2010
Total Physicians	100.0	100.0	100.0	100.0	100.0	100.0	100.0
Aerospace Medicine	0.2	0.1	0.1	0.1	0.1	0.1	0.0
Allergy/Immunology	0.4	0.3	0.6	0.6	0.5	0.5	0.4
Anesthesiology	3.3	3.4	4.0	4.2	4.6	4.4	4.4
Cardiovascular Dis.	1.8	2.1	2.4	2.6	2.6	2.6	2.3
Child Psychiatry	0.7	0.7	0.7	0.7	0.8	0.8	0.8
Colon/Rectal Surgery	0.2	0.2	0.1	0.1	0.1	0.1	0.2
Dermatology	1.2	1.2	1.2	1.2	1.2	1.2	1.1
Diagnostic Radiology	0.9	1.5	2.3	2.5	2.7	2.6	2.6
Emergency Medicine*	*	1.2	2.0	2.3	2.7	2.8	3.4
Family Medicine	3.1	5.9	7.2	7.7	8.2	8.8	8.9
Forensic Pathology	0.0	0.1	0.1	0.1	0.1	0.1	0.1
Gastroenterology	0.6	0.9	1.1	1.2	1.3	1.3	1.3
General Practice	10.8	7.0	4.9	3.7	2.3	1.9	0.9
Gen. Preventive Med.	0.2	0.2	0.2	0.2	0.2	0.2	0.2
General Surgery	8.0	7.3	6.9	6.2	5.2	4.5	3.8
Internal Medicine	13.8	15.3	16.1	16.0	16.0	16.5	16.4
Medical Genetics**	**	**	**	**	0.0	0.0	0.1
Neurological Surgery	0.7	0.7	0.7	0.7	0.7	0.6	0.6
Neurology	1.0	1.2	1.4	1.5	1.6	1.5	1.6
Nuclear Medicine*	*	*	0.2	0.2	0.2	0.2	0.1
Obstetrics/Gynecology	5.5	5.6	5.6	5.5	5.2	4.9	4.3
Occupational Medicine	0.6	0.5	0.5	0.4	0.4	0.4	0.2
Ophthalmology	2.8	2.8	2.7	2.6	2.4	2.2	1.9
Orthopedic Surgery	2.9	3.0	3.1	3.1	3.1	2.7	2.6
Otolaryngology	1.5	1.4	1.3	1.3	1.3	1.2	1.0
Path.-Anatomic/Clin.	3.0	2.9	2.8	2.6	2.5	2.2	1.9
Pediatric Cardiology	0.1	0.1	0.1	0.2	0.2	0.2	0.2
Pediatrics	5.6	6.2	6.5	6.6	7.0	7.7	7.8
Physical Med./Rehab.	0.4	0.5	0.6	0.7	0.8	0.8	0.9
Plastic Surgery	0.6	0.6	0.7	0.7	0.8	0.8	0.8
Psychiatry	6.1	5.9	5.8	5.7	5.3	4.8	4.0
Public Health	0.7	0.5	0.4	0.3	0.2	0.2	0.1
Pulmonary Diseases	0.6	0.8	0.9	1.0	1.0	1.1	1.1
Radiation Oncology	0.3	0.3	0.4	0.5	0.5	0.5	0.5
Radiology	2.9	2.5	1.6	1.4	1.1	1.1	1.0
Thoracic Surgery	0.5	0.5	0.4	0.3	0.3	0.6	0.5
Urological Surgery	1.7	1.7	1.6	1.5	1.4	1.3	1.1
Other Specialty	1.8	1.2	1.2	1.2	1.0	0.7	0.6
Unspecified	1.9	2.6	1.5	1.3	1.2	1.0	1.0
Inactive	5.4	5.5	7.0	8.6	10.0	9.2	12.8
Not Classified	6.6	4.4	2.5	2.1	2.9	5.5	6.5
Address Unknown	1.5	1.4	0.5	0.5	0.3	0.1	0.0

Note: Data for 1990 are as of January 1; data for all other years, December 31.

**Data were not available for Emergency Medicine prior to 1980 and Nuclear Medicine prior to 1985.*

***Data on Medical Genetics were not available prior to 1994.*

Table 6.4

Percent Change of Physicians by Self-Designated Specialty, 1975-2010

Specialty	1975-2010	1975-1985	1985-1995	1975-1980	1980-1985	1985-1990	1990-2010
Total Physicians	150.3	40.4	30.3	18.8	18.2	11.3	60.1
Aerospace Medicine	–39.6	–1.5	–14.7	–14.2	14.8	1.9	–39.9
Allergy/Immunology	151.3	78.3	23.4	–11.5	101.6	10.7	27.3
Anesthesiology	237.1	71.2	49.2	24.1	38.0	18.0	66.9
Cardiovascular Dis.	230.1	90.7	43.7	41.7	34.6	19.9	44.3
Child Psychiatry	188.2	46.6	46.5	26.7	15.7	14.8	71.3
Colon/Rectal Surgery	125.6	23.6	21.2	8.8	13.6	8.0	69.0
Dermatology	142.8	41.2	30.1	21.4	16.3	14.8	49.7
Diagnostic Radiology	635.2	263.6	53.7	98.9	82.8	19.6	69.1
Emergency Medicine*	*	*	69.4	*	98.0	26.2	133.6
Family Medicine	619.2	228.5	48.3	126.0	45.4	19.0	83.9
Forensic Pathology	252.6	63.7	59.5	26.3	29.6	33.1	61.8
Gastroenterology	454.8	148.5	61.4	69.9	46.2	26.6	76.3
General Practice	–79.7	–36.2	–37.6	–23.3	–16.9	–15.5	–62.4
Gen. Preventive Med.	182.3	18.3	36.0	2.7	15.2	11.0	115.0
General Surgery	18.2	20.9	–1.6	7.8	12.1	0.5	–2.8
Internal Medicine	196.8	63.6	29.6	31.7	24.2	10.7	64.0
Medical Genetics**	**	**	**	**	**	**	**
Neurological Surgery	97.6	37.4	21.6	14.2	20.3	8.4	32.7
Neurology	283.7	88.2	46.6	37.6	36.8	18.8	71.6
Nuclear Medicine*	*	*	6.1	*	*	-0.9	8.7
Obstetrics/Gynecology	96.9	42.0	22.0	21.0	17.3	9.2	27.0
Occupational Medicine	3.0	12.1	14.8	0.1	12.0	3.9	–11.6
Ophthalmology	65.8	33.7	17.4	16.6	14.7	8.0	14.8
Orthopedic Surgery	121.8	50.9	28.4	23.0	22.6	11.5	31.9
Otolaryngology	79.7	26.5	25.0	14.1	10.9	12.0	26.9
Path.-Anatomic/Clin.	62.3	31.9	15.3	14.4	15.3	4.6	17.7
Pediatric Cardiology	290.5	51.1	64.3	22.5	23.4	23.7	108.8
Pediatrics	244.3	62.3	40.5	29.8	25.1	13.5	86.8
Physical Med./Rehab.	443.6	95.8	70.8	29.0	51.8	26.0	120.3
Plastic Surgery	231.8	76.7	39.0	33.3	32.6	16.2	61.6
Psychiatry	66.1	34.8	18.1	14.9	17.4	9.0	13.0
Public Health	-51.9	–22.7	–14.6	–13.1	–11.1	–2.2	–36.3
Pulmonary Diseases	376.5	117.7	46.6	59.1	36.8	19.6	83.0
Radiation Oncology	301.9	94.4	59.8	35.2	43.7	24.2	66.5
Radiology	–18.6	–24.0	–8.2	1.1	–24.9	–3.0	10.5
Thoracic Surgery	132.7	10.3	5.8	7.8	2.3	–5.5	123.2
Urological Surgery	60.5	32.5	11.9	16.1	14.1	6.1	14.2
Other Specialty	–24.3	–12.1	14.2	–20.2	10.1	13.4	–24.0
Unspecified	25.4	9.4	2.7	62.9	–32.9	–2.3	17.4
Inactive	487.1	80.2	87.2	20.0	50.1	36.2	139.2
Not Classified	145.4	–46.6	47.5	–21.1	–32.4	–9.1	406.0
Address Unknown	–92.6	–49.2	–33.7	8.9	–53.4	–6.7	–84.5

Note: Data for 1990 are as of January 1; data for all other years, December 31.

**Data were not available for Emergency Medicine prior to 1980 and Nuclear Medicine prior to 1985.*

***Data on Medical Genetics were not available prior to 1994.*

Table 6.5

Physicians by Age and Sex, 1975-2010

Year and Sex	Total Physicians	< 35	35-44	45-54	55-64	≥ 65
			Number			
1975						
Total Physicians	393,742	108,393	96,368	82,166	55,822	50,993
Male	358,106	94,863	87,687	76,027	52,190	47,339
Female	35,636	13,530	8,681	6,139	3,632	3,654
1980						
Total Physicians	467,679	128,506	118,840	88,063	68,239	64,031
Male	413,395	105,507	104,160	81,106	63,278	59,344
Female	54,284	22,999	14,680	6,957	4,961	4,687
1985						
Total Physicians	552,716	141,622	154,752	99,692	78,987	77,663
Male	471,991	107,357	130,148	89,786	72,859	71,841
Female	80,725	34,265	24,604	9,906	6,128	5,822
1990						
Total Physicians	615,421	134,872	184,743	116,803	83,614	95,389
Male	511,227	96,856	147,545	102,052	76,833	87,941
Female	104,194	38,016	37,198	14,751	6,781	7,448
2000						
Total Physicians	813,770	136,704	211,873	201,646	118,608	144,939
Male	618,233	81,473	145,043	156,782	102,522	132,413
Female	195,537	55,231	66,830	44,864	16,086	12,526
2010						
Total Physicians	985,375	165,544	214,468	220,858	189,648	194,857
Male	688,468	86,505	128,445	152,102	149,078	172,338
Female	296,907	79,039	86,023	68,756	40,570	22,519
			Percent			
1975						
Total Physicians	100.0%	100.0%	100.0%	100.0%	100.0%	100.0%
Male	90.9%	87.5%	91.0%	92.5%	93.5%	92.8%
Female	9.1%	12.5%	9.0%	7.5%	6.5%	7.2%
1980						
Total Physicians	100.0%	100.0%	100.0%	100.0%	100.0%	100.0%
Male	88.4%	82.1%	87.6%	92.1%	92.7%	92.7%
Female	11.6%	17.9%	12.4%	7.9%	7.3%	7.3%
1985						
Total Physicians	100.0%	100.0%	100.0%	100.0%	100.0%	100.0%
Male	85.4%	75.8%	84.1%	90.1%	92.2%	92.5%
Female	14.6%	24.2%	15.9%	9.9%	7.8%	7.5%
1990						
Total Physicians	100.0%	100.0%	100.0%	100.0%	100.0%	100.0%
Male	83.1%	71.8%	79.9%	87.4%	91.9%	92.2%
Female	16.9%	28.2%	20.1%	12.6%	8.1%	7.8%
2000						
Total Physicians	100.0%	100.0%	100.0%	100.0%	100.0%	100.0%
Male	6.0%	59.6%	68.5%	77.8%	86.4%	91.4%
Female	24.0%	40.4%	31.5%	22.2%	13.6%	8.6%
2009						
Total Physicians	100.0%	100.0%	100.0%	100.0%	100.0%	100.0%
Male	69.9%	52.3%	59.9%	68.9%	78.6%	88.4%
Female	30.1%	47.7%	40.1%	31.1%	21.4%	11.6%

Note: Data for 1990 are as of January 1; data for all other years, December 31.

Table 6.6

International Medical Graduates by Self-Designated Specialth, 1975-2010

Specialty	1975	1980	1985	1990	1995	2000	2010
Total Physicians	80,848	97,726	118,875	131,764	165,498	196,961	254,396
Aerospace Medicine	40	40	41	52	47	43	32
Allergy/Immunology	205	189	218	682	855	999	1,000
Anesthesiology	4,585	5,886	7,558	7,863	9,182	10,844	11,423
Cardiovascular Dis.	1,383	2,248	3,343	4,085	5,249	6,178	7,089
Child Psychiatry	580	749	973	1,107	1,318	1,630	2,231
Colon/Rectal Surgery	89	128	194	212	225	247	281
Dermatology	414	468	541	560	587	638	605
Diagnostic Radiology	626	1,299	2,090	2,185	2,378	2,873	2,871
Emergency Medicine*	*	*	1,768	1,997	2,225	2,296	2,843
Family Medicine	1,007	3,192	5,443	6,743	9,662	11,920	20,105
Forensic Pathology	53	65	85	114	128	136	144
Gastroenterology	437	796	1,298	1,630	2,192	2,735	3,675
General Practice	6,748	5,970	6,510	6,569	6,215	6,108	4,308
Gen. Preventive Med.	99	96	137	148	171	252	320
General Surgery	6,786	6,729	7,831	7,692	7,783	7,354	6,636
Internal Medicine	10,538	13,065	18,713	21,423	34,730	42,762	60,935
Medical Genetics**	**	**	**	**	23	76	154
Neurological Surgery	477	552	658	682	720	722	749
Neurology	933	1,180	1,784	2,153	3,077	3,606	5,201
Nuclear Medicine*	*	*	*	400	479	480	559
Obstetrics/Gynecology	4,209	5,268	6,504	6,844	7,048	7,159	6,981
Occupational Medicine	182	228	310	332	404	407	349
Ophthalmology	950	1,173	1,358	1,382	1,432	1,493	1,343
Orthopedic Surgery	1,095	1,500	1,734	1,759	1,842	1,709	1,512
Otolaryngology	777	955	1,121	1,120	1,061	1,007	811
Path.-Anatomic/Clin.	3,848	3,933	4,659	4,806	5,468	6,003	6,157
Pediatric Cardiology	164	180	213	238	337	382	507
Pediatrics	5,137	6,597	9,419	10,849	15,123	17,115	20,442
Physical Med./Rehab.	675	950	1,473	1,559	1,740	2,154	2,629
Plastic Surgery	319	469	680	755	794	816	804
Psychiatry	6,122	6,793	8,763	9,344	11,255	12,009	12,591
Public Health	287	271	274	249	203	220	142
Pulmonary Diseases	563	858	1,143	1,390	1,945	2,527	3,926
Radiation Oncology	354	481	695	727	775	833	727
Radiology	1,991	2,095	1,996	1,539	1,461	1,505	1,679
Thoracic Surgery	442	496	536	522	507	1,065	953
Urological Surgery	1,050	1,447	1,781	1,805	1,782	1,731	1,412
Other Specialty	1,420	2,201	1,280	1,465	1,515	1,100	1,057
Unspecified	2,112	3,044	2,009	1,444	2,368	3,303	3,771
Inactive	2,131	2,731	4,827	7,651	11,127	13,244	29,608
Not Classified	10,087	10,235	7,527	8,397	9,486	18,913	25,748
Address Unknown	1,933	3,169	1,388	1,290	579	367	86

Note: Data for 1990 are as of January 1; data for all other years, December 31.

**Data were not available for Emergency Medicine prior to 1980 and Nuclear Medicine prior to 1985.*

***Data on Medical Genetics were not available prior to 1994.*

Table 6.7

Percent Distribution of International Medical Graduates by Self-Designated Specialty, 1975-2010

Specialty	1975	1980	1985	1990	1995	2000	2010
Total Physicians	100.0	100.0	100.0	100.0	100.0	100.0	100.0
Aerospace Medicine	0.0	0.0	0.0	0.0	0.0	0.0	0.0
Allergy/Immunology	0.3	0.2	0.2	0.5	0.5	0.5	0.4
Anesthesiology	5.7	6.0	6.4	6.0	5.5	5.5	4.5
Cardiovascular Dis.	1.7	2.3	2.8	3.1	3.2	3.1	2.8
Child Psychiatry	0.7	0.8	0.8	0.8	0.8	0.8	0.9
Colon/Rectal Surgery	0.1	0.1	0.2	0.2	0.1	0.1	0.1
Dermatology	0.5	0.5	0.5	0.4	0.4	0.3	0.2
Diagnostic Radiology	0.8	1.3	1.8	1.7	1.4	1.5	1.1
Emergency Medicine*	*	*	1.5	1.5	1.3	1.2	1.1
Family Medicine	1.2	3.3	4.6	5.1	5.8	6.1	7.9
Forensic Pathology	0.1	0.1	0.1	0.1	0.1	0.1	0.1
Gastroenterology	0.5	0.8	1.1	1.2	1.3	1.4	1.4
General Practice	8.3	6.1	5.5	5.0	3.8	3.1	1.7
Gen. Preventive Med.	0.1	0.1	0.1	0.1	0.1	0.1	0.1
General Surgery	8.4	6.9	6.6	5.8	4.7	3.7	2.6
Internal Medicine	13.0	13.4	15.7	16.3	21.0	21.7	24.0
Medical Genetics**	**	**	**	**	0.0	0.0	0.1
Neurological Surgery	0.6	0.6	0.6	0.5	0.4	0.4	0.3
Neurology	1.2	1.2	1.5	1.6	1.9	1.8	2.0
Nuclear Medicine*	*	*	*	0.3	0.3	0.2	0.2
Obstetrics/Gynecology	5.2	5.4	5.5	5.2	4.3	3.6	2.7
Occupational Medicine	0.2	0.2	0.3	0.3	0.2	0.2	0.1
Ophthalmology	1.2	1.2	1.1	1.0	0.9	0.8	0.5
Orthopedic Surgery	1.4	1.5	1.5	1.3	1.1	0.9	0.6
Otolaryngology	1.0	1.0	0.9	0.9	0.6	0.5	0.3
Path.-Anatomic/Clin.	4.8	4.0	3.9	3.6	3.3	3.0	2.4
Pediatric Cardiology	0.2	0.2	0.2	0.2	0.2	0.2	0.2
Pediatrics	6.4	6.8	7.9	8.2	9.1	8.7	8.0
Physical Med./Rehab.	0.8	1.0	1.2	1.2	1.1	1.1	1.0
Plastic Surgery	0.4	0.5	0.6	0.6	0.5	0.4	0.3
Psychiatry	7.6	7.0	7.4	7.1	6.8	6.1	4.9
Public Health	0.4	0.3	0.2	0.2	0.1	0.1	0.1
Pulmonary Diseases	0.7	0.9	1.0	1.1	1.2	1.3	1.5
Radiation Oncology	0.4	0.5	0.6	0.6	0.5	0.4	0.3
Radiology	2.5	2.1	1.7	1.2	0.9	0.8	0.7
Thoracic Surgery	0.5	0.5	0.5	0.4	0.3	0.5	0.4
Urological Surgery	1.3	1.5	1.5	1.4	1.1	0.9	0.6
Other Specialty	1.8	2.3	1.1	1.1	0.9	0.6	0.4
Unspecified	2.6	3.1	1.7	1.1	1.4	1.7	1.5
Inactive	2.6	2.8	4.1	5.8	6.7	6.7	11.6
Not Classified	12.5	10.5	6.3	6.4	5.7	9.6	10.1
Address Unknown	2.4	3.2	1.2	1.0	0.3	0.2	0.0

Note: Data for 1990 are as of January 1; data for all other years, December 31.

**Data were not available for Emergency Medicine prior to 1980 and Nuclear Medicine prior to 1985.*

***Data on Medical Genetics were not available prior to 1994.*

Table 6.8

Percent Change of International Medical Graduates by Self-Designated Specialty, 1975-2010

Specialty	1975-2010	1975-1985	1985-1995	1975-1980	1980-1985	1985-1990	1990-2010
Total Physicians	214.7	47.0	39.2	20.9	21.6	10.8	93.1
Aerospace Medicine	–20.0	2.5	14.6	0.0	2.5	26.8	–38.5
Allergy/Immunology	387.8	6.3	292.2	–7.8	15.3	212.8	46.6
Anesthesiology	149.1	64.8	21.5	28.4	28.4	4.0	45.3
Cardiovascular Dis.	412.6	141.7	57.0	62.5	48.7	22.2	73.5
Child Psychiatry	284.7	67.8	35.5	29.1	29.9	13.8	101.5
Colon/Rectal Surgery	215.7	118.0	16.0	43.8	51.6	9.3	32.5
Dermatology	46.1	30.7	8.5	13.0	15.6	3.5	8.0
Diagnostic Radiology	358.6	233.9	13.8	107.5	60.9	4.5	31.4
Emergency Medicine*	*	*	25.8	*	*	13.0	42.4
Family Medicine	1896.5	440.5	77.5	217.0	70.5	23.9	198.2
Forensic Pathology	171.7	60.4	50.6	22.6	30.8	34.1	26.3
Gastroenterology	741.0	197.0	68.9	82.2	63.1	25.6	125.5
General Practice	–36.2	–3.5	–4.5	–11.5	9.0	0.9	–34.4
Gen. Preventive Med.	223.2	38.4	24.8	–3.0	42.7	8.0	116.2
General Surgery	–2.2	15.4	–0.6	–0.8	16.4	–1.8	–13.7
Internal Medicine	478.2	77.6	85.6	24.0	43.2	14.5	184.4
Medical Genetics**	**	**	**	**	**	**	**
Neurological Surgery	57.0	37.9	9.4	15.7	19.2	3.6	9.8
Neurology	457.4	91.2	72.5	26.5	51.2	20.7	141.6
Nuclear Medicine*	*	*	*	*	*	*	39.8
Obstetrics/Gynecology	65.9	54.5	8.4	25.2	23.5	5.2	2.0
Occupational Medicine	91.8	70.3	30.3	25.3	36.0	7.1	5.1
Ophthalmology	41.4	42.9	5.4	23.5	15.8	1.8	–2.8
Orthopedic Surgery	38.1	58.4	6.2	37.0	15.6	1.4	–14.0
Otolaryngology	4.4	44.3	–5.4	22.9	17.4	–0.1	–27.6
Path.-Anatomic/Clin.	60.0	21.1	17.4	2.2	18.5	3.2	28.1
Pediatric Cardiology	209.1	29.9	58.2	9.8	18.3	11.7	113.0
Pediatrics	297.9	83.4	60.6	28.4	42.8	15.2	88.4
Physical Med./Rehab.	289.5	118.2	18.1	40.7	55.1	5.8	68.6
Plastic Surgery	152.0	113.2	16.8	47.0	45.0	11.0	6.5
Psychiatry	105.7	43.1	28.4	11.0	29.0	6.6	34.7
Public Health	–50.5	–4.5	–25.9	–5.6	1.1	–9.1	–43.0
Pulmonary Diseases	597.3	103.0	70.2	52.4	33.2	21.6	182.4
Radiation Oncology	105.4	96.3	11.5	35.9	44.5	4.6	0.0
Radiology	-15.7	0.3	–26.8	5.2	–4.7	–22.9	9.1
Thoracic Surgery	115.6	21.3	–5.4	12.2	8.1	–2.6	82.6
Urological Surgery	34.5	69.6	0.1	37.8	23.1	1.3	–21.8
Other Specialty	–25.6	–9.9	18.4	55.0	–41.8	14.5	–27.8
Unspecified	78.6	–4.9	17.9	44.1	–34.0	–28.1	161.1
Inactive	1289.4	126.5	130.5	28.2	76.7	58.5	287.0
Not Classified	155.3	–25.4	26.0	1.5	–26.5	11.6	206.6
Address Unknown	–95.6	–28.2	–58.3	63.9	–56.2	–7.1	–93.3

Note: Data for 1990 are as of January 1; data for all other years, December 31.

**Data were not available for Emergency Medicine prior to 1980 and Nuclear Medicine prior to 1985.*

***Data on Medical Genetics were not available prior to 1994.*

Table 6.9

International Medical Graduates by Activity, 1975-2010

Activity	1975	1980	1985	1990	1995	2000	2010
			Number				
Total Physicians	80,848	97,726	118,875	131,764	165,498	196,961	254,396
Patient Care	61,416	72,935	95,362	106,515	136,812	156,810	192,046
Office-Based Practice	32,796	45,764	66,076	74,824	94,920	113,936	140,246
Hospital-Based Practice	28,620	27,171	29,286	31,691	41,892	42,874	51,800
Residents/Fellows*	16,447	11,424	12,837	13,496	22,552	22,419	28,434
Full-Time Staff	12,173	15,747	16,449	18,195	19,340	20,455	23,366
Other Prof. Activity	5,248	8,656	9,771	7,911	7,494	7,627	6,908
Administration	1,319	1,533	1,743	1,936	2,217	1,718	1,812
Medical Teaching	1,317	1,569	1,443	1,438	1,672	2,164	1,654
Research**	2,071	4,918	5,768	3,683	2,835	2,901	2,462
Other	541	636	817	854	770	844	980
Inactive	2,131	2,731	4,827	7,651	11,127	18,913	29,608
Not Classified	10,120	10,235	7,527	8,397	9,486	13,244	25,748
Address Unknown	1,933	3,169	1,388	1,290	579	367	86
			Percent Distribution				
Total Physicians	100.0	100.0	100.0	100.0	100.0	100.0	100.0
Patient Care	76.0	74.6	80.2	80.8	82.7	79.6	75.5
Office-Based Practice	40.6	46.8	55.6	56.8	57.4	57.8	55.1
Hospital-Based Practice	35.4	27.8	24.6	24.1	25.3	21.8	20.4
Residents/Fellows*	20.3	11.7	10.8	10.2	13.6	11.4	11.2
Full-Time Staff	15.1	16.1	13.8	13.8	11.7	10.4	9.2
Other Prof. Activity	6.5	8.9	8.2	6.0	4.5	3.9	2.7
Administration	1.6	1.6	1.5	1.5	1.3	0.9	0.7
Medical Teaching	1.6	1.6	1.2	1.1	1.0	1.1	0.7
Research**	2.6	5.0	4.9	2.8	1.7	1.5	1.0
Other	0.7	0.7	0.7	0.6	0.5	0.4	0.4
Inactive	2.6	2.8	4.1	5.8	6.7	9.6	11.6
Not Classified	12.5	10.5	6.3	6.4	5.7	6.7	10.1
Address Unknown	2.4	3.2	1.2	1.0	0.3	0.2	0.0
			Percent Change				
	1975-2010	1975-1985	1985-1995	1975-1980	1980-1985	1985-1990	1990-2010
Total Physicians	214.7	47.0	39.2	20.9	21.6	10.8	93.1
Patient Care	212.7	55.3	43.5	18.8	30.7	11.7	80.3
Office-Based Practice	327.6	101.5	43.7	39.5	44.4	13.2	87.4
Hospital-Based Practice	81.0	2.3	43.0	-5.1	7.8	8.2	63.5
Residents/Fellows*	72.9	-21.9	75.7	-30.5	12.4	5.1	110.7
Full-Time Staff	91.9	35.1	17.6	29.4	4.5	10.6	28.4
Other Prof. Activity	31.6	86.2	-23.3	64.9	12.9	-19.0	-12.7
Administration	37.6	32.1	27.2	16.2	13.7	11.1	26.0
Medical Teaching	25.4	9.6	15.9	19.1	-8.0	-0.3	-14.6
Research**	18.9	178.5	-50.8	137.5	17.3	-36.1	-33.2
Other	81.1	51.0	-5.8	17.6	28.5	4.5	14.8
Inactive	1289.4	126.5	130.5	28.2	76.7	58.5	287.0
Not Classified	154.4	-25.6	26.0	1.1	-26.5	11.6	206.6
Address Unknown	-95.6	-28.2	-58.3	63.9	-56.2	-7.1	-93.3

Note: Data for 1990 are as of January 1; all other years, December 31.

**Includes all years of Residency and Clinical Fellows.*

***Includes physicians in research activities and Research Fellows.*

Table 6.10

Female Physicians by Self-Designated Specialty, 1975-2010

Specialty	1975	1980	1985	1990	1995	2000	2010
Total Physicians	35,626	54,284	80,725	104,194	149,404	195,537	296,907
Aerospace Medicine	7	13	32	35	32	31	35
Allergy/Immunology	124	116	138	506	736	883	1,356
Anesthesiology	1,819	2,388	3,710	4,608	6,422	7,343	10,437
Cardiovascular Dis.	185	327	598	839	1,293	1,623	2,594
Child Psychiatry	659	896	1,193	1,489	2,146	2,504	3,595
Colon/Rectal Surgery	5	5	15	31	52	91	246
Dermatology	375	628	1,082	1,641	2,453	3,189	4,931
Diagnostic Radiology	228	656	1,781	2,418	3,757	4,129	6,135
Emergency Medicine*			1,348	2,058	3,297	4,351	8,300
Family Medicine	590	2,638	5,657	8,248	13,971	20,401	32,376
Forensic Pathology	10	26	53	92	130	168	230
Gastroenterology	52	118	269	456	729	927	1,851
General Practice	2,276	2,039	2,339	2,354	2,361	2,338	1,856
Gen. Preventive Med.	98	109	199	249	399	586	893
General Surgery	567	1,150	1,987	2,406	3,302	4,024	6,660
Internal Medicine	4,006	8,130	14,716	19,171	27,609	37,073	54,182
Medical Genetics**					75	162	283
Neurological Surgery	18	48	91	139	213	233	430
Neurology	341	580	1,059	1,462	2,166	2,609	4,535
Nuclear Medicine*			168	184	254	248	322
Obstetrics/Gynecology	1,777	3,243	5,597	7,551	11,231	14,124	20,820
Occupational Medicine	79	118	210	291	482	490	526
Ophthalmology	395	657	1,120	1,550	2,227	2,628	3,896
Orthopedic Surgery	60	144	293	421	677	774	1,437
Otolaryngology	69	141	287	426	693	838	1,547
Path.-Anatomic/Clin.	1,674	2,215	3,217	3,716	4,891	5,408	7,013
Pediatric Cardiology	99	125	146	199	324	390	643
Pediatrics	5,135	8,189	12,440	15,675	22,646	30,322	43,079
Physical Med./Rehab.	322	515	920	1,193	1,767	2,143	3,009
Plastic Surgery	62	120	219	309	478	610	1,029
Psychiatry	3,144	4,361	6,539	8,170	10,392	11,648	14,264
Public Health	533	470	440	471	458	516	404
Pulmonary Diseases	166	239	352	501	826	1,097	1,878
Radiation Oncology	103	191	360	498	786	857	1,198
Radiology	675	895	680	842	953	1,136	1,567
Thoracic Surgery	4	14	26	25	50	132	221
Urological Surgery	16	39	98	134	244	334	790
Other Specialty	615	1,027	734	961	1,111	902	1,377
Unspecified	930	2,136	1,767	1,968	2,571	2,937	3,315
Inactive	3,440	3,773	5,267	7,438	8,755	9,406	18,856
Not Classified	4,173	4,030	2,894	2,844	5,924	15,621	28,655
Address Unknown	795	1,775	684	625	521	311	136

Note: Data for 1990 are as of January 1; data for all other years, December 31.

**Data were not available for Emergency Medicine prior to 1980 and Nuclear Medicine prior to 1985.*

***Data on Medical Genetics were not available prior to 1994.*

Table 6.11

Percent Distribution of Female Physicians by Self-Designated Specialty, 1975-2010

Specialty	1975	1980	1985	1990	1995	2000	2010
Total Physicians	100.0	100.0	100.0	100.0	100.0	100.0	100.0
Aerospace Medicine	0.0	0.0	0.0	0.0	0.0	0.0	0.0
Allergy/Immunology	0.3	0.2	0.2	0.5	0.5	0.5	0.5
Anesthesiology	5.1	4.4	4.6	4.4	4.3	3.8	3.5
Cardiovascular Dis.	0.5	0.6	0.7	0.8	0.9	0.8	0.9
Child Psychiatry	1.8	1.7	1.5	1.4	1.4	1.3	1.2
Colon/Rectal Surgery	0.0	0.0	0.0	0.0	0.0	0.0	0.1
Dermatology	1.1	1.2	1.3	1.6	1.6	1.6	1.7
Diagnostic Radiology	0.6	1.2	2.2	2.3	2.5	2.1	2.1
Emergency Medicine*	*	*	1.7	2.0	2.2	2.2	2.8
Family Medicine	1.7	4.9	7.0	7.9	9.4	10.4	10.9
Forensic Pathology	0.0	0.0	0.1	0.1	0.1	0.1	0.1
Gastroenterology	0.1	0.2	0.3	0.4	0.5	0.5	0.6
General Practice	6.4	3.8	2.9	2.3	1.6	1.2	0.6
Gen. Preventive Med.	0.3	0.2	0.2	0.2	0.3	0.3	0.3
General Surgery	1.6	2.1	2.5	2.3	2.2	2.1	2.2
Internal Medicine	11.2	15.0	18.2	18.4	18.5	19.0	18.2
Medical Genetics**	**	**	**	**	0.1	0.1	0.1
Neurological Surgery	0.1	0.1	0.1	0.1	0.1	0.1	0.1
Neurology	1.0	1.1	1.3	1.4	1.4	1.3	1.5
Nuclear Medicine*	*	*	*	0.2	0.2	0.1	0.1
Obstetrics/Gynecology	5.0	6.0	6.9	7.2	7.5	7.2	7.0
Occupational Medicine	0.2	0.2	0.3	0.3	0.3	0.3	0.2
Ophthalmology	1.1	1.2	1.4	1.5	1.5	1.3	1.3
Orthopedic Surgery	0.2	0.3	0.4	0.4	0.5	0.4	0.5
Otolaryngology	0.2	0.3	0.4	0.4	0.5	0.4	0.5
Path.-Anatomic/Clin.	4.7	4.1	4.0	3.6	3.3	2.8	2.4
Pediatric Cardiology	0.3	0.2	0.2	0.2	0.2	0.2	0.2
Pediatrics	14.4	15.1	15.4	15.0	15.2	15.5	14.5
Physical Med./Rehab.	0.9	0.9	1.1	1.1	1.2	1.1	1.0
Plastic Surgery	0.2	0.2	0.3	0.3	0.3	0.3	0.3
Psychiatry	8.8	8.0	8.1	7.8	7.0	6.0	4.8
Public Health	1.5	0.9	0.5	0.5	0.3	0.3	0.1
Pulmonary Diseases	0.5	0.4	0.4	0.5	0.6	0.6	0.6
Radiation Oncology	0.3	0.4	0.4	0.5	0.5	0.4	0.4
Radiology	1.9	1.6	0.8	0.8	0.6	0.6	0.5
Thoracic Surgery	0.0	0.0	0.0	0.0	0.0	0.1	0.1
Urological Surgery	0.0	0.1	0.1	0.1	0.2	0.2	0.3
Other Specialty	1.7	1.9	0.9	0.9	0.7	0.5	0.5
Unspecified	2.6	3.9	2.2	1.9	1.7	1.5	1.1
Inactive	9.7	7.0	6.5	7.1	5.9	4.8	6.4
Not Classified	11.7	7.4	3.6	2.7	4.0	8.0	9.7
Address Unknown	2.2	3.3	0.8	0.6	0.3	0.2	0.0

Note: Data for 1990 are as of January 1; data for all other years, December 31.

**Data were not available for Emergency Medicine prior to 1980 and Nuclear Medicine prior to 1985.*

***Data on Medical Genetics were not available prior to 1994.*

Table 6.12

Percent Change of Female Physicians by Self-Designated Specialty, 1975-2010

Specialty	1975-2010	1975-1985	1985-1995	1975-1980	1980-1985	1985-1990	1990-2010
Total Physicians	733.4	126.6	85.1	52.4	48.7	29.1	185.0
Aerospace Medicine	400.0	357.1	0.0	85.7	146.2	9.4	0.0
Allergy/Immunology	993.5	11.3	433.3	–6.5	19.0	266.7	168.0
Anesthesiology	473.8	104.0	73.1	31.3	55.4	24.2	126.5
Cardiovascular Dis.	1302.2	223.2	116.2	76.8	82.9	40.3	209.2
Child Psychiatry	445.5	81.0	79.9	36.0	33.1	24.8	141.4
Colon/Rectal Surgery	4820.0	200.0	246.7	0.0	200.0	106.7	693.5
Dermatology	1214.9	188.5	126.7	67.5	72.3	51.7	200.5
Diagnostic Radiology	2590.8	681.1	110.9	187.7	171.5	35.8	153.7
Emergency Medicine*	*	*	144.6	*	*	52.7	303.3
Family Medicine	5387.5	858.8	147.0	347.1	114.4	45.8	292.5
Forensic Pathology	2200.0	430.0	145.3	160.0	103.8	73.6	150.0
Gastroenterology	3459.6	417.3	171.0	126.9	128.0	69.5	305.9
General Practice	–18.5	2.8	0.9	–10.4	14.7	0.6	–21.2
Gen. Preventive Med.	811.2	103.1	100.5	11.2	82.6	25.1	258.6
General Surgery	1074.6	250.4	66.2	102.8	72.8	21.1	176.8
Internal Medicine	1252.5	267.3	87.6	102.9	81.0	30.3	182.6
Medical Genetics**	**	**	**	**	**	**	**
Neurological Surgery	2288.9	405.6	134.1	166.7	89.6	52.7	209.4
Neurology	1229.9	210.6	104.5	70.1	82.6	38.1	210.2
Nuclear Medicine*	*	*	51.2	*	*	9.5	75.0
Obstetrics/Gynecology	1071.6	215.0	100.7	82.5	72.6	34.9	175.7
Occupational Medicine	565.8	165.8	129.5	49.4	78.0	38.6	80.8
Ophthalmology	886.3	183.5	98.8	66.3	70.5	38.4	151.4
Orthopedic Surgery	2295.0	388.3	131.1	140.0	103.5	43.7	241.3
Otolaryngology	2142.0	315.9	141.5	104.3	103.5	48.4	263.1
Path.-Anatomic/Clin.	318.9	92.2	52.0	32.3	45.2	15.5	88.7
Pediatric Cardiology	549.5	47.5	121.9	26.3	16.8	36.3	223.1
Pediatrics	738.9	142.3	82.0	59.5	51.9	26.0	174.8
Physical Med./Rehab.	834.5	185.7	92.1	59.9	78.6	29.7	152.2
Plastic Surgery	1559.7	253.2	118.3	93.5	82.5	41.1	233.0
Psychiatry	353.7	108.0	58.9	38.7	49.9	24.9	74.6
Public Health	-24.2	–17.4	4.1	–11.8	–6.4	7.0	–14.2
Pulmonary Diseases	1031.3	112.0	134.7	44.0	47.3	42.3	274.9
Radiation Oncology	1063.1	249.5	118.3	85.4	88.5	38.3	140.6
Radiology	132.1	0.7	40.1	32.6	–24.0	23.8	86.1
Thoracic Surgery	5425.0	550.0	92.3	250.0	85.7	–3.8	784.0
Urological Surgery	4837.5	512.5	149.0	143.8	151.3	36.7	489.6
Other Specialty	123.9	19.3	51.4	67.0	–28.5	30.9	43.3
Unspecified	256.5	90.0	45.5	129.7	–17.3	11.4	68.4
Inactive	448.1	53.1	66.2	9.7	39.6	41.2	153.5
Not Classified	586.7	–30.6	104.7	–3.4	–28.2	–1.7	907.6
Address Unknown	–82.9	–14.0	–23.8	123.3	–61.5	–8.6	–78.2

Note: Data for 1990 are as of January 1; data for all other years, December 31.

**Data were not available for Emergency Medicine prior to 1980 and Nuclear Medicine prior to 1985.*

***Data on Medical Genetics were not available prior to 1994.*

Table 6.13

Female Physicians by Activity, 1975-2010

Activity	1975	1980	1985	1990	1995	2000	2010
				Number			
Total Physicians	35,626	54,284	80,725	104,194	149,404	195,537	296,907
Patient Care	24,345	39,969	64,424	86,376	126,583	161,837	238,980
Office-Based Practice	12,497	20,609	36,526	49,249	79,843	108,120	165,595
Hospital-Based Practice	11,848	19,360	27,898	37,127	46,740	53,717	73,385
Residents/Fellows*	7,512	13,322	19,778	26,838	32,797	37,363	49,053
Full-Time Staff	4,336	6,038	8,120	10,289	13,943	16,354	24,332
Other Prof. Activity	2,873	4,737	7,456	6,911	7,621	8,362	10,280
Administration	1,020	1,178	1,484	1,816	2,399	2,310	2,973
Medical Teaching	795	1,090	1,319	1,584	2,142	2,580	2,775
Research**	743	2,077	4,062	2,856	2,442	2,700	3,094
Other	315	392	591	655	638	772	1,438
Inactive	3,440	3,773	5,267	7,438	8,755	9,406	18,856
Not Classified	4,173	4,030	2,894	2,844	5,924	15,621	28,655
Address Unknown	795	1,775	684	625	521	311	136
				Percent Distribution			
Total Physicians	100.0	100.0	100.0	100.0	100.0	100.0	100.0
Patient Care	68.3	73.6	79.8	82.9	84.7	82.8	80.5
Office-Based Practice	35.1	38.0	45.2	47.3	53.4	55.3	55.8
Hospital-Based Practice	33.3	35.7	34.6	35.6	31.3	27.5	24.7
Residents/Fellows*	21.1	24.5	24.5	25.8	22.0	19.1	16.5
Full-Time Staff	12.2	11.1	10.1	9.9	9.3	8.4	8.2
Other Prof. Activity	8.1	8.7	9.2	6.6	5.1	4.3	3.5
Administration	2.9	2.2	1.8	1.7	1.6	1.2	1.0
Medical Teaching	2.2	2.0	1.6	1.5	1.4	1.3	0.9
Research**	2.1	3.8	5.0	2.7	1.6	1.4	1.0
Other	0.9	0.7	0.7	0.6	0.4	0.4	0.5
Inactive	9.7	7.0	6.5	7.1	5.9	4.8	6.4
Not Classified	11.7	7.4	3.6	2.7	4.0	8.0	9.7
Address Unknown	2.2	3.3	0.8	0.6	0.3	0.2	0.0
				Percent Change			
	1975-2010	1975-1985	1985-1995	1975-1980	1980-1985	1985-1990	1990-2010
Total Physicians	733.4	126.6	85.1	52.4	48.7	29.1	185.0
Patient Care	881.6	164.6	96.5	64.2	61.2	34.1	176.7
Office-Based Practice	1225.1	192.3	118.6	64.9	77.2	34.8	236.2
Hospital-Based Practice	519.4	135.5	67.5	63.4	44.1	33.1	97.7
Residents/Fellows*	553.0	163.3	65.8	77.3	48.5	35.7	82.8
Full-Time Staff	461.2	87.3	71.7	39.3	34.5	26.7	136.5
Other Prof. Activity	257.8	159.5	2.2	64.9	57.4	-7.3	48.7
Administration	274.0	45.5	61.7	15.5	26.0	22.4	87.7
Medical Teaching	172.1	65.9	62.4	37.1	21.0	20.1	52.8
Research**	316.4	446.7	-39.9	179.5	95.6	-29.7	8.3
Other	356.5	87.6	8.0	24.4	50.8	10.8	119.5
Inactive	448.1	53.1	66.2	9.7	39.6	41.2	153.5
Not Classified	586.7	-30.6	104.7	-3.4	-28.2	-1.7	907.6
Address Unknown	-82.9	-14.0	-23.8	123.3	-61.5	-8.6	-78.2

Note: Data for 1990 are as of January 1; all other years, December 31.

**Includes all years of Residency and Clinical Fellows.*

***Includes physicians in research activities and Research Fellows.*

Table 6.14

Physicians, Population, and Physician/Population Ratios, 1965-2010

Year	Total Physicians*	Total Population (in Thousands	Physicians/ 100,000 Population	Pop/One Physician	Patient Care Physicians**	Patient Care Phy/100,00 Population	Pop/One Patient Care Physician
1965	292,088	197,147	148	675	259,418	132	760
1970	334,028	208,066	161	623	278,535	134	747
1975	393,742	219,272	180	557	311,937	142	703
1980	467,679	231,266	202	494	376,512	163	614
1981	485,123	233,459	208	481	389,369	167	600
1982	501,958	235,691	213	470	408,663	173	577
1983	519,546	238,139	218	458	423,361	178	562
1984	536,986	240,543	223	448	437,089	182	550
1985	552,716	242,946	228	440	448,820	185	541
1986	569,160	245,163	232	431	462,126	188	531
1987	585,597	247,488	237	423	478,511	193	517
1989	600,789	249,876	240	416	493,159	197	507
1990	615,421	252,164	244	410	503,870	200	500
1992	653,062	256,570	255	393	535,220	209	479
1993	670,336	259,250	259	387	550,448	212	471
1994	684,414	260,341	263	380	562,456	216	463
1995	720,325	262,755	274	365	582,131	222	451
2000	813,770	282,217	288	347	647,430	229	436
2010	985,375	309,051	319	314	752,572	244	411

Note: Data for 1989-1994 are as of January 1. Data for 1995, 2000, 2002, and prior to 1989 are as of December 31.

**Includes Active and Inactive Physicians in the US. Excludes physicians located in the Possessions (Pacific Islands, Puerto Rico, Virgin Islands, and Canal Zone prior to 1980).*

***Includes Office-Based Practice, Residents, and Hospital Staff physicians.*

Sources: US Bureau of the Census, Current Population Reports, Series P-25, No. St-99-2, 1044, 1045, 1106, and 1127. US Government Printing Office, Washington, DC, March 1990 and 1992, November 1993, and March 1994 and 1995. Also prior nos. 460, 876, 911. Also, US Census Bureau, Population Division, Annual Population Estimates and Estimated Components of Change for the United States and States: April 1, 2000 to July 1, 2009; Source: Population Division, US Census Bureau. Physician Characteristics and Distribution in the US, *Dept. of Physician Practice and Communications Information, Division of Survey and Data Resources, American Medical Association, 2011 and prior editions.*

Table 6.15

Physicians, Population, and Physician/Population Ratios, 1980-2010

	1980			1985		
State	Total Nonfed	Civilian Pop. (000)	Physician/ Population Ratio	Total Nonfed	Civilian Pop. (000)	Physician/ Population Ratio
Total*	439,301	225,552	195	542,343	237,924	228
Alabama	5,039	3,871	130	6,335	3,973	159
Alaska	509	380	134	845	532	159
Arizona	5,535	2,706	205	7,323	3,184	230
Arkansas	2,939	2,289	128	3,698	2,327	159
California	58,368	23,499	248	72,089	26,441	273
Colorado	5,999	2,863	210	7,347	3,209	229
Connecticut	8,177	3,100	264	9,725	3,201	304
Delaware	1,001	591	169	1,299	618	210
Dist. Of Col.	3,626	629	576	4,157	635	655
Florida	20,374	9,786	208	27,534	11,351	243
Georgia	8,060	5,414	149	10,851	5,963	182
Hawaii	2,020	911	222	2,743	1,040	264
Idaho	1,089	942	116	1,382	994	139
Illinois	21,740	11,392	191	25,503	11,400	224
Indiana	7,415	5,483	135	8,667	5,459	159
Iowa	3,847	2,912	132	4,420	2,830	156
Kansas	3,893	2,342	166	4,546	2,427	187
Kentucky	5,059	3,628	139	6,134	3,695	166
Louisiana	6,752	4,190	161	8,541	4,408	194
Maine	1,865	1,117	167	2,302	1,163	198
Maryland	11,745	4,183	281	16,053	4,413	364
Massachusetts	16,342	5,730	285	19,693	5,881	335
Michigan	15,347	9,244	166	17,456	9,076	192
Minnesota	8,150	4,080	200	9,517	4,184	227
Mississippi	2,797	2,500	112	3,551	2,588	137
Missouri	8,331	4,903	170	10,011	5,000	200
Montana	1,100	784	140	1,337	822	163
Nebraska	2,442	1,560	157	2,815	1,585	178
Nevada	1,171	797	147	1,679	951	177
New Hampshire	1,655	920	180	2,117	997	212
New Jersey	14,799	7,353	201	18,617	7,566	246
New Mexico	2,143	1,290	166	2,822	1,438	196
New York	49,105	17,549	280	57,492	17,792	323
North Carolina	9,354	5,791	162	11,810	6,254	189
North Dakota	919	643	143	1,190	677	176
Ohio	18,342	10,790	170	21,838	10,735	203
Oklahoma	4,031	3,008	134	5,107	3,271	156
Oregon	5,119	2,635	194	5,923	2,673	222
Pennsylvania	23,347	11,868	197	28,185	11,771	239
Rhode Island	2,102	943	223	2,478	969	256
South Carolina	4,362	3,061	143	5,637	3,303	171
South Dakota	809	684	118	1,089	698	156
Tennessee	7,460	4,574	163	9,252	4,715	196
Texas	22,571	14,182	159	30,238	16,273	186
Utah	2,492	1,466	170	3,130	1,643	191
Vermont	1,185	512	231	1,471	530	278
Virginia	9,682	5,216	186	12,756	5,715	223
Washington	7,921	4,098	193	10,319	4,400	235
West Virginia	2,745	1,950	141	3,417	1,907	179
Wisconsin	7,859	4,727	166	9,151	4,748	193
Wyoming	567	471	120	751	500	150

** Excludes physicians located in the Possessions (Pacific Islands, Puerto Rico, Virgin Islands, and Canal Zone prior to 1980), and physicians whose address is unknown.*

Note: 1980 figures are for nonfederal physicians only. All other figures include both federal and nonfederal physicians. Federal status is defined as full time employment by the federal government, including the Army, Navy, Air Force, Veterans' Administration, Public Health Service, and other federally funded agencies.

Table 6.15

Physicians, Population, and Physician/Population Ratios, 1980-2010, continued

	1990			1995		
State	Total Nonfed	Civilian Pop. (000)	Physician/ Population Ratio	Total Nonfed	Civilian Pop. (000)	Physician/ Population Ratio
Total*	604,089	249,464	242	708,951	262,803	270
Alabama	7,246	4,049	179	8,793	4,263	206
Alaska	915	553	165	1,092	601	182
Arizona	8,560	3,679	233	10,383	4,307	241
Arkansas	4,120	2,354	175	4,921	2,480	198
California	80,874	29,950	270	88,553	31,494	281
Colorado	8,037	3,304	243	9,999	3,738	267
Connecticut	10,892	3,289	331	12,278	3,265	376
Delaware	1,500	669	224	1,804	718	251
Dist. Of Col.	4,318	604	715	4,296	551	779
Florida	32,425	13,018	249	38,918	14,185	274
Georgia	12,689	6,507	195	16,120	7,189	224
Hawaii	3,097	1,113	278	3,562	1,180	302
Idaho	1,495	1,012	148	1,936	1,165	166
Illinois	27,140	11,447	237	31,845	11,885	268
Indiana	9,693	5,555	174	11,743	5,792	203
Iowa	4,831	2,780	174	5,463	2,841	192
Kansas	5,037	2,481	203	5,865	2,587	227
Kentucky	6,878	3,693	186	8,259	3,855	214
Louisiana	8,929	4,219	212	10,616	4,328	245
Maine	2,604	1,231	211	2,956	1,237	239
Maryland	18,291	4,797	381	21,345	5,024	425
Massachusetts	21,904	6,019	364	25,831	6,062	426
Michigan	18,872	9,310	203	22,404	9,660	232
Minnesota	10,661	4,387	243	12,512	4,605	272
Mississippi	3,956	2,577	153	4,482	2,691	167
Missouri	11,057	5,126	216	12,781	5,325	240
Montana	1,513	800	189	1,896	869	218
Nebraska	3,063	1,581	194	3,679	1,635	225
Nevada	2,006	1,219	165	2,806	1,526	184
New Hampshire	2,582	1,112	232	2,908	1,146	254
New Jersey	20,882	7,757	269	24,236	7,966	304
New Mexico	3,289	1,520	216	4,030	1,682	240
New York	61,628	18,003	342	71,637	18,151	395
North Carolina	13,990	6,657	210	17,527	7,185	244
North Dakota	1,246	637	195	1,475	642	230
Ohio	23,729	10,862	218	27,435	11,155	246
Oklahoma	5,310	3,147	169	5,929	3,266	182
Oregon	6,756	2,859	236	8,000	3,141	255
Pennsylvania	31,369	11,896	264	36,780	12,045	305
Rhode Island	2,822	1,005	281	3,302	989	334
South Carolina	6,415	3,499	183	7,999	3,700	216
South Dakota	1,159	697	166	1,437	728	197
Tennessee	10,643	4,891	218	13,301	5,241	254
Texas	33,357	17,045	196	40,243	18,680	215
Utah	3,511	1,730	203	4,320	1,977	219
Vermont	1,673	565	296	1,878	583	322
Virginia	14,656	6,214	236	17,423	6,601	264
Washington	11,955	4,901	244	14,609	5,431	269
West Virginia	3,490	1,792	195	4,066	1,821	223
Wisconsin	10,258	4,902	209	12,399	5,137	241
Wyoming	766	453	169	879	478	184

** Excludes physicians located in the Possessions (Pacific Islands, Puerto Rico, Virgin Islands, and Canal Zone prior to 1980), and physicians whose address is unknown.*

Table 6.15

Physicians, Population, and Physician/Population Ratios, 1980-2010, continued

	2000			2010		
State	Total Nonfed	Civilian Pop. (000)	Physician/ Population Ratio	Total Nonfed	Civilian Pop. (000)	Physician/ Population Ratio
Total*	802,156	282,217	284	971,307	309,051	314
Alabama	9,887	4,452	222	11,613	4,730	246
Alaska	1,362	628	217	1,823	709	257
Arizona	12,250	5,167	237	16,944	6,677	254
Arkansas	5,711	2,679	213	6,771	2,910	233
California	97,213	34,008	286	118,110	37,267	317
Colorado	11,692	4,327	270	15,595	5,095	306
Connecticut	13,279	3,413	389	15,270	3,527	433
Delaware	2,099	787	267	2,550	891	286
Dist. Of Col.	4,488	571	786	5,776	611	946
Florida	46,013	16,050	287	58,026	18,678	311
Georgia	19,324	8,231	235	24,496	9,908	247
Hawaii	3,887	1,212	321	4,866	1,300	374
Idaho	2,370	1,300	182	3,215	1,560	206
Illinois	35,943	12,441	289	41,724	12,944	322
Indiana	13,461	6,092	221	15,898	6,445	247
Iowa	5,927	2,929	202	6,677	3,023	221
Kansas	6,486	2,693	241	7,558	2,841	266
Kentucky	9,468	4,049	234	11,417	4,339	263
Louisiana	12,207	4,470	273	13,587	4,529	300
Maine	3,598	1,277	282	4,426	1,313	337
Maryland	23,449	5,312	441	27,334	5,737	476
Massachusetts	28,886	6,363	454	35,334	6,631	533
Michigan	25,209	9,957	253	29,331	9,931	295
Minnesota	14,257	4,934	289	18,143	5,290	343
Mississippi	5,399	2,849	190	6,149	2,960	208
Missouri	14,061	5,607	251	16,802	6,012	279
Montana	2,188	904	242	2,658	980	271
Nebraska	4,300	1,713	251	5,150	1,811	284
Nevada	4,025	2,018	199	5,899	2,655	222
New Hampshire	3,438	1,241	277	4,563	1,324	345
New Jersey	27,462	8,434	326	30,976	8,733	355
New Mexico	4,565	1,822	251	5,759	2,034	283
New York	78,524	19,000	413	86,293	19,578	441
North Carolina	21,118	8,079	261	27,850	9,459	294
North Dakota	1,603	641	250	1,832	654	280
Ohio	30,229	11,364	266	35,925	11,532	312
Oklahoma	6,565	3,455	190	7,619	3,724	205
Oregon	9,312	3,432	271	13,007	3,856	337
Pennsylvania	39,603	12,287	322	44,988	12,633	356
Rhode Island	3,814	1,051	363	4,622	1,057	437
South Carolina	9,689	4,024	241	12,240	4,597	266
South Dakota	1,708	756	226	2,098	820	256
Tennessee	15,360	5,703	269	19,035	6,338	300
Texas	46,904	20,952	224	60,991	25,213	242
Utah	5,041	2,243	225	6,865	2,831	243
Vermont	2,318	610	380	2,752	622	442
Virginia	20,362	7,105	287	25,571	7,952	322
Washington	16,693	5,912	282	21,795	6,746	323
West Virginia	4,442	1,808	246	4,922	1,826	270
Wisconsin	13,954	5,375	260	17,220	5,669	304
Wyoming	1,013	494	205	1,242	548	227

** Excludes physicians located in the Possessions (Pacific Islands, Puerto Rico, Virgin Islands, and Canal Zone prior to 1980), and physicians whose address is unknown.*

Sources: US Bureau of the Census, Current Population Reports, Series P-25, No. St-99-2, 1044, 1045, 1106, and 1127. US Government Printing Office, Washington, DC, March 1990 and 1992, November 1993, and March 1994 and 1995. Also prior nos. 460, 876, 911. Also, US Census Bureau, Population Division, Preliminary Annual Estimates of the Resident Population for the United States, Regions, States, and Puerto Rico : April 1, 2000 to July 1, 2010; Source: Population Division, US Census Bureau. Physician Characteristics and Distribution in the US, *Dept. of Physician Practice and Communications Information, Division of Survey and Data Resources, American Medical Association, 2011 and prior editions.*

Table 6.16

Population Ratios per One Physician by State, 1980-2010

State	1980	1985	1990	1995	2000	2010
	Individuals per One Physician					
Total*	513	439	413	371	352	318
Alabama	768	627	559	485	450	407
Alaska	747	630	605	551	461	389
Arizona	489	435	430	415	422	394
Arkansas	779	629	571	504	469	430
California	403	367	370	356	350	316
Colorado	477	437	411	374	370	327
Connecticut	379	329	302	266	257	231
Delaware	590	476	446	398	375	350
Dist. Of Col.	173	153	140	128	127	106
Florida	480	412	401	364	349	322
Georgia	672	550	513	446	426	404
Hawaii	451	379	359	331	312	267
Idaho	865	719	677	602	548	485
Illinois	524	447	422	373	346	310
Indiana	739	630	573	493	453	405
Iowa	757	640	575	520	494	453
Kansas	602	534	492	441	415	376
Kentucky	717	602	537	467	428	380
Louisiana	621	516	473	408	366	333
Maine	599	505	473	419	355	297
Maryland	356	275	262	235	227	210
Massachusetts	351	299	275	235	220	188
Michigan	602	520	493	431	395	339
Minnesota	501	440	412	368	346	292
Mississippi	894	729	652	600	528	481
Missouri	589	499	464	417	399	358
Montana	713	615	529	458	413	369
Nebraska	639	563	516	444	398	352
Nevada	681	566	607	544	501	450
New Hampshire	556	471	431	394	361	290
New Jersey	497	406	371	329	307	282
New Mexico	602	510	462	417	399	353
New York	357	309	292	253	242	227
North Carolina	619	530	476	410	383	340
North Dakota	700	569	512	435	400	357
Ohio	588	492	458	407	376	321
Oklahoma	746	641	593	551	526	489
Oregon	515	451	423	393	369	296
Pennsylvania	508	418	379	327	310	281
Rhode Island	449	391	356	300	276	229
South Carolina	702	586	545	463	415	376
South Dakota	845	641	601	507	443	391
Tennessee	613	510	460	394	371	333
Texas	628	538	511	464	447	413
Utah	588	525	493	458	445	412
Vermont	432	360	337	310	263	226
Virginia	539	448	424	379	349	311
Washington	517	426	410	372	354	310
West Virginia	710	558	514	448	407	371
Wisconsin	601	519	478	414	385	329
Wyoming	831	665	591	544	488	441

** Excludes physicians located in the Possessions (Pacific Islands, Puerto Rico, Virgin Islands, and Canal Zone prior to 1980), and physicians whose address is unknown.*

Note: 1980 and 1990 figures are for nonfederal physicians only. 2009 figures include both federal and nonfederal physicians. Federal status is defined as full time employment by the federal government, including the Army, Navy, Air Force, Veterans' Administration, Public Health Service, and other federally funded agencies.

Sources: US Bureau of the Census, Current Population Reports, Series P-25, No. St-99-2, 1044, 1045, 1106, and 1127. US Government Printing Office, Washington, DC, March 1990 and 1992, November 1993, and March 1994 and 1995. Also prior nos. 460, 876, 911. Also, US Census Bureau, Population Division, Preliminary Annual Estimates of the Resident Population for the United States, Regions, States, and Puerto Rico : April 1, 2000 to July 1, 2010; Source: Population Division, US Census Bureau. Physician Characteristics and Distribution in the US, *Dept. of Physician Practice and Communications Information, Division of Survey and Data Resources, American Medical Association, 2011 and prior editions.*

Table 6.17

Physician/Population Ratios and Rank by State, 2010

	Physicians Per 100,000 Population		Rank By Physician/ Population Ratio		Individuals Per One Physician	
State	Total	Patient Care	Total	Patient Care	Total	Patient Care
Total*	314	240			318	416
Alabama	246	198	42	40	407	504
Alaska	257	212	37	33	389	472
Arizona	254	192	39	43	394	521
Arkansas	233	185	45	45	430	539
California	317	237	18	22	316	422
Colorado	306	234	21	23	327	427
Connecticut	433	325	7	6	231	308
Delaware	286	223	27	29	350	448
Dist. Of Col.	946	674	1	1	106	148
Florida	311	229	20	26	322	437
Georgia	247	194	40	41	404	516
Hawaii	374	282	8	8	267	354
Idaho	206	163	50	50	485	615
Illinois	322	249	16	15	310	401
Indiana	247	200	41	39	405	501
Iowa	221	169	48	48	453	591
Kansas	266	207	35	36	376	483
Kentucky	263	212	36	34	380	473
Louisiana	300	242	24	17	333	414
Maine	337	254	14	13	297	393
Maryland	476	339	3	3	210	295
Massachusetts	533	390	2	2	188	257
Michigan	295	229	25	25	339	436
Minnesota	343	272	12	10	292	368
Mississippi	208	166	49	49	481	604
Missouri	279	219	31	30	358	456
Montana	271	203	32	38	369	493
Nebraska	284	224	28	28	352	446
Nevada	222	172	47	47	450	582
New Hampshire	345	264	11	12	290	379
New Jersey	355	272	10	9	282	368
New Mexico	283	212	29	32	353	472
New York	441	327	5	5	227	305
North Carolina	294	228	26	27	340	438
North Dakota	280	232	30	24	357	432
Ohio	312	240	19	20	321	416
Oklahoma	205	162	51	51	489	618
Oregon	337	253	13	14	296	396
Pennsylvania	356	266	9	11	281	376
Rhode Island	437	333	6	4	229	301
South Carolina	266	214	34	31	376	467
South Dakota	256	206	38	37	391	485
Tennessee	300	239	23	21	333	419
Texas	242	193	44	42	413	519
Utah	243	188	43	44	412	531
Vermont	442	324	4	7	226	309
Virginia	322	249	17	16	311	401
Washington	323	241	15	18	310	415
West Virginia	270	209	33	35	371	478
Wisconsin	304	241	22	19	329	415
Wyoming	227	176	46	46	441	568

** Excludes physicians located in the Possessions (Pacific Islands, Puerto Rico, Virgin Islands, and Canal Zone prior to 1980), and physicians whose address is unknown.*

Source: US Census Bureau, Population Division, Preliminary Annual Estimates of the Resident Population for the United States, Regions, States, and Puerto Rico : April 1, 2000 to July 1, 2010; Physician Characteristics and Distribution in the US, *Dept. of Physician Practice and Communications Information, Division of Survey and Data Resources, American Medical Association, 2011 and prior editions.*

Table 6.18

Total and Office-Based Physicians by Self-Designated Specialty, 1980-2010

	1980		1990		2010	
	Fed & Nonfed Physicians		Fed & Nonfed Physicians		Fed & Nonfed Physicians	
Specialty	Total	Office Based	Total	Office Based	Total	Office Based
Total Physicians	467,679	272,000	615,421	360,995	985,375	563,742
Allergy/Immunology	1,518	1,371	3,388	2,453	4,312	3,391
Anesthesiology	15,958	11,338	25,981	17,803	43,359	31,714
Cardiovascular Dis.	9,823	6,729	15,862	10,680	22,888	17,447
Child Psychiatry	3,271	1,961	4,343	2,615	7,438	5,355
Dermatology	5,660	4,378	7,557	6,006	11,316	9,262
Diagnostic Radiology	7,048	4,191	15,412	9,815	26,054	17,423
Emergency Medicine	5,699	3,362	14,243	8,420	33,278	20,576
Family Practice	27,530	18,378	47,639	37,476	87,618	69,680
Gastroenterology	4,046	2,737	7,493	5,200	13,210	10,456
General Practice	32,519	29,642	22,841	20,517	8,591	7,172
General Surgery	34,034	22,426	38,376	24,520	37,291	24,410
Internal Medicine	71,531	40,616	98,349	57,950	161,276	110,428
Neurological Surgery	3,341	2,468	4,358	3,092	5,781	3,988
Neurology	5,685	3,253	9,237	5,595	15,850	10,535
Obstetrics/Gynecology	26,305	19,513	33,697	25,485	42,797	34,025
Ophthalmology	12,974	10,603	16,073	13,068	18,457	15,715
Orthopedic Surgery	13,996	10,728	19,138	14,199	25,241	19,305
Otolaryngology	6,553	5,266	8,138	6,367	10,326	7,961
Pathology-1	13,642	6,081	16,584	7,494	19,697	11,034
Pediatrics-2	29,462	18,209	41,899	27,073	78,502	54,156
Physical Med./Rehab.	2,146	1,014	4,105	2,183	9,045	6,449
Plastic Surgery	2,980	2,438	4,590	3,835	7,418	6,180
Psychiatry	27,481	16,004	35,163	20,146	39,738	25,568
Pulmonary Diseases	3,715	2,048	6,080	3,662	11,126	7,838
Radiation Oncology	1,581	1,027	2,821	1,968	4,698	3,358
Radiology	11,653	7,802	8,492	6,060	9,386	7,001
Urological Surgery	7,743	6,228	9,372	7,398	10,701	8,598
Other Specialty	5,810	2,418	7,254	2,656	5512	2,172
Other Surgical Spec.-3	2,852	2,261	2,945	2,389	6,096	4,872
Other Remaining Spec.-4	6,071	2,549	7,822	3,316	8,402	4,070
Unspecified	12,289	4,959	8,058	1,554	9,458	3,603
Not Classified	20,629		12,678		64,153	
Other Categories-5	32,134		55,433		126,360	

Note: Data for 1990 are as of January 1. Data for 1980 and 2009 are as of December 31.

1 - Includes Pathology and Forensic Pathology

2 - Includes Pediatrics and Pediatric Cardiology. Also includes Pediatric Allergy for 1980.

3 - Includes Colon and Rectal Surgery and Thoracic Surgery.

4 - Includes Aerospace Medicine, General Preventive Medicine, Nuclear Medicine, Occupational Medicine, Medical Genetics, and Public Health.

5 - Includes Inactive and Address Unknown. These categories are included in Total Physicians only, not in Office-Based Practice.

Table 6.19

Physician/Population Ratios for Total and Office-Based Physicians by Self-Designated Specialty, 2010

	1980 Physicians Per 100,000 Population		1990 Physicians Per 100,000 Population		2010 Physicians Per 100,000 Population	
Specialty	Total	Office Based	Total	Office Based	Total	Office Based
Total Physicians	207.3	120.6	249.6	146.4	326.7	186.9
Allergy/Immunology	0.7	0.6	1.4	1.0	1.4	1.1
Anesthesiology	7.1	5.0	10.5	7.2	14.4	10.5
Cardiovascular Dis.	4.4	3.0	6.4	4.3	7.6	5.8
Child Psychiatry	1.5	0.9	1.8	1.1	2.5	1.8
Dermatology	2.5	1.9	3.1	2.4	3.8	3.1
Diagnostic Radiology	3.1	1.9	6.3	4.0	8.6	5.8
Emergency Medicine	2.5	1.5	5.8	3.4	11.0	6.8
Family Practice	12.2	8.1	19.3	15.2	29.0	23.1
Gastroenterology	1.8	1.2	3.0	2.1	4.4	3.5
General Practice	14.4	13.1	9.3	8.3	2.8	2.4
General Surgery	15.1	9.9	15.6	9.9	12.4	8.1
Internal Medicine	31.7	18.0	39.9	23.5	53.5	36.6
Neurological Surgery	1.5	1.1	1.8	1.3	1.9	1.3
Neurology	2.5	1.4	3.7	2.3	5.3	3.5
Obstetrics/Gynecology	11.7	8.7	13.7	10.3	14.2	11.3
Ophthalmology	5.8	4.7	6.5	5.3	6.1	5.2
Orthopedic Surgery	6.2	4.8	7.8	5.8	8.4	6.4
Otolaryngology	2.9	2.3	3.3	2.6	3.4	2.6
Pathology-1	6.0	2.7	6.7	3.0	6.5	3.7
Pediatrics-2	13.1	8.1	17.0	11.0	26.0	18.0
Physical Med./Rehab.	1.0	0.4	1.7	0.9	3.0	2.1
Plastic Surgery	1.3	1.1	1.9	1.6	2.5	2.0
Psychiatry	12.2	7.1	14.3	8.2	13.2	8.5
Pulmonary Diseases	1.6	0.9	2.5	1.5	3.7	2.6
Radiation Oncology	0.7	0.5	1.1	0.8	1.6	1.1
Radiology	5.2	3.5	3.4	2.5	3.1	2.3
Urological Surgery	3.4	2.8	3.8	3.0	3.5	2.9
Other Specialty	2.6	1.1	2.9	1.1	1.8	0.7
Other Surgical Spec.-3	1.3	1.0	1.2	1.0	2.0	1.6
Other Remaining Spec.-4	2.7	1.1	3.2	1.3	2.8	1.3
Unspecified	5.4	2.2	3.3	0.6	3.1	1.2
Not Classified	9.1		5.1		21.3	
Other Categories-5	14.2		22.5		41.9	

Note: Data for 1990 are as of January 1. Data for 1980 and 2009 are as of December 31.

1 - Includes Pathology and Forensic Pathology

2 - Includes Pediatrics and Pediatric Cardiology. Also includes Pediatric Allergy for 1980.

3 - Includes Colon and Rectal Surgery and Thoracic Surgery.

4 - Includes Aerospace Medicine, General Preventive Medicine, Nuclear Medicine, Occupational Medicine, Medical Genetics, and Public Health.

5 - Includes Inactive and Address Unknown. These categories are included in Total Physicians only, not in Office-Based Practice.

Source: US Census Bureau, Population Division, Annual Population Estimates and Estimated Components of Change for the United States and States: April 1, 2000 to July 1, 2010; Physician Characteristics and Distribution in the US, *Dept. of Physician Practice and Communications Information, Division of Survey and Data Resources, American Medical Association, 2010 and prior editions.*

Appendix A

Self-Designated Practice Specialties

Allergy & Immunology (AI)
Allergy (A)
Allergy & Immunology/Clinical & Laboratory Immunology (ALI)
Immunology (IG)

Aerospace Medicine (AM)

Anesthesiology (AN)
Adult Cardiothoracic Anesthesiology (ACA)
Pain Medicine (Anesthesiology) (APM)
Critical Care (Anesthesiology) (CCA)
Pain Management (PME)

Cardiovascular Disease (CD)

Child & Adolescent Psychiatry (CHP)

Colon & Rectal Surgery (CRS)
Proctology (PRO)

Dermatology (D)
Clinical & Laboratory Dermatological Immunology (DDL)
Procedural Dermatology (PRD)

Diagnostic Radiology (DR)
Cardiothoracic Radiology (CTR)

Emergency Medicine (EM)
Sports Medicine (Emergency Medicine) (ESM)
Medical Toxicology (Emergency Medicine) (ETX)
Hospice & Palliative Medicine (Emergency Medicine) (HPE)
Pediatric Emergency Medicine (Emergency Medicine) (PE)
Urgent Care Medicine (UCM)
Underseas Medicine (Emergency Medicine) (UME)

Forensic Pathology (FOP)

Family Medicine (FM)
Adolescent Medicine for Family Practice (AMF)
Family Medicine/Preventive Medicine (FMP)
Geriatric Medicine (Family Medicine) (FPG)
Sports Medicine (Family Medicine) (FSM)
Hospice and Palliative Medicine (Family Medicine) (HPF)

Gastroenterology (GE)

General Practice (GP)

General Preventive Medicine (GPM)
Medical Toxicology (Preventive Medicine) (PTX)
Underseas Medicine (Preventive Medicine) (UM)

General Surgery (GS)
Abdominal Surgery (AS)
Surgical Critical Care (Surgery) (CCS)
Craniofacial Surgery (CFS)
Dermatologic Surgery (DS)
Head & Neck Surgery (HNS)
Hand Surgery (HS)
Hand Surgery (Surgery) (HSS)
Oral & Maxillofacial Surgery (OMF)
Pediatric Cardiothoracic Surgery (PCS)
Pediatric Surgery (Surgery) (PDS)
Surgical Oncology (SO)
Trauma Surgery (TRS)
Vascular Surgery (VS)

Internal Medicine (IM)
Adolescent Medicine (AMI)
Critical Care Medicine (Internal Medicine)(CCM)
Diabetes (DIA)
Endocrinology, Diabetes & Metabolism (END)
Hematology (Internal Medicine) (HEM)
Hepatology (HEP)
Hematology/Oncology (HO)
Hospitalist (HOS)
Hospice & Palliative Medicine (Internal Medicine) (HPI)
Interventional Cardiology (IC)
Cardiac Electrophysiology (ICE)

Infectious Diseases (ID)
Clinical & Laboratory Immunology (Internal Medicine) (ILI)
Geriatric Medicine (IMG)
Internal Medicine/Nuclear Medicine (INM)
Sports Medicine (Internal Medicine) (ISM)
Nuclear Cardiology (NC)
Nephrology (NEP)
Nutrition (NTR)
Medical Oncology (ON)
Rheumatology (RHU)
Sleep Medicine (Internal Medicine) (SMI)
Transplant Hepatology (Internal Medicine) (THP)

Medical Genetics (MG)
Clinical Biochemical Genetics (CBG)
Clinical Cytogenetics (CCG)
Clinical Genetics (CG)
Clinical Molecular Genetics (CMG)
Medical Biochemical Genetics (MBG)
Molecular Genetic Pathology (Medical Genetics) (MGG)

Neurology (N)
Child Neurology (CHN)
Clinical Neurophysiology (CN)
Endovascular Surgical Neuroradiology (Neurology) (ENR)
Hospice & Palliative Medicine (Psychiatry & Neurology) (HPN)
Pain Medicine (Neurology) (PMN)
Sleep Medicine (Psychiatry & Neurology) (SMN)
Vascular Neurology (VN)

Nuclear Medicine (NM)

Neurological Surgery (NS)
Endovascular Surgical Neuroradiology (ES)
Endovascular Surgical Neuroradiology (ESN)
Pediatric Surgery (Neurology) (NSP)

Obstetrics & Gynecology (OBG)
Gynecological Oncology (GO)
Gynecology (GYN)
Hospice & Palliative Medicine (Obstetrics & Gynecology) (HPO)
Maternal & Fetal Medicine (MFM)
Obstetrics (OBS)
Critical Care Medicine (Obstetrics & Gynecology) (OCC)
Reproductive Endocrinology (REN)

Occupational Medicine (OM)

Ophthalmology (OPH)
Ophthalmic Plastic and Reconstructive Surgery (OPR)
Pediatric Ophthalmology (PO)

Orthopedic Surgery (ORS)
Hand Surgery (Orthopedic Surgery) (HSO)
Adult Reconstructive Orthopedics (OAR)
Orthopedics, Foot & Ankle (OFA)
Osteopathic Manipulative Medicine (OMM)
Musculoskeletal Oncology (OMO)
Pediatric Orthopedics (OP)
Sports Medicine (Orthopedic Surgery) (OSM)
Orthopedic Surgery of the Spine (OSS)
Orthopedic Trauma (OTR)

Other Specialty (OS)
Addiction Medicine (ADM)
Pediatric Psychiatry/Child Psychiatry (CPP)
Emergency Medicine/Family Medicine (EFM)
Pediatrics/Emergency Medicine (EMP)
Epidemiology (EP)
Family Medicine/Psychiatry (FPP)
Hospice & Palliative Medicine (HPM)
Internal Medicine/Emergency Medicine/Critical Care Medicine (IEC)
Internal Medicine/Family Medicine (IFP)
Internal Medicine/Dermatology (IMD)
Internal Medicine (Preventive Medicine) (IPM)
Legal Medicine (LM)
Internal Medicine/Medical Genetics (MDG)
Medical Management (MDM)
Internal Medicine (Emergency Medicine) (MEM)
Internal Medicine & Neurology (MN)
Internal Medicine/Psychiatry (MP)
Internal Medicine/Physical Medicine and Rehabilitation (MPM)
Neurology/Diagnostic Radiology/Neuroradiology (NRN)
Clinical Pharmacology (PA)
Pediatrics/Dermatology (PDM)
Phlebology (PHL)
Pharmaceutical Medicine (PHM)
Palliative Medicine (PLM)
Pediatrics/Medical Genetics (PMG)
Pediatrics/Physical Medicine & Rehabilitation (PPM)
Psychiatry/Neurology (PYN)
Sleep Medicine (SME)

Otolaryngology (OTO)
Otology/Neurotology (NO)
Pediatric Otolaryngology (PDO)
Plastic Surgery within the Head and Neck (Otolaryngology) (PSO)

Sleep Medicine (Otolaryngology) (SMO)

Psychiatry (P)

Addiction Psychiatry (ADP)

Neurodevelopmental Disabilities (Psychiatry & Neurology) (NDN)

Neuropsychiatry (NUP)

Forensic Psychiatry (PFP)

Pain Medicine (Psychiatry) (PPN)

Psychoanalysis (PYA)

Geriatric Psychiatry (PYG)

Psychosomatic Medicine (PYM)

Pediatrics (PD)

Adolescent Medicine (ADL)

Child Abuse Pediatrics (CAP)

Pediatric Critical Care Medicine (CCP)

Developmental/Behavioral Pediatrics (DBP)

Hospice and Palliative Medicine (Pediatrics) (HPP)

Internal Medicine/Pediatrics (MPD)

Neurodevelopmental Disabilities (Pediatrics) (NDP)

Neonatal-Perinatal Medicine (NPM)

Pediatric Anesthesiology (PAN)

Pediatric Allergy (PDA)

Pediatric Dermatology (PDD)

Pediatric Endocrinology (PDE)

Pediatric Infectious Disease (PDI)

Pediatric Pulmonology (PDP)

Medical Toxicology (Pediatrics) (PDT)

Pediatric Emergency Medicine (Pediatrics) (PEM)

Pediatric Gastroenterology (PG)

Pediatric Hematology/Oncology (PHO)

Clinical & Laboratory Immunology (Pediatrics) (PLI)

Pain Management (Physical Medicine & Rehabilitation) (PMP)

Pediatric Nephrology (PN)

Pediatric Rheumatology (PPR)

Sports Medicine (Pediatrics) (PSM)

Pediatric Rehabilitation Medicine (RPM)

Sleep Medicine (Pediatrics) (SMP)

Pediatric Cardiology (PDC)

Public Health & General Preventive Medicine (PHP)

Physical Medicine & Rehabilitation (PM)

Hospice and Palliative Medicine (Physical Medicine & Rehabilitation) (HPR)

Neuromuscular Medicine (NMN)

Neuromuscular Medicine (Physical Medicine & Rehabilitation) (NMP)

Pain Medicine (PMM)

Sports Medicine (Physical Medicine & Rehabilitation) (PRS)

Spinal Cord Injury (SCI)

Plastic Surgery (PS)

Cosmetic Surgery (CS)

Facial Plastic Surgery (FPS)

Surgery of the Hand (Plastic Surgery) (HSP)

Plastic Surgery Within the Head & Neck (PSH)

Plastic Surgery - Integrated (PSI)

Plastic Surgery Within the Head & Neck (Plastic Surgery) (PSP)

Anatomic/Clinical Pathology (PTH)

Anatomic Pathology (ATP)

Blood Banking/Transfusion Medicine (BBK)

Clinical Pathology (CLP)

Dermatopathology (DMP)

Hematology (HMP)

Molecular Genetic Pathology (MGP)

Medical Microbiology (MM)

Neuropathology (NP)

Chemical Pathology (PCH)

Cytopathology (PCP)

Pediatric Pathology (PP)

Selective Pathology (SP)

Pulmonary Disease (PUD)

Pulmonary Critical Care Medicine (PCC)

Radiology (R)

Abdominal Radiology (AR)

Hospice and Palliative Medicine (Radiology) (HPD)

Musculoskeletal Radiology (MSR)

Nuclear Radiology (NR)

Pediatric Radiology (PDR)

Neuroradiology (RNR)

Radiological Physics (RP)

Vascular & Interventional Radiology (VIR)

Radiation Oncology (RO)

Thoracic Surgery (TS)

Congenital Cardiac Surgery (Thoracic Surgery) (CHS)

Thoracic Surgery - Integrated (TSI)

Transplant Surgery (TTS)

Urology (U)

Pediatric Urology (UP)

Vascular Medicine (VM)

Unspecified (US)

Appendix B

American Specialty Boards

American Board of	Certifies in Specialties of
Allergy and Immunology	Allergy and Immunology,*
Anesthesiology	Anesthesiology,* Critical Care Medicine,** Hospice & Palliative Medicine,** Pain Medicine,** Pediatric Anesthesiology,** Sleep Medicine**
Colon and Rectal Surgery	Colon & Rectal Surgery*
Dermatology	Dermatology,* Dermatopathology,** Pediatric Dermatology**
Emergency Medicine	Emergency Medicine,* Hospice & Palliative Medicine,** Medical Toxicology,** Pediatric Emergency Medicine,** Sports Medicine,** Undersea & Hyperbaric Medicine**
Family Medicine	Family Medicine,* Adolescent Medicine,** Geriatric Medicine,** Hospice & Palliative Medicine,** Sleep Medicine,** Sports Medicine**
Internal Medicine	Internal Medicine,* Adolescent Medicine,** Advanced Heart Failure and Transplant Cardiology,** Cardiovascular Disease,** Cardiac Electrophysiology, ** Critical Care Medicine,** Endocrinology, Diabetes & Metabolism,** Gastroenterology,** Geriatric Medicine,** Hematology,** Hospice & Palliative Medicine,** Infectious Disease,** Interventional Cardiology,** Medical Oncology,** Nephrology,** Pulmonary Disease,** Rheumatology,** Sleep Medicine,** Sports Medicine,** Transplant Hepatology**
Medical Genetics	Clinical Biochemical Genetics,* Clinical Cytogenetics,* Clinical Genetics — MD,* Clinical Molecular Genetics,* Medical Biochemical Genetics,** Molecular Genetic Pathology**
Neurological Surgery	Neurological Surgery*
Nuclear Medicine	Nuclear Medicine*
Obstetrics and Gynecology	Obstetrics & Gynecology,* Critical Care Medicine,** Gynecologic Oncology,** Hospice & Palliative Medicine,** Maternal & Fetal Medicine,** Reproductive Endocrinology**
Ophthalmology	Ophthalmology*
Orthopaedic Surgery	Orthopaedic Surgery,* Hand Surgery,** Sports Medicine**
Otolaryngology	Otolaryngology,* Neurotology,** Pediatric Otolaryngology,** Plastic Surgery Within the Head & Neck,** Sleep Medicine**
Pathology	Anatomic & Clinical Pathology,* Anatomic Pathology,* Clinical Pathology,* Blood Banking,** Chemical Pathology,** Cytopathology,** Dermatopathology,** Forensic Pathology,** Hematology,** Medical Microbiology,** Molecular Genetic Pathology, ** Neuropathology,** Pediatric Pathology**

American Board of	Certifies in Specialties of
Pediatrics	Pediatrics,* Adolescent Medicine,** Child Abuse Pediatrics,** Developmental-Behavioral Pediatrics,** Hospice & Palliative Medicine,** Medical Toxicology,** Neonatal-Perinatal Medicine,** Neurodevelopmental Disabilities,** Pediatric Cardiology,** Pediatric Critical Care Medicine,** Pediatric Emergency Medicine,** Pediatric Endocrinology,** Pediatric Gastroenterology,** Pediatric Hematology-Oncology,** Pediatric Infectious Disease,** Pediatric Nephrology,** Pediatric Pulmonology,** Pediatric Rheumatology,** Pediatric Transplant Hepatology,** Sleep Medicine,** Sports Medicine**
Physical Medicine and Rehabilitation	Physical Medicine & Rehabilitation,* Hospice & Palliative Medicine,** Pain Medicine,** Neuromuscular Medicine,** Pain Medicine,** Pediatric Rehabilitation Medicine,** Spinal Cord Injury Medicine,** Sports Medicine **
Plastic Surgery	Plastic Surgery,* Plastic Surgery Within the Head and Neck, ** Surgery of the Hand**
Preventive Medicine	Aerospace Medicine,* Occupational Medicine,* Public Health & General Preventive Medicine,* Medical Toxicology,** Undersea & Hyperbaric Medicine**
Psychiatry and Neurology	Neurology,* Neurology With Special Qualifications in Child Neurology,* Psychiatry,* Addiction Psychiatry,** Child & Adolescent Psychiatry,** Clinical Neurophysiology,** Forensic Psychiatry,** Geriatric Psychiatry,** Hospice & Palliative Medicine,** Neurodevelopmental Disabilities,** Neuromuscular Medicine,** Pain Medicine,** Psychosomatic Medicine,** Sleep Medicine,** Vascular Neurology**
Radiology	Diagnostic Radiology,* Radiation Oncology,* Medical Physics,* Hospice & Palliative Medicine,** Neuroradiology,** Nuclear Radiology,** Pediatric Radiology, ** Vascular & Interventional Radiology**
Surgery	Surgery,* Vascular Surgery,* Hospice & Palliative Medicine,** Pediatric Surgery,** Surgery of the Hand,** Surgical Critical Care**
Thoracic Surgery	Thoracic Surgery* Congenital Cardiac Surgery
Urology	Urology*, Pediatric Urology**

Note: Includes current name of certificate. Excludes certificates that were issued during selected years prior to 1990.

Source: Annual Report and Reference Handbook–1994. The American Board of Medical Specialties Research & Education Foundation.

** General Certification*

*** Subspecialty Certification*

Appendix C

Metropolitan Statistical Areas (MSAs)

The 374 Metropolitan Statistical Areas in this publication are comprised of the following counties:

Abilene, TX - Callahan, Jones, Taylor
Aguadilla-Isabela-San Sebastián, PR - Aguada, Aguadilla, Anasco, Isabela, Lares, Moca, Rincon, San Sebastian
Akron, OH - Portage, Summit
Albany, GA - Dougherty, Lee, Terrell, Worth
Albany-Schenectady-Troy, NY - Albany, Rensselaer, Saratoga, Schenectady, Schoharie
Albuquerque, NM - Bernalillo, Sandoval, Torrance, Valencia
Alexandria, LA - Grant, Rapides
Allentown-Bethlehem-Easton, PA-NJ -
New Jersey Portion - Warren
Pennsylvania Portion - Carbon, Lehigh, Northampton
Altoona, PA - Blair
Amarillo, TX - Potter, Randall
Ames, IA - Story
Anchorage, AK - Anchorage, Matanuska-Susitna
Anderson, IN - Madison
Anderson, SC - Anderson
Ann Arbor, MI - Washtenaw
Anniston-Oxford, AL - Calhoun
Appleton, WI - Calumet, Outagamie
Asheville, NC - Buncombe, Haywood, Henderson, Madison
Athens-Clarke County, GA - Clarke, Madison, Oconee, Oglethorpe
Atlanta-Sandy Springs-Marietta, GA - Barrow, Bartow, Butts, Carroll, Cherokee, Clayton, Cobb, Coweta, Dawson, Dekalb, Douglas, Fayette, Forsyth, Fulton, Gwinnett, Haralson, Heard, Henry, Jasper, Lamar, Meriwether, Newton, Paulding, Pickens, Pike, Rockdale, Spalding, Walton
Atlantic City-Hammonton, NJ - Atlantic
Auburn-Opelika, AL - Lee
Augusta-Richmond County, GA-SC -
Georgia Portion - Burke, Columbia, Mcduffie, Richmond
South Carolina Portion - Aiken, Edgefield
Austin-Round Rock, TX - Bastrop, Caldwell, Hays, Travis, Williamson
Bakersfield, CA - Kern
Baltimore-Towson, MD - Anne Arundel, Baltimore, Baltimore City, Carroll, Harford, Howard, Queen Annes
Bangor, ME - Penobscot
Barnstable Town, MA - Barnstable
Baton Rouge, LA - Ascension, East Baton Rouge, East Feliciana, Iberville, Livingston, Pointe Coupee, Saint Helena, West Baton Rouge, West Feliciana
Battle Creek, MI - Calhoun
Bay City, MI - Bay
Beaumont-Port Arthur, TX - Hardin, Jefferson, Orange
Bellingham, WA - Whatcom
Bend, OR - Deschutes
Billings, MT - Carbon, Yellowstone
Binghamton, NY - Broome, Tioga
Birmingham-Hoover, AL - Bibb, Blount, Chilton, Jefferson, Saint Clair, Shelby, Walker
Bismarck, ND - Burleigh, Morton
Blacksburg-Christiansburg-Radford, VA - Giles, Montgomery, Pulaski, Radford
Bloomington, IN - Greene, Monroe, Owen
Bloomington-Normal, IL - Mclean
Boise City-Nampa, ID - Ada, Boise, Canyon, Gem, Owyhee
Boston-Cambridge-Quincy, MA-NH -
Massachusetts Portion - Essex, Middlesex, Norfolk, Plymouth, Suffolk
New Hampshire Portion - Rockingham, Strafford
Boulder, CO - Boulder
Bowling Green, KY - Edmonson, Warren
Bradenton-Sarasota-Venice, FL - Manatee, Sarasota
Bremerton-Silverdale, WA - Kitsap
Bridgeport-Stamford-Norwalk, CT - Fairfield
Brownsville-Harlingen, TX - Cameron
Brunswick, GA - Brantley, Glynn, Mcintosh
Buffalo-Niagara Falls, NY - Erie, Niagara
Burlington, NC - Alamance
Burlington-South Burlington, VT - Chittenden, Franklin, Grand Isle
Canton-Massillon, OH - Carroll, Stark
Cape Coral-Fort Myers, FL - Lee
Cape Girardeau-Jackson, MO-IL -
Missouri Portion - Cape Girardeau, Bollinger
Illinois Portion - Alexander
Carson City, NV - Carson City
Casper, WY - Natrona
Cedar Rapids, IA - Benton, Jones, Linn

Champaign-Urbana, IL - Champaign, Ford, Piatt
Charleston, WV - Boone, Clay, Kanawha, Lincoln, Putnam
Charleston-North Charleston-Summerville, SC - Berkeley, Charleston, Dorchester
Charlotte-Gastonia-Concord, NC-SC -
North Carolina Portion - Anson, Cabarrus, Gaston, Mecklenburg, Union
South Carolina Portion - York
Charlottesville, VA - Albemarle, Charlottesville City, Fluvanna, Greene, Nelson
Chattanooga, TN-GA -
Georgia Portion - Catoosa, Dade, Walker
Tennessee Portion - Hamilton, Marion, Sequatchie
Cheyenne, WY - Laramie
Chicago-Naperville-Joliet, IL-IN-WI -
Illinois Portion - Cook, DeKalb, DuPage, Grundy, Kane, Kendall, Lake, McHenry, Will
Indiana Portion - Jasper, Lake, Newton, Porter
Wisconsin Portion - Kenosha
Chico, CA - Butte
Cincinnati-Middletown, OH-KY-IN -
Indiana Portion - Dearborn, Franklin, Ohio
Kentucky Portion - Boone, Bracken, Campbell, Gallatin, Grant, Kenton, Pendleton
Ohio Portion - Brown, Butler, Clermont, Hamilton, Warren
Clarksville, TN-KY -
Kentucky Portion - Christian, Trigg
Tennessee Portion - Montgomery, Stewart
Cleveland, TN - Bradley, Polk
Cleveland-Elyria-Mentor, OH - Cuyahoga, Geauga, Lake, Lorain, Medina
Coeur d'Alene, ID - Kootenai
College Station-Bryan, TX - Brazos, Burleson, Robertson
Colorado Springs, CO - El Paso, Teller
Columbia, MO - Boone, Howard
Columbia, SC - Calhoun, Fairfield, Kershaw, Lexington, Richland, Saluda
Columbus, GA-AL -
Alabama Portion - Russell
Georgia Portion - Chattahoochee, Harris, Marion, Muscogee
Columbus, IN - Bartholomew
Columbus, OH - Delaware, Fairfield, Franklin, Licking, Madison, Morrow, Pickaway, Union
Corpus Christi, TX - Aransas, Nueces, San Patricio
Corvallis, OR - Benton
Cumberland, MD-WV -
Maryland Portion - Allegany
West Virginian Portion - Mineral
Dallas-Fort Worth-Arlington, TX - Collin, Dallas, Delta, Denton, Ellis, Hunt, Johnson, Kaufman, Parker, Rockwall, Tarrant, Wise
Dalton, GA - Murray, Whitfield
Danville, IL - Vermilion
Danville, VA - Danville City, Pittsylvania
Davenport-Moline-Rock Island, IA-IL -
Iowa Portion - Scott
Illinois - Henry, Mercer, Rock Island
Dayton, OH - Greene, Miami, Montgomery, Preble
Decatur, AL - Lawrence, Morgan
Decatur, IL - Macon
Deltona-Daytona Beach-Ormond Beach, FL - Volusia
Denver-Aurora-Broomfield, CO - Adams, Arapahoe, Broomfield, Clear Creek, Denver, Douglas, Elbert, Gilpin, Jefferson, Park
Des Moines-West Des Moines, IA - Dallas, Guthrie, Madison, Polk, Warren
Detroit-Warren-Livonia, MI - Lapeer, Livingston, Macomb, Oakland, Saint Clair, Wayne
Dothan, AL - Geneva, Henry, Houston
Dover, DE - Kent
Dubuque, IA - Dubuque
Duluth, MN-WI -
Minnesota Portion - Carlton, Saint Louis
Wisconsin Portion - Douglas
Durham-Chapel Hill, NC - Chatham, Durham, Orange, Person
Eau Claire, WI - Chippewa, Eau Claire
El Centro, CA - Imperial
El Paso, TX - El Paso
Elizabethtown, KY - Hardin, Larue
Elkhart-Goshen, IN - Elkhart
Elmira, NY - Chemung
Erie, PA - Erie
Eugene-Springfield, OR - Lane
Evansville, IN-KY -
Indiana Portion - Gibson, Posey, Vanderburgh, Warrick
Kentucky Portion - Henderson, Webster
Fairbanks, AK - Fairbanks North Star
Fajardo, PR - Ceiba, Fajardo, Luquillo
Fargo, ND-MN -
Minnesota Portion - Clay
North Dakota Portion - Cass
Farmington, NM - San Juan
Fayetteville, NC - Cumberland, Hoke
Fayetteville-Springdale-Rogers, AR-MO -
Arkansas Portion - Benton, Madison, Washington
Missouri Portion - McDonald
Flagstaff, AZ - Coconino
Flint, MI - Genesee
Florence, SC - Darlington, Florence
Florence-Muscle Shoals, AL - Colbert, Lauderdale
Fond du Lac, WI - Fond Du Lac
Fort Collins-Loveland, CO - Larimer
Fort Smith, AR-OK -
Arkansas Portion - Crawford, Franklin, Sebastian
Oklahoma Portion - Le Flore, Sequoyah
Fort Walton Beach-Crestview-Destin, FL - Okaloosa
Fort Wayne, IN - Allen, Wells, Whitley
Fresno, CA - Fresno
Gadsden, AL - Etowah
Gainesville, FL - Alachua, Gilchrist

Gainesville, GA - Hall
Glens Falls, NY - Warren, Washington
Goldsboro, NC - Wayne
Grand Forks, ND-MN -
Minnesota Portion - Polk
North Dakota Portion - Grand Forks
Grand Junction, CO - Mesa
Grand Rapids-Wyoming, MI - Barry, Ionia, Kent, Newaygo
Great Falls, MT - Cascade
Greeley, CO - Weld
Green Bay, WI - Brown, Kewaunee, Oconto
Greensboro-High Point, NC - Guilford, Randolph, Rockingham
Greenville, NC - Greene, Pitt
Greenville-Mauldin-Easley, SC - Greenville, Laurens, Pickens
Guayama, PR - Arroyo, Guayama, Patillas
Gulfport-Biloxi, MS - Hancock, Harrison, Stone
Hagerstown-Martinsburg, MD-WV -
Maryland Portion - Washington
West Virginia Portion - Berkeley, Morgan
Hanford-Corcoran, CA - Kings
Harrisburg-Carlisle, PA - Cumberland, Dauphin, Perry
Harrisonburg, VA - Harrisonburg City, Rockingham
Hartford-West Hartford-East Hartford, CT - Hartford, Middlesex, Tolland
Hattiesburg, MS - Forrest, Lamar, Perry
Hickory-Lenoir-Morganton, NC - Alexander, Burke, Caldwell, Catawba
Hinesville-Fort Stewart, GA - Liberty
Holland-Grand Haven, MI - Ottawa
Honolulu, HI - Honolulu
Hot Springs, AR - Garland
Houma-Bayou Cane-Thibodaux, LA - Lafourche, Terrebonne
Houston-Sugar Land-Baytown, TX - Austin, Brazoria, Chambers, Fort Bend, Galveston, Harris, Liberty, Montgomery, San Jacinto, Waller
Huntington-Ashland, WV-KY-OH -
Kentucky Portion - Boyd, Greenup
Ohio Portion - Lawrence
West Virginia Portion - Cabell, Wayne
Huntsville, AL - Limestone, Madison
Idaho Falls, ID - Bonneville, Jefferson
Indianapolis-Carmel, IN - Boone, Brown, Hamilton, Hancock, Hendricks, Johnson, Marion, Morgan, Putnam, Shelby
Iowa City, IA - Johnson, Washington
Ithaca, NY - Tompkins
Jackson, MI - Jackson
Jackson, MS - Copiah, Hinds, Madison, Rankin, Simpson
Jackson, TN - Chester, Madison
Jacksonville, FL - Baker, Clay, Duval, Nassau, Saint Johns
Jacksonville, NC - Onslow
Janesville, WI - Rock
Jefferson City, MO - Callaway, Cole, Moniteau, Osage
Johnson City, TN - Carter, Unicoi, Washington
Johnstown, PA - Cambria
Jonesboro, AR - Craighead, Poinsett
Joplin, MO - Jasper, Newton
Kalamazoo-Portage, MI - Kalamazoo, Van Buren
Kankakee-Bradley, IL - Kankakee
Kansas City, MO-KS
Kansas Portion - Franklin, Johnson, Leavenworth, Linn, Miami, Wyandotte
Missouri Portion - Bates, Caldwell, Cass, Clay, Clinton, Jackson, Lafayette, Platte, Ray
Kennewick-Pasco-Richland, WA - Benton, Franklin
Killeen-Temple-Fort Hood, TX - Bell, Coryell, Lampasas
Kingsport-Bristol-Bristol, TN-VA
Tennessee Portion - Hawkins, Sullivan
Virginia Portion - Bristol, Scott, Washington
Kingston, NY - Ulster
Knoxville, TN - Anderson, Blount, Knox, Loudon, Union
Kokomo, IN - Howard, Tipton
La Crosse, WI-MN
Minnesota Portion - Houston
Wisconsin Portion - La Crosse
Lafayette, IN - Benton, Carroll, Tippecanoe
Lafayette, LA - Lafayette, Saint Martin
Lake Charles, LA - Calcasieu, Cameron
Lake Havasu City-Kingman, AZ - Mohave
Lakeland-Winter Haven, FL - Polk
Lancaster, PA - Lancaster
Lansing-East Lansing, MI - Clinton, Eaton, Ingham
Laredo, TX - Webb
Las Cruces, NM - Dona Ana
Las Vegas-Paradise, NV - Clark
Lawrence, KS - Douglas
Lawton, OK - Comanche
Lebanon, PA - Lebanon
Lewiston, ID-WA -
Idaho Portion - Nez Perce
Washington Portion - Asotin
Lewiston-Auburn, ME - Androscoggin
Lexington-Fayette, KY - Bourbon, Clark, Fayette, Jessamine, Scott, Woodford
Lima, OH - Allen
Lincoln, NE - Lancaster, Seward
Little Rock-North Little Rock-Conway, AR - Faulkner, Grant, Lonoke, Perry, Pulaski, Saline
Logan, UT-ID -
Idaho Portion - Franklin
Utah Portion - Cache
Longview, TX - Gregg, Rusk, Upshur
Longview, WA - Cowlitz
Los Angeles-Long Beach-Santa Ana, CA - Los Angeles, Orange
Louisville/Jefferson County, KY-IN -
Indiana Portion - Clark, Floyd, Harrison, Washington
Kentucky Portion - Bullitt, Henry, Jefferson, Meade, Nelson, Oldham, Shelby, Spencer, Trimble
Lubbock, TX - Crosby, Lubbock
Lynchburg, VA - Amherst, Appomattox, Bedford, Campbell, Lynchburg City

Macon, GA - Bibb, Crawford, Jones, Monroe, Twiggs
Madera-Chowchilla, CA - Madera
Madison, WI - Columbia, Dane, Iowa
Manchester-Nashua, NH - Hillsborough
Manhattan, KS - Geary, Pottawatomie, Riley
Mankato-North Mankato, MN - Blue Earth, Nicollet
Mansfield, OH - Richland
Mayagüez, PR - Hormigueros, Mayaguez
McAllen-Edinburg-Mission, TX - Hidalgo
Medford, OR - Jackson
Memphis, TN-MS-AR -
Arkansas Portion - Crittenden
Mississippi Portion - Desoto, Marshall, Tate, Tunica
Tennessee Portion - Fayette, Shelby, Tipton
Merced, CA, Merced
Miami-Fort Lauderdale-Pompano Beach, FL - Broward, Miami-Dade, Palm Beach
Michigan City-La Porte, IN - La Porte
Midland, TX - Midland
Milwaukee-Waukesha-West Allis, WI - Milwaukee, Ozaukee, Washington, Waukesha
Minneapolis-St. Paul-Bloomington, MN-WI -
Minnesota Portion - Anoka, Carver, Chisago, Dakota, Hennepin, Isanti, Ramsey, Scott, Sherburne, Washington, Wright
Wisconsin Portion - Pierce, Saint Croix
Missoula, MT - Missoula
Mobile, AL - Mobile
Modesto, CA - Stanislaus
Monroe, LA - Ouachita, Union
Monroe, MI - Monroe
Montgomery, AL - Autauga, Elmore, Lowndes, Montgomery
Morgantown, WV - Monongalia, Preston
Morristown, TN - Grainger, Hamblen, Jefferson
Mount Vernon-Anacortes, WA - Skagit
Muncie, IN - Delaware
Muskegon-Norton Shores, MI - Muskegon
Myrtle Beach-North Myrtle Beach-Conway, SC - Horry
Napa, CA - Napa
Naples-Marco Island, FL - Collier
Nashville-Davidson--Murfreesboro--Franklin, TN - Cannon, Cheatham, Davidson, Dickson, Hickman, Macon, Robertson, Rutherford, Smith, Sumner, Trousdale, Williamson, Wilson
New Haven-Milford, CT - New Haven
New Orleans-Metairie-Kenner, LA - Jefferson, Orleans, Plaquemines, Saint Bernard, Saint Charles, Saint Tammany, St John The Baptist
New York-Northern New Jersey-Long Island, NY-NJ-PA -
New Jersey Portion - Bergen, Essex, Hudson, Hunterdon, Middlesex, Monmouth, Morris, Ocean, Passaic, Somerset, Sussex, Union
New York Portion - Bronx, Kings, Nassau, New York, Putnam, Queens, Richmond, Rockland, Suffolk, Westchester
Pennsylvania Portion - Pike
Niles-Benton Harbor, MI - Berrien
Norwich-New London, CT - New London
Ocala, FL - Marion
Ocean City, NJ - Cape May
Odessa, TX - Ector
Ogden-Clearfield, UT - Davis, Morgan, Weber
Oklahoma City, OK - Canadian, Cleveland, Grady, Lincoln, Logan, McClain, Oklahoma
Olympia, WA - Thurston
Omaha-Council Bluffs, NE-IA -
Iowa Portion - Harrison, Mills, Pottawattamie
Nebraska Portion - Cass, Douglas, Sarpy, Saunders, Washington
Orlando-Kissimmee, FL - Lake, Orange, Osceola, Seminole
Oshkosh-Neenah, WI - Winnebago
Owensboro, KY - Daviess, Hancock, Mclean
Oxnard-Thousand Oaks-Ventura, CA - Ventura
Palm Bay-Melbourne-Titusville, FL - Brevard
Palm Coast, FL - Flagler
Panama City-Lynn Haven-Panama City Beach, FL - Bay
Parkersburg-Marietta-Vienna, WV-OH -
Ohio Portion - Washington
West Virginia Portion - Pleasants, Wirt, Wood
Pascagoula, MS - George, Jackson
Pensacola-Ferry Pass-Brent, FL - Escambia, Santa Rosa
Peoria, IL - Marshall, Peoria, Stark, Tazewell, Woodford
Philadelphia-Camden-Wilmington, PA-NJ-DE-MD -
Delware Portion - New Castle
Maryland Portion - Cecil
New Jersey Portion - Burlington, Camden, Gloucester, Salem
Pennsylvania - Bucks, Chester, Delaware, Montgomery, Philadelphia
Phoenix-Mesa-Scottsdale, AZ - Maricopa, Pinal
Pine Bluff, AR - Cleveland, Jefferson, Lincoln
Pittsburgh, PA - Allegheny, Armstrong, Beaver, Butler, Fayette, Washington, Westmoreland
Pittsfield, MA - Berkshire
Pocatello, ID - Bannock, Power
Ponce, PR - Juana Diaz, Ponce, Villalba
Port St. Lucie, FL - Martin, Saint Lucie
Portland-South Portland-Biddeford, ME - Cumberland, Sagadahoc, York
Portland-Vancouver-Beaverton, OR-WA -
Oregon Portion - Clackamas, Columbia, Multnomah, Washington, Yamhill
Washington Portion - Clark, Skamania
Poughkeepsie-Newburgh-Middletown, NY - Dutchess, Orange
Prescott, AZ - Yavapai
Providence-New Bedford-Fall River, RI-MA -
Massachusetts Portion - Bristol
Rhode Island Portion - Bristol, Kent, Newport, Providence, Washington
Provo-Orem, UT - Juab, Utah
Pueblo, CO - Pueblo
Punta Gorda, FL - Charlotte

Racine, WI - Racine
Raleigh-Cary, NC - Franklin, Johnston, Wake
Rapid City, SD - Meade, Pennington
Reading, PA - Berks
Redding, CA - Shasta
Reno-Sparks, NV - Storey, Washoe
Richmond, VA - Amelia, Caroline, Charles City, Chesterfield, Colonial Heights City, Cumberland, Dinwiddie, Goochland, Hanover, Henrico, Hopewell City, King And Queen, King William, Louisa, New Kent,
Petersburg City, Powhatan, Prince George, Richmond City, Sussex
Riverside-San Bernardino-Ontario, CA - Riverside, San Bernardino
Roanoke, VA - Botetourt, Craig, Franklin, Roanoke, Roanoke City, Salem
Rochester, MN - Dodge, Olmsted, Wabasha
Rochester, NY - Livingston, Monroe, Ontario, Orleans, Wayne
Rockford, IL - Boone, Winnebago
Rocky Mount, NC - Edgecombe, Nash
Rome, GA - Floyd
Sacramento-Arden-Arcade-Roseville, CA - El Dorado, Placer, Sacramento, Yolo
Saginaw-Saginaw Township North, MI - Saginaw
Salem, OR - Marion, Polk
Salinas, CA - Monterey
Salisbury, MD - Somerset, Wicomico
Salt Lake City, UT - Salt Lake, Summit, Tooele
San Angelo, TX - Tom Green
San Antonio, TX - Atascosa, Bandera, Bexar, Comal, Guadalupe, Kendall, Medina, Wilson
San Diego-Carlsbad-San Marcos, CA - San Diego
San Francisco-Oakland-Fremont, CA - Alameda, Contra Costa, Marin, San Francisco, San Mateo
San Germán-Cabo Rojo, PR - Cabo Rojo, Lajas, Sabana Grande, San German
San Jose-Sunnyvale-Santa Clara, CA - San Benito, Santa Clara
San Juan-Caguas-Guaynabo, PR - Aguas Buenas, Aibonito, Arecibo, Barceloneta, Barranquitas, Bayamon, Caguas, Camuy, Canovanas, Carolina, Catano, Cayey, Ciales, Cidra, Comerio, Corozal, Dorado, Florida, Guaynabo, Gurabo, Hatillo, Humacao, Juncos, Las Piedras, Loiza, Manati, Maunabo, Morovis, Naguabo, Naranjito, Orocovis, Quebradillas, Rio Grande, San Juan, San Lorenzo, Toa Alta, Toa Baja, Trujillo Alto, Vega Alta, Vega Baja, Yabucoa
San Luis Obispo-Paso Robles, CA - San Luis Obispo
Sandusky, OH - Erie
Santa Barbara-Santa Maria-Goleta, CA - Santa Barbara
Santa Cruz-Watsonville, CA - Santa Cruz
Santa Fe, NM - Santa Fe
Santa Rosa-Petaluma, CA - Sonoma
Savannah, GA - Bryan, Chatham, Effingham
Scranton-Wilkes-Barre, PA - Lackawanna, Luzerne, Wyoming
Seattle-Tacoma-Bellevue, WA - King, Pierce, Snohomish
Sebastian-Vero Beach, FL - Indian River
Sheboygan, WI - Sheboygan
Sherman-Denison, TX - Grayson
Shreveport-Bossier City, LA - Bossier, Caddo, De Soto
Sioux City, IA-NE-SD -
  Iowa Portion - Woodbury
  Nebraska Portion - Dakota, Dixon
  South Dakota Portion - Union
Sioux Falls, SD - Lincoln, McCook, Minnehaha, Turner
South Bend-Mishawaka, IN-MI -
  Indiana Portion - St Joseph
  Michigan Portion - Cass
Spartanburg, SC - Spartanburg
Spokane, WA - Spokane
Springfield, IL - Menard, Sangamon
Springfield, MA - Franklin, Hampden, Hampshire
Springfield, MO - Christian, Dallas, Greene, Polk, Webster
Springfield, OH - Clark
St. Cloud, MN - Benton, Stearns
St. George, UT - Washington
St. Joseph, MO-KS -
  Kansas Portion - Doniphan
  Missouri - Andrew, Buchanan, Dekalb
St. Louis, MO-IL -
  Illinois Portion - Bond, Calhoun, Clinton, Jersey, Macoupin, Madison, Monroe, Saint Clair
Missouri Portion - Franklin, Jefferson, Lincoln, Saint Charles, Saint Louis, Saint Louis City, Warren, Washington
State College, PA - Centre
Stockton, CA - San Joaquin
Sumter, SC - Sumter
Syracuse, NY - Madison, Onondaga, Oswego
Tallahassee, FL - Gadsden, Jefferson, Leon, Wakulla
Tampa-St. Petersburg-Clearwater, FL - Hernando, Hillsborough, Pasco, Pinellas
Terre Haute, IN - Clay, Sullivan, Vermillion, Vigo
Texarkana, TX-Texarkana, AR - Miller, Bowie
Toledo, OH - Fulton, Lucas, Ottawa, Wood
Topeka, KS - Jackson, Jefferson, Osage, Shawnee, Wabaunsee
Trenton-Ewing, NJ - Mercer
Tucson, AZ - Pima
Tulsa, OK - Creek, Okmulgee, Osage, Pawnee, Rogers, Tulsa, Wagoner
Tuscaloosa, AL - Greene, Hale, Tuscaloosa
Tyler, TX - Smith
Utica-Rome, NY - Herkimer, Oneida
Valdosta, GA - Brooks, Lanier, Lowndes
Vallejo-Fairfield, CA - Solano
Victoria, TX - Calhoun, Goliad, Victoria
Vineland-Millville-Bridgeton, NJ - Cumberland
Virginia Beach-Norfolk-Newport News, VA-NC -
  North Carolina Portion - Currituck

Virginia Portion - Chesapeake City, Gloucester, Hampton City, Isle Of Wight, James City, Mathews, Newport News City, Norfolk City, Poquoson City, Portsmouth City, Suffolk City, Surry, Virginia Beach City, Williamsburg City, York

Visalia-Porterville, CA - Tulare

Waco, TX - McLennan

Warner Robins, GA - Houston

Washington-Arlington-Alexandria, DC-VA-MD-WV

DC Portion - District Of Columbia

Maryland Portion - Calvert, Charles, Frederick, Montgomery, Prince Georges

Virginia Portion - Alexandria City, Arlington, Clarke, Fairfax, Fairfax City, Falls Church City, Fauquier, Fredericksburg City, Loudoun, Manassas City, Prince William, Spotsylvania, Stafford, Warren

West Virginia Portion - Jefferson

Waterloo-Cedar Falls, IA - Black Hawk, Bremer, Grundy

Wausau, WI - Marathon

Weirton-Steubenville, WV-OH -

Ohio Portion - Jefferson

West Virginia Portion - Brooke, Hancock

Wenatchee-East Wenatchee, WA - Chelan, Douglas

Wheeling, WV-OH -

Ohio Portion - Belmont

West Virginia Portion - Marshall, Ohio

Wichita Falls, TX - Archer, Clay, Wichita

Wichita, KS - Butler, Harvey, Sedgwick, Sumner

Williamsport, PA - Lycoming

Wilmington, NC - Brunswick, New Hanover, Pender

Winchester, VA-WV -

Virginia Portion - Frederick, Winchester City

West Virginia Portion - Hampshire

Winston-Salem, NC - Davie, Forsyth, Stokes, Yadkin

Worcester, MA - Worcester

Yakima, WA - Yakima

Yauco, PR - Guanica, Guayanilla, Penuelas, Yauco

York-Hanover, PA - York

Youngstown-Warren-Boardman, OH-PA -

Ohio Portion - Mahoning, Trumbull

Pennsylvania Portion - Mercer

Yuba City, CA - Sutter, Yuba

Yuma, AZ - Yuma

Appendix D

Regions, Divisions, and States

Census Region
Census Division
State

Northeast
Middle Atlantic
New Jersey
New York
Pennsylvania

New England
Connecticut
Maine
Massachusetts
New Hampshire
Rhode Island
Vermont

North Central
East North Central
Illinois
Indiana
Michigan
Ohio
Wisconsin

West North Central
Iowa
Kansas
Minnesota
Missouri
Nebraska
North Dakota
South Dakota

South
East South Central
Alabama
Kentucky
Mississippi
Tennessee

South Atlantic
Delaware
District of Columbia
Florida
Georgia
Maryland
North Carolina
South Carolina
Virginia
West Virginia

West South Central
Arkansas
Louisiana
Oklahoma
Texas

West
Mountain
Arizona
Colorado
Idaho
Montana
Nevada
New Mexico
Utah
Wyoming

Pacific
Alaska
California
Hawaii
Oregon
Washington

Possessions
Puerto Rico
Virgin Islands
Pacific Islands

Index

D

I

N

R

U

W

Y